Promoting Healthy and Supportive Acoustic Environments

Promoting Healthy and Supportive Acoustic Environments

Going beyond the Quietness

Special Issue Editors

Francesco Aletta
Jian Kang

MDPI • Basel • Beijing • Wuhan • Barcelona • Belgrade • Manchester • Tokyo • Cluj • Tianjin

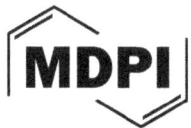

Special Issue Editors

Francesco Aletta
Institute for Environmental
Design and Engineering,
University College London
UK

Jian Kang
Institute for Environmental
Design and Engineering,
University College London
UK

Editorial Office
MDPI
St. Alban-Anlage 66
4052 Basel, Switzerland

This is a reprint of articles from the Special Issue published online in the open access journal *International Journal of Environmental Research and Public Health* (ISSN 1660-4601) (available at: https://www.mdpi.com/journal/ijerph/special_issues/PHSAE).

For citation purposes, cite each article independently as indicated on the article page online and as indicated below:

LastName, A.A.; LastName, B.B.; LastName, C.C. Article Title. *Journal Name* **Year**, *Article Number*, Page Range.

ISBN 978-3-03928-272-2 (Hbk)
ISBN 978-3-03928-273-9 (PDF)

Cover image courtesy of Tin Oberman.

© 2020 by the authors. Articles in this book are Open Access and distributed under the Creative Commons Attribution (CC BY) license, which allows users to download, copy and build upon published articles, as long as the author and publisher are properly credited, which ensures maximum dissemination and a wider impact of our publications.

The book as a whole is distributed by MDPI under the terms and conditions of the Creative Commons license CC BY-NC-ND.

Contents

About the Special Issue Editors vii

Francesco Aletta and Jian Kang
Promoting Healthy and Supportive Acoustic Environments: Going beyond the Quietness
Reprinted from: *Int. J. Environ. Res. Public Health* **2019**, *16*, 4988, doi:10.3390/ijerph16244988 . . . 1

Angel M. Dzhambov, Iana Markevych, Boris Tilov, Zlatoslav Arabadzhiev, Drozdstoj Stoyanov, Penka Gatseva and Donka D. Dimitrova
Lower Noise Annoyance Associated with GIS-Derived Greenspace: Pathways through Perceived Greenspace and Residential Noise
Reprinted from: *Int. J. Environ. Res. Public Health* **2018**, *15*, 1533, doi:10.3390/ijerph15071533 . . . 5

Marcus Hedblom, Bengt Gunnarsson, Martin Schaefer, Igor Knez, Pontus Thorsson and Johan N Lundström
Sounds of Nature in the City: No Evidence of Bird Song Improving Stress Recovery
Reprinted from: *Int. J. Environ. Res. Public Health* **2019**, *16*, 1390, doi:10.3390/ijerph16081390 . . . 21

Sarah R. Payne and Neil Bruce
Exploring the Relationship between Urban Quiet Areas and Perceived Restorative Benefits
Reprinted from: *Int. J. Environ. Res. Public Health* **2019**, *16*, 1611, doi:10.3390/ijerph16091611 . . . 33

Shilun Zhang, Xiaolong Zhao, Zixi Zeng and Xuan Qiu
The Influence of Audio-Visual Interactions on Psychological Responses of Young People in Urban Green Areas: A Case Study in Two Parks in China
Reprinted from: *Int. J. Environ. Res. Public Health* **2019**, *16*, 1845, doi:10.3390/ijerph16101845 . . . 59

Gunnar Cerwén
Listening to Japanese Gardens: An Autoethnographic Study on the Soundscape Action Design Tool
Reprinted from: *Int. J. Environ. Res. Public Health* **2019**, *16*, 4648, doi:10.3390/ijerph16234648 . . . 73

Gunnar Cerwén and Frans Mossberg
Implementation of Quiet Areas in Sweden
Reprinted from: *Int. J. Environ. Res. Public Health* **2019**, *16*, 134, doi:10.3390/ijerph16010134 . . . 103

Karmele Herranz-Pascual, Itziar Aspuru, Ioseba Iraurgi, Álvaro Santander, Jose Luis Eguiguren and Igone García
Going beyond Quietness: Determining the Emotionally Restorative Effect of Acoustic Environments in Urban Open Public Spaces
Reprinted from: *Int. J. Environ. Res. Public Health* **2019**, *16*, 1284, doi:10.3390/ijerph16071284 . . . 121

Francesco Aletta and Jian Kang
Towards an Urban Vibrancy Model: A Soundscape Approach
Reprinted from: *Int. J. Environ. Res. Public Health* **2018**, *15*, 1712, doi:10.3390/ijerph15081712 . . . 141

Daniel Steele, Edda Bild, Cynthia Tarlao and Catherine Guastavino
Soundtracking the Public Space: Outcomes of the Musikiosk Soundscape Intervention
Reprinted from: *Int. J. Environ. Res. Public Health* **2019**, *16*, 1865, doi:10.3390/ijerph16101865 . . . 159

Jieling Xiao and Andrew Hilton
An Investigation of Soundscape Factors Influencing Perceptions of Square Dancing in Urban Streets: A Case Study in a County Level City in China
Reprinted from: *Int. J. Environ. Res. Public Health* **2019**, *16*, 840, doi:10.3390/ijerph16050840 . . . 197

Luis Hermida, Ignacio Pavón, Antonio Carlos Lobo Soares and J. Luis Bento-Coelho
On the Person-Place Interaction and Its Relationship with the Responses/Outcomes of Listeners of Urban Soundscape (Compared Cases of Lisbon and Bogotá): Contextual and Semiotic Aspects
Reprinted from: *Int. J. Environ. Res. Public Health* **2019**, *16*, 551, doi:10.3390/ijerph16040551 . . . 213

Francesco Aletta, Tin Oberman and Jian Kang
Associations between Positive Health-Related Effects and Soundscapes Perceptual Constructs: A Systematic Review
Reprinted from: *Int. J. Environ. Res. Public Health* **2018**, *15*, 2392, doi:10.3390/ijerph15112392 . . . 235

Mercede Erfanian, Andrew J. Mitchell, Jian Kang and Francesco Aletta
The Psychophysiological Implications of Soundscape: A Systematic Review of Empirical Literature and a Research Agenda
Reprinted from: *Int. J. Environ. Res. Public Health* **2019**, *16*, 3533, doi:10.3390/ijerph16193533 . . . 251

Armin Taghipour, Tessa Sievers and Kurt Eggenschwiler
Acoustic Comfort in Virtual Inner Yards with Various Building Facades
Reprinted from: *Int. J. Environ. Res. Public Health* **2019**, *16*, 249, doi:10.3390/ijerph16020249 . . . 271

Sonja Di Blasio, Louena Shtrepi, Giuseppina Emma Puglisi and Arianna Astolfi
A Cross-Sectional Survey on the Impact of Irrelevant Speech Noise on Annoyance, Mental Health and Well-being, Performance and Occupants' Behavior in Shared and Open-Plan Offices
Reprinted from: *Int. J. Environ. Res. Public Health* **2019**, *16*, 280, doi:10.3390/ijerph16020280 . . . 291

Shan Shu and Hui Ma
Restorative Effects of Classroom Soundscapes on Children's Cognitive Performance
Reprinted from: *Int. J. Environ. Res. Public Health* **2019**, *16*, 293, doi:10.3390/ijerph16020293 . . . 309

About the Special Issue Editors

Francesco Aletta, AFHEA has been Research Associate at the Institute for Environmental Design and Engineering, The Bartlett, University College London since 2018. He was Postdoctoral Research Fellow at the Department of Information Technology of Ghent University from 2016 to 2018 and Research Associate at the School of Architecture of the University of Sheffield, working on the soundscapes of both indoor and outdoor spaces. He has been Visiting Lecturer at Birmingham City University and Visiting Professor at the Polytechnic Institute of Turin and the University of Roma Tre. His work on soundscape descriptors and predictive models has informed policy documents and international standards. He is Secretary of the Technical Committee for Noise of the European Acoustics Association. He serves on the editorial board of several peer-reviewed international journals in the fields of building and environmental acoustics, environmental psychology, and urban studies. Dr. Aletta has worked in soundscape studies for 10 years, with 70+ publications. He is the recipient of several research awards and funding for research equipment. He serves as a reviewer for 50+ journals and works as a referee for research projects for the Italian Ministry for Education, University, and Research.

Jian Kang, FREng, FIOA, FASA, FIIAV, CEng has been Chair in Acoustics at the Institute for Environmental Design and Engineering, The Bartlett, University College London since 2018. He was Professor of Acoustics at the School of Architecture of the University of Sheffield from 2003 and is now Visiting Professor. He has also worked at the University of Cambridge, the Fraunhofer Institute of Building Physics in Germany, and Tsinghua University in China. He chairs the Technical Committee for Noise of the European Acoustics Association and the EU COST Action on Soundscape of European Cities and Landscapes. He was awarded the IOA Tyndall Medal in 2008, the Peter Lord Award in 2014, the NAS Lifetime Achievement Award in 2014, and the CIBSE Napier Shaw Bronze Medal in 2013. In addition, he is Fellow of the Royal Academy of Engineering. Professor Kang has worked in environmental and architectural acoustics for 30+ years, with 70+ research projects, 800+ publications, 90+ engineering/consultancy projects, and 20+ patents. His work on acoustic theories, design guidance, and products has brought major improvements to noise control in underground stations/tunnels and soundscape design in urban areas. He was the recipient of the prestigious Advanced ERC Grant Award and is currently working internationally on developing soundscape indices.

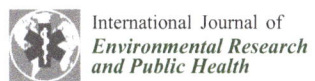

Editorial

Promoting Healthy and Supportive Acoustic Environments: Going beyond the Quietness

Francesco Aletta * and Jian Kang *

UCL Institute for Environmental Design and Engineering, The Bartlett, University College London (UCL), Central House, 14 Upper Woburn Place, WC1H 0NN London, UK
* Correspondence: francesco.aletta@virgilio.it (F.A.); j.kang@ucl.ac.uk (J.K.); Tel.: +44-(0)20-3108-7338 (J.K.)

Received: 22 November 2019; Accepted: 30 November 2019; Published: 8 December 2019

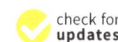

When confronted with the topic of the quality of the acoustic environments, society and communities around the world tend to consider "sound" mainly in its negative facet of "noise". This approach is reflected in a number of recommendations and prescriptions to reduce people's exposure to excessive sound levels from transportation and industry, promoted by international institutions and authorities, such as the World Health Organization or the European Union [1,2]. Notwithstanding, such a strategy is not always effective in delivering the desired enhancements in terms of health and quality of life, and this is because "quietness" and the pursuit of "silence" are not necessarily enough to define an acoustic environment of high quality [3]. Indeed, environmental sounds often have positive effects on people, as they provide information, communicate safety, enable certain desirable activities, and, more generally, contribute to people's appeasement and psychophysical well-being [4,5]. With the rapid increase of urbanization, more research is needed towards alternative approaches for the characterization, management, and design of urban acoustic environments that support (and not only allow) restoration, health, and better quality of life, as well as basic research on the mechanisms underpinning the perception of environmental sounds in context and how their experience might affect health-related outcomes.

Researchers in the environmental acoustics and soundscape domains are addressing these challenges by exploring new inter- and trans-disciplinary approaches to the characterization of the quality of the acoustic environments, new prediction and modeling methodologies for the acoustic environments and their qualities, and the relationships between sound, space, and behaviors in the built environment. From the 16 contributions published in this Special Issue, three main research themes were identified, which are briefly discussed below.

1. Rethinking Quiet Areas and Their Restorative Potential for Health and Well-Being

The concept of perceived quietness has been thoroughly investigated over the years, partly also due to the emphasis put on this topic by major environmental agencies and policymakers. However, clear criteria that go beyond setting a mere sound level threshold for identifying areas where quietness can be experienced have not been internationally agreed on so far. The connection with natural elements and the experience of greenery seem to be prerequisites for quietness and similarly related perceptual constructs (e.g., tranquillity, calmness), and this applies at different urban scales; however, many aspects still need to be clarified, as some of the contributions of this Special Issue highlighted.

Dzhambov et al. [6] show that more green areas in residential environments are associated with lower noise annoyance, whereas higher tree cover is similarly effective only in small-radius buffer zones. Hedblom and colleagues [7] question a relatively well-established concept in soundscape studies, that birdsong typically facilitates stress recovery, by reporting that in their listening experiment, such effect was, in fact, not observed. This more generally raises the point about what sound sources one would expect to contribute more to quietness perception, as well as supporting health and well-being. To some extent, the work by Payne and Bruce [8] also claims that the type of sounds heard and other aspects of a site experience are likely to be related to a non-linear relationship between sound levels and perceived restoration of an acoustic environment. Other contextual aspects might indeed play a role, such as audio–visual interactions in environmental perception, as suggested in the work by Zhang et al. [9]. Cerwén [10] explores new autoethnographic approaches to propose possible actions, which are organized into three main categories (i.e., localization of functions, reduction of unwanted sounds, and introduction of wanted sounds) that designers can take into account when managing quiet areas in the urban realm. Finally, Cerwén and Mossberg [11] report on a study about the implementation of quiet areas in accordance with the EU Environmental Noise Directive (END) of 2002, conducted with several municipalities in Sweden. They find out that at the local authority level, many initiatives have dealt with mapping and identification of quiet areas, but less has been done regarding their maintenance and enforcement, and this is likely to be a common issue for other (European) countries too.

2. Extending the Research Scope to More Soundscape Quality Dimensions, Contextual, and Physiological Factors

While quietness is certainly a key theme in the current discourse about community noise, other dimensions might be relevant in different contexts to characterize the acoustic quality of public spaces. It is fair to assume that non-quiet spaces might still have the potential to promote positive user experiences of an urban environment, or that quietness cab not necessarily always match less "loud" acoustic environments. Herranz-Pascual and colleagues [12] indeed suggest that lively and vibrant urban soundscapes may also enhance people's restoration. Aletta and Kang [13] propose a model to predict urban "vibrancy" using a soundscape approach. Perceived vibrancy can be predicted by a set of (psycho)acoustic parameters, the number of visible people on site, and the presence of music in the auditory scene. Music is indeed a key component of modern urban soundscapes: Whether designed or not, it has the potential to enhance the social experience of a place. Steele and colleagues [14] carried out an interventional study with an unsupervised installation in a public pocket park allowing users to play audio content from personal devices over publicly provided speakers and they found out that the soundscape was experienced as more pleasant for both users and non-users, and the calmness and appropriateness of the place were not affected. Xiao and Hilton [15] investigate the factors influencing sound environments perception in relation to "square dancing", a growing social phenomenon in many Chinese cities. A better understanding of contextual factors and aspects related to the interactions between people and places is required to characterize soundscapes holistically, as pointed out by Hermida and colleagues [16] in their case studies in Lisbon and Bogotá. For this purpose, it is certainly useful to review the corpus of literature looking at the positive effects that soundscapes and environmental sounds more generally can have on people's quality of life and well-being [17,18].

3. Supportive Indoor Soundscapes—A Perceptual Perspective on Building and Room Acoustics

The quality of outdoor acoustic environments is, of course, a mainstream dimension in the narrative of soundscape studies. However, considering that people spend the vast majority of their time in indoor environments, addressing the acoustic quality of such spaces is of paramount importance. It is, therefore, right to question how we expect buildings to "sound like" in order to promote supportive indoor soundscapes. While the acoustics in buildings has typically been dealing with sound insulation and room acoustics performances, a new perceptual perspective on the topic is gradually finding its way in. Taghipour et al. [19] look at how different building facades are likely to affect the perceived acoustic quality of inner yards of residential complexes. Di Blasio and colleagues [20] focus on the overall comfort and performance of open-plan office workers when affected by undue noise coming from irrelevant speech. Similarly, looking at cognitive performance, Shu and Ma [21] carry out a study to explore the restorative effects of different soundscapes on children's sustained attention and short-term memory.

Overall, the works published in this special issue reflect an active and engaged research community, which is exploring the connections between human well-being and the acoustic quality of the built environment from a broad range of methodologies and perspectives in terms of quietness and other dimensions. This is promising, as more efforts are required to address the challenges we face in promoting positive acoustic environments beyond noise control and acoustically "sanitized" spaces.

Author Contributions: Conceptualization, F.A. and J.K.; methodology, F.A. and J.K.; writing—original draft preparation, F.A.; writing—review and editing, F.A. and J.K.; funding acquisition, J.K.

Funding: This work was funded through the European Research Council (ERC) Advanced Grant (No. 740696) on "Soundscape Indices" (SSID).

Acknowledgments: The Editors would like to thank all authors for their submissions and all reviewers for their thorough work on the manuscripts. Furthermore, the Editors are grateful to all IJERPH Editorial staff, in particular to Lin Li and Florence Wang for their professionalism and patient support throughout this process.

Conflicts of Interest: The Editors declare no conflict of interest.

References

1. World Health Organization. *Environmental Noise Guidelines for the European Region*; WHO Regional Office for Europe: Copenhagen, Denmark, 2018.
2. European Parliament and Council. *Directive 2002/49/EC Relating to the Assessment and Management of Environmental Noise*; Publications Office of the European Union: Brussels, Bergium, 2002.
3. Kang, J.; Aletta, F.; Gjestland, T.T.; Brown, L.A.; Botteldooren, D.; Schulte-Fortkamp, B.; Lavia, L. Ten questions on the soundscapes of the built environment. *Build. Environ.* **2016**, *108*, 284–294. [CrossRef]
4. Kang, J. *Urban Sound Environment*; Taylor Francis incorporating Spon: London, UK, 2007.
5. Kang, J.; Schulte-Fortkamp, B. (Eds.) *Soundscape and the Built Environment*; CRC Press: Boca Raton, FL, USA, 2015.
6. Dzhambov, A.M.; Markevych, I.; Tilov, B.; Arabadzhiev, Z.; Stoyanov, D.; Gatseva, P.; Dimitrova, D.D. Lower Noise Annoyance Associated with GIS-Derived Greenspace: Pathways through Perceived Greenspace and Residential Noise. *Int. J. Environ. Res. Public Health* **2018**, *15*, 1533. [CrossRef] [PubMed]
7. Hedblom, M.; Gunnarsson, B.; Schaefer, M.; Knez, I.; Thorsson, P.; Lundström, J.N. Sounds of Nature in the City: No Evidence of Bird Song Improving Stress Recovery. *Int. J. Environ. Res. Public Health* **2019**, *16*, 1390. [CrossRef] [PubMed]
8. Payne, S.R.; Bruce, N. Exploring the Relationship between Urban Quiet Areas and Perceived Restorative Benefits. *Int. J. Environ. Res. Public Health* **2019**, *16*, 1611. [CrossRef] [PubMed]
9. Zhang, S.; Zhao, X.; Zenz, Z.; Qiu, X. The Influence of Audio-Visual Interactions on Psychological Responses of Young People in Urban Green Areas: A Case Study in Two Parks in China. *Int. J. Environ. Res. Public Health* **2019**, *16*, 1845. [CrossRef] [PubMed]
10. Cerwén, G. Listening to Japanese Gardens: An Autoethnographic Study on a Tool for Soundscape Design. *Int. J. Environ. Res. Public Health* **2019**, *16*, 4648. [CrossRef]
11. Cerwén, G.; Mossberg, F. Implementation of Quiet Areas in Sweden. *Int. J. Environ. Res. Public Health* **2019**, *16*, 134. [CrossRef]
12. Herranz-Pascual, K.; Aspuru, I.; Iraurgi, I.; Santander, Á.; Eguiguren, J.L.; Garcia, I. Going beyond Quietness: Determining the Emotionally Restorative Effect of Acoustic Environments in Urban Open Public Spaces. *Int. J. Environ. Res. Public Health* **2019**, *16*, 1284. [CrossRef] [PubMed]
13. Aletta, F.; Kang, J. Towards an Urban Vibrancy Model: A Soundscape Approach. *Int. J. Environ. Res. Public Health* **2018**, *15*, 1712. [CrossRef] [PubMed]
14. Steele, D.; Bild, E.; Tarlao, C.; Guastavino, C. Soundtracking the Public Space: Outcomes of the Musikiosk Soundscape Intervention. *Int. J. Environ. Res. Public Health* **2019**, *16*, 1865. [CrossRef] [PubMed]
15. Xiao, J.; Hilton, A. An Investigation of Soundscape Factors Influencing Perceptions of Square Dancing in Urban Streets: A Case Study in a County Level City in China. *Int. J. Environ. Res. Public Health* **2019**, *16*, 840. [CrossRef] [PubMed]

16. Hermida, L.; Pavón, I.; Lobo Soares, A.C.; Bento-Coelho, J.L. On the Person-Place Interaction and Its Relationship with the Responses/Outcomes of Listeners of Urban Soundscape (Compared Cases of Lisbon and Bogotá): Contextual and Semiotic Aspects. *Int. J. Environ. Res. Public Health* **2019**, *16*, 551. [CrossRef] [PubMed]
17. Aletta, F.; Oberman, T.; Kang, J. Associations between Positive Health-Related Effects and Soundscapes Perceptual Constructs: A Systematic Review. *Int. J. Environ. Res. Public Health* **2018**, *15*, 2392. [CrossRef] [PubMed]
18. Erfanian, M.; Mitchell, A.J.; Kang, J.; Aletta, F. The Psychophysiological Implications of Soundscape: A Systematic Review of Empirical Literature and a Research Agenda. *Int. J. Environ. Res. Public Health* **2019**, *16*, 3533. [CrossRef] [PubMed]
19. Taghipour, A.; Sievers, T.; Eggenschwiler, K. Acoustic Comfort in Virtual Inner Yards with Various Building Facades. *Int. J. Environ. Res. Public Health* **2019**, *16*, 249. [CrossRef] [PubMed]
20. Di Blasio, S.; Shtrepi, L.; Puglisi, G.E.; Astolfi, A. A Cross-Sectional Survey on the Impact of Irrelevant Speech Noise on Annoyance, Mental Health and Well-being, Performance and Occupants' Behavior in Shared and Open-Plan Offices. *Int. J. Environ. Res. Public Health* **2019**, *16*, 280. [CrossRef] [PubMed]
21. Shu, S.; Ma, H. Restorative Effects of Classroom Soundscapes on Children's Cognitive Performance. *Int. J. Environ. Res. Public Health* **2019**, *16*, 293. [CrossRef] [PubMed]

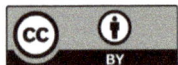

© 2019 by the authors. Licensee MDPI, Basel, Switzerland. This article is an open access article distributed under the terms and conditions of the Creative Commons Attribution (CC BY) license (http://creativecommons.org/licenses/by/4.0/).

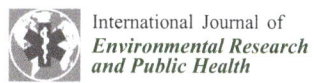

Article

Lower Noise Annoyance Associated with GIS-Derived Greenspace: Pathways through Perceived Greenspace and Residential Noise

Angel M. Dzhambov [1,*], Iana Markevych [2,3], Boris Tilov [4], Zlatoslav Arabadzhiev [5], Drozdstoj Stoyanov [5], Penka Gatseva [1] and Donka D. Dimitrova [6]

1. Department of Hygiene and Ecomedicine, Faculty of Public Health, Medical University of Plovdiv, 4002 Plovdiv, Bulgaria; gatseva_p@mail.bg
2. Institute and Clinic for Occupational, Social and Environmental Medicine, University Hospital, LMU Munich, 80336 Munich, Germany; iana.markevych@helmholtz-muenchen.de
3. Institute of Epidemiology, Helmholtz Zentrum München—German Research Center for Environmental Health, 85764 Neuherberg, Germany
4. Medical College, Medical University of Plovdiv, 4000 Plovdiv, Bulgaria; btilov@abv.bg
5. Department of Psychiatry and Medical Psychology, Faculty of Medicine, Medical University of Plovdiv, 4002 Plovdiv, Bulgaria; zlatolini@gmail.com (Z.A.); stojanovpisevski@gmail.com (D.S.)
6. Department of Health Management and Healthcare Economics, Faculty of Public Health, Medical University of Plovdiv, 4002 Plovdiv, Bulgaria; donka_d@hotmail.com
* Correspondence: angelleloti@gmail.com; Tel.: +359-897-950-802

Received: 1 July 2018; Accepted: 19 July 2018; Published: 19 July 2018

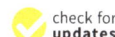

Abstract: Growing amounts of evidence support an association between self-reported greenspace near the home and lower noise annoyance; however, objectively defined greenspace has rarely been considered. In the present study, we tested the association between objective measures of greenspace and noise annoyance, with a focus on underpinning pathways through noise level and perceived greenspace. We sampled 720 students aged 18 to 35 years from the city of Plovdiv, Bulgaria. Objective greenspace was defined by several Geographic Information System (GIS)-derived metrics: Normalized Difference Vegetation Index (NDVI), tree cover density, percentage of green space in circular buffers of 100, 300 and 500 m, and the Euclidean distance to the nearest structured green space. Perceived greenspace was defined by the mean of responses to five items asking about its quantity, accessibility, visibility, usage, and quality. We assessed noise annoyance due to transportation and other neighborhood noise sources and daytime noise level (L_{day}) at the residence. Tests of the parallel mediation models showed that higher NDVI and percentage of green space in all buffers were associated with lower noise annoyance, whereas for higher tree cover this association was observed only in the 100 m buffer zone. In addition, the effects of NDVI and percentage of green space were mediated by higher perceived greenspace and lower L_{day}. In the case of tree cover, only perceived greenspace was a mediator. Our findings suggest that the potential for greenspace to reduce noise annoyance extends beyond noise abatement. Applying a combination of GIS-derived and perceptual measures should enable researchers to better tap individuals' experience of residential greenspace and noise.

Keywords: green space; greenness; noise exposure; noise perception; soundscape

1. Introduction

Residential noise is a ubiquitous environmental stressor that has been linked to a wide range of non-auditory health outcomes, including cardiometabolic diseases, adverse pregnancy outcomes, and mental ill-health, to name a few [1]. Reduction of noise annoyance, which serves as a proxy for noise exposure and is itself detrimental to health, is one of the possible explanations why people residing in green neighborhoods have better health compared to their counterparts [2]. Greener neighborhoods have less artificial noise-emitting sources [2]; moreover, vegetation can reduce noise levels by physical disruption of sound waves propagated from the source to the receiver [3]. Nevertheless, existing elements in the urban green network, such as street trees, have limited capacity as noise barriers and may even increase pedestrian noise exposure, for instance, in street canyons, where tree canopies can reflect sound waves to the level of pedestrian's ears [4,5]. Additionally, a large proportion of the variation in residents' annoyance is caused by non-acoustic factors [1,6]. Therefore, changes in annoyance may be disproportionate to the actual reduction in noise level [1,4].

Accumulating evidence is showing that greenspace can reduce traffic-related annoyance via psychological mechanisms, including visual screening of the noise source, increased restorative quality of the residential environment, and masking of unwanted noise with pleasant nature sounds [4]. Additionally, green spaces near the home may strengthen residents' feeling of control over their acoustic environment by allowing respite from traffic noise, thereby diminishing their noise annoyance [7]. Investigating the latter hypothesis, Riedel et al. observed an indirect effect of near-dwelling greenspace on noise annoyance through perceived noise control [7]. Residing in quiet green areas has been associated with higher health-related quality of life, and that could be due in part to the "quietness" characteristic that people ascribe to greener areas [8]. Even if green spaces are not actively visited, the very knowledge that the residential environment has such natural areas may enhance residential satisfaction and possibly improve noise perception [4,9]. These psychological effects could explain findings that living in a neighborhood with more trees seemed to buffer the negative effect of traffic noise on mental health [10].

Most previous studies on psychological buffering of noise annoyance employed self-reported measures of greenspace and mostly considered only annoyance due to road traffic noise [11]. Van Renterghem and Botteldooren's study was one of the prominent exceptions, as they examined the effect of both objectively-measured and self-reported green view from home on general and traffic noise annoyance [12]. Another such example is the study by Riedel et al. who used land use maps to assess residential greenspace [7]. Spatial and perceived indices should be used together to better understand the effect of greenspace on health, including noise perception [2]. Metrics derived from Geographic Information Systems (GIS) would be useful when investigating the indirect path linking objective greenspace to noise annoyance through reduced noise levels, whereas self-reports would better highlight residents' greenspace experience [2]. Another issue that should be considered is that both objective and perceived greenspace can be defined differently, and these metrics may be related differently to noise annoyance [13]. Consistent with this idea, a meta-analysis showed lower odds of high noise annoyance in people who had a green view from their home, whereas the overall greenness (i.e., vegetation degree) in the neighborhood did not reduce noise annoyance [11]. Another study examined the effect of different objective greenspace measures and observed a beneficial effect only for tree cover density in the 100 m buffer zone, but not for overall greenness [14].

To our knowledge, no previous study has investigated whether the effect of greenspace on noise annoyance is mediated by a reduction in noise level and higher perceived greenspace. Such knowledge could help us understand whether relying on objective measures in urban planning and forestry is sufficient to gain insight into these human-environment interactions. In the present study, we examined the association between objectively-measured greenspace and noise annoyance, with a focus on underpinning pathways through residential noise and perceived greenspace in the neighborhood. We tested the model shown in Figure 1 using different measures of greenspace.

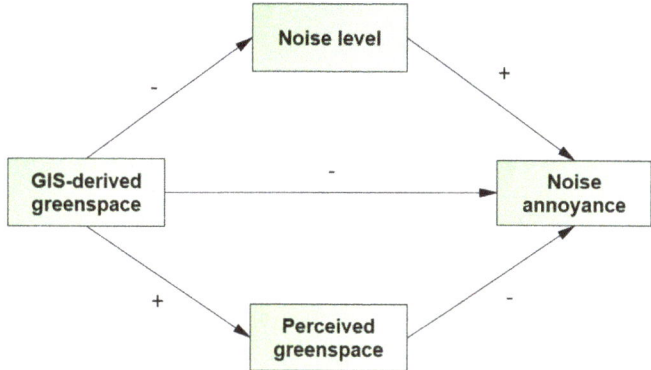

Figure 1. Conceptual diagram showing theoretically-indicated pathways linking Geographic Information System (GIS)-derived greenspace to noise annoyance. (Positive associations are marked with "+", and negative associations, with "−".)

2. Materials and Methods

2.1. Study Design and Sampling

We used data from a cross-sectional survey conducted between October and November 2017 in students from the Medical University of Plovdiv, Bulgaria. Plovdiv is the second largest city in the country with a population of around 342,000 and a territory of around 102 km². Public green spaces in the city account for 75.3% (381.5 ha) of all green areas, which is 11.2 m² per capita. The distribution of these green spaces is scattered, and in some parts of Plovdiv, there are less than 4 m² of green space per capita [15]. At the same time, the 2016 noise mapping campaign indicated that 77% of residents were exposed to day-evening-night road traffic noise above 60 dB(A) [16].

The aim of our study was to investigate the mental health-supporting effects of residential greenspace. To be included in the study, students had to be aged from 18 to 35 years and reside in Plovdiv or its surroundings for the last six months. We targeted potential participants with different ethnic and cultural backgrounds, ages, and program enrollments to ensure sufficient variation in the data. During a class or lecture, members of the research group advertised the study, informing the students about its general objectives, and asked them to complete a questionnaire. In addition to questions on sociodemographic factors and residential environment, participants were asked to report their current living address for subsequent assignment of geographic variables. The study was conducted in accordance with the Declaration of Helsinki, and the protocol was approved by the Ethics Committee of the Medical University of Plovdiv (1/02.02.2017). All participants provided their informed consent for inclusion before they participated in the study. No incentives were offered. A more detailed account of the survey design has been reported previously [17].

Of the 1000 students invited, 823 (82%) agreed to participate. Residential addresses were manually converted into geocodes with the help of Google maps. Of the 823 students, 720 provided sufficient data, including residential addresses, to be included in the study. The majority of them (n = 642, 89.2%) lived in the city of Plovdiv (Figure 2).

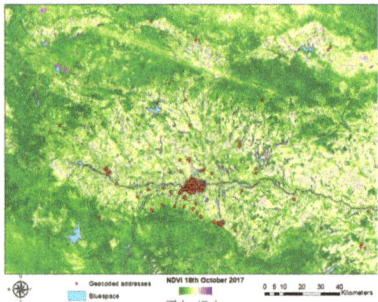

Figure 2. Map of residential addresses superimposed over Normalized Difference Vegetation Index (NDVI) geographic layer.

2.2. Greenspace

Based on previous evidence that different types and properties of greenspace may have different potential to reduce noise annoyance [14], objective greenspace was defined by several GIS-derived metrics: Normalized Difference Vegetation Index (NDVI), percentage of green space, tree cover density, and the Euclidean distance to the nearest structured green space. NDVI [18] served as a measure of surrounding greenness. NDVI is commonly used as a proxy for overall vegetation level and ranges from −1 to +1, with positive values close to 1 indicating dense vegetation [19]. The NDVI equation is based on the difference in surface reflectance in two vegetation-informative wavelengths: visible red and near infrared light. For these calculations, we used six Sentinel 2 MultiSpectral Instrument satellite images with a resolution of 10 × 10 m for the needed bands, obtained on 16 and 18 October 2017. Because bluespace is thought to share the capacity of greenspace to improve noise perception, we wanted to differentiate the effect of greenspace from the effect of bluespace. So, we removed all water pixels from the satellite images prior to assigning NDVI to the geocodes by using the Open Street Maps (OSM) water layer [20]. Tree cover density was calculated based on the Tree Cover Density 2012 map developed by the European Environmental Agency at a resolution of 20 × 20 m. Percentage of structured green space was calculated from the Urban Atlas 2012 land use map. Mean NDVI, mean tree cover density, and percentage of structured green space were abstracted in circular buffers of 100, 300 and 500 m around the residence [17,20]. Euclidean distance to the edge of the nearest structured urban green space was calculated based on the OSM data, and included parks, allotments, and recreation grounds. Geographic data management and calculations were performed using ArcGIS 10.3–10.4 Geographical Information System (GIS) (ESRI, Redlands, CA, USA).

Perceived greenspace was assessed with five items asking respondents about different aspects of their experience of, and interaction with, greenspace in their neighborhood [17]. Specifically, we considered the overall perceived neighborhood greenness, visible greenery from home, accessibility to the nearest structured green space, time spent in green space, and quality of green space. Items could be answered on a 6-point scale. The score for this measure was the mean of item responses, with higher values indicating greater perceived greenspace in the living environment. Cronbach's alpha for this scale was 0.81.

2.3. Noise Level

Noise level was calculated by a combination of measurements and modelling at each participant's address with the help of a land use regression (LUR) model. The LUR was developed specifically for this study and was based on noise measurements recorded by the Regional Health Inspection at 40 locations in Plovdiv in 2016. Measurements were conducted over a 12-hour period from 7:00 a.m. to 7:00 p.m. (L_{day}) according to ISO 1996-2:1987. Predictor variables derived from GIS were considered in the regression equation, following a supervised forward stepwise selection procedure, as described by Aguilera et al. [21]. The final LUR had an adjusted correlation coefficient (R^2) of 0.72 and leave-one-out cross validation R^2 of 0.65. More details about model development have been reported previously [17].

2.4. Noise Annoyance

Noise annoyance was calculated by the mean of responses to two items. Items asked about annoyance/disturbance by traffic noise and other neighborhood noise sources included: "How much does road traffic noise bother, disturb, or annoy you?" and "How much does noise from neighbors/construction/recreational establishments bother, disturb, or annoy you?". The response scale ranged from "0 = Not at all" to "4 = Extremely" and followed the recommendation by the International Commission on Biological Effects of Noise [22]. The correlation between the two items was strong enough to justify their combination into one scale, r = 0.47 ($p < 0.001$). The mean of the responses served as a measure of noise annoyance in the living environment.

2.5. Confounders

We also considered several potential confounding factors, including participants' age, sex, ethnicity, duration of residence at the address, and average time spent at home per day. Individual-level economic status was assessed by a single item: "Having in mind your monthly income, how easy is it for you to "make ends meet", meet your expenses without depriving yourself?". Responses could range from "0 = Very difficult" to "5 = Very easy". Recently experienced stressful life events were assessed with the item "Have you lately experienced a stressful life event, such as death/illness of a relative, separation from a loved one, or being fired?". The geocodes were used to assess population density in a 500 m buffer zone around the address from the 2011 Census population grid of Bulgaria and whether participants lived in Plovdiv or any other settlement nearby. We also considered the presence of bluespace in circular buffers of 100 m, 300 m and 500 m, and the Euclidean distance to the edge of bluespace nearest to the residence. For these calculations, we extracted data on all types of water bodies and wetlands from the Urban Atlas 2012. Given seasonal variations in noise annoyance [23], we also considered the month of data collection.

2.6. Statistical Analysis

Most variables in the dataset had less than 5% missing values, except L_{day} (11.3% missing) because the LUR for noise was only applied to address points in Plovdiv, where its validity was confirmed. All missing data were replaced using the expectation maximization algorithm [24,25]. Interrelations between the variables were examined with Pearson correlations. Given the robustness of parametric analyses to deviations from the normal distribution and that Likert scales with five or more categories can be treated as continuous variables [26,27], noise annoyance and perceived greenspace were included in the parametric tests.

For the main analysis, we tested mediation models linking greenspace to noise annoyance. According to mediation theory, the total effect of greenspace is the sum of the direct effect of greenspace on annoyance, controlling for perceived greenspace and L_{day}, and the two indirect paths through perceived greenspace and L_{day} working in parallel. We employed the pre-specified Model 4 of PROCESS v. 2.16 [28]. PROCESS is a free macro for SPSS that simplifies the implementation of mediation analysis with observed variables, based on a set of preprogrammed conceptual and statistical models. It uses ordinary least squares regression to estimate the parameters of each of the equations, including all the path coefficients, standard errors, t- and p-values, and confidence intervals [29]. In our case, the bias-corrected 95% confidence intervals (CIs) of indirect paths were computed using bootstrapping (5000 samples). The model was applied to each of the objective greenspace metrics. All models were adjusted for a priori selected confounders: age, sex, ethnicity (Bulgarian vs. other), economic status, duration of residence (<5 vs. ≥5 years), time spent at home per day (<8 vs. ≥8 h), stressful life events (no vs. yes), population in the 500 m buffer, settlement

(Plovdiv vs. other), presence of bluespace in the respective buffer (or distance to bluespace in the model with distance to green space), and month of data collection (October vs. November). Coefficients for NDVI and distance to green space were rescaled to an interquartile range increment, and for tree cover density and percentage of green space, to a 5% increment. In a sensitivity analysis, the model was fitted separately for annoyances due to traffic noise and other neighborhood sources.

Results were considered statistically significant at the $p < 0.05$ level, and mediation was considered present when the indirect path significantly exceeded zero, regardless of the significance of the total effect [30].

3. Results

Participants' age was not normally distributed, with a median of 21.00 years (interquartile range = 3.0). The sample included substantially more women than men (66% vs. 34%), and most were Bulgarian (74%). The majority of the sample was from the city of Plovdiv (89%), lived in their home for less than five years (62%), and spent at least eight hours at home per day (55%). Correlations between the key variables were in line with theory (Table 1). That is, higher noise level at the residence was associated with higher noise annoyance, whereas those living in a greener neighborhood, or perceiving their neighborhood as greener, reported lower annoyance. In addition, higher residential greenspace was related to lower noise level and higher perceived greenspace.

Tests of the total effect of greenspace showed that higher NDVI and percentage of green space were associated with lower noise annoyance across all buffers (Table 2). For tree cover density, this association was significant only in the 100 m buffer zone. Distance to green space had no effect. Further, only NDVI in the larger buffers (300 m and 500 m) had a direct effect on noise annoyance, and for all other buffers and metrics, the effect was only indirect. More specifically, the associations between NDVI and percentage of green space and noise annoyance were mediated by higher perceived greenspace and lower L_{day}, and the coefficients associated with these paths did not differ significantly. Perceived greenspace accounted for around 20–25% of these total effects. In terms of tree cover, only perceived greenspace was a mediator, explaining from 14 to 75% of the total effect depending on the buffer.

A similar overall trend was revealed when we fitted the mediation model separately to traffic and neighborhood noise annoyances. However, associations between greenspace and neighborhood noise annoyance appeared to be stronger and more consistent than for traffic noise annoyance. (Appendix A, Table A1). Conversely, the path through L_{day} was significant only in the model with traffic noise annoyance.

Table 1. Pearson correlations of the main variables in the analysis ($N = 720$).

Variable	(1)	(2)	(3)	(4)	(5)	(6)	(7)	(8)	(9)	(10)	(11)	(12)	(13)	(14)	(15)
(1) Traffic NA	1	0.47	**0.85**	**0.17**	−**0.15**	−0.07	−0.08	−**0.11**	−0.04	0.01	0.04	−0.08	−0.07	−**0.10**	−0.07
(2) Neighborhood NA		1	**0.86**	**0.11**	−**0.18**	−**0.18**	−**0.18**	−**0.15**	−**0.10**	−0.03	0.03	−**0.10**	−0.07	−0.04	−**0.09**
(3) Total NA			1	**0.16**	−**0.19**	−**0.14**	−**0.15**	−**0.15**	−**0.08**	−0.01	0.04	−**0.10**	−**0.08**	−**0.08**	−**0.09**
(4) L_{day}				1	−**0.15**	−**0.28**	−**0.26**	−**0.17**	−0.07	0.02	0.07	−**0.17**	−**0.25**	−**0.25**	−**0.15**
(5) Perceived GS					1	**0.29**	**0.24**	**0.20**	**0.13**	**0.09**	0.06	**0.14**	**0.12**	0.08	**0.10**
(6) NDVI 100m						1	**0.75**	**0.53**	**0.47**	**0.17**	0.04	**0.21**	**0.34**	**0.26**	**0.12**
(7) NDVI 300m							1	**0.83**	**0.25**	**0.14**	0.05	**0.20**	**0.58**	**0.49**	**0.13**
(8) NDVI 500m								1	**0.15**	**0.18**	**0.16**	**0.22**	**0.42**	**0.48**	**0.23**
(9) Tree cover 100m									1	**0.73**	**0.56**	**0.16**	−0.02	−0.04	−**0.12**
(10) Tree cover 300m										1	**0.88**	**0.10**	−**0.16**	−**0.15**	−**0.19**
(11) Tree cover 500m											1	0.04	−**0.14**	−**0.11**	−**0.27**
(12) GS% 100m												1	**0.49**	**0.34**	0.05
(13) GS% 300m													1	**0.86**	−0.03
(14) GS% 500m														1	0.05
(15) Distance to GS															1
Mean	1.58	1.54	1.56	67.05	2.98	0.35	0.36	0.36	6.03	6.31	6.56	2.71	11.42	13.37	398.15
Standard deviation	1.09	1.13	0.95	1.73	1.10	0.08	0.06	0.05	6.66	4.44	3.48	8.66	12.86	12.16	1024.64

Notes: GS: greenspace, L_{day}: day average noise level, NA: noise annoyance, NDVI: Sentinel-derived Normalized Difference Vegetation Index. Boldface indicates statistically significant coefficients ($p < 0.05$).

Table 2. Parallel mediation models linking Geographic Information System (GIS)-derived greenspace to noise annoyance (N = 720).

GIS-Metrics	Total Effect	Direct Effect	Indirect Paths (% of the Total Effect Explained)	
			L_{day}	Perceived GS
NDVI$_{100m}$	−0.16 (−0.26, −0.06)[1]	−0.08 (−0.19, 0.02)	−0.04 (−0.07, −0.02)[1] (25%)	−0.04 (−0.08, −0.01)[1] (25%)
NDVI$_{300m}$	−0.26 (−0.39, −0.13)[1]	−0.18 (−0.31, −0.05)[1]	−0.04 (−0.07, −0.01)[1] (15%)	−0.05 (−0.09, −0.02)[1] (20%)
NDVI$_{500m}$	−0.16 (−0.25, −0.07)[1]	−0.12 (−0.21, −0.03)[1]	−0.01 (−0.03, −0.002)[1] (6%)	−0.03 (−0.06, −0.01)[1] (19%)
Tree cover$_{100m}$	−0.07 (−0.12, −0.01)[1]	−0.05 (−0.10, 0.001)	−0.003 (−0.01, 0.004) (4%)	−0.01 (−0.03, −0.003)[1] (14%)
Tree cover$_{300m}$	−0.05 (−0.14, 0.03)	−0.04 (−0.12, 0.05)	0.003 (−0.01, 0.02) (−6%)	−0.02 (−0.04, −0.01)[1] (40%)
Tree cover$_{500m}$	−0.04 (−0.15, 0.07)	−0.02 (−0.13, 0.09)	0.01 (−0.003, 0.03) (−25%)	−0.03 (−0.06, −0.01)[1] (75%)
GS%$_{100m}$	−0.05 (−0.09, −0.01)[1]	−0.03 (−0.07, 0.01)	−0.01 (−0.03, −0.004)[1] (20%)	−0.01 (−0.02, −0.003)[1] (20%)
GS%$_{300m}$	−0.04 (−0.07, −0.01)[1]	−0.02 (−0.05, 0.01)	−0.01 (−0.02, −0.003)[1] (25%)	−0.01 (−0.01, −0.002)[1] (25%)
GS%$_{500m}$	−0.04 (−0.07, −0.004)[1]	−0.03 (−0.06, 0.01)	−0.01 (−0.01, −0.002)[1] (25%)	−0.004 (−0.01, <0.001) (10%)
Distance to GS	−0.01 (−0.03, 0.01)	−0.002 (−0.02, 0.02)	−0.01 (−0.02, 0.00) (100%)	−0.002 (−0.01, 0.001) (20%)

Notes: GS: greenspace, L_{day}: day average noise level, NDVI: Sentinel-derived Normalized Difference Vegetation Index. Models adjusted for age, sex, ethnicity (Bulgarian vs. other), individual-level economic status, duration of residence (<5 vs. ≥5 years), time spent at home/day (<8 vs. ≥8 h), stressful life events (no vs. yes), population in 500 m buffer, settlement (Plovdiv vs. other), presence of bluespace in the respective buffer (Distance to green space is adjusted for distance to bluespace) and month of data collection (October vs. November); in addition, L_{day} and Perceived GS are mutually adjusted for each other. Coefficients for NDVI and Distance to green space are rescaled to an interquartile range increment, and for Tree cover and GS%, to a 5% increment. Effect size coefficient is unstandardized regression coefficient with its 95% confidence interval. [1] Coefficient is statistically significant at $p < 0.05$.

4. Discussion

4.1. General Discussion

This study examined associations between GIS-derived greenspace and noise annoyance in Bulgarian students. Higher surrounding greenness and percentage of green space in the residential environment were associated with lower noise annoyance across all buffers, whereas greater tree cover density seemed beneficial only in the 100 m buffer zone. Proximity to green space had no effect. The effects of surrounding greenness and percentage of green space were mediated by higher perceived greenspace and lower noise level, and these paths were equally important. In the case of tree cover, only perceived greenspace was a mediator.

Overall, our results are in line with a substantial body of literature on residential greenspace and its capacity to reduce noise annoyance [12,13,31–35]. To the best of our knowledge, only our earlier study in Plovdiv [14] examined this relationship across different definitions of greenspace, as measured by different remotely-sensed vegetation indices. However, in that earlier study, results were diametrically opposite, as NDVI and percentage of green space (in the 100 m and 300 m buffers) were associated with higher road traffic noise annoyance [14]. Although such contrasting findings cannot be fully understood here, we offer an angle to these differences. In the present study, participants were older (18–35 vs. 15–25 years), some were foreigners, and the two items used tackled noise annoyance both at home and in the neighborhood, as opposed to noise annoyance at home only, in our previous study. The difference in definitions of annoyance deserves specific consideration because, depending on the spatial context, different mechanisms could explain the effect of greenspace on annoyance. Conceivably, having a green view from the home windows may be more beneficial for noise perception at home than the overall greenness in the neighborhood [11]. From this perspective, tree cover in the 100 m buffer zone possibly served as a proxy for visible greenery from home [2]. This effect may be attributed to visual screening of the noise source by street trees, stress reduction, or reinforcing the notion that noise levels are actually lowered by street trees [4]. Further, living in a green environment and having dwelling-related green might be associated with lower noise annoyance via increased perceived control over the acoustic environment [11]. That is, a person's feeling of being unable to escape and retaliate against the noise source might be suppressed by the knowledge that their home has tranquil green spaces in its vicinity [7]. However, NDVI and percentage of green space in larger buffers represent general availability of greenspace in the neighborhood, which may be relevant for noise annoyance experienced outside of the home. Green areas typically serve as places of a high restorative quality where people can find refuge from noise and also engage in social contacts and physical activity [2,36]. In smaller buffers, tree cover is a more precise measure considering only trees, which are observable from afar owing to their height, whereas NDVI can grasp vegetation not visible from home (on roofs, herbaceous vegetation, etc.). Percentage of green space is based on land use data; hence, it can encompass green spaces with varying, sometimes scarce, vegetation levels. As for distance to urban green space, no association was observed here, in contrast with previous reports [31,32] that found that having access to green space within 200–400 m from home is beneficial. Non-linearity in the effect or the urban fabric of Plovdiv may explain such findings.

Tests of the mediation models showed that only NDVI in the 300 m and 500 m buffers had a direct effect on noise annoyance, and for all other combinations and metrics, the effect was only indirect. That is, higher greenspace is related to lower noise level and higher perceived greenspace, and in turn to lower annoyance. These two mediators worked in parallel and seemed equally important, explaining some 20–25% of the total effect. Our findings that both perceived greenspace and lower noise level were equally important mediators imply that greenspace may support noise perception beyond reduction in noise level. This could have value for the planning and management of urban green systems. Installation of solid noise barriers, albeit associated with a considerable reduction in noise exposure, is one of the least cost-efficient noise abatement approaches [37,38]. Street trees also have limited potential to block sound propagation despite what residents might believe [4]. Conversely, urban green systems could be retrofitted, such as by rejuvenation, installing water features, and attracting songbirds, to improve the acoustic and restorative quality in residential areas at a relatively low cost. Such interventions to enhance residents' satisfaction with the neighborhood and to reduce their noise annoyance seem more feasible than changing the existing urban fabric, such as by changing traffic-related infrastructure. To understand the personal factors that could affect soundscape appraisal beyond physical features of green spaces, case studies and noise-related social surveys in areas where noise has been identified as an issue could be a useful tool for policy-makers and planners [39]. In any case, improving the acoustic comfort of residents is just one of the many benefits delivered by urban green infrastructure, and this evidence should be heralded to increase the awareness of stakeholders and narrow the gap between science and greenspace policy [40].

In the sensitivity analysis, we found a stronger effect of greenspace on neighborhood noise annoyance than on traffic noise annoyance. We think this effect could be due to the fact that, for some residents, other noise sources may be more annoying than road traffic, possibly due to differences in spectral characteristics, residents' learned helplessness, or other psychoacoustic, social, and cognitive determinants of noise perception [1,41]. We also found that noise level was a mediator only in the traffic noise annoyance model, possibly because the L_{day} variable, for the most part, captured variations in outdoor traffic noise. However, noise originating from within the residential building or from neighbors and recreational activities should be more relevant for neighborhood noise annoyance.

Our findings encourage the consideration of both objective and perceptual measures of greenspace. Self-reports may better account for the actual interaction with greenspace, and therefore reduce misclassification in remote sensing exposure assessments, which is due to some well-known issues with GIS-derived metrics like the NDVI and land use indices (e.g., poor discrimination between types of greenspace and disregarding their actual quality, accessibility, and visibility from pedestrian's point of view) [2,19]. Some remedies include new indices capturing multiple aspects of greenspace by integrating information from different sources, including remote sensing, local land use databases, private ownership data, and quality appraisals [42]; using GPS technology to track participants' movement and assess greenspace along their actual travel routes [43]; and calculating visible vegetation from geotagged eye-level panoramic images [44]. However, perceptual measures not only compensate for the lack of precision of vegetation indices and land use-derived green space metrics, but also access the mental representation of residents' living environment, considering individual differences, such as the attention that people pay to their surroundings, their preference for specific attributes involved in the appraisal of greenspace quality, personal salience, and intentions to engage in particular greenspace-related behaviors (e.g., "green sport") [45,46]. Given the mismatch between GIS-derived and perceptual measures [46,47] and the sporadic use of more sophisticated exposure assessment techniques, applying a combination of objective and self-reported greenspace measures should enable researchers to better capture individuals' experience of greenspace and to understand how it may relate to noise annoyance [45,46,48].

4.2. Strengths and Limitations

As a novel contribution here, we collected data on various objective and perceived greenspace measures and employed state of the art exposure assessment—e.g., NDVI's resolution was higher than in most greenspace research (10×10 m vs. 30×30 m) [2], and noise level was assessed by a specifically developed and up-to-date LUR model. Another novel feature of this study is that we assessed noise annoyance due to neighborhood sources other than road traffic. We focused on an understudied age group from South-East Europe. By sampling students from one university, we reduced overdispersion in the data and also controlled for environmental influences (e.g., traffic noise, greenness) on campus. The high response rate (>80%) is also a strength.

However, several limitations should be discussed. First, this study was of cross-sectional design like all earlier studies in the field [11]. This precludes us from drawing causal inferences about revealed associations. Additionally, cross-sectional tests of mediation might entail bias and produce overconfident results [49]. Recall bias cannot be ruled out either. Therefore, our findings should be replicated in longitudinal analyses. It is important to know the length of time a person needs to be "exposed" to greenspace for noise perception to be improved. Also of interest would be describing how the effect of greenspace varies throughout the year depending on seasonal variations in residential vegetation and in different geographic contexts.

Second, the inclusion of foreigners and sampling from a medical school means that our sample was very specific and not representative of the general population of Plovdiv of that age range. Still, this lack of external validity does not have an effect on the internal validity of our study, because we controlled for a wide range of sociodemographic and residential factors.

Third, we likely overestimated noise level at addresses located near minor roads and in smaller settlements, due to the limited observed range of measurements used to construct the LUR. Even though that should have diminished the real association between L_{day} and noise annoyance, we still detected significant mediation through L_{day}.

Forth, concerns that single noise annoyance questions do not adequately reflect the whole experience of noise have been expressed [50,51]. That prompted us to combine the two annoyance items, but the resulting scale was rather crude [52] because our study was not specifically designed to investigate noise perception.

Finally, data were collected in October and November, when people spend less time outdoors than in summer. That could have diminished the associations, at least for larger buffers. Therefore, we adjusted the models for month of data collection. Limitations notwithstanding, the associations we found were significant, lending support to our hypothesis.

5. Conclusions

Higher greenness and more green space in the residential environment were associated with lower noise annoyance, whereas for higher tree cover, this association was observed only in the 100 m buffer zone. Observed associations between greenspace and noise annoyance were mediated by higher perceived greenspace and lower noise level, and these paths seemed equally important. In the case of tree cover, only perceived greenspace was a mediator. Our findings suggest that the potential of greenspace to reduce noise annoyance extends beyond noise abatement. Applying a combination of GIS-derived and perceptual measures should enable researchers to better capture individual experiences of greenspace and to understand how it may relate to noise annoyance.

Author Contributions: Conceptualization, data curation, and formal analysis, A.M.D.; Investigation, A.M.D., B.T., Z.A., D.S. and P.G.; Methodology, A.M.D., I.M. and D.D.D.; Project administration, D.D.D.; Resources, B.T., Z.A., D.S. and P.G.; Supervision, I.M. and D.D.D.; Visualization, I.M.; Writing—original draft, A.M.D.; Writing—review and editing, I.M., B.T., Z.A., D.S., P.G. and D.D.D.

Funding: This research received no external funding.

Acknowledgments: We are grateful to the participating students for making this study possible. We would also like to thank our colleagues at the Department of Anatomy, Histology and Embryology (Medical University of Plovdiv) for their help with collection of questionnaire data.

Conflicts of Interest: The authors declare no conflict of interest.

Appendix A

Table A1. Parallel mediation models linking Geographic Information System (GIS)-derived greenspace to traffic- and neighborhood noise annoyances ($N = 720$).

GIS-Metrics	Total Effect	Direct Effect	Indirect Paths	
			L_{day}	Perceived GS
Traffic Noise Annoyance				
NDVI $_{100m}$	−0.11 (−0.22, 0.01)	0.002 (−0.12, 0.12)	−0.06 (−0.10, −0.03) [1]	−0.05 (−0.09, −0.02) [1]
NDVI $_{300m}$	−0.18 (−0.33, −0.03) [1]	−0.06 (−0.22, 0.09)	−0.05 (−0.10, −0.02) [1]	−0.06 (−0.11, −0.02) [1]
NDVI $_{500m}$	−.13 (−0.23, −0.02) [1]	−0.07 (−0.18, 0.03)	−0.02 (−0.05, −0.002) [1]	−0.03 (−0.07, −0.01) [1]
Tree cover $_{100m}$	−0.04 (−0.10, 0.02)	−0.02 (−0.08, 0.04)	−0.005 (−0.02, 0.005)	−0.01 (−0.03, −0.005) [1]
Tree cover $_{300m}$	−0.01 (−0.11, 0.09)	0.01 (−0.08, 0.11)	0.004 (−0.01, 0.02)	−0.02 (−0.05, −0.01) [1]
Tree cover $_{500m}$	0.01 (−0.12, 0.14)	0.03 (−0.10, 0.16)	0.02 (−0.004, 0.05)	−0.04 (−0.07, −0.01) [1]
GS% $_{100m}$	−0.04 (−0.08, 0.01)	−0.01 (−0.06, 0.04)	−0.02 (−0.03, −0.01) [1]	−0.01 (−0.02, −0.004) [1]
GS% $_{300m}$	−0.04 (−0.07, −0.003) [1]	−0.02 (−0.06, 0.01)	−0.01 (−0.02, −0.004) [1]	−0.01 (−0.02, −0.002) [1]
GS% $_{500m}$	−0.05 (−0.09, −0.02) [1]	−0.04 (−0.08, −0.002) [1]	−0.01 (−0.02, −0.003) [1]	−0.005 (−0.01, <0.001)
Distance to GS	−0.01 (−0.03, 0.02)	0.003 (−0.02, 0.03)	−0.01 (−0.03, −0.0003) [1]	−0.002 (−0.01, 0.002)
Neighborhood Noise Annoyance				
NDVI $_{100m}$	−0.22 (−0.34, −0.10) [1]	−0.17 (−0.30, −0.05) [1]	−0.02 (−0.05, 0.01)	−0.03 (−0.07, −0.002) [1]
NDVI $_{300m}$	−0.35 (−0.50, −0.19) [1]	−0.30 (−0.46, −0.14) [1]	−0.02 (−0.05, 0.005)	−0.03 (−0.08, 0.004)
NDVI $_{500m}$	−0.20 (−0.30, −0.09) [1]	−0.17 (−0.28, −0.06) [1]	−0.01 (−0.02, 0.001)	−0.02 (−0.05, −0.001) [1]
Tree cover $_{100m}$	−0.10 (−0.16, −0.03) [1]	−0.08 (−0.15, −0.02) [1]	−0.002 (−0.01, 0.001)	−0.01 (−0.03, −0.001) [1]
Tree cover $_{300m}$	−0.10 (−0.20, −0.001) [1]	−0.08 (−0.18, 0.01)	0.002 (−0.004, 0.01)	−0.02 (−0.04, −0.003) [1]
Tree cover $_{500m}$	−0.09 (−0.23, 0.04)	−0.08 (−0.21, 0.06)	0.01 (−0.001, 0.03)	−0.03 (−0.06, −0.01) [1]
GS% $_{100m}$	−0.06 (−0.10, −0.01) [1]	−0.04 (−0.09, 0.004)	−0.01 (−0.02, 0.0004)	−0.01 (−0.02, −0.002) [1]
GS% $_{300m}$	−0.03 (−0.07, 0.001) [1]	−0.03 (−0.06, 0.01)	−0.004 (−0.01, 0.001)	−0.01 (−0.01, −0.001) [1]
GS% $_{500-m}$	−0.02 (−0.06, 0.02)	−0.01 (−0.05, 0.03)	−0.003 (−0.01, 0.0004)	−0.004 (−0.01, 0.0001)
Distance to urban GS	−0.01 (−0.04, 0.01)	−0.01 (−0.03, 0.02)	−0.003 (−0.01, 0.001)	−0.002 (−0.01, 0.001)

Notes: GS: greenspace, L_{day}: day average noise level, NDVI: Sentinel-derived Normalized Difference Vegetation Index. Models adjusted for age, sex, ethnicity (Bulgarian vs. other), individual-level economic status, duration of residence (<5 vs. ≥5 years), time spent at home/day (<8 vs. ≥8 h), stressful life events (no vs. yes), population in 500 m buffer, settlement (Plovdiv vs. other), presence of bluespace in the respective buffer (Distance to green space is adjusted for distance to bluespace) and month of data collection (October vs. November); in addition, L_{day} and Perceived GS are mutually adjusted for each other. Coefficients for NDVI and Distance to green space are rescaled to an interquartile range increment, and for Tree cover and GS%, to a 5% increment. Effect size coefficient is unstandardized regression coefficient with its 95% confidence interval. [1] Coefficient is statistically significant at $p < 0.05$.

References

1. Lercher, P. Noise in Cities: Urban and Transport Planning Determinants and Health in Cities. In *Integrating Human Health into Urban and Transport Planning*; Nieuwenhuijsen, M., Khries, H., Eds.; Springer: Cham, Switzerland, 2018; pp. 443–481.
2. Markevych, I.; Schoierer, J.; Hartig, T.; Chudnovsky, A.; Hystad, P.; Dzhambov, A.M.; de Vries, S.; Triguero-Mas, M.; Brauer, M.; Nieuwenhuijsen, M.; et al. Exploring pathways linking greenspace to health: Theoretical and methodological guidance. *Environ. Res.* **2017**, *158*, 301–317. [CrossRef] [PubMed]
3. Van Renterghem, T.; Forssén, J.; Attenborough, K.; Jean, P.; Defrance, J.; Hornikx, M.; Kang, J. Using natural means to reduce surface transport noise during propagation outdoors. *Appl. Acoust.* **2015**, *92*, 86–101. [CrossRef]
4. Van Renterghem, T. Towards explaining the positive effect of vegetation on the perception of environmental noise. *Urban For. Urban Green.* **2018**, in press. [CrossRef]
5. Jang, H.S.; Lee, S.C.; Jeon, J.Y.; Kang, J. Evaluation of road traffic noise abatement by vegetation treatment in a 1:10 urban scale model. *J. Acoust. Soc. Am.* **2015**, *138*, 3884–3895. [CrossRef] [PubMed]
6. Guski, R.; Felscher-Suhr, U.; Schuemer, R. The concept of noise annoyance: How international experts see it. *J. Sound Vib.* **1999**, *223*, 513–527. [CrossRef]

7. Riedel, N.; Köckler, H.; Scheiner, J.; van Kamp, I.; Erbel, R.; Loerbroks, A.; Claßen, T.; Bolte, G. Home as a Place of Noise Control for the Elderly? A Cross-Sectional Study on Potential Mediating Effects and Associations between Road Traffic Noise Exposure, Access to a Quiet Side, Dwelling-Related Green and Noise Annoyance. *Int. J. Environ. Res. Public Health.* **2018**, *15*, 1036. [CrossRef] [PubMed]
8. Shepherd, D.; Welch, D.; Dirks, K.N.; McBride, D. Do Quiet Areas Afford Greater Health-Related Quality of Life than Noisy Areas? *Int. J. Environ. Res. Public Health* **2013**, *10*, 1284–1303. [CrossRef] [PubMed]
9. Kaplan, R.; Kaplan, S. *The Experience of Nature: A Psychological Perspective*; Cambridge University Press: New York, NY, USA, 1989.
10. Dzhambov, A.M.; Markevych, I.; Tilov, B.G.; Dimitrova, D.D. Residential greenspace might modify the effect of road traffic noise exposure on general mental health in students. *Urban For. Urban Green.* **2018**, *34*, 233–239. [CrossRef]
11. Dzhambov, A.M. More residential greenspace is associated with lower noise annoyance: Results from a quantitative synthesis of the literature. In *Traffic Noise: Exposure, Health Effects and Mitigation*; Łucjan, C., Gérard, D., Eds.; Nova Science Publishers: New York, NY, USA, 2017; pp. 77–104.
12. Van Renterghem, T.; Botteldooren, D. View on outdoor vegetation reduces noise annoyance for dwellers near busy roads. *Landsc. Urban Plan.* **2016**, *148*, 203–215. [CrossRef]
13. Li, H.N.; Chau, C.K.; Tang, S.K. Can surrounding greenery reduce noise annoyance at home? *Sci. Total Environ.* **2010**, *408*, 4376–4384. [CrossRef] [PubMed]
14. Dzhambov, A.; Dimitrova, D.; Markevych, I.; Tilov, B. Association between different indices of greenspace "exposure" and noise annoyance in youth. In Proceedings of the 12th ICBEN Congress on Noise as a Public Health Problem, Zurich, Switzerland, 18–22 June 2017.
15. Shalamanov, S.; Stamov, S.; Kodzhamanov, S.; Margov, N.; Petrova, R.; Marinov, V.; Raicheva, K.; Radeva, S.; Pandeva, N.; Sokolov, R. *Program for Development, Maintenance and Protection of the Green System of Plovdiv City*; Art Plan: Plovdiv, Bulgaria, 2013; Available online: http://www.plovdiv.bg/proekt-programa-zelena-sistema/ (accessed on 17 July 2018). (In Bulgarian)
16. SPECTRI. Development of Updated Strategic Noise Maps of Plovdiv Agglomeration. *Sofia*, 2017. Available online: http://www.plovdiv.bg/item/ecology/noise/ (accessed on 17 July 2018). (In Bulgarian)
17. Dzhambov, A.M.; Markevych, I.; Hartig, T.; Tilov, B.; Arabadzhiev, Z.; Stoyanov, D.; Gatseva, P.; Dimitrova, D.D. Multiple pathways link urban green- and bluespace to mental health in young adults. *Environ Res.* **2018**, *166*, 223–233. [CrossRef] [PubMed]
18. Tucker, C.J. Red and Photographic Infrared Linear Combinations for Monitoring Vegetation. *Remote Sens. Environ.* **1979**, *8*, 127–150. [CrossRef]
19. Gascon, M.; Cirach, M.; Martínez, D.; Dadvand, P.; Valentín, A.; Plasència, A.; Nieuwenhuijsen, M.J. Normalized difference vegetation index (NDVI) as a marker of surrounding greenness in epidemiological studies: The case of Barcelona city. *Urban For. Urban Green.* **2016**, *19*, 88–94. [CrossRef]
20. Gascon, M.; Sánchez-Benavides, G.; Dadvand, P.; Martínez, D.; Gramunt, N.; Gotsens, X.; Cirach, M.; Vert, C.; Molinuevo, J.L.; Crous-Bou, M.; Nieuwenhuijsen, M. Long-term exposure to residential green and blue spaces and anxiety and depression in adults: A cross-sectional study. *Environ. Res.* **2018**, *162*, 231–239. [CrossRef] [PubMed]
21. Aguilera, I.; Foraster, M.; Basagaña, X.; Corradi, E.; Deltell, A.; Morelli, X.; Phuleria, HC.; Ragettli, MS.; Rivera, M.; Thomasson, A.; et al. Application of land use regression modelling to assess the spatial distribution of road traffic noise in three European cities. *J. Expo. Sci. Environ. Epidemiol.* **2015**, *25*, 97–105. [CrossRef] [PubMed]
22. Fields, J.M.; de Jong, R.G.; Gjestland, T.; Flindell, I.H.; Job, R.F.S.; Kurra, S.; Lercher, P.; Vallet, M.; Yano, T.; Guski, R.; et al. Standardized general-purpose noise reaction questions for community noise surveys: Research and a recommendation. *J. Sound Vib.* **2001**, *242*, 641–679. [CrossRef]
23. Brink, M.; Schreckenberg, D.; Vienneau, D.; Cajochen, C.; Wunderli, J.M.; Probst-Hensch, N.; Röösli, M. Effects of Scale, Question Location, Order of Response Alternatives, and Season on Self-Reported Noise Annoyance Using ICBEN Scales: A Field Experiment. *Int. J. Environ. Res. Public Health.* **2016**, *13*, 1163. [CrossRef] [PubMed]
24. Dempster, A.P.; Laird, N.M.; Rubin, D.B. Maximum likelihood estimation from incomplete data via the EM algorithm (with discussion). *J. R. Stat. Soc. Ser. B* **1977**, *39*, 1–38.
25. Pigott, T.D. A review of methods for missing data. *Educ. Res. Eval.* **2001**, *7*, 353–383. [CrossRef]

26. Norman, G. Likert scales, levels of measurement and the "laws" of statistics. *Adv. Health Sci. Educ. Theory Pract.* **2010**, *15*, 625–632. [CrossRef] [PubMed]
27. Rhemtulla, M.; Brosseau-Liard, P.É.; Savalei, V. When can categorical variables be treated as continuous? A comparison of robust continuous and categorical SEM estimation methods under suboptimal conditions. *Psychol. Methods* **2012**, *17*, 354–373. [CrossRef] [PubMed]
28. Hayes, A. *Introduction to Mediation, Moderation, and Conditional Process Analysis: A Regression-Based Approach*; Guilford Press: New York, NY, USA, 2013.
29. Hayes, A.F.; Montoya, A.K.; Rockwood, N.J. The analysis of mechanisms and their contingencies: PROCESS versus structural equation modeling. *Australas. Market. J.* **2017**, *25*, 76–81. [CrossRef]
30. Zhao, X.; Lynch, J.G.; Chen, Q. Reconsidering Baron and Kenny: Myths and truths about mediation analysis. *J. Consum. Res.* **2010**, *37*, 197–206. [CrossRef]
31. Gidlöf-Gunnarsson, A.; Öhrström, E. Noise and well-being in urban residential environments: The potential role of perceived availability to nearby green areas. *Landsc. Urban Plan.* **2007**, *8*, 115–126. [CrossRef]
32. Gidlöf-Gunnarsson, A.; Öhrström, E.; Ögren, M.; Jerson, T. Good sound environment in green areas modify road-traffic noise annoyance at home. In Processing of 8th European Conference on Noise Control 2009 (EURONOISE 2009). Edinburgh, Scotland, UK, 26–28 October 2009; pp. 1579–1587.
33. Bodin, T.; Björk, J.; Ardö, J.; Albin, M. Annoyance, sleep and concentration problems due to combined traffic noise and the benefit of quiet side. *Int. J. Environ. Res. Public Health* **2015**, *12*, 1612–1628. [CrossRef] [PubMed]
34. Dzhambov, A.M.; Dimitrova, D.D. Green spaces and environmental noise perception. *Urban For. Urban Green.* **2015**, *14*, 1000–1008. [CrossRef]
35. Li, H.N.; Chau, C.K.; Tse, M.S.; Tang, S.K. On the study of the effects of sea views, greenery views and personal characteristics on noise annoyance perception at homes. *J. Acoust. Soc. Am.* **2012**, *131*, 2131–2140. [CrossRef] [PubMed]
36. Hartig, T.; Mitchell, R.; de Vries, S.; Frumkin, H. Nature and Health. *Annu. Rev. Public Health* **2014**, *35*, 207–228. [CrossRef] [PubMed]
37. Science Communication Unit. *Noise Abatement Approaches. Future Brief 17. Produced for the European Commission DG Environment by the Science Communication Unit, UWE, Bristol. Science for Environment Policy*; Science Communication Unit, UWE: Bristol, UK, 2017.
38. Münzel, T.; Schmidt, FP.; Steven, S.; Herzog, J.; Daiber, A.; Sørensen, M. Environmental Noise and the Cardiovascular System. *J. Am. Coll. Cardiol.* **2018**, *71*, 688–697. [CrossRef] [PubMed]
39. Aletta, F.; Van Renterghem, T.; Botteldooren, D. Influence of Personal Factors on Sound Perception and Overall Experience in Urban Green Areas. A Case Study of a Cycling Path Highly Exposed to Road Traffic Noise. *Int. J. Environ. Res. Public Health* **2018**, *15*, 1118. [CrossRef] [PubMed]
40. Van den Bosch, M.; Nieuwenhuijsen, M. No time to lose-Green the cities now. *Environ Int.* **2017**, *99*, 343–350. [CrossRef] [PubMed]
41. Riedel, N.; van Kamp, I.; Köckler, H.; Scheiner, J.; Loerbroks, A.; Claßen, T.; Bolte, G. Cognitive-Motivational Determinants of Residents' Civic Engagement and Health (Inequities) in the Context of Noise Action Planning: A Conceptual Model. *Int. J. Environ. Res. Public Health* **2017**, *14*, 578. [CrossRef] [PubMed]
42. Rugel, E.J.; Henderson, S.B.; Carpiano, R.M.; Brauer, M. Beyond the Normalized Difference Vegetation Index (NDVI): Developing a Natural Space Index for population-level health research. *Environ Res.* **2017**, *159*, 474–483. [CrossRef] [PubMed]
43. Triguero-Mas, M.; Donaire-Gonzalez, D.; Seto, E.; Valentín, A.; Martínez, D.; Smith, G.; Hurst, G.; Carrasco-Turigas, G.; Masterson, D.; van den Berg, M.; et al. Natural outdoor environments and mental health: Stress as a possible mechanism. *Environ. Res.* **2017**, *159*, 629–638. [CrossRef] [PubMed]
44. Li, X.; Zhang, Z.; Li, W.; Ricard, R.; Meng, O.; Zhang, W. Assessing street-level urban greenery using Google Street view and a modified green view index. *Urban For. Urban Green.* **2015**, *14*, 675–685. [CrossRef]
45. Leslie, E.; Sugiyama, T.; Ierodiaconou, D.; Kremer, P. Perceived and objectively measured greenness of neighbourhoods: Are they measuring the same thing? *Landsc. Urban Plan.* **2010**, *95*, 28–33. [CrossRef]
46. Dzhambov, A.; Hartig, T.; Markevych, I.; Tilov, B.; Dimitrova, D. Urban residential greenspace and mental health in youth: Different approaches to testing multiple pathways yield different conclusions. *Environ. Res.* **2018**, *160*, 47–59. [CrossRef] [PubMed]

47. Jiang, B.; Deal, B.; Pan, H.; Larsen, L.; Hsieh, C.-H.; Chang, C.-Y.; Sullivan, W.C. Remotely-sensed imagery vs. eye-level photography: Evaluating associations among measurements of tree cover density. *Landsc. Urban Plan.* **2017**, *157*, 270–281. [CrossRef]
48. Tilt, J.H.; Unfried, T.M.; Roca, B. Using objective and subjective measures of neighborhood greenness and accessible destinations for understanding walking trips and BMI in Seattle, Washington. *Am. J. Health Promot.* **2007**, *21*, 371–379. [CrossRef] [PubMed]
49. Maxwell, S.E.; Cole, D.A.; Mitchell, M.A. Bias in cross-sectional analyses of longitudinal mediation: Partial and complete mediation under an autoregressive model. *Multivar. Behav. Res.* **2011**, *46*, 816–841. [CrossRef] [PubMed]
50. Job, R.F.S.; Hatfield, J.; Carter, N.L.; Peploe, P.; Taylor, R.; Morrell, S. General scales of community reaction to noise (dissatisfaction and perceived affectedness) are more reliable than scales of annoyance. *J. Acoust. Soc. Am.* **2001**, *110*, 939–946. [CrossRef] [PubMed]
51. Lercher, P.; De Coensel, B.; Dekonink, L.; Botteldooren, D. Community Response to Multiple Sound Sources: Integrating Acoustic and Contextual Approaches in the Analysis. *Int. J. Environ. Res. Public Health* **2017**, *14*, 663. [CrossRef] [PubMed]
52. Schreckenberg, D.; Belke, C.; Spilski, J. The Development of a Multiple-Item Annoyance Scale (MIAS) for Transportation Noise Annoyance. *Int. J. Environ. Res. Public Health* **2018**, *15*, 971. [CrossRef] [PubMed]

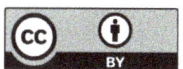

© 2018 by the authors. Licensee MDPI, Basel, Switzerland. This article is an open access article distributed under the terms and conditions of the Creative Commons Attribution (CC BY) license (http://creativecommons.org/licenses/by/4.0/).

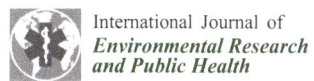

Article

Sounds of Nature in the City: No Evidence of Bird Song Improving Stress Recovery

Marcus Hedblom [1,2,*], Bengt Gunnarsson [3], Martin Schaefer [4], Igor Knez [5], Pontus Thorsson [6] and Johan N. Lundström [4,7,8,9]

1. Department of Forest Resource Management, Swedish University of Agricultural Sciences, 901 83 Umeå, Sweden
2. Department of Ecology, Swedish University of Agricultural Sciences, 750 07 Uppsala, Sweden
3. Department of Biological and Environmental Sciences, University of Gothenburg, 405 30 Gothenburg, Sweden; bengt.gunnarsson@bioenv.gu.se
4. Department of Clinical Neuroscience, Karolinska Institutet, 171 77 Stockholm, Sweden; martin.schaefer@ki.se
5. Department of Social Work and Psychology, University of Gävle, 801 76 Gävle, Sweden; igor.knez@hig.se
6. Division of Applied Acoustics, Chalmers University of Technology, 412 96 Gothenburg, Sweden; pontus.thorsson@akustikverkstan.se
7. Monell Chemical Senses Center, Philadelphia, PA 19104-3308, USA; johan.lundstrom@ki.se
8. Department of Psychology, University of Pennsylvania, Philadelphia, PA 191 04, USA
9. Stockholm University Brain Imaging Centre, Stockholm University, 106 91 Stockholm, Sweden
* Correspondence: marcus.hedblom@slu.se; Tel.: +46-18-671041

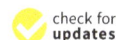

Received: 23 March 2019; Accepted: 13 April 2019; Published: 17 April 2019

Abstract: Noise from city traffic is one of the most significant environmental stressors. Natural soundscapes, such as bird songs, have been suggested to potentially mitigate or mask noise. All previous studies on masking noise use self-evaluation data rather than physiological data. In this study, while respondents (n = 117) watched a 360° virtual reality (VR) photograph of a park, they were exposed to different soundscapes and mild electrical shocks. The soundscapes—"bird song", "bird song and traffic noise", and "traffic noise"—were played during a 10 min recovery period while their skin conductance levels were assessed as a measure of arousal/stress. No significant difference in stress recovery was found between the soundscapes although a tendency for less stress in "bird song" and more stress in "traffic noise" was noted. All three soundscapes, however, significantly reduced stress. This result could be attributed to the stress-reducing effect of the visual VR environment, to the noise levels being higher than 47 dBA (a level known to make masking ineffective), or to the respondents finding bird songs stressful. Reduction of stress in cities using masking with natural sounds requires further studies with not only larger samples but also sufficient methods to detect potential sex differences.

Keywords: stress; experiment; virtual reality; soundscape; bird song; noise

1. Introduction

The health and well-being of an urban population are strongly influenced by the characteristics of the urban systems where factors such as density of houses, the presence of green spaces, urban heat island effects, population densities, traffic, air pollution, and noise pollution all have an impact [1]. However, when it comes to environmental stressors associated with disease, noise pollution has been identified as one of the most significant factors [2–7]. In larger European cities, half the population is likely to be exposed to noise levels that produce physiological and psychological stresses that affect health and well-being (The European Directive COM 2002/49/EC), a problem that has been predicted to increase, leading to even higher societal costs [8,9]. Whereas research into this topic has traditionally focused on mechanical ways to reduce noise, few studies have assessed whether other environmental factors, such as the presence of nature or green areas, might reduce stress by their mere presence.

Urbanization naturally leads to a decreased availability to urban green areas [10], the very urban green areas that promote general human health and stress recovery [11]. Urban green areas can generate cognitive, affective, and psychophysiological benefits, reducing stress and attention fatigue [11–13]. However, the literature vaguely describes the concept of "green" areas and how "green" areas are linked to human well-being and mechanisms of stress reduction [14,15].

Most literature on perceived and actual attention restoration and stress recovery as the result of exposure to nature has focused on visual stimuli [11]. However, few studies have examined how sound in outdoor environments, such as urban green areas, influences stress reduction. Evaluating outdoor environments (compared to indoor environments) for their psycho-acoustic properties is a non-trivial task due to interactions between various sound sources and other acoustical and non-acoustical factors [16]. Studies conducted in outdoor environments commonly adopt a theoretical framework of soundscapes, which includes the total acoustic environment in which respondents perceive a sound [16,17]. Earlier studies that define well-being in general (self-reported well-being) and not stress reduction per se have emphasized the interdependence of visual and acoustic stimuli [18,19]. Individuals respond negatively to the lack of non-visual natural stimuli when observing nature through a video-only feed [20]. For example, participants reported missing "the smells and sounds" of nature and described the setting as "too quiet". This observation suggests that natural sounds may contribute to the restorative experience of being in nature, perhaps because natural sounds signify a living or vital natural environment. Similarly, several self-evaluation studies have found that traffic noise is considered more stressful than natural sounds [19,21].

Urban noise can be reduced by using barriers [22], by enhancing certain sounds through architectural design strategies, and by masking noise using other sounds [16]. The least studied strategy for reducing urban noise is perhaps the masking strategy, which uses common sound sources from outdoor environments, such as bird songs and traffic noise [23], rather than masking speech with speech [24]. Investigating these relationships may help urban planners understand how natural sounds influence human well-being and health. According to Hao et al. masking is a "hearing phenomenon through which soundscape characteristics are altered by the presence of interfering sound event(s)" [23]. They further emphasize the importance of the specific context, such as real-life sound environments linked to birds chirping at different times of day, bird density, and visibility of sound sources. Most studies evaluating the impact of non-natural sounds are based on sounds that residents consider annoying [16]. However, natural sounds such as bird songs increase positive perceptions as well as reduce stress [25–27]. Few studies have investigated the physiological effects of positive soundscapes (cf. [28,29]), and previous experiments assessing the effects of masking noise with natural sounds rely on self-evaluations rather than physiological responses [16,30,31].

In this study, we investigate the physiological effects (stress reduction) of masking noise with a natural sound using an experimental design. We conducted the study in a laboratory to avoid bias linked to possible self-evaluation confounding factors in complex soundscape environments, personal elements such as expectation, preconception, and familiarity, as well as the need to control stimuli [32]. By using a laboratory setup, we controlled the soundscape environment as well as the visual environment, which relied on a multisensory virtual reality (VR) 360° setup.

This study aims to determine whether natural sounds from birds, presented at an ecologically valid sound level, reduce physical stress by masking noise from urban traffic. We hypothesize that when respondents are exposed to a stressor (mild electrical shocks), the type of soundscape they are exposed to will have a differential effect on their stress recovery. We predict that natural sounds will have the greatest effect on stress reduction, masked sounds from natural sources will have the second greatest effect on stress reduction, and noise from traffic will have the least effect on stress reduction.

2. Materials and Methods

2.1. Participants

This between n-group study included 117 participants (73 females and 44 males). Each participant was exposed to one of three types of soundscapes ("bird song", "traffic noise", and "bird song and traffic noise") and one visual environment (360° VR photograph of a Swedish urban park). That is, the experiment included one soundscape environment for each participant, who were pseudo-randomly assigned a soundscape based on the order of participant entry: "traffic noise" (n = 38, 25 women, mean age 27.2 years, SD = 5.4), "bird song and traffic noise" (n = 39, 21 women, mean age 26.8 years, SD = 6.2), and "bird song" (n = 40, 27 women, mean age 27.5 years, SD = 4.9). The following inclusion criteria were used: self-declared health, age between 18 and 50 years, normal to corrected eye-sight and hearing, self-declared as not being currently pregnant, and no prescription medication use. Before enrolment, all participants provided signed informed consent. All research activities were performed in accordance with relevant guidelines/regulations as well as approved by the regional ethical review board in Uppsala (*Etikprövningsnämnden*, Dnr: 2016/175).

2.2. Virtual Reality Photograph

The experiment included one 360° virtual reality (VR) photograph of an urban park in Uppsala (Figure 1). The 360° photograph was presented using a VR mask (Oculus Rift). A Samsung Gear 360 SM-R210 camera was used to photograph a common park setting with an expansive lawn, some trees, distant buildings, paths, and a distant road. The camera was placed on a tripod at a height of 1.75 m. The photograph purposely lacked any elements of major commercial signs and was taken early in the morning to avoid pedestrians. In total, respondents spent 13 minutes in this environment (three minutes during the stress-inducing phase and ten minutes during the relaxation phase).

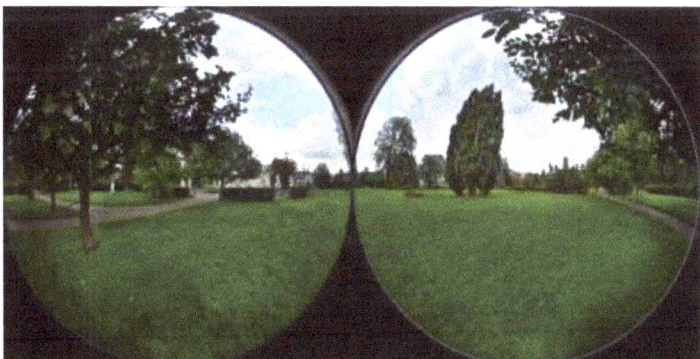

Figure 1. Illustrating the park photograph used in the experiment. The Oculus Rift provides a 360° view, but this photo only provides an approximation of the setting rather than how it would be perceived using the gear.

2.3. Soundscapes

The soundscapes (auditory stimuli) were presented through headphones integrated in the VR mask. The respondents were placed in a separate room with a closed door to minimize outside sound from entering the room. This closed door provided access to another room where a laboratory assistant was located. The door leading out of this room was also closed during the experiment, providing yet another sound barrier. To provide a soundscape with high positive perception, we used bird songs (highest rated natural sound in [26] and [22]) and the same number of species and abundance as the highest rated bird song combination in Hedblom et al. [25]. Although abundance and species number ($n = 7$) were equal (same number of strophes during the 30 s) to Hedblom et al. [33], the species composition in this study resembled the species composition heard in an urban park (the previously mentioned article used an urban woodlands soundscape). The species included in the present soundscape were willow warbler (*Phylloscopus trochilus*), chaffinch (*Fringilla coelebs*), blackbird (*Turdus merula*), blue tit (*Cyanistes caeruleus*), European robin (*Erithacus rubecula*), common swift (*Apus apus*), and common wood pigeon (*Columba palumbus*). The bird songs were downloaded from open sources on the internet and mixed using Audacity 2.1.2. To make the sound more realistic, the sound of a slight breeze was also mixed into the soundscapes. The bird songs were played in stereo, mimicking the way they are heard in nature, and the songs were heard in the left and right ears at different strengths (resembling a bird either far or near). The same bird song combination was used for the conditions "bird song" and "bird song and traffic noise".

The condition "traffic noise" was recorded in the vicinity of a Swedish road in the city of Mariestad, which has a traffic intensity of 8000–10,000 vehicles a day (*Akustikverkstaden*). The recording was done from an open space at a distance of 20 m from the road. Human voices and bird songs were removed using the software program Audacity 2.1.2, leaving only the noise of vehicles. The noise from the traffic varied, including noise peaks when motorcycles or trucks passed by and less noise when the flow of traffic was less (but never absent).

When played through the headphones, the sounds had an intensity variation during the exposure at the level of the participant's ears: "traffic noise"—L_p = 50–62 dBA; "bird song"—L_p = 45–80 dBA; and "bird song and traffic noise"—L_p = 50–77 dBA. The sounds and their corresponding A-weighted sound were chosen to resemble a realistic soundscape as if a respondent were standing in the park hearing noise at a distance and birds nearby and distant.

2.4. Experimental Procedure

These multisensory experiments, conducted in a laboratory at Karolinska Institutet in Stockholm, were specifically designed for using soundscape and visual stimuli. Upon arrival, the respondents provided signed informed consent and were informed about the experiment. In addition, they were told that they would be exposed to a virtual reality (VR) environment, mild electrical shocks, and skin conductance measurements. As the experiments were a between-group design, each participant was exposed to only one visual stimulus and one soundscape. We used mild electrical shocks instead of stressful social situations [34] or movies [13] to elicit a mild physical stress response. After an initial shock of 0.5 amperes was delivered, subsequent shocks were increased gradually by 0.3 amperes. The respondent rated the experienced shock of each increase on a 0–10 scale: 1 = "does not feel at all" and 10 = "hurts". When the respondent perceived a 7 ("uncomfortable but not painful"), the intensity was considered to be proper and that intensity was then used throughout the experiment. That is, the intensity of the electrical shock was determined by the individual. Electrical shocks were generated via a Powerlab system (ADInstruments, Boulder, CO, USA) at different time intervals (see below). The shocks were delivered through electrodes on the middle phalanx of the index and middle fingers on the non-dominant hand. Skin conductance levels (SCL) were measured throughout the whole experiment using Ag/AgCl electrodes on the index and middle fingers of the dominant hand. Data were acquired at a 1000 Hz rate and then filtered offline using a 0.1 Hz high-pass filter.

While experiencing the virtual park, the participants received five shocks in total. The first shock started after 30 s and the last after 150 s. After 150 s, no more shocks were used although the participants were not aware that the stress induction period was over. After 180 s, the sound started and continued for 780 s (in total, ten minutes in one soundscape).

2.5. Statistical Analyses

Skin conductance levels were recorded continuously for the full duration that the participants spent in the virtual environment. The first 30 s of recording (before the initiation of the shock stimuli) were used to obtain baseline measurements for each participant. All subsequent values were adjusted by the mean value of the first 30 s of the experiment, creating a "baseline-adjusted skin conductance value". For each participant, an average of the SCL values was taken every 30 s to remove spontaneous fluctuations and to reduce the resolution of subsequent statistical analyses. This technique resulted in 21 unique data points for each participant. Individuals with a mean value (within each experimental phase) more than three standard deviations from the mean had their value, within the phase in question, replaced with the group mean to limit data skew yet remain in the dataset.

To assess statistical effects, analyses were performed within the R environment (R Core Team, 2018), we used non-parametric tests where assumptions of normal distributions and equal variance were not met, otherwise, parametric tests were used. First, we assessed whether our paradigm could induce stress responses by performing a one-sample, one-tailed Student's t-test against 0 (no change) on mean SCL values within the stress period with all three groups merged. Second, we assessed whether the three soundscapes produced different recovery effects during the relaxation period using ANOVA with the between-group factor "soundscape" (i.e., "bird song", "traffic noise", and "bird song and traffic noise") and with the dependent variable SCL change (difference between the mean of the first 30 s and the mean of the last 30 s of the relaxation period). Third, we assessed whether there were differences between the soundscapes in their ability to reduce stress over time by dividing the SCL levels across the full ten minutes of the relaxation period into four-time segments. To this end, we created mean SCL values for the following periods: 180–330 s, 330–480 s, 480–630 s, and 630–780 s. These mean SCL values within each of the four periods were then entered into a mixed-ANOVA with the three soundscapes ("traffic noise", "bird song", and "bird song and traffic noise"), creating a 3 × 4 ANOVA model.

We further tested whether there were differences between sexes in stress reduction using a similar approach as above with ANOVA (the difference between the mean of the first 30 s and the mean of the last 30 s of the relaxation period) and mixed-ANOVA (sexes and four periods).

3. Results

3.1. Stress Induction

First, we assessed whether our paradigm successfully induced a stress response among participants. As predicted, compared to baseline, there was a significant increase in SCL in response to the weak electric shocks—t (9.48); df = 116, $p < 2.2\text{e-}16$. This increase indicated that our paradigm successfully induced a weak but reliable physical stress response.

3.2. Soundscapes and Stress

We then assessed whether there was a difference between the soundscapes in their ability to reduce stress following the stress induction period. We found no difference in stress reduction, F (2,114) = 0.187, $p = 0.83$, between the three soundscapes, as indicated by ANOVA (Figure 2).

A mixed-ANOVA comparing four periods with that of the three soundscapes revealed that there was a significant effect of period across all three soundscapes. In other words, SCL were reduced over the recovery period independent of soundscape ($p < 0.001$) (Table 1) (Figure 3). There were, however, no differences between the soundscapes ($p = 0.181$) nor an interaction between period and soundscapes ($p = 0.995$).

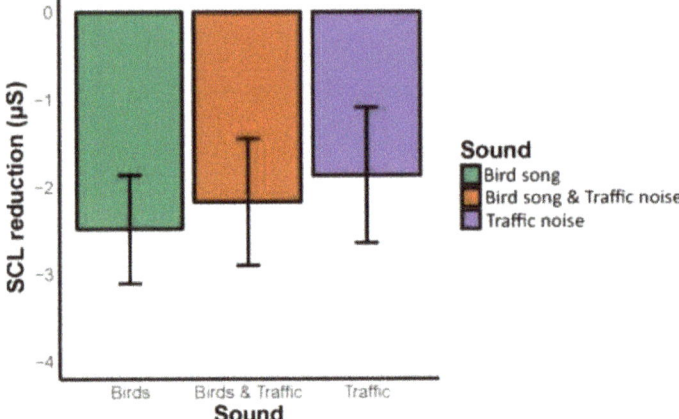

Figure 2. Average reduction change in skin conductance levels (μSiemens) during the relaxation period (from onset to end) for the three soundscape conditions. Errors bars indicate standard error of the mean (SEM).

Table 1. Mixed-ANOVA comparing soundscapes, recovery period (only soundscapes in the recovery period and no stress for ten minutes), and the combination of sounds and period.

	Df	Sum Sq	Mean Sq	F Value	Pr (>F)
Soundscape	2	33	16.25	1.715	0.181107
Recovery period	3	176	58.61	6.185	0.000399 *
Sound:period	6	6	1.04	0.110	0.995304
Residuals	456	4321	9.48		

* indicates a significant result.

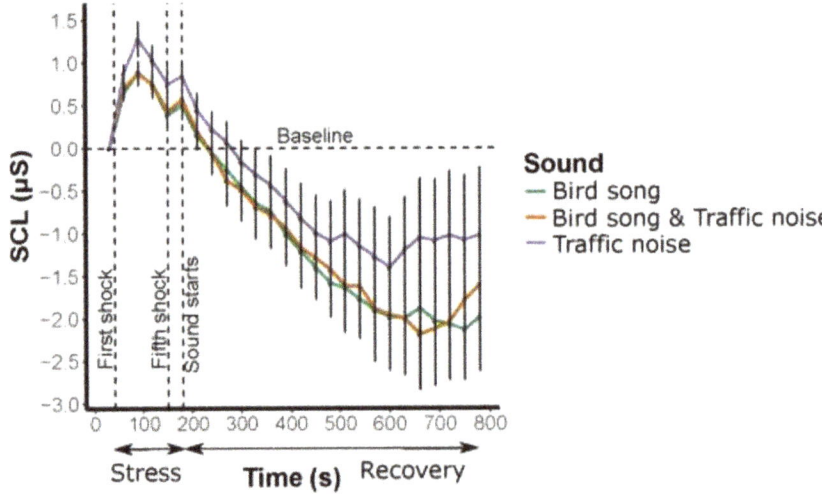

Figure 3. Skin conductance levels (SCL) responses (μSiemens) over time between the three soundscapes in the stress period (five minor electrical shocks) and the recovery period. Errors bars indicate the standard error of the mean (SEM).

3.3. Sex and Stress

We found no significant differences (except for a decrease of stress) between the sexes, but, surprisingly, we found a tendency of differences between sexes during the relaxation period (Figure 4).

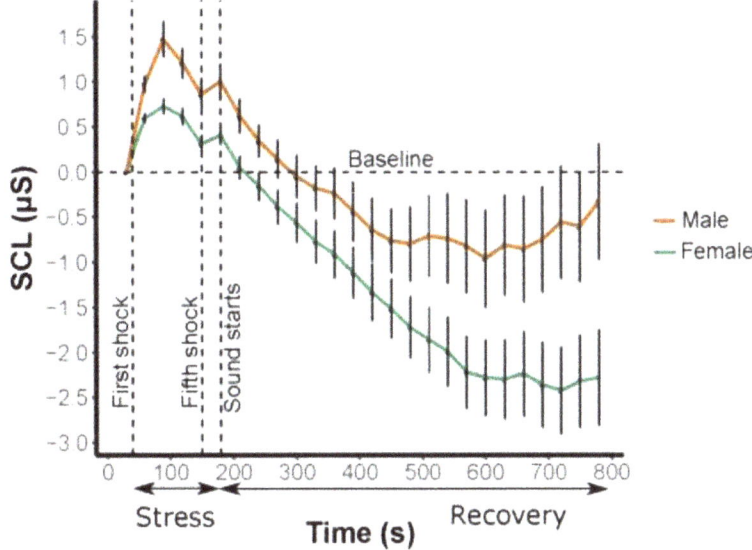

Figure 4. Illustrating non-significant differences in stress reduction (μSiemens) between male and female respondents during the stress period (five minor electrical shocks) and the recovery period (pooled values). Errors bars indicate standard error of the mean (SEM).

During the stress period (30–180 s), there was a significant difference in stress between sexes (Figure 4) as shown in the Student's t-test based on the average SCL during the stress period, t (63) = 3.3021, p = 0.001575. The men chose slightly higher ampere values on average than women in the set up for the experiment (male average: 2.9; female average: 2.4). During the recovery, no differences were found in stress reduction between the sexes, t (87.42) = 1.6086, p = 0.1113.

There was stress reduction during the recovery period for both sexes (p < 0.001) (Table 2). When comparing stress recovery and sex for the four periods (1st: 180–330 s; 2nd: 330–480 s; 3rd: 480–630 s; and 4th: 630–780 s), there was a tendency of differences between sexes (p = 0.08523) (Table 2) although this was not statistically significant. No statistical significance was found between the interaction of sex and period.

Table 2. Mixed-ANOVA comparing recovery period between sexes for ten minutes, four stress recovery periods, and the combination of sex and recovery period.

	Df	Sum Sq	Mean Sq	F value	Pr (>F)
Sex	1	26	25.63	2.973	0.085323
Recovery period	3	176	58.61	6.800	0.000171 *
Sex period	3	23	7.80	0.904	0.438825
Residuals	460	3965	8.62		

* indicates a significant result.

4. Discussion

No statistically significant difference in stress reduction was found between the three soundscapes—"bird song", "traffic noise", and "bird song and traffic noise". Although non-significant, there seems to be a pattern linked to our hypothesis that "traffic noise" would have the least reduction in stress and "bird song" would the greatest reduction in stress (Figures 2 and 3). However, these results may be linked to the small sample size and potential large individual variation. Our hypotheses, however, were based on previous findings from studies that used self-evaluations to conclude that bird songs compared to other noises such as traffic noise reduce stress (cf. [16,35]). Understanding why our study found no statistically significant differences should help urban planners understand how to use natural sounds to mask urban noise to reduce noise-associated stress. Below, we discuss the importance of the context of the physiological responses to the soundscapes: (i) the link (interdependent) to the visual feature of urban green (in this case a park); (ii) masking sounds; (iii) dBA levels; (iv) demography, such as sex aspects and dose-response for the setting, for example, the time spent in the experimental setup; (v) the physiological tests of stress in the experimental set up; and (vi) the conclusions with recommendations based on results.

4.1. Interdependence of Soundscape and Visual Features

Overall, the induced stress decreased significantly during the ten minutes of the stress-recovery period irrespective of the soundscape. This decrease could be linked to visual features, such as urban green (or green in general) has been shown to be associated with stress reduction [36,37]. However, the link between sound and visual features are sometimes arbitrary and context dependent. In a self-evaluation experiment, Hong and Jeon [22] found that visual aspects were more important than auditory aspects of an experience. Other studies, however, such as Hedblom et al. [25], found that natural sounds of birds increase positive ratings of visual settings. Moreover, Viollon et al. [19] found that traffic noises and bird songs were significantly influenced by the visual degree of urbanization (self-evaluations). Thus, the results from Viollon et al. [19] support our results: a pleasant visual urban green environment increases the positive perception regardless of whether the soundscape contains traffic noise or bird songs, or both. We used a virtual reality photograph where the respondent was placed in the middle of an urban park with the possibility to view the scene from a 360° perspective, enabling the respondent to view the scene as if they were in the actual park, with the ability, for example, to look up trees, to look at the ground, and to look at the sky. This VR experience potentially provided a more visually relaxing (and realistic) environment than a conventional photograph of a green environment on a screen, which previous studies use to elicit responses, as VR increases the influence of visual features [19,25]. Nevertheless, it is not clear if it is the visual dominance of the VR photograph that provides the stress recovery or if people find all three sounds relaxing (possibly with bird songs being more relaxing than the other soundscapes) (Figure 3).

4.2. Masking of Sounds

In this study, we used bird songs to mask the noise because it is a common soundscape found globally in cities [38]. Typically, bird songs [23] and moving or running water [16,17,21,30,31] are the natural sounds used to mask noise. People's perceptions of which sound is the most pleasant (or the most stress-reducing) vary between individuals and studies. In Hong and Jeon [22], bird songs are preferred to falling water, which was found to decrease the soundscape quality. Similarly, Ratcliffe et al. [26] found that bird songs were preferred to the sound of moving water; however, Jeon et al. [16] found that the sound of streams and lake waves were preferred over the sound of birds in a forest. Overall, soundscapes are rather vaguely defined and do not identify or describe the birds other than using the phrase "chirps of birds" although more than 10,000 bird species and even more bird songs exist. The type of species, abundance of species, and the combination of species affect people's perceptions of an urban setting [25]. Furthermore, bird songs and water sounds are important features for masking noise when respondents are self-evaluating a soundscapes [21,35]. One explanation for the results in this study might be that differences detected in self-evaluations are not reflected in physiological responses; the differences are simply too small. Medvedev et al. [29] failed to reveal statistical differences between soundscapes and physiological responses, although not for self-evaluations. Therefore, it might be that subjective self-evaluation, or self-perception, of soundscapes are perceived as strong differences while actual physiological effects are not very large, at least not in the context of the soundscapes presented in this study (and in [29]). However, there might be a rather large individual variation in perception of a soundscape that impacts the overall results. Future studies should include recovery periods without any stimuli as well as only visual or only sound stimuli.

4.3. dBA Levels

Numerous studies assessing masking emphasize the importance of context where the dBA level is important [21,23]. Urban planning should consider specific dBA levels because individuals exposed to high noise levels commonly suffer from poorer health, including poor cardiovascular effects [39]. Regardless of dBA levels, respondents perceive an environment as more natural if they can hear bird songs [23]. Nonetheless, small differences have shown to influence self-evaluated perceptions of the masking effects that natural sounds have on noise. When traffic noise is lower ($L_{eq} < 52.5$ dBA, e.g., when the traffic noise is greater than 19 m away), the masking effects are more significant than if the noise is louder or the distance is shorter [23]. The results from Hao et al. [23] might contribute to our non-significant findings because our span of sound level for road traffic noise was as high as 62 dBA, a level that reduces the potential for bird song masking. Hao et al. [23] indeed show that when traffic noise exceeds 47.5 dBA, the pleasantness decreases sharply. As for bird songs in a real city park situation, the sound level of the bird songs is often low compared to the traffic. In this study, we wanted the bird songs to be audible in the mixed sound, so there is a risk that some of the bird song strophes reached an unrealistic level of 80 dBA on some occasions. A sound at this level can be a stressor due to its strength [40] rather than its subjectively interpreted content. This is something that should be tested in future experiments.

4.4. Demography and Time of Experiment

We found some tendencies of differences between sexes. Men showed higher stress initially during the stress period, a finding that is confirmed in other studies [41]. During the recovery period, there was a tendency that women, compared to men, had greater reductions in stress ($p = 0.0853$), but no significant difference was found. After eight minutes, women seemed to continue to experience stress reduction, whereas men seemed to increase stress (Figure 4). Previous experiments found that participants experience two minutes of stress reduction and four minutes of stress recovery. For example, it is important to study longer exposure times to include ecological validity and habituation effects [29]. We hypothesize that the tendency of men to experience a reduced recovery can be linked to previous results showing that men have less appreciation for urban green areas than women [42]. Previous studies of soundscapes reveal differences between the sexes where women, more than men, preferred natural sounds from birds [43]. Thus, a potential future replication of this study should provide a design that systematically assesses potential differences between men and women.

4.5. Measuring Stress in an Experimental Setup

We used electrical shocks to induce reliable physiological stress responses from all participants within an experimental setup and operationalized stress levels such as skin conductance levels (SCL). Other studies have used amylase enzyme [44] or heart rate [29] and each method has its advantages and disadvantages. How the physiological stress response is specifically linked to psychological or social stress is not known, although social stress seems to be one of the leading causes of impaired well-being in modern societies [45]. The direct link between environmental stimuli and long-term stress is difficult to assess using an experimental design without undue burden on the research participants. More studies are needed to fully understand the potential of natural sounds as masking sounds and their potential for reducing psychological stress.

5. Conclusions

We found no significant results for a reduction in physiological stress when masking traffic noise with bird songs. Stress levels during the recovery period were reduced below baseline levels for all soundscapes (although less so for traffic noise and least for bird songs), which could be due to the strong preferences for the visual 360° VR environment of a green park. It could also be that respondents, who were mostly urban dwellers, expected an urban park to have traffic noise and thus did not experience any impedance to their stress recovery from its presence. Our results further illustrate an example where bird songs do not have any physical effect on stress. Adding bird songs to a noisy traffic environment (above 47 dBA) might not reduce people's stress but might lower noisy environments.

Author Contributions: M.H., B.G. and J.N.L. conceptualized the research. M.H. wrote the original draft. M.H., B.G. and J.N.L. contributed to the writing. M.H., B.G., J.N.L., M.S., I.K. and P.T. helped review and edit. M.S. and J.N.L. provided formal analyses and M.S. provided figures and conducted the laboratory experiments.

Funding: This research was funded by the Swedish Research Council for Environment, Agricultural Sciences and Spatial Planning (FORMAS) project number: 942-2015-610. Johan N Lundström was funded by grants from the Knut and Alice Wallenberg Foundation (KAW 2018.0152) and the Swedish Research Council (2014-01346).

Acknowledgments: We would like to thank psychology students Mikael Billfors Gustavsson and Michael Borgert for providing support in the laboratory tests.

Conflicts of Interest: The authors declare no conflicts of interest.

References

1. Lakes, T.; Bruckner, M.; Kramer, A. Development of an environmental justice index to determine socio-economic disparities of noise pollution and green space in residential areas in Berlin. *J. Environ. Plan. Manag.* **2014**, *57*, 538–556. [CrossRef]
2. Miedema, H.M.E.; Vos, H. Exposure-response relationships for transportation noise. *J. Acoust. Soc. Am.* **1998**, *104*, 3432–3445. [CrossRef] [PubMed]
3. Munzel, T.; Gori, T.; Babisch, W.; Basner, M. Cardiovascular effects of environmental noise exposure. *Eur. Heart J.* **2014**, *35*, 829–836. [CrossRef] [PubMed]
4. Raggam, R.B.; Cik, M.; Holdrich, R.R.; Fallast, K.; Gallasch, E.; Fend, M.; Lackner, A.; Marth, E. Personal noise ranking of road traffic: Subjective estimation versus physiological parameters under laboratory conditions. *Int. J. Hyg. Environ. Health* **2007**, *210*, 97–105. [CrossRef] [PubMed]
5. Babisch, W. Cardiovascular effects of noise. *Noise Health* **2011**, *13*, 201–204. [CrossRef]
6. Van Kempen, E.E.M.M.; Kruize, H.; Boshuizen, H.C.; Ameling, C.B.; Staatsen, B.A.M.; de Hollander, A.E.M. The association between noise exposure and blood pressure and ischemic heart disease: A meta-analysis. *Environ. Health Perspect.* **2002**, *110*, 307–317. [CrossRef]
7. An, R.P.; Wang, J.J.; Ashrafi, S.A.; Yang, Y.; Guan, C.H. Chronic Noise Exposure and Adiposity: A Systematic Review and Meta-analysis. *Am. J. Prev. Med.* **2018**, *55*, 403–411. [CrossRef] [PubMed]
8. Passchier-Vermeer, W.; Passchier, W.F. Noise exposure and public health. *Environ. Health Perspect.* **2000**, *108*, 123–131.
9. Luck, G.W.; Davidson, P.; Boxall, D.; Smallbone, L. Relations between Urban Bird and Plant Communities and Human Well-Being and Connection to Nature. *Conserv. Biol.* **2011**, *25*, 816–826. [CrossRef]
10. Seto, K.C.; Guneralp, B.; Hutyra, L.R. Global forecasts of urban expansion to 2030 and direct impacts on biodiversity and carbon pools. *Proc. Natl. Acad. Sci. USA* **2012**, *109*, 16083–16088. [CrossRef]
11. Hartig, T.; Evans, G.W.; Jamner, L.D.; Davis, D.S.; Garling, T. Tracking restoration in natural and urban field settings. *J. Environ. Psychol.* **2003**, *23*, 109–123. [CrossRef]
12. Berman, M.G.; Jonides, J.; Kaplan, S. The Cognitive Benefits of Interacting With Nature. *Psychol. Sci.* **2008**, *19*, 1207–1212. [CrossRef] [PubMed]

13. Ulrich, R.S.; Simons, R.F.; Losito, B.D.; Fiorito, E.; Miles, M.A.; Zelson, M. Stress Recovery during Exposure to Natural and Urban Environments. *J. Environ. Psychol.* **1991**, *11*, 201–230. [CrossRef]
14. Joye, Y.; van den Berg, A. Is love for green in our genes? A critical analysis of evolutionary assumptions in restorative environments research. *Urban For. Urban Green.* **2011**, *10*, 261–268. [CrossRef]
15. Taylor, L.; Hochuli, D.F. Defining greenspace: Multiple uses across multiple disciplines. *Landsc. Urban Plan* **2017**, *158*, 25–38. [CrossRef]
16. Jeon, J.Y.; Lee, P.J.; You, J.; Kang, J. Perceptual assessment of quality of urban soundscapes with combined noise sources and water sounds. *J. Acoust. Soc. Am.* **2010**, *127*, 1357–1366. [CrossRef] [PubMed]
17. Axelsson, O.; Nilsson, M.E.; Hellstrom, B.; Lunden, P. A field experiment on the impact of sounds from a jet-and-basin fountain on soundscape quality in an urban park. *Landsc. Urban Plan* **2014**, *123*, 49–60. [CrossRef]
18. Carles, J.L.; Barrio, I.L.; de Lucio, J.V. Sound influence on landscape values. *Landsc. Urban Plan* **1999**, *43*, 191–200. [CrossRef]
19. Viollon, S.; Lavandier, C.; Drake, C. Influence of visual setting on sound ratings in an urban environment. *Appl. Acoust.* **2002**, *63*, 493–511. [CrossRef]
20. Kjellgren, A.; Buhrkall, H. A comparison of the restorative effect of a natural environment with that of a simulated natural environment. *J. Environ. Psychol.* **2010**, *30*, 464–472. [CrossRef]
21. Nilsson, M.E.; Berglund, B. Soundscape quality in suburban green areas and city parks. *Acta Acust. United Acust.* **2006**, *92*, 903–911.
22. Hong, J.Y.; Jeon, J.Y. Designing sound and visual components for enhancement of urban soundscapes. *J. Acoust. Soc. Am.* **2013**, *134*, 2026–2036. [CrossRef]
23. Hao, Y.Y.; Kang, J.; Wortche, H. Assessment of the masking effects of birdsong on the road traffic noise environment. *J. Acoust. Soc. Am.* **2016**, *140*, 978–987. [CrossRef] [PubMed]
24. Brungart, D.S.; Scott, K.R. The effects of production and presentation level on the auditory distance perception of speech. *J. Acoust. Soc. Am.* **2001**, *110*, 425–440. [CrossRef] [PubMed]
25. Hedblom, M.; Heyman, E.; Antonsson, H.; Gunnarsson, B. Bird song diversity influences young people's appreciation of urban landscapes. *Urban For. Urban Green.* **2014**, *13*, 469–474. [CrossRef]
26. Ratcliffe, E.; Gatersleben, B.; Sowden, P.T. Bird sounds and their contributions to perceived attention restoration and stress recovery. *J. Environ. Psychol.* **2013**, *36*, 221–228. [CrossRef]
27. Ratcliffe, E.; Gatersleben, B.; Sowden, P.T. Associations with bird sounds: How do they relate to perceived restorative potential? *J. Environ. Psychol.* **2016**, *47*, 136–144. [CrossRef]
28. Hume, K.; Ahtamad, M. Physiological responses to and subjective estimates of soundscape elements. *Appl. Acoust.* **2013**, *74*, 275–281. [CrossRef]
29. Medvedev, O.; Shepherd, D.; Hautus, M.J. The restorative potential of soundscapes: A physiological investigation. *Appl. Acoust.* **2015**, *96*, 20–26. [CrossRef]
30. Galbrun, L.; Ali, T.T. Acoustical and perceptual assessment of water sounds and their use over road traffic noise. *J. Acoust. Soc. Am.* **2013**, *133*, 227–237. [CrossRef] [PubMed]
31. Radsten-Ekman, M.; Axelsson, O.; Nilsson, M.E. Effects of Sounds from Water on Perception of Acoustic Environments Dominated by Road-Traffic Noise. *Acta Acust. United Acust.* **2013**, *99*, 218–225. [CrossRef]
32. Aletta, F.; Kang, J. Towards an Urban Vibrancy Model: A Soundscape Approach. *Int. J. Environ. Res. Public Health* **2018**, *15*, 1712. [CrossRef]
33. Aronson, M.F.J.; La Sorte, F.A.; Nilon, C.H.; Katti, M.; Goddard, M.A.; Lepczyk, C.A.; Warren, P.S.; Williams, N.S.G.; Cilliers, S.; Clarkson, B.; et al. A global analysis of the impacts of urbanization on bird and plant diversity reveals key anthropogenic drivers. *Proc. R. Soc. B Biol. Sci.* **2014**, *281*, 20133330. [CrossRef] [PubMed]
34. Annerstedt, M.; Jonsson, P.; Wallergard, M.; Johansson, G.; Karlson, B.; Grahn, P.; Hansen, A.M.; Wahrborg, P. Inducing physiological stress recovery with sounds of nature in a virtual reality forest—Results from a pilot study. *Physiol. Behav.* **2013**, *118*, 240–250. [CrossRef]
35. Coensel, B.D.; Vanwetswinkel, S.; Botteldooren, D. Effects of natural sounds on the perception of road traffic noise. *J. Acoust. Soc. Am.* **2011**, *129*, EL148–EL153. [CrossRef]
36. Tyrvainen, L.; Ojala, A.; Korpela, K.; Lanki, T.; Tsunetsugu, Y.; Kagawa, T. The influence of urban green environments on stress relief measures: A field experiment. *J. Environ. Psychol.* **2014**, *38*, 1–9. [CrossRef]

37. Thompson, C.W.; Roe, J.; Aspinall, P.; Mitchell, R.; Clow, A.; Miller, D. More green space is linked to less stress in deprived communities: Evidence from salivary cortisol patterns. *Landsc. Urban Plan* **2012**, *105*, 221–229. [CrossRef]
38. Hedblom, M.; Knez, I.; Gunnarsson, B. Bird diversity improves the well-being of city residents. In *Ecology and Conservation of Birds in Urban Environments*; Enrique Murgui, M.H., Ed.; Springer: Cham, Switzerland, 2017; pp. 287–306.
39. Tetreault, L.F.; Perron, S.; Smargiassi, A. Cardiovascular health, traffic-related air pollution and noise: Are associations mutually confounded? A systematic review. *Int. J. Public Health* **2013**, *58*, 649–666. [CrossRef] [PubMed]
40. Bjork, E.A. Laboratory Annoyance and Skin-Conductance Responses to Some Natural Sounds. *J. Sound Vib.* **1986**, *109*, 339–345. [CrossRef]
41. Krantz, G.; Forsman, M.; Lundberg, U. Consistency in physiological stress responses and electromyographic activity during induced stress exposure in women and men. *Integr. Physiol. Behav. Sci.* **2004**, *39*, 105–118. [CrossRef] [PubMed]
42. Sang, A.O.; Knez, I.; Gunnarsson, B.; Hedblom, M. The effects of naturalness, gender, and age on how urban green space is perceived and used. *Urban For. Urban Green.* **2016**, *18*, 268–276. [CrossRef]
43. Hedblom, M.; Knez, I.; Sang, A.O.; Gunnarsson, B. Evaluation of natural sounds in urban greenery: Potential impact for urban nature preservation. *R. Soc. Open. Sci.* **2017**, *4*, 170037. [CrossRef] [PubMed]
44. Ewert, A.; Chang, Y. Levels of Nature and Stress Response. *Behav. Sci.* **2018**, *8*, 49. [CrossRef] [PubMed]
45. Wilkinson, R.; Pickett, K. The Inner Level. How more equal societies reduce stress, restore sanity and improve everybody's wellbeing. Allen Lane: London, UK, 2018; p. 35.

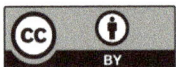

© 2019 by the authors. Licensee MDPI, Basel, Switzerland. This article is an open access article distributed under the terms and conditions of the Creative Commons Attribution (CC BY) license (http://creativecommons.org/licenses/by/4.0/).

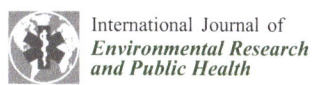

Article

Exploring the Relationship between Urban Quiet Areas and Perceived Restorative Benefits

Sarah R. Payne * and Neil Bruce

The Urban Institute, Heriot-Watt University, Edinburgh EH14 4AS, UK; N.Bruce@hw.ac.uk
* Correspondence: S.R.Payne@hw.ac.uk

Received: 29 March 2019; Accepted: 5 May 2019; Published: 8 May 2019

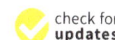

Abstract: To help mitigate the adverse health impacts of environmental noise, European cities are recommended to identify urban quiet areas for preservation. Procedures for identifying urban quiet areas vary across cities and between countries, and little is known of the strength of the salutogenic (health-promoting) benefits they may provide. Taking a multi-site approach, this study examines the potential of three sites as urban quiet areas and their associated health benefits, particularly in relation to perceived restorative benefits. Across three cities in the United Kingdom, an urban garden, urban park, and an urban square had sound pressure levels measured. Responses from 151 visitors to these sites evaluated the place as quiet, calm, and tranquil, and assessed their experience of the place in terms of perceived sounds, its benefits, how it made them feel, and perceived restoration. Depending on the criteria used, the sites varied in their suitability as urban quiet areas, although all provided perceived health benefits. Relationships between sound levels (subjective and objective) and perceived restoration were not linear, with the type of sounds heard and other aspects of the place experience believed to affect the relationship. Building on this work, a future experimental approach based on the study sites is planned to manipulate the multiple variables involved. This will provide a clearer understanding of the relationship between urban quiet areas and perceived restorative benefits.

Keywords: perceived restoration; public health; quiet area; soundscape; environmental noise; urban park; urban square

---

1. Introduction

The relationship between poor environmental acoustics, rising sound levels within urban environments, and its negative impacts on human health have long been documented [1], with the World Health Organization (WHO) concluding "there is overwhelming evidence that exposure to environmental noise has adverse effects on the health of the population" [2] (p. 105). Furthermore, the burden of traffic-related environmental noise in Western Europe has been quantified as "at least one million healthy life years are lost every year" [2] (p. 5). Since then, the WHO has updated its Environmental Noise Guidelines for the European Region exploring both prevention and intervention opportunities for environmental noise to reduce its "public health burden" [3]. Broadly, the guidelines cover transportation noise (e.g., road, rail, air), wind turbine noise, and leisure noise (listening to music through headphones or at various venues). It explores their cognitive effects (annoyance, mental health, cognitive impairments), physical effects (cardiovascular and metabolic, sleep disturbances, hearing impairments, adverse birth outcomes) and impact on overall quality of life and wellbeing.

Examination of environmental noise and its health impacts has predominantly been studied through exposure–response relationships (e.g., [4]). In recent years, a slightly different approach to studying "noise" has developed, which also offers opportunities for examining health impacts through less traditional means than quantified exposure–response relationships. Moreover, the starting point in this approach is a consideration of the acoustic environment in terms of sound rather than noise, recognising that individuals may evaluate sounds differently, thereby only utilising the term noise after public evaluations. This approach is termed soundscapes, which are defined as "acoustic environments as perceived or experienced, and/or understood by a person or people, in context" [5] (p. 1). Soundscape research draws on multiple methods [6], although a recently developed international standard which notes common methodological criteria to be used should increase the ability to compare results across studies [7]. The soundscape approach also enables the consideration of acoustic environments in positive terms, with soundscapes evaluated either positively or negatively, rather than a pure focus on environmental noise.

The potential for positively evaluated acoustic environments aligns with the recommendations from the Environmental Noise Directive (END 2002/49/EC), which despite originating from a noise perspective, require action plans which aim to identify and preserve quiet areas in urban outdoor environments (agglomerations with more than 250,000 inhabitants) to mitigate environmental noise [8]. This infers a potential health value derived from lower sound levels, but only in relation to alleviating the impacts of negative acoustic environments. For example, access to a quiet side of a house may reduce noise annoyance [9] and sleep disturbance [10]. This has resulted in the first of the five WHO environmental noise guiding principles to be "reduce exposure to noise, while conserving quiet areas" [3] (p. 15). Quiet areas, however, may have their own positive beneficial health effects, beyond those of mitigation [11]. For example, they may provide access to hearing other sounds in the city, such as children playing or birds singing, which might perhaps evoke positive feelings, memories, or cognitive improvements.

Currently there is no set definition on what an urban quiet area is, with each European country choosing their own definition and criteria to meet the environmental noise directive [12]. In addition to this, researchers and agencies have also highlighted the importance of other, potentially related, terms for these areas, such as "calm areas" and "tranquil areas" [12,13]. The END, however, suggests the possibility of using averaged day and night sound pressure levels (SPLs) as a way of defining an area as quiet: "an area, ... for instance which is not exposed to a value of L_{den} or of another appropriate noise indicator greater than a certain value set by the Member State, from any noise source" [8] (p. L189/14). From this and within the UK, Scotland chose to examine public gardens, open spaces and open land datasets, before applying to those results the specification that the Candidate Quiet Area (CQA) needs to be bigger than 9 hectares, and have L_{day} levels of below 55 dB(A) across 75% of the place [14]. They later adopted the rule that local authorities could also include other areas if justifiable [15]. In contrast in England, CQAs are identified first as outstanding and tranquil local green spaces (or open land if in London), which are "quiet or relatively quiet, and generate significant benefits (in terms of health, wellbeing, and quality of life) for the communities they serve" and could include public gardens, city parks, or urban squares [16] (p. 23). In contrast to Scotland, SPL or land size criteria are not provided, only that the CQAs have a wide appreciation across the city, and as such are accessible. Both countries, however, have chosen to use public green or open spaces as their starting point for defining urban quiet areas "because Local Green Spaces are green areas that have already been identified as demonstrably special to the local community". Therefore, the beneficial value that these places provide is of importance to their definition.

Indeed, the health benefits of nature and urban green spaces are widely reported across academia, policy, public media, and the World Health Organization [17–19]. One of these benefits is psychological restoration, either affectively, cognitively, or physiologically, which helps mitigate against reduced functioning levels (productively, emotionally, or physically) and is related to stress alleviation [20,21]. Generally, natural environments are perceived as more restorative and have higher restorative outcomes, than built environments with limited green or blue (water) features (e.g., [21,22]). Evidenced pathways between natural environments and health benefits include stress reduction, as well as improved air quality, opportunities for physical activity, and increased social connectivity [23]. Reduced sound levels or improved soundscapes may be an additional pathway between the impact of green spaces on health. For example, living near green areas reduces road traffic annoyance and the researchers suggested this could be because they provided a comparatively quieter space nearby (similar to having a quiet side to a house) [24]. Urban park soundscapes are also perceived as having higher levels of restorative components than urban soundscapes predominated by traffic and construction work [25], with perceived restorativeness increasing for more natural urban park soundscapes [26]. Similarly, certain bird sounds are perceived as higher in their restorative potential [27]. However, further research is needed to associate the role of soundscapes as a mechanism for green spaces providing health benefits. Moreover, evidence is so far limited on how to achieve these salutogenic (health-promoting) urban soundscapes with only a few studies examining the positive health effects of soundscapes [24,28].

Therefore, the aim of this project was to take a multi-site approach to explore the restorative and other self-reported health benefits of public urban spaces that could fall into the remit of Candidate Quiet Areas. To meet the aim, first the objective and subjective place characteristics are assessed to determine their suitability as urban "quiet areas". Secondly, the role of psychological restoration in visiting these places is explored alongside other perceived health benefits gained from being in the place. Finally, the necessity of "quiet" for restoration in urban spaces is examined.

2. Methods

Fieldwork was conducted in public urban outdoor places, located in three UK cities in the summer of 2018. Fieldwork consisted of questionnaires with people in the three places and taking acoustic measurements in each place during the same period as the questionnaires.

2.1. Environment

Due to their varied geographical locations (South England on the coast, North England in the middle of the country, and Central Scotland on a coast line), the three UK cities chosen for this study were Brighton and Hove, Sheffield, and Edinburgh. Three cities were chosen across the UK as they vary in their architectural style, planning systems (at different stages in identifying candidate quiet areas and using different criteria) and potentially their sound sources (e.g., seagulls in Brighton and Hove). This widens the implications of the findings rather than potentially the results being limited to one city. An urban garden, urban park and urban square were chosen as the study sites. These three types of urban spaces were chosen as they fit within the underlying definitions for CQAs in England (Defra 2018) and the original CQA dataset in Scotland (the Scottish Government 2009). The three chosen places vary in size and are located in city centres, thus accessible to the city population. The choice of places was in part guided by results from a connected study on Project DeStress, where the public identified their quiet areas in these three cities [29]. The Garden was identified as a quiet area by the public and the Park was adjacent to a place identified as a quiet area and was considered part of the same connecting green spaces.

The urban gardens in Edinburgh was Dunbar's Close Garden (from herein referred to as the Garden) in the city centre, only 0.19 Ha and just off the famous Royal Mile. The Garden (Figure 1) is landscaped to replicate a 17th century garden, and has distinctive zones consisting of a gravel courtyard with a tree in the middle surrounded by low shrub patterns, two parterres (symmetrically patterned planting beds), yew bush square borders, a square lawn, a wild area, and a long flower border. The gravel path can be followed on a circular loop through the garden. One or two stone or wooden benches are located in each zone except the long border. To the east of the long border are single-storey and multi-storey residential buildings and to the south-east another gated archway through to the Royal Mile. At the north of the garden behind the square lawn there is no exit and a steep slope down which is covered in trees hiding the high-rise apartment blocks. On the west is a large churchyard behind a high stonewall, while the entrance to the garden is off the royal mile down an archway (close) cut into a large five storey stone building which shields the garden from the cars, coaches, buses and pedestrians on the Royal Mile.

The urban park in Brighton and Hove was Palmeira Lawns (from here in referred to as the Park), which is a rectangular green park of 0.72 Ha. The park (Figure 2) contains a number of crisscrossing pathways across the mowed lawns, with benches and waste bins frequently placed alongside the paths. The park is largely open mowed grass with a few clusters of shrubs and flowers. Mature trees line the westerly side of the park, with a few more on the easterly side. On the south side there are numerous trees and bushes delimiting the edge of the park, while to the north, the park is completely open to the adjacent street, with a bus stop at the top and a busy minor (B) road. The park has two residential roads running along the east and west, with cars parked all the way along each side of the park. Five-storey white Victorian town houses overlook the park on the west and east side, whilst the sea can be seen in the near distance when looking to the south.

The urban square in Sheffield was Tudor Square, in the city centre (from here in referred to as the Square), which is 0.27 Ha. The Square (Figure 3) is known for its cultural activities due to the two theatres and library/gallery flanking two sides of the square (NE and SE). Opposite these stone buildings is a pub and two cafes, both with outside seating areas, with the final side of the square overlooked by a large glass greenhouse with a small cobbled side street (dead end for traffic) in between. The square is paved throughout with 9 stone "pods" of various sizes which contain wooden benches on their sides and are topped by trees or grassy shrubs. There are also three steel pods that can be sat on if not too hot. In two corners, either side of one of the theatres, are street canyons to a side road or a major inner-city carriageway with many bus stops located just behind the theatre.

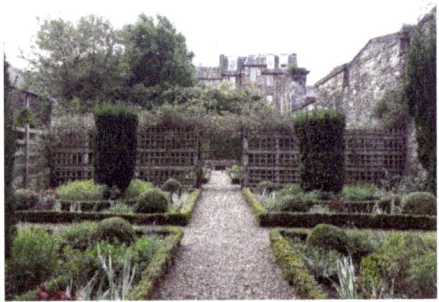

Figure 1. The urban Garden, Dunbar's Close Garden, Edinburgh, UK, as viewed from the North-West looking South-East within the parterre zone.

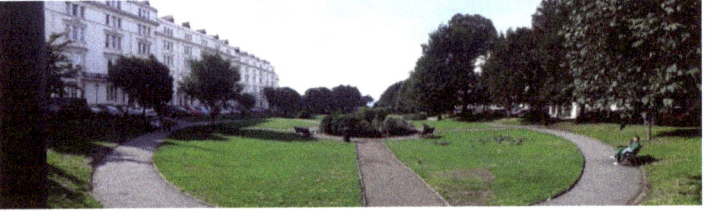

Figure 2. The urban Park, Palmeira Lawns, Edinburgh, UK, as viewed from the North looking South.

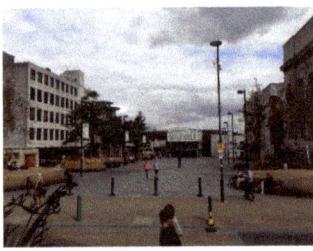

Figure 3. The urban Square, Tudor Square, Sheffield, UK, as viewed from the South-West looking North-East.

2.2. Participants

Two-hundred-and-sixty-four people in the three places were asked to participate. The positive response rate was 60%, resulting in 159 initial participants. Those under 16 years old ($n = 1$), or whose duration in the place was less than 5 min ($n = 4$) or was unknown ($n = 3$) were removed from all analysis, resulting in a total of 151 participants. There were no significant differences in the response rate depending on the type of day (week or weekend), gender, or if alone or with company ($\chi^2 = 0.17, 0.11, 0.79, p > 0.05$, respectively). There were significant differences in the response rate depending on the place ($\chi^2 = 13.24, p < 0.001$), with more people saying no than yes in the Square ($n = 70$ and 66, respectively), while more people said yes than no in the Garden ($n = 47$ to 18) and Park ($n = 38$ to 17). All participants gave their informed consent for inclusion before they participated in the study. The study was conducted in accordance with the Declaration of Helsinki, and the protocol was approved by the Ethics Committee of the School of Energy, Geoscience, Infrastructure and Society at Heriot-Watt University (Project 316249).

The Park and Square had similar participant demographics. The majority of participants lived in the city (60% and 62% respectively, with 32% and 28% visiting), had a fairly equal gender representation (55% and 52%, female respectively), a median age group of 30 to 39 years olds (varying from 16 years to over 75 years), and a slight urban identity ($\bar{x} = 3.92$, SD = 1.09 and $\bar{x} = 3.51$, SD = 1.35 respectively). In contrast, the Garden participants were more frequently visitors to the city (53% compared to 38% living there), were often female participants (72%), had a median age group of 40 to 49 years old (varying from 20 years to over 80 years) and were neutral in their urban to rural identity ($\bar{x} = 3.06$, SD = 1.37). In total, 81 participants were questioned between 10:00 and 13:59, and 70 participants were questioned between 14:00 and 18:00. Far more participants were questioned on a weekday than at the weekend ($n = 117$ and 34, respectively).

Despite some differences identified above, gender did not significantly differ across the three places ($\chi = 4.73, p > 0.05$), and the sample size for age and live/work/visit was too small to be confident of the non-significant results. Urban–rural identity did significantly differ across the three sites with a significantly lower urban identity rating in the Garden than in the Park (F = 4.53, df = 2, $p = 0.01$). Participants answering on the weekend or weekdays did not significantly differ in gender ($\chi = 0.45, p > 0.05$), rural–urban identity (F = 0.35, df = 1, $p > 0.05$), or if they lived, worked, or were visiting the city ($\chi = 2.37, p > 0.05$), while samples size for age was too small to be confident of the non-significant results.

2.3. Measures

To assess the objective acoustic characteristics of the place, 15 min sound pressure level measurements were taken to determine, $L_{Aeq,15}$ (averaged A-weighted level), $L_{A,max}$ (maximum A-weighted level reached), as well as L_{A10}, L_{A50}, and L_{A90} (L_{A10} level exceeded for 10% of measurement time; L_{A50} statistical average; L_{A90} ambient or background level). Although L_{den} and L_{night} are common measures used when assessing health impacts [3], night-time measurements were not considered necessary for this study, as the study interest was on the health impacts relating to time spent within the places, which are used by the majority of the population in the daytime. To assess the perceived characteristics of the place, participants were asked when "thinking about describing this place, to what extent would you agree with these descriptors", followed by ten descriptors (Section 3.2.3), and a scale ranging from Disagree (1) to Agree (7). The two authors also made evaluations of the place characteristics using the criteria and parameters listed in the European project Quadmap's tool for expert assessments [30]. However, neither authors are ecological experts but could make a fair estimation across the three sites.

To understand the use and general experience of the place, participants were first asked two open-ended questions "Why did you come to or pass through this place today?", "Roughly how long have you been in the place just now?", followed by closed-ended questions of "Were you with anyone while in this place?" (No, Yes – 1 other, 2 others, more than 2), and "What activity did you do

MOST while in this place?" (please tick one). For the activity question, participants were provided with a variety of response options that reflected the Urban, Social, and Aquatic categories previously identified [31] and reflect those utilised in the Monitor of Engagement with the Natural Environment UK surveys [32]. These are depicted in Section 3.1, aside from "energetic physical activities", "aquatic activities", and "other" which were not chosen by any participant. The open-ended question 'please name some sounds you have heard in this place today' helped determine the soundscape, along with three of the perceived place characteristics (quiet, calm, and tranquil).

To understand the health outcomes from being in the place, participants were asked the open-ended question "What do you think the *benefits* are that you gain from walking through or stopping in this place?", and "How do you feel in this place?". In between these, perceived restoration was assessed using existing items [33,34], slightly adapted to prevent an assumption or need for prior fatigue levels (e.g., using "increase" or "improve" rather than "regain" or "renew"). The items asked participants "On a scale from 1 to 7, to what extent do you agree that after having spent some time in this place today, you have now been able to ... ". This was followed by eight items, each with a numerical scale alongside ranging from "Disagree 1" through to "7 Agree". The items consisted of "improve your energy levels", "increase the ability to concentrate", "reduce any tension", "become yourself again", "ponder over your daily experiences", "think about your relationships with others", "think about important issues", and "see things in a new perspective". Principal Component Analysis with direct oblimin rotation, and adequate Kaiser's sample measure (0.89) confirmed a one factor structure (56% variance explained), rather than a separation into two factors representing recovery and reflection. The eight perceived psychological restorative outcomes had high reliability as a set of items that are measuring a similar concept ($\alpha = 0.89$). This is also the case when the three sites were considered separately ($\alpha = 0.91, 0.91, 0.84$, for the Garden, Park, and Square, respectively). A perceived restoration score was calculated from the average of participants' scores for the eight items. Small values reflect low levels of perceived restoration; large values reflect high levels of perceived restoration.

Participants rated their rural or urban identity on a five point scale from rural (1) to urban (5), in line with previous studies [34,35]. They were also asked to indicate if they lived in, worked in, or were a visitor to the city, as well as noting their gender and age.

2.4. Equipment

For the acoustic measurements a Casella CEL 246 Sound Level Meter and CEL-120/2 acoustic calibrator (Class 2) were utilised. The CEL 246 is a data logging sound level meter, which stores a time history of the noise levels set to a 1 s interval for the recording period. The CEL 246 also displays the time history as a histogram on the screen and maximum ($L_{A,max}$) and average levels (L_{Aeq}). The meter was set to measure A-weighted levels. A windshield was applied to the microphone to reduce wind noise. The CEL246 was mounted on a tripod at 1.5 metres high as necessary for outdoor acoustic measurements [36]. Calibration of the sound level meter to 114db was conducted using the CEL at the beginning of each measurement session.

2.5. Procedure

Fieldwork was completed in three sessions (10:00–11:30; 12:30–14:30; 16:00–18:00) on eight days (Tuesday × 3, Wednesday × 3, Saturday × 2), over a three-week period (mid-August 2018 to early September 2018). These days and hours were chosen to ensure the data reflected the range of activities, usage patterns and sonic environments that can occur in and around the three study sites. Additional, ambient sound level measurements were taken on one weekday early morning (05:00 to 07:00) in each city during the fieldwork. During fieldwork hours, temperatures were a chillier 9 to 18 °C ($\bar{x} = 15$) with wind speeds of 1 to 14mph ($\bar{x} = 6$) for the Garden, but ranged from 18 to 22 °C ($\bar{x} = 20$) with wind speeds of 10 to 24 mph ($\bar{x} = 16$) for the Park, and 18 to 24 °C ($\bar{x} = 21$) with wind speeds of 2 to 20 mph ($\bar{x} = 12$) for the Square [37].

For the acoustic measurements, each study site was measured at three to five locations. There were four locations for the Garden (top (S), centre in the Partrees, bottom in the lawn (N), and to the side in the long border (SE)); three locations for the Park (top (N), centre and bottom (S)); and four locations for the Square (top left (N), top right (NE), centre, and bottom (SW)). These selected locations gathered data from distinctly different parts of the sites, to ensure representative measurements for the whole site. Measurements were recorded in each location for each time period, rotating between the locations within each time period. During the measurements, notes were made of any sound events including any interruptions from the public, or weather issues (such as strong gusts of wind). Additional measurements on the pavements by the adjacent major roads for the Garden (the Royal Mile), the Park (busy bus stop street), and the Square (busy bus stop street) were conducted. These were once on a weekday and once at the weekend for the Gardens, once on a weekday for the Park, but at all the same time as the four locations in the Square.

People who had been seen sitting or walking through the places for a period of time were asked to participate in a study about people's use and experiences of urban outdoor places. Participants were informed that all responses would be treated anonymously, and they could withdraw at any time. Participants were first asked about their general place experience, followed by the benefits gained, their perceived restoration, how they felt, what sounds they had heard, before ending on demographic questions. All questions relating to sound were after questions on the benefits and feelings of being in the place. Upon completion, participants were thanked, debriefed and any questions answered. Questionnaires took an average of 10 min to complete (ranging from 5 to 25 min).

2.6. Analysis

Data was collected over three sessions, but at times are analysed here in two sessions, morning/lunchtime (10 am to 13:59 pm) and afternoon/early evening (14:00–18:00). A logarithmic average of the sound pressure level data collected in each of the measurement locations, was calculated using the follow averaging equation where n = number of measurements being averaged.

$$Average\ L_{aeq,15min} = 10log_{10}\left[\frac{1}{n}\sum_{i=1}^{n}10^{(\frac{L_{aeq,15mon}}{10})}\right] \quad (1)$$

The data was averaged for the time periods of 10:00–13:59, 14:00–18:00, and a daily average. To calculate the weekday and weekend average, the daily results were averaged together to form an overall result for the location. The time logged data from the CEL sound level meter enabled calculations of the L_{A10}, L_{A50} and L_{A90}.

Participants with missing data from items used to calculate a composite score (e.g., missing a response for perceived restoration items, particularly "become yourself again") are excluded from that individual analysis. Although participants were asked to name one activity, they did the most, some provided multiple answers, and were thus coded as "multiple" activities.

Content Analysis was conducted on all the open-ended questions. The first author initially generated themes by examining responses. Based on frequency counts of these themes, adaptations were made merging or separating some themes. A research assistant then independently coded all responses into the identified themes. Differences were examined and after typing errors were corrected, inter-rater agreement measured by Cohen's Kappa was 0.74 ($p < 0.001$) for reasons in place, 0.64 ($p < 0.001$) for benefits, 0.83 ($p < 0.001$) for feelings and 0.87 ($p < 0.001$) for sounds heard. These are interpreted as substantial agreement for reasons in place and benefits, and almost perfect agreement for feelings and sounds [38]. Final decisions on the coding were derived by discussing the context of the response and to seek consensus the second author independently coded remaining items that differed, with items finally coded based on the majority response.

3. Results

3.1. Activity and Social Experience

The Park' and Square's participants reported similar activities and social situations (Table 1). The majority of participants main activity was resting, they were by themselves, and had spent around a quarter of an hour in the place (median = 17.5 min and 15 min; both ranging from 5 min to 180 min). The second most frequent activity in both places was doing multiple activities, which were predominantly resting and being social. In contrast, in the Garden although most participants' main activity had also been resting, a large number had also been doing light physical activities (walking around the gardens). Participants generally spent a much shorter time in the Garden compared to the two other places, ranging from 5 to 60 min (median = 10 min).

Participants not alone in the Park were split between being with 1, 2 or more than 3 other people, while most participants not alone in the Square were only with one other person. A similar proportion of participants were visiting the Garden by themselves as those with one other person, but overall more people were with someone else than alone.

Table 1. Percentage of participants reporting their main activity whilst in the Garden (N = 47 participants), Park (N = 38), Square (N = 66) and if they were with someone.

		Garden	Park	Square	Overall
Activity	Resting	44.7	55.3	62.1	55.0
	Social	4.3	7.9	10.6	7.9
	Cognitive	8.5	10.5	9.1	9.3
	Light Physical	31.9	10.5	1.5	13.2
	Multiple	10.6	15.8	16.7	14.6
Social Situation	Alone	40.4	52.6	50.0	47.7
	With 1 person	42.6	21.1	40.9	36.4
	With 2 people	14.9	10.5	6.1	9.9
	With 3 or more	2.1	15.8	3.0	6.0

Examining the data across each place and by time of day, the modal activity was still resting in all three places for morning/lunch and afternoon. The modal social situation was being alone, except in the Garden in the afternoon. The median time spent in the place was the same in the morning and afternoon for the Square (15 min), but slightly decreased in the afternoon for the Garden (from 12.5 min to 10 min). In the Park, participants spent on average double the time than of the morning/lunch participants (median is 20 min compared to 10 min), due to the maximum time spent there increasing from 35 min to 180 min.

3.2. Suitability of Places as Urban Quiet Areas

To assess the suitability of the three study sites as potential urban quiet areas, the objective acoustic measurements and subjective evaluations of the place and its soundscapes are presented.

3.2.1. Acoustic Measurements

Across all measurements, the Garden had the lowest averaged sound pressure level (L_{Aeq15}) of 49 dB(A), while the Park and Square were substantially higher at 58 dB(A) and 60 dB(A) respectively. There were little differences between averaged sound pressure levels ($L_{Aeq,15}$) for the weekday and weekend in the Garden (51 dB(A) and 48 dB(A) respectively) and in the Square (59 dB(A) and 60 dB(A) respectively) (only weekdays were measured in the Park; Table 2). Similarly, there are little differences between averaged sound pressure levels (L_{Aeq15}) for the time of day (morning/lunchtime or afternoon) the measurements were made (Figure 4). In contrast to the daytime variation between the places, the early morning sound levels of each site were much lower and very similar across the three sites ($L_{Aeq,15}$ 52, 52, 54 dB(A) and $L_{A,max}$ 69, 67, 69 dB(A) for the Garden, Park, and Square, respectively). Overall there is little variance within each site during the daytime hours, but greater variation between each site.

Table 2. Average acoustic measurements at the weekday and weekend in each site.

	Week Day Average					Weekend Average				
	$L_{Aeq,15}$	$L_{A,max}$	L_{A10}	L_{A50}	L_{A90}	$L_{Aeq,15}$	$L_{A,max}$	L_{A10}	L_{A50}	L_{A90}
Garden	51	69	59	51	46	48	60	61	52	47
Park	58	63	61	57	52	-	-	-	-	-
Square	59	74	63	58	54	60	74	62	58	55

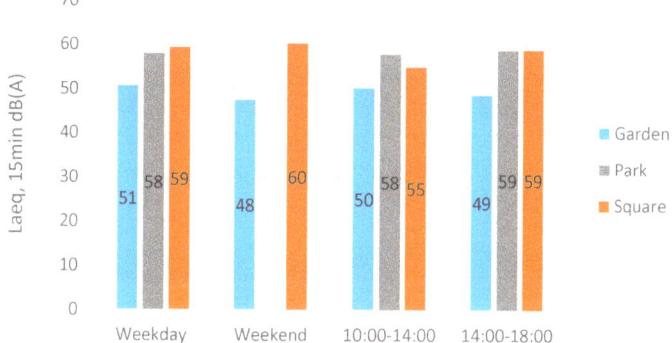

Figure 4. Bar chart of averaged $L_{Aeq,15}$ across different types of day (weekday and weekend) and times of day (morning/lunchtime and afternoon) for the three sites.

The additional road measurements for the Garden averaged at $L_{Aeq,15}$ 66 dB(A), and an $L_{A,max}$ of 80, for the Park they averaged $L_{Aeq,15}$ 61 dB(A), and an $L_{A,max}$ of 70, while the additional main road measurements for the Square averaged at LA_{eq15} 64 dB(A) and an $L_{A,max}$ of 73. For the gardens, this means there was a 17 dB(A) reduction within the Garden compared to on the pavement by the road, while for the Park and Square there was only a 3 and 4 dB(A) reduction respectively compared to near their respective roadsides.

3.2.2. "Expert" Place Characteristic Assessments

Landscape views for the urban Park and Square were similar, with the authors identifying views of the sea, hills, or pleasant architectural structures in three or four directions. In contrast, only two directions from the urban Garden provides a clear landscape view to hills and the adjacent large church. Within the Garden and Park, natural elements were visible in all directions, but were only present on two sides of the Square. The researchers estimated that 95% of the surface area in the Garden was natural compared to 5% artificial materials for the paths, with the natural surfaces consisting of 20% tree canopy, 5% amenity turf, and 70% amenity planting. Similarly, in the Park 85% was estimated to be natural surfaces, but this time consisting of 5% tree canopy, 15% amenity planting, and 65% amenity turf. In contrast, the Square was estimated as only having 10% natural surfaces and 90% artificial, with tree canopy comprising 1%, amenity planting 8%, and amenity turf (on top of the seating pods) 2%. These differences in amount and type of natural surfaces was also reflected in the estimated biodiversity levels, with around 40 habitat types and 6 singing bird species in the Garden, 10 habitat types and four or five singing bird species in the Park, and only eight habitat types and three singing bird species in the Square.

All three sites were regularly maintained and clean, and appeared safe during the daytime, although some drug taking activity was observed in two of the sites. Accessibility was rated high for all three sites, as they were located close to key points, had good transportation networks close by, and were near to residential properties. The Garden had the lowest number of users during the survey hours, with less than 1 user per 9 m^2 with most areas well used (often as people walked around the place). The larger Park had between 1 and 2 users per 9 m^2 with more people using the top (near the road and bus stop) and middle of the park, than the more secluded bottom end. The Square was the busiest site, with more than 2 users per 9 m^2 estimated, with most sitting at the SE end, away from the main road.

3.2.3. Perceived Place Characteristics

A one-way ANOVA test was conducted to assess significant differences between participants' descriptions of the three places. Significant differences were found for all characteristics, except for the perception of crowded and safety (although the latter was significant, but Bonferroni post-hoc comparisons found no significant differences between each paired place). Depending on the significance results of Levene's test of homogeneity, Bonferroni or Tamhane's post-hoc comparisons were examined. Notably the Garden was perceived as significantly quieter, more tranquil, less built up, and slightly less accessible than both the Park and the Square (Table 3). In contrast the Square was perceived as significantly less quiet, less calm, less tranquil, less natural, less biodiverse and a lower feeling of being alone than both the Park and the Square.

Table 3. Mean, standard deviations (brackets), and significance testing of participants extent of agreement with each place descriptor (1 = disagree, 7 = agree) in the Garden, Park and Square.

	Garden	Park	Square	Significance
Quiet	6.23 (0.96)	5.51 (1.39)	4.78 (1.53)	$F(2,144) = 16.21$ ***
Calm	6.64 (0.57)	6.17 (0.85)	**5.49 (1.2)**	$F(2,143) = 20.02$ ***
Tranquil	6.34 (0.84)	5.42 (1.32)	4.22 (1.59)	$F(2,143) = 35.17$ ***
Built Up	**2.50 (1.55)**	4.11 (1.47)	4.41 (1.63)	$F(2,142) = 21.24$ *** [a]
Natural	5.51 (1.57)	5.62 (1.34)	**3.97 (1.69)**	$F(2,144) = 18.47$ *** [a]
Biodiverse	4.87 (1.54)	4.89 (1.58)	**3.54 (1.55)**	$F(2,144) = 13.38$ ***
Crowded	2.40 (1.65)	2.86 (1.53)	3.05 (1.54)	$F(2,144) = 2.30$
Alone	4.49 (1.50)	4.03 (1.48)	**3.03 (1.65)**	$F(2,142) = 12.28$ *** [a]
Accessible	**5.72 (1.46)**	6.38 (0.86)	6.32 (0.93)	$F(2,144) = 4.96$ **
Safe	6.00 (0.98)	6.03 (0.97)	5.52 (1.26)	$F(2,143) = 3.50$ *

* $p < 0.05$, ** $p < 0.01$, *** $p < 0.001$, [a] Tamhane's post-hoc comparisons were utilised. Bold numericals indicate the place that significantly differs to the two other places.

Perceived ratings of quiet, calm and tranquil across all three sites had significant moderate positive correlations ($r = 0.62$ for quiet and calm; $r = 0.59$ for quiet and tranquil; and $r = 0.69$ for calm and tranquil; $p < 0.01$). There were also weak to moderate strength positive significant correlations between natural and biodiverse descriptors ($r = 0.54$, $p < 0.01$), natural with quiet, calm and tranquil ($r = 0.43$, 0.47, 0.47, respectively; $p < 0.01$), and natural with alone ($r = 0.49$, $p < 0.01$). Alone also had weak but significant correlations with quiet, calm and tranquil ($r = 0.45$, 0.47, 0.51, respectively; $p < 0.01$), but surprisingly no significant relationship with crowded.

3.2.4. Sounds Heard

Participants named between one and seven sounds they heard while in the place, resulting in 371 sounds, with a similar number named per person in each place (Garden = 2.53 sounds per person, Park = 2.18, Square = 2.56). These were coded into 11 sound categories, ranging from natural sounds (e.g., "*birds*", "*wind*"), people - other sounds (e.g., "*people*", "*children*", where the specifics of the sound being made is unclear and could be vocal or movement based), construction work, traffic sounds, and comments about the sound level (e.g., "*quietness*") with a few noticing an absence of sounds (e.g., "*no sounds*") (Table 4). Overall, participants equally mentioned nature (n = 85), people's vocal sounds (n = 84; e.g., "*conversations*", "*people chatting*", "*laughing*"), and vehicles/traffic (n = 77; e.g., "*cars*", "*traffic*", "*buses*"), although the number mentioned varied between the three places. In the Garden, the most frequently mentioned sounds were nature, followed by people's vocal sounds and vehicles/traffic. The most frequently mentioned sounds in the Park were natural sounds, followed by vehicles/traffic. In the Square, the most frequently mentioned sounds were people's vocal sounds, followed by vehicles/traffic. Dogs were not present in the Garden, people's footsteps (e.g., "*footsteps on gravel*", "*people walking by*") could not be heard in the Park, and neither was distant traffic (e.g., "*cars in the distance*") due to the proximity of the road, while in the Square no one commented on an absence of sounds.

Table 4. Percentage of times each sound category was mentioned by participants whilst in the Garden (n = 119 sounds), Park (n = 83) and Square (n = 169).

	Garden	Park	Square	Overall
Nature	31.9	37.3	9.5	22.9
Dogs	0.0	8.4	0.6	2.2
People - Vocal	18.5	12.0	30.8	22.6
People - Other	1.7	7.2	8.3	5.9
People - Footsteps/Walking	9.2	0.0	3.6	4.6
Recreational or Cultural artefacts	5.9	1.2	10.7	7.0
Mechanical or Construction work	6.7	3.6	10.7	7.8
Vehicles or Traffic	17.6	26.5	20.1	20.8
Distant Traffic	1.7	0.0	3.0	1.9
Sound Level/Acoustics Comment	5.0	1.2	3.0	3.2
Absence of Sounds/Noises	1.7	2.4	0.0	1.1

Pearson Chi square tests with 1 degree of freedom were calculated and assessed with two tailed probability levels for the presence or absence of each sound type being mentioned by a participant, within a place, depending on the time of day (morning/lunch or afternoon) or type of day (weekday or weekend). Only three significant differences were noted for across the time of day, and only two for the type of day (Table 5). In the Garden, vehicles or traffic were more likely reported in the afternoon than in the morning, while recreational or cultural artefacts were more likely reported at the weekend (e.g., an occurrence of music from a residential house) than in the weekday. These were moderate and relatively strong associations respectively as interpreted using existing criteria [39]. In the Park, people, other sounds and dogs were more likely to be reported in the afternoon than morning (moderate associations). While in the Square, recreational or cultural artefacts were more likely heard on a weekday (e.g., the quarterly hour clock bells and pub music) than at the weekend (moderate association).

Table 5. Chi square tests of associations between time of day or type of day and sound types heard in the Garden, Park or Square.

Sound Type	Type of Day or Time of Day	Observed Count (Expected Count)			χ^2	p	ϕ_c
		Garden	Park	Square			
Dogs	Morning		1 (3.7)		5.29 [a]	0.021 *	0.39
	Afternoon		6 (3.3)				
People - Other	Morning		1 (3.2)		3.85 [a]	0.050 *	0.34
	Afternoon		5 (2.8)				
Vehicles or Traffic	Morning	9 (12.4)			4.18	0.041 *	0.30
	Afternoon	13 (9.6)					
Recreational or Cultural artefacts	Weekday	1 (4.6)			13.39 [a]	0.000 ***	0.54
	Weekend	5 (1.4)					
	Weekday			13 (8.6)	7.52	0.006 **	0.35
	Weekend			1 (5.4)			

[a] Caution should be taken as low expected cell counts. * $p < 0.05$, ** $p < 0.01$ *** $p < 0.001$.

3.3. Psychological Restoration as a Motivator and Perceived Health Outcomes

The reasons for being in the place highlight the role of psychological restoration in motivating people to visit a place. Perceived benefits from visiting the place, how they felt and their perceived restorative outcomes are presented to highlight the perceived health outcomes from visiting the place.

3.3.1. Reasons for Being in the Place

Participants provided 184 reasons why they were in the place (as a few people provided multiple reasons). These were represented by 10 themes, ranging from purposely visiting the place, for the ambient qualities (sun and fresh air, or peace and quiet), because of its location (near to where work/live or another nearby event) or to be able to relax or have food (Table 6). Although the most frequently mentioned reason overall ($n = 34$) was to visit the place (e.g., "to enjoy the park"; "heard about it and was in [travel guide book]"), the reasons largely differed across the three sites, with purposely visiting the place only for a strong reason for the Garden ($n = 24$). For the Square, its location was the most frequently mentioned reason for being there ($n = 19$), with it commonly used as a stopping point while on the way to another nearby event or place (e.g., "just been to the library", "come after church", "kill some time before catching train"). Eating food and drink in the Square was similarly frequently mentioned ($n = 18$), while meeting or spending time with friends/family or just being around other people was also an important reason for a number of participants ($n = 10$; e.g., "it's our time together before head off in different directions", "meeting my daughter", "because lonely"). In the Park, there was a slightly more even distribution of reasons provided, with the most frequently mentioned reason of relaxing or reading accounting for 21% of responses ($n = 9$; $n = 8$ in the Square; and $n = 5$ in the Garden). Interestingly, seeking peace and quiet (e.g., Garden: "knew it was a nice peaceful place", Square: "nice place to sit and quiet") was the 5th most frequently referred to reason (excluding "other") across all sites ($n = 14$), but was the second most frequently mentioned reason in the Garden ($n = 9$).

Table 6. Percentage of times each type of reason was provided by participants for being in the Garden (n = 62 reasons), Park (n = 43) and Square (n = 79).

	Garden	Park	Square	Overall
For the Place	38.7	9.3	7.6	18.5
Food or Drink	6.5	14.0	22.8	15.2
Event or Place Nearby	4.8	14.0	24.1	15.2
Relax or Read	8.1	20.9	10.1	12.0
Peace and Quiet	14.5	2.3	5.1	7.6
Be with Friends, Family or Around People	1.6	2.3	12.7	6.5
On a Break	11.3	4.7	2.5	6.0
Sun or Fresh Air	8.1	4.7	3.8	5.4
Live or Work in the Place	0.0	11.6	5.1	4.9
Other	6.5	16.3	6.3	8.7

3.3.2. Benefits from Being in the Place

Participants named between one and eight benefits gained from being in or walking through the place, resulting in 336 benefits, with the most benefits mentioned in the Square (Table 7). These were coded into 19 types of benefits, ranging from resting, relaxing, feeling good, being in nature, and being with or avoiding people or traffic. Seven types of benefits referred to the place; these benefits described characteristics of the place that they thought were beneficial rather than describing a personal benefit. Overall, participants most commonly mentioned benefit was the place was peaceful, quiet, or calm (n = 53; e.g., *"calm place to sit"*, *"quiet"* *"bit of peace and calm from city"* *"relative quiet"*). This was also the most common benefit in the Square and Garden, and the second most common benefit in the Park. In the Garden, some way behind referring to the benefit of the place as being peaceful (n = 26), participants frequently referred to gaining a positive feeling (n = 14), and that the place felt very different to other places (n = 13; e.g., *"switch off from main road"*, *"work in busy environment"*, *"nice feels more comfortable than on streets"*). For the Park, relaxing was the most frequently mentioned benefit (n = 14), followed by the place being peaceful (n = 9), and then themselves benefiting from gaining a positive feeling (n = 8), which included *"its calming"* and *"sense of peace"*. In the Square, being able to rest was the second most common benefit (n = 17), only one behind the place being peaceful (n = 18). Overall, restorative benefits of resting, relaxing, recovering, and reflecting accounted for 26% of the total responses, but was only 19% of the Garden's responses, and 31% of the Park's, and 29% of Square's.

3.3.3. Feelings in the Place

Some participants already referred to how they felt when they provided the benefits, they gained from being in the place. However, a total of 242 feelings were reported by participants (between one and four per participant) when asked specifically about how they felt in the place (Table 8). A similar number of feelings were reported in the Garden and Square, with fewer in the Park (partly due to the lower sample size). Ten types of feelings were identified, ranging from feeling relaxed, calm, peaceful, happy, good, safe, and supported. A few participants again commented on the place rather than on how they felt (n = 15 overall; e.g., *"like it"*, *"nice little garden, cute"*).

Overall, participants most commonly reported feeling was of relaxation (n = 83; *"relaxed"*, *"chilled out"*) and this was the most frequently reported feeling in each of the places (n = 25, 17 and 41 for the Garden, Park, and Square respectively). In the Garden, a large number of participants reported feeling *"peaceful"*, *"quiet"*, or *"tranquil"* (n = 22). In the Park, the second most frequently mentioned benefit was feeling "*happy*" or "*great*" ($n = 10$), while in the Square it was feeling "*good*" or "*okay*" ($n = 11$) closely followed by feeling "*calm*" ($n = 10$).

Table 7. Percentage of times each type of benefit was experienced whilst in the Garden ($n = 115$ benefits), Park ($n = 75$) and Square ($n = 146$).

	Garden	Park	Square	Total
Rest	6.1	5.3	11.6	8.3
Relax or Read	7.8	18.7	8.9	10.7
Recover	1.7	4.0	4.8	3.6
Think or Reflect	3.5	2.7	3.4	3.3
Food or Drink	0.9	1.3	2.7	1.8
Positive Feeling	12.2	10.7	2.7	7.7
Being in Nature	7.8	4.0	0.0	3.6
Being Outside in Sunshine or fresh Air	5.2	8.0	9.6	7.7
People - Be with or around	0.9	8.0	8.2	5.7
People - Avoid being around	3.5	1.3	0.0	1.5
Traffic - Avoid being by it	0.9	1.3	5.5	3.0
Place - Peaceful/calm	22.6	12.0	12.3	15.8
Place - Beautiful/nice	7.8	4.0	6.8	6.5
Place - Landscape description	5.2	6.7	4.8	5.4
Place - Built environment description	0.9	2.7	4.1	2.7
Place – Clean, tidy and safe	0.9	4.0	4.1	3.0
Place - Location	0.0	1.3	3.4	1.8
Place - Different to another place	11.3	1.3	4.8	6.3
Other	0.9	2.7	2.1	1.8

Table 8. Percentage of times each feeling was experienced whilst in the Garden ($n = 94$ feelings), Park ($n = 53$) and Square ($n = 95$).

	Garden	Park	Square	Total
Relaxed /Comfortable	26.6	32.1	43.2	34.3
Peaceful /Quiet /Tranquil	23.4	13.2	7.4	14.9
Calm	14.9	7.5	10.5	11.6
Happy /Great	6.4	18.9	9.5	10.3
Good /Okay /content	6.4	3.8	11.6	7.9
Place Comment	9.6	3.8	4.2	6.2
Restored	1.1	11.3	1.1	3.3
Safe	2.1	1.9	4.2	2.9
Supported (by others)	0.0	1.9	3.2	1.7
Other	9.6	5.7	5.3	7.0

3.3.4. Perceived Restoration

Participants, on average only perceived themselves as being slightly restored when leaving the places ($\bar{x} = 4.76$, SD = 1.31, on a 7-point scale). A one way ANOVA comparing participants' perceived restoration in the three places, showed significant differences ($F(2,129) = 4.64$, $p = 0.011$). Bonferroni post-hoc comparisons (homogeneity of variance was not violated) identified participants in the Park ($\bar{x}$ = 5.38, SD = 1.22, n = 30) perceived higher levels of restoration than participants in the Garden ($\bar{x}$ = 4.57, SD = 1.41, n = 42) and Square ($\bar{x}$ = 4.57, SD = 1.29, n = 60).

A one-way ANOVA for the Park showed significant differences between participants' perceived restoration at different times of day ($F(1,29) = 7.31$, $p = 0.012$) with higher perceived restoration in the afternoon (Table 9). A between-subjects ANOVA for the Garden and for the Square, showed significant differences between participants' perceived restoration at different times of day but not between the weekdays and weekend (Table 10) (Garden: $F(1,38) = 4.13$, $p = 0.049$ for time of day; $F(1,38) = 0.71$, $p > 0.05$ for type of day; $F(1,38) = 0.39$, $p > 0.05$ for interaction of time and type of day), (Square: $F(1,56) = 5.61$, $p = 0.021$ for time of day; $F(1,56) = 0.55$, $p > 0.05$ for type of day; $F(1,56) = 0.05$, $p > 0.05$ for interaction of time and type of day). Participants in the Garden had higher perceived restoration in the morning/lunch, while those in the Square had higher perceived restoration in the afternoon, which is the same as for the Park participants.

Table 9. Participants' mean perceived restoration for the Park at different times of day.

	Mean	Standard Deviation	N
Morning/Lunchtime (10:00 to 13:59)	**4.87**	1.16	16
Afternoon/Early evening (14:00 to 18:00)	**5.96**	1.05	14
All day (10:00 to 18:00)	5.38	1.22	30

Bold numericals indicate the variables with significant differences.

Table 10. Participants' mean perceived restoration for the Garden and Square at different times and types of day.

Time and Type of Day		Garden			Square		
		Mean	Standard Deviation	N	Mean	Standard Deviation	N
Morning/Lunchtime (10:00 to 13:59)	Weekday	4.95	1.15	17	4.36	1.28	22
	Weekend	4.88	0.73	7	4.06	1.03	11
	Total	**4.93**	1.03	24	**4.26**	1.19	33
Afternoon/Early evening (14:00 to 18:00)	Weekday	4.28	1.79	14	5.03	0.98	15
	Weekend	3.50	1.62	4	4.86	1.27	12
	Total	**4.10**	1.74	18	**4.95**	1.10	27
All day (10:00 to 18:0)	Weekday	4.65	1.49	31	4.63	1.20	37
	Weekend	4.38	1.26	11	4.48	1.21	23
	Total	4.57	1.42	42	4.57	1.19	60

Bold numericals indicate the variables with significant differences.

4. Discussion

This study took a multi-site approach to explore the restorative and other self-reported health benefits of public urban spaces that could fall into the remit of a Candidate Quiet Area (CQA). To address the aim, each of the main objectives are discussed in turn. First, objective and subjective place characteristics are assessed to determine the chosen sites suitability as urban "quiet areas". Second, the role of psychological restoration in visiting these places is explored alongside the perceived health benefits gained from being in the places. Finally, the necessity of "quiet" for restoration in urban places is discussed.

4.1. Suitability of Places as Urban Quiet Areas

Given their land type, the study sites of an urban Garden, Park, and Square all have the potential for being defined as an urban quiet area in the UK. If the Scottish guidelines are applied for defining a CQA as having L_{day} levels of below 55 dB(A) across 75% of the place [14], only the Garden would meet this criteria (49 dB(A)). The Garden was substantially quieter than the two other places which were both above the Scottish level; however, all three sites were smaller than their additional recommendation of the place being larger than 9 hectares. For CQA requirements in England, the Square would not be included as only green spaces are permissible outside of London. The Square also only had a small difference between measurements taken on an adjacent road and with the square itself, suggesting it was not "relatively quiet". Furthermore, participants only slightly rated it above neutral, rather than quiet. In contrast, both the Garden and Park were subjectively rated by their visitors as quiet, and the Garden could be acoustically described as relatively quiet, given the 17 dB(A) difference between the measurements inside and outside of the Garden. A summary table mapping the study sites against English and Scottish CQA criteria [14,16] is presented in Table 11.

Table 11. Study sites mapped against England and Scotland Candidate Quiet Area criteria.

	L_{day} <55 dB(A)	> 9 hectares	(Perceived) Quiet	Relatively Quiet	(Perceived) Tranquil	Health and Wellbeing Benefits
Garden	✓		✓	✓	✓	✓
Park			✓		✓	✓
Square						✓

Although the sound levels differed between the three places in the daytime, there was no difference in the early morning, confirming the need to take sound level measurements at appropriate times to be able to differentiate between places. Interestingly within each place, there was also very little variation between sound levels taken in the morning/lunchtime and those in the afternoon, nor between weekday and weekend measurements. Given human activities within and around those places (including traffic levels) is expected to vary, the stableness of the measurements is quite surprising.

Sound level measurements alone are not representative soundscape indicators as they do not incorporate perceptions [5,36] and were shown to be unable to distinguish between the variety of sounds heard in this study. Indeed, there was some variation in the types of sounds heard by visitors to the three sites at different times, with significantly more vehicles and traffic sounds heard in the afternoon in the Garden, despite the averaged sound levels remaining similar. Likewise, recreational and cultural artefact sounds were significantly heard more in the weekdays in the Square but more in the Weekend in the Garden. For the Garden, this was largely due to an adjacent residential building playing music when a number of participants were surveyed. Although this did little to the average sound levels, it affected those individuals' experience of the place, and hence, their assessment of it as quiet and or restorative, possibly due to prior expectation [40]. Thus, it is imperative to ask people about their perception and experience of a place rather than relying on sound level characteristics or criteria chosen by councils, which cannot be agreed upon across cities and countries. This coincides with the European Quadmap project conclusions that quiet area identification should include surveys with the public on their experiences of the place [30].

The sound level also did not relate to the number of sounds heard within the sites. Participants in the Garden and Square noted a similar number per person, suggesting the raised sound levels in the Square were not from one sound source, such as traffic, masking all the other sounds and creating a cacophonic experience but from a combination of sounds. From the freely recalled sounds, eleven categories of perceived sound were identified that were similar to those used in prior urban park studies [34,41], but with people sounds being split into "vocal", "footsteps/walking" and "other". Despite the increasing methods for automatic sensor recognition of environmental sounds [42], asking visitors to identify sounds is currently still likely to produce more reliable results, particularly if interested in *perceived* sounds. Moreover, perceived sounds are more important for understanding soundscapes and its impact on people than just the physical presence of a sound source. People's attendance to the presence of a sound source varies, thus using an automated process of establishing which sounds are present will make it harder to associate health outcomes with experiences, which are influenced by people's environmental perception.

Associations between objective and subjective sound level measures do exist though [43], and similarly in this study the lower the objectively measured sound level, the subjectively quieter the place was perceived. This suggests sound level measurements can be a good proxy to help identify places (perceived) as *quiet*, but it cannot determine the *quality* of the acoustic environment. To determine the quality, further measures are necessary to indicate the types of sounds that are perceived which importantly shape people's experience of a place. For example, the process of determining quiet areas in a Greek Island city involved, amongst other processes, informed academics identifying quiet areas and acoustically determining the level of biological and anthropogenic sounds in each of these places [44]. This resulted in proposing two quiet areas, both of which were fairly small, were over L_{den} 55 dB(A) and were the few sites that contained more biological than anthropogenic sounds. Preserving high acoustic quality environments rather than acoustically defined "quiet" environments is increasingly supported [45], suggesting the approach taken by England rather than Scotland to define CQAs may be more appropriate as it incorporates additional criteria than objective physical measurements [14,16]. Therefore, an important aspect highlighted by the England criteria may indeed be the ability of the place to "generate significant benefits (in terms of health, wellbeing and quality of life) for the communities they serve" [16] (p. 23). These issues are explored further in the discussions of the results for the second objective.

The substantial reduction in sound levels for the Garden compared to by the roadside is due to the five-storey thick stone terraced buildings that separates the road from the Garden with only a 2 by 3.5 metre archway (close) providing access. These buildings block the sound waves from directly travelling into the Garden resulting in much lower sound levels, and potentially resulting in the greater perceived quiet and tranquillity compared to the other sites. Prior research has also concluded that secluded backyards and courtyards provide increased tranquillity than urban parks, as the latter tend to be exposed to traffic noise [46], which was the case for this study's Park. Similarly, it has been recommended that "a good placement of buildings is much more efficient in creating high-quality soundscapes than remediating measures such as placing noise barriers or absorbing materials" [47] (p. 274). Although, the Square also had a few large three-to-five-storey stone buildings between the road and Square, they are completely separate from each other and with a wider gap between the buildings that act as a street canyon. In addition, the Square has very few absorbent surfaces with only a few vegetated raised pods, and the rest of the material is reflective (stone floor, stone or glass building facades). Therefore, the sound of the traffic is reflected into one section of the Square, whilst all other sounds in the Square are also reflected around, increasing the sound levels. The surface material of a place may be just as important as the building facade material in influencing soundscape evaluations. In this study, hearing footsteps in the gravel was frequently commented on in the Garden, whereas no reference to footsteps or the surface material were made in the stone tiled Square, or grass and tarmac pathed Park. One laboratory study has also highlighted the importance of surface material that urban park users walk on in influencing soundscape quality ratings (although conversely they found gravel to be rated significantly lower in quality than grass or wood) [48]. Therefore, in addition to a consideration of the sound sources that are present in a place, the surface material and surrounding façades should also be considered when hoping to create a quiet or high acoustic quality place.

Vegetation and its substrate, is a more absorptive material than stone or glass, with fewer higher frequency sound waves reflected into the surrounding space and reducing sound levels [49]. Indeed, the more vegetation and more biodiverse the study site (as assessed by the authors), the lower the sound levels and the perceived quiet ratings. Similarly, the place with the lower perceived built up ratings (Garden) received the quietest ratings, while the place with the lower perceived (and "expert") evaluated) natural and biodiverse ratings (Square) received the most neutral ratings for perceived quiet. These place differences were again reflected in the most frequently perceived sounds in each place, with natural sounds frequently recalled in the Garden and Park, while people's vocal sounds were frequently recalled in the Square, reflecting the greater social activities happening there. Although natural sounds were more frequently recalled in the Park, vehicle sounds were the second most frequently recalled sounds, potentially explaining the increased sound levels and lower perceived quiet and tranquillity rating compared to the Garden. Whereas in the Garden, the second most frequently perceived sound was people's vocal sounds, which are generally at a lower sound level than traffic and were unlikely to reduce perceived quiet and tranquillity levels as much as traffic sounds. In this study, tranquillity ratings varied in line with the differences in perceived vegetation, biodiversity levels and types of sounds heard. Although caution needs to be applied in interpreting these results, given contextual differences across the three sites, the results are supportive of prior research definitions of tranquillity using a mix of physical characteristics (presence of natural views) and sound levels of types of sounds (presence of natural sounds) [13]. It also supports the predominant choice of green spaces as urban quiet areas in England and Scotland [15,16].

Perceived tranquillity ratings were moderately correlated with perceived quiet ratings, suggesting the inclusion of tranquillity in the England criteria [16] is helpful for identifying CQAs. Perceived calm, however, had a stronger correlation with perceived quiet and tranquillity ratings, and "calm" has been suggested by the European Environment Agency [11,12] as an alternative to "quiet" for choosing places to preserve. All three places were rated positively for perceived calm, suggesting that if this alternative criterion is used, they may all be worth protecting, despite the Square not being as natural, nor as quiet. However, perceived calm ratings only significantly separated the Square from the two other places, suggesting additional criteria would still be necessary to help further distinguish between sites. Additional research into public perceptions and use of the terms quiet, calm, and tranquil areas has been conducted in a connected study on Project DeStress [29] and will be fully reported at a later date.

The accessibility of a site is used as CQA criteria by some European nations [12]. In this study, perceived accessibility was rated highly in all three places. Decisions on how accessibility is defined needs consideration though, as alternative objective measurements such as the Euclidean distance (as a crow flies) or by network distance vary in their resulting distances. This has implications on whether an accessible quiet space would be related to beneficial health outcomes, as found when considering nearby (accessible) nature outcomes [19]. A summary table mapping the study sites against alternative CQA criteria is presented in Table 12.

Table 12. Study sites mapped against alternative Candidate Quiet Area criteria.

	Perceived Natural	Perceived Built up	Perceived Calm	Accessible	Sounds Most Frequently Perceived	Sounds Least Frequently Perceived
Garden	✓	X	✓	✓	Nature	Dogs
Park	✓		✓	✓	Nature	People – Footsteps
Square			✓	✓	People - Vocal	Absence of sounds

4.2. Psychological Restoration as a Motivator and Perceived Health Outcomes

Across all participants, the main reason for being in one of the places was "for the place" itself. To relax or read was the fourth biggest reason (out of 19 categorised reasons), and to have some peace and quiet was the fifth biggest reason overall. This shows the value of restoring and importance of low sound levels for people's motivation in using these places, although many other reasons also exist for visiting a place. Reasons for the visits also varied substantially across the three places, showing the different benefits the types of spaces can bring. For the Garden, the majority of visitors were tourists who had heard of the place (hence visiting "for the place"), but for those more familiar with the place, they sought the peace and quiet it offered while on a break. This could be interpreted as the place providing a feeling of "Being Away", which is one of the four components that contribute to a restorative environment in Attention Restoration Theory [20,50]. Indeed, even a travel guide describes it as, "Tucked away at the end of an Old Town close, this walled garden has been laid out in the style of the 17th century, with gravel paths, neatly trimmed shrubs, herbs, flowers and mature trees. A hidden gem, and an oasis of tranquillity amid the bustle of the Royal Mile" [51]. Thus, even the tourists may visit as an opportunity to "be away" from other environment types and hints at the importance of relative quiet or tranquillity (which the Garden was acoustically assessed to have). For the Park, the opportunity to relax was the most frequently mentioned reason for being in the place, with relaxation commonly associated with restoring, restorative components, and little need for restoration [33,52]. The convenience of the place also seemed to be important to many participants as they could stop to rest there as it was near to another event or place they were going to/from, or lived in the surrounding accommodation. This can relate to the place's "Compatibility" with what an individual wants to do, another component of restorative environments [20,50], as it offers the chance to relax in a convenient location given the time available to them. Similarly, the location of the Square was the main reason for use, particularly for eating food and drink, and then for providing an opportunity to be in a social environment. Thus, the place was compatible with their needs, but this time from a food and social perspective rather than necessarily the need to relax.

The differences in users' reasons for visiting each place and their potential relationship to components considered necessary in creating a restorative environment, is also reflected by the variance in the perceived restorative outcomes of the users from being in these places. Park respondents had higher perceived restorative outcomes than both the Garden and Square respondents. This reflects the desired intention of the Park users to relax, while many in the Garden were there to "see it" while with a companion, and for the Square it was convenience and the social atmosphere that the users came for, rather than relaxation per se. Being with others can influence optimal restoration levels, as the opportunity to reflect on things can be reduced [53]; therefore, the social experience of the users in the Garden and Park may have lowered their perceived restorative outcomes.

Although perceived restorative outcomes were minimal, as assessed by standard items relating to aspects of Attention Restoration Theory [33,34], a quarter of participants freely stated restorative related terms (rest, relax, recover and reflect). This suggests restorative benefits are gained or at least expected to occur from visiting these places. This was particularly true for the Park and Square respondents (31 and 29% or benefits listed respectively), and less so for the Garden respondents (19%), despite the average perceived restorative outcomes being the same in the Garden and Square. Similarly, feeling relaxed was also the most frequently reported feeling overall from being in the places and for each individual place, accounting for nearly half of participants' feelings in the Square. In contrast the word restored was used a lot less, although did occur more frequently with Park participants, who reported the higher perceived restorative outcomes. Feeling restored however is not necessarily a term that lay people may use compared to academics familiar with Attention Restoration Theory, thus determining restoration based solely on examining phrases for similar terminology is not necessarily appropriate. Instead, these results indicate that people visited these places in part due to the desire to "restore" and gained feelings that could be associated with restoration. The differences in results between the rated restorative outcomes data and the freely stated benefits and feelings gained from a place, however, does raise issues with the way subjective restoration is currently assessed. Similarities and differences in the terminology used by laypeople and experts for assessing a concept such as restoration and restorative outcomes may need further exploration, as has started with a scale designed to assess the perceived restorativeness of soundscapes [54] which examines lay people's interpretation of items used to assess perceived restorativeness. Additionally, Attention Restoration Theory and the perceived restorative outcome items focus on cognitive recovery and reflection, but emotional restoration is just as important and can occur rapidly [21]. As people spent less time in the Garden than the other two sites, this may help explain the lower perceived restorative outcomes and reduced use of terms such as relaxing, recovering, and reflecting for benefits, but the increased use of positive feelings and feeling peaceful and calm.

Other health benefits gained from visiting these places included an increase in positive emotions, which can be associated with emotional restoration and improved wellbeing. In general, the language used by participants was positive, referring to increases in, or more of, a positive attribute rather than less of a negative attribute. Unlike much of the environmental noise literature which talks about quiet areas or green spaces as helping to prevent and mitigate from negative feelings [3], the public instead focus on the positive attributes, and salutogenic (health-promoting) benefits. The concept of instoration—which is the improvement of mood or attention without a prior negative or fatigued state above a beneficial value [55]—may also be relevant here as people may not have needed to "recover" (hence the neutral perceived restorative outcomes) but still improved on their already positive, or neutral mood. As prior fatigue levels or emotional states were not assessed beforehand, this study cannot confirm what changes were made and whether their prior emotion was negative or positive, thus caution should be noted in the interpretation of these results in relation to restoration theory. However, the study does highlight the language the public use to describe the perceived health outcomes they gain from visiting these places, which can help future experimental studies assess health outcomes by using terminology with which the public associate.

Many respondents also recognized other positive states, of feeling peaceful, quiet, tranquil and calm. These comments were clearly about how *they* felt from being in the place, rather than a description of the *place*. These terms were the second and third most frequently described feelings after relaxed. Indeed, even the Square which was rated significantly lower in its description of calm than the other two sites, still had "calm" as a frequently used term to describe the users emotional state. This raises questions about using the phraseology of candidate calm areas instead of CQA as suggested by the European Environment Agency [11,12]; should the users *emotional state* of calm be incorporated, or is it only an assessment of the *place* as calm? The same could be applied to the terms "quiet" and "peaceful" which was used both to describe the place (its sound levels) and themselves (emotional state). The complexities of these terms was also explored in a study in Amsterdam where the difference between "quiet" as a mental state, an experienced place and as a situation was examined [56].

The social experience of being with or around other people was also seen as a benefit from visiting these places. Prior research has highlighted the relationship between social relationships and wellbeing and the social value of public urban spaces [19], and this was echoed again in this study. For a few, it helped them feel better and less lonely, thus the busyness of the place was appreciated. A number of people also enjoyed the opportunity to be outdoors in the sunshine, fresh air, and in nature which have all been shown to help people's wellbeing [19].

Alongside listing benefits to themselves, many people described characteristics of the place. It seems the benefit to the people was the existence of the place itself rather than the benefits it directly derived *them*, or at least they found it easier to describe these benefits. This shows high levels of appreciation of all three places and highlights the value of good quality urban spaces, either involving nature or architectural features, which are well maintained. Appreciated places will subsequently benefit its visitors, and are associated with perceived restorative outcomes directly [34] or via preference [57]. Additionally, the most frequent benefits listed overall was the places being peaceful or calm, and this was before any questions about sound had been mentioned. Even in the Square, which had the highest objective sound level ratings and the lowest subjective rating for quiet, calm, and tranquil, the most frequently mentioned benefit of being in the place was its peacefulness and calmness. Together, these results support the idea that criteria for choosing candidate quiet or calm areas should incorporate both the public perception of the place and objective values [30], and should have a measurable beneficial impact on its users [16]. This currently differs to the process that Scotland use to identify CQAs.

4.3. Exploring the Necessity of Quiet for Restoration

Despite the Park and Square having similar sound levels, albeit above the recommended level that Scotland uses to identify CQAs, visitors' perceived restorative outcomes significantly differed between the two places. Similarly, the Garden's sound levels were much lower than the Square, yet on average, visitors' perceived restorative outcomes were the same in these two places. Clearly, with these three sites, there was no clear correlation between sound levels and perceived restorative outcomes. Furthermore, as perceived sound levels varied in line with objective sound levels, there was also no clear relationship between perceived sound levels (quiet) or ratings of calm and tranquillity, with perceived restorative outcomes. Additionally, all places produced frequent feelings of relaxation, and a visitor benefit of feeling at peace and calm. Therefore, the relationship between perceived restoration and subjective and objective assessments of sound level was not a simple one, yet restoration is an important health and wellbeing outcome that is often associated with the benefit of CQAs [11].

The amount of time people spent in the places was a varying factor between the sites, with people spending a shorter time in the Garden than the other sites, and people spending longer in the Park in the afternoon than in the morning. Temporal factors could explain the perceived restorative outcomes between these two sites and between ratings in the Park for the morning and afternoon. The longer someone stays in a restorative environment, the greater the chance for restoration to occur (perhaps to a certain point) and prior fatigue levels will also influence this relationship.

Finally the type of sounds perceived, rather than just the sound levels are important in creating a restorative experience [26]. For example, natural soundscapes are more restorative than urban soundscapes dominated by traffic [25,26,45,58] and individual natural sounds of birds singing are rated highly in their perceived restorative potential [27]. Natural sounds were more frequently recalled in the Garden and Park than in the Square, and fewer vehicle sounds were heard in the morning in the Garden, when higher perceived restorative outcomes were rated. Therefore, despite visitors spending similar amount of times in the Park and Square and experiencing similar sound levels (both subjectively and objectively), the differences in sound types and the level of vegetation and biodiversity between the sites could in part explain the differences in perceived restorative outcomes. Further exploration of all these factors together is necessary, and only through controlling for the differing variables or systematically varying these variables, can a clearer relationship between the soundscape and restoration be established before being applied, if appropriately, as important criteria for identifying candidate quiet or calm areas.

5. Conclusions

Typically, much environmental acoustics research and policy focus has been reactive, trying to mitigate negative health outcomes from urban noise exposure. In contrast, preventative health research involving positive health outcomes from exposure to urban sounds is limited. A reconsideration of acoustic environments in terms of soundscapes, rather than environmental noise, helps readdress this imbalance and enables exploring positive health outcomes. Practically, public urban environments need designing in a manner that prevents environmental noise exposure and supports acoustic environments, which are positively evaluated and potentially provide restorative experiences.

Taking a multi-site approach, this work identified the positive benefits people hoped to achieve and felt from visiting an urban garden, park and square, and how a desire for restoration alongside a peaceful, calm and quiet soundscape were valuable for many. These aspects were discussed alongside the study sites match with criteria for identifying urban Candidate Quiet Areas (CQAs) across the United Kingdom. Despite the public perceiving two of the sites as quiet, the local authorities did not recognize them as CQAs, highlighting disparities between criteria used by authorities to identify CQAs and what the public may consider as quiet. Further reflection on suitable CQA criteria may still be necessary, including a greater understanding of public perception of quiet and its value. As part of Project DeStress, an online survey is currently exploring these issues to help identify key physical and social characteristics of places the public identify as quiet, to help determine relevant CQA criteria to use in future UK noise action plans.

The use of three different types of urban public spaces in three different cities, means local contextual variations may have influenced participants' responses, making it more difficult to draw conclusive results from comparisons across the sites. Similarly, different people were evaluating different sites, thus individual variations (e.g., ages, familiarity with sites) will exist in how people perceived and evaluated the places due to differing preferences and needs, although the averaging of results should help reduce such issues. The sample size in this study does limit the conclusions that can be drawn from the work, as further statistical analysis to control for variance across all the factors could not occur, thus the interpretation of the results is discursive rather than conclusive. For example, in line with existing research, other factors such as the presence of nature, people and available time were likely to influence perceived restoration ratings in this study, but quiet also seemed to be associated with the desire and ability to restore. Future work is planned as part of Project DeStress involving larger sample sizes and virtual simulations of the study sites where variables can be systematically manipulated to establish clearer relationships between sound levels, perceived quiet, sound sources, type of place and the subsequent health benefits, including restoration. Further understanding of the relationships between environmental sound, psychological restoration, and other health benefits will help policy makers and planners to continue their goals in preserving and identifying urban quiet areas that not only help mitigate the adverse health impacts from environmental noise, but also establish salutogenic environments that create healthy, sustainable societies.

Author Contributions: S.P. conceptualized the study and collaborated with N.B. on the study methodology and development of the paper. S.P. collected and analysed the participant data while N.B. collected and analysed the acoustic data. Both authors contributed to the paper writing, with S.P. contributing the majority. Conceptualization, S.P.; Formal analysis, S.P. and N.B.; Funding acquisition, S.P.; Methodology, S.P. and N.B.; Writing—original draft, S.P. and N.B.; Writing—review and editing, S.P. and N.B.

Funding: This research is part of Project DeStress, which was funded by the Engineering and Physical Sciences Research Council (EPSRC) in the United Kingdom, grant number EP/R003467/1. The APC was funded by Heriot–Watt University.

Acknowledgments: We thank the participants for their help in making this work possible. We thank research assistant Jordan Greenhorn for being the second coder and for the weather data analysis. We also thank our Project Partners who helped make this work possible, Jack Harvie-Clark of Apex Acoustics, Clive Bentley of Sharps Redmore, Lisa Lavia of the Noise Abatement Society, and Professor Marketta Kyttä of Aalto University, Finland.

Conflicts of Interest: The authors declare no conflict of interest. The funders had no role in the design of the study; in the collection, analyses, or interpretation of data; in the writing of the manuscript, or in the decision to publish the results.

Data Availability: Data used in this paper is openly available from Heriot–Watt University archive system from 12th September 2019 when the project ends. Any use of the data must include attributions to the paper authors who collected the data. It can be found at https://doi.org/10.17861/3ca48e2d-7a6e-4553-ac3c-3b08a6612d19.

References

1. World Health Organisation. *Guidelines for Community Noise*; World Health Organisation: Geneva, Switzerland, 2000.
2. World Health Organisation Regional Office for Europe JRC. *Burden of Environmental Noise. Quantification of Healthy Life Years Lost in Europe*; WHO Regional Office for Europe: Copenhagen, Denmark, 2011.
3. World Health Organisation Regional Office for Europe. *Environmental Noise Guidelines for the European Region*; World Health Organisation Regional Office for Europe: Copenhagen, Denmark, 2018.
4. Babisch, W. Updated exposure-response relationship between road traffic noise and coronary heart diseases: A meta analysis. *Noise Health* **2014**, *16*, 1–9. [CrossRef] [PubMed]
5. ISO (International Organization for Standardization). 12913-1:2014 Acoustics–Soundscape–Part 1: Definition & Conceptual Framework. 2014. Available online: https://www.iso.org/standard/52161.html (accessed on 4 January 2019).

6. Payne, S.R.; Davies, W.J.; Adams, M.D. *Research into the Practical and Policy Applications of Soundscape Concepts and Techniques in Urban Areas*; Department of Environment Food and Rural Affairs, HMSO: London, UK, 2009.
7. ISO (International Organization for Standardization). *ISO/TS12913-2. Acoustics–Soundscape–Part 2: Data Collection and Reporting Requirements*; International Organization for Standardization: Geneva, Switzerland, 2018; Available online: https://www.iso.org/standard/75267.html (accessed on 4 January 2019).
8. European Parliament and Council. Directive 2002/49/EC of the European Parliament and of the Council of 25th June 2002, relating to the assessment and management of environmental noise. *Off. J. Eur. Communities* **2002**, *L189*, 0012–0026.
9. de Kluizenaar, Y.; Janssen, S.A.; Vos, H.; Salomons, E.M.; Zhou, H.; van den Berg, F. Road traffic noise and annoyance: A quantification of the effect of quiet side exposure at dwellings. *Int. J. Environ. Res. Public Health* **2013**, *10*, 2258–2270. [CrossRef] [PubMed]
10. van Renterghem, T.; Botteldooren, D. Focused study on the quiet side effect in dwellings highly exposed to road traffic noise. *Int. J. Environ. Res. Public Health* **2012**, *9*, 4293–4310. [CrossRef]
11. European Environment Agency. *Quiet Areas in Europe. The Environment Unaffected by Noise Pollution*; EEA Report No.14; Publications Office of the European Union: Luxembourg, 2016.
12. European Environment Agency. *Good Practice Guide on quiET AREas*; EEA technical report No. 4; Publications Office of the European Union: Luxembourg, 2014.
13. Pheasant, R.J.; Fisher, M.N.; Watts, G.R.; Whitaker, D.J.; Horoshenkov, K. The importance of auditory-visual interaction in the construction of 'tranquil space'. *J. Environ. Psychol.* **2010**, *30*, 501–509. [CrossRef]
14. The Scottish Government. *Technical Guidance. Noise Action Plans. Candidate Quiet Areas to Quiet Areas*; Scottish Government: Edinburgh, Scotland, 2009.
15. The Scottish Government. *Consultation on the Noise Directive Action Plan: Strategic Noise Action Plan for the Edinburgh Agglomeration*; Scottish Government: Edinburgh, Scotland, 2018.
16. Defra. Consultation on Draft noise action plan: Agglomerations (urban areas). In *Environmental Noise (England) Regulations 2006, as Amended October 2018*; Department for Environment, Food, & Rural Affairs: London, UK, 2018.
17. Bowler, D.; Buyung-Ali, L.; Knight, T.; Pullin, A. A systematic review of evidence for the added benefits to health of exposure to natural environments. *BMC Public Health* **2010**, *10*, 456. [CrossRef] [PubMed]
18. Houses of Parliament Parliamentary office of Science and technology. *Green space and Health*; POST note 538, Oct 2016; Parliamentary offfice of Science and technology: London, UK, 2016.
19. World Health Organisation Regional Office for Europe. *Urban Green Space Interventions and Health: A Review of Impacts and Effectiveness*; WHO Regional Office for Europe: Copenhagen, Denmark, 2017.
20. Kaplan, S. The restorative benefits of nature: Toward an integrative framework. *J. Environ. Psychol.* **1995**, *15*, 169–182. [CrossRef]
21. Ulrich, R.S.; Simons, R.F.; Losito, B.D.; Fiorito, E.; Miles, M.A.; Zelson, M. Stress recovery during exposure to natural and urban environments. *J. Environ. Psychol.* **1991**, *11*, 201–230. [CrossRef]
22. Van den Berg, A.E.; Jorgensen, A.; Wilson, E.R. Evaluating restoration in urban green spaces: Does setting type make a difference? *Landsc. Urban Plan.* **2014**, *127*, 173–181. [CrossRef]
23. Hartig, T.; Mitchell, R.; de Vries, S.; Frumkin, H. Nature and health. *Annu. Rev. Public Health* **2014**, *35*, 207–228. [CrossRef]
24. Gidlöf-Gunnarsson, A.; Öhrström, E. Noise and well-being in urban residential environments: The potential role of perceived availability to nearby green areas. *Landsc. Urban Plan.* **2007**, *83*, 115–126. [CrossRef]
25. Payne, S.R. The production of a Perceived Restorativeness Soundscape Scale. *Appl. Acoust.* **2013**, *74*, 255–263. [CrossRef]
26. Payne, S.R. Urban park soundscapes and their perceived restorativeness. *Proc. Inst. Acoust. Belg. Acoust. Soc.* **2010**, *32*, 264–271.
27. Ratcliffe, E.; Gatersleben, B.; Sowden, P.T. Associations with bird sounds: How do they relate to perceived restorative potential? *J. Environ. Psychol.* **2016**, *47*, 136–144. [CrossRef]
28. Aletta, F.; Oberman, T.; Kang, J. Associations between positive health-related effects and soundscapes perceptual constructs: A systematic review. *Int. J. Environ. Res. Public Health* **2018**, *15*, 2392. [CrossRef]
29. Payne, S.R.; Bruce, N. DeStress: Soundscapes, quiet areas and restorative environments. *Proc. Inst. Acoust.* **2019**, *41*. In press.

30. Bartalucci, C.; Borchi, F.; Carfacni, M.; Governi, L.; Zonfrillo, G.; Aspuru, I.; Garcia, I.; Herranz, K.; Weber, M.; Wolfert, H.; et al. Guidelines for the Identification, Selection, Analysis, and Managaement of Quiet Urban Areas. Ver 2.0. 2015. Available online: http://www.quadmap.eu/wp-content/uploads/2012/01/Guidelines_QUADMAP_ver2.0.pdf (accessed on 4 January 2019).
31. Axelsson, O. How to measure soundscape quality. In Proceedings of the Euronoise, Maastricht, The Netherlands, 31 May–3 June 2015; pp. 1477–1481.
32. Natural England. *Monitor of Engagement with the Natural Environment. The National Survey on People and the Natural Environment*; Technical report to the 2009-2018 surveys; Natural England: Worcester, UK, 2018.
33. Staats, H.; Kieviet, A.; Hartig, T. Where to recover from attentional fatigue: An expectancy-value analysis of environmental preference. *J. Environ. Psychol.* **2003**, *23*, 147–157. [CrossRef]
34. Payne, S.R. Are perceived soundscapes within urban parks restorative? In Proceedings of the Euronoise, Acoustics '08, Paris, France, 30 June–4 July 2008; pp. 5519–5524.
35. Knez, I. Attachment and identity as related to a place and its perceived climate. *J. Environ. Psychol.* **2005**, *25*, 207–218. [CrossRef]
36. ISO (International Organization for Standardization). *1996-2:2017. Acoustics—Description, Measurement and Assessment of Environmental Noise. Part 2: Determination of Sound Pressure Levels*; International Organization for Standardization: Geneva, Switzerland, 2017; Available online: https://www.iso.org/standard/59766.html (accessed on 4 January 2019).
37. Weather Underground. Available online: https://www.wunderground.com (accessed on 14 February 2019).
38. Landis, J.R.; Koch, G.G. The measurement of observer agreement for categorical data. *Biometrics* **1977**, *33*, 159–174. [CrossRef]
39. Rea, L.M.; Parker, R.A. *Designing and Conducting Survey Research*; Jossey-Bass: San Francisco, CA, USA, 1992.
40. Bruce, N.; Davies, W.J. The effect of expectation on the perception of soundscapes. *Appl. Acoust.* **2014**, *85*, 1–22. [CrossRef]
41. Payne, S.R. The classification, semantics, and perception of urban park sounds: Methodological issues. *Inst. Acoust.* **2008**, *30*, 560–567.
42. Chu, S.; Narayanan, S.; Jay Kuo, C.-C. Environmental Sound Recognition with Time-Frequency Audio Features. *IEEE Trans. Audio Speech Lang. Process.* **2009**, *17*, 1142–1158. [CrossRef]
43. Yang, W.; Kang, J. Acoustic comfort evaluation in urban open public spaces. *Appl. Acoust.* **2005**, *66*, 211–229. [CrossRef]
44. Tsaligopoulos, A.; Economou, C.; Matsinos, Y.G. Identification, Prioritization, and Assessment of Urban Quiet Areas. In *Handbook of Research on Perception-Driven Approaches to Urban Assessment and Design*; Aletta, F., Xiao, J., Eds.; IGI Global: Hershey, PA, USA, 2018; pp. 150–180.
45. Van Kamp, I.; Klæboe, R.; Brown, A.L.; Lercher, P. Soundscapes, Human Restoration, and Quality of Life. In *Soundscape and the Built Environment*; Kang, J., Schulte-Fortkamp, B., Eds.; CRC Press: Boca Raton, FL, USA, 2016; pp. 43–68.
46. De Coensel, B.; Botteldooren, D. Acoustic design for early stage urban planning. *Des. Soundscape Sustain. Urban Dev.* **2010**, 17–20.
47. Lavia, L.; Dixon, M.; Witchel, H.; Goldsmith, M. Applied Soundscape Practices. In *Soundscape and the Built Environment*; Kang, J., Schulte-Fortkamp, B., Eds.; CRC Press: Boca Raton, FL, USA, 2016; pp. 243–301.
48. Aletta, F.; Kang, J.; Fuda, S.; Astolfi, A. The effect of walking sounds from different walked-on materials on the soundscape of urban parks. *J. Environ. Eng. Landsc. Manag.* **2016**, *24*, 165–175. [CrossRef]
49. HOSANNA project. *Novel Solutions for Quieter and Greener Cities*; European Union Seventh Framework Programme: Stockholm, Sweden, 2013.
50. Kaplan, R.; Kaplan, S. *The Experience of Nature: A Psychological Perspective*; Cambridge University Press: Cambridge, UK, 1989.
51. Lonely Planet. Lonely Planet Guide. Available online: https://www.lonelyplanet.com/scotland/edinburgh/attractions/dunbar-s-close-garden/a/poi-sig/399269/360630 (accessed on 23 March 2019).
52. Laumann, K.; Gärling, T.; Stormark, K.M. Rating scale measures of restorative components of environments. *J. Environ. Psychol.* **2001**, *21*, 31–44. [CrossRef]
53. Staats, H.; Hartig, T. Alone or with a friend: A social context for psychological restoration and environmental preferences. *J. Environ. Psychol.* **2004**, *24*, 199–211. [CrossRef]

54. Payne, S.R.; Guastavino, C. Exploring the validity of the Perceived Restorativeness Soundscape Scale: A psycholinguistic approach. *Front. Psychol.* **2018**, *9*, 1–17. [CrossRef]
55. Hartig, T.; Böök, A.; Garvill, J.; Olsson, T.; Gärling, T. Environmental influences on psychological restoration. *Scand. J. Psychol.* **1996**, *37*, 378–393. [CrossRef]
56. Booi, H.; van den Berg, F. Quiet areas and the Need for Quietness in Amsterdam. *Int. J. Environ. Res. Public Health* **2012**, *9*, 1030–1050. [CrossRef]
57. van den Berg, A.E.; Koole, S.L.; van der Wulp, N.Y. Environmental preference and restoration: (How) are they related? *J. Environ. Psychol.* **2003**, *23*, 135–146. [CrossRef]
58. Alvarsson, J.J.; Wiens, S.; Nilsson, M.E. Stress Recovery during Exposure to Nature Sound and Environmental Noise. *Int. J. Environ. Res. Public Health* **2010**, *7*, 1036–1046. [CrossRef]

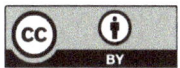

© 2019 by the authors. Licensee MDPI, Basel, Switzerland. This article is an open access article distributed under the terms and conditions of the Creative Commons Attribution (CC BY) license (http://creativecommons.org/licenses/by/4.0/).

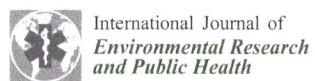

Article

The Influence of Audio-Visual Interactions on Psychological Responses of Young People in Urban Green Areas: A Case Study in Two Parks in China

Shilun Zhang [1,*], Xiaolong Zhao [1,2,*], Zixi Zeng [1] and Xuan Qiu [1]

1. Key Laboratory of Cold Region Urban and Rural Human Settlement Environment Science and Technology, Ministry of Industry and Information Technology, School of Architecture, Harbin Institute of Technology, Harbin 150001, China; zixi_zeng@outlook.com (Z.Z.); qiux.x@outlook.com (X.Q.)
2. School of Architecture and Urban Planning, Suzhou University of Science and Technology, Suzhou 215009, China
* Correspondence: zhang.sl@outlook.com (S.Z.); zhaoxiaolong@hit.edu.cn (X.Z.); Tel.: +86-155-4082-9333 (S.Z.); +86-188-4679-3560 (X.Z.)

Received: 29 March 2019; Accepted: 22 May 2019; Published: 24 May 2019

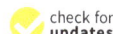

Abstract: Audio-visual interactions in green spaces are important for mental health and wellbeing. However, the influence of audio-visual interactions on psychological responses is still less clear. This study introduced a new method, namely the audio-visual walk (AV-walk), to obtain data on the audio-visual context, audio-visual experiences, and psychological responses in two typical parks, namely Cloves Park and Music Park in Harbin, China. Some interesting results are as follows: First, based on Pearson's correlation analysis, sound pressure level and roughness were significantly correlated with psychological responses in Cloves Park ($p < 0.05$). Second, the results of stepwise regression models showed the impact intensity of acoustic comfort was 1.64–1.68 times higher than that of visual comfort on psychological responses of emotion dimension, while visual comfort was 1.35–1.37 times higher than acoustic comfort on psychological responses of cognition dimension in Music Park. In addition, an orthogonal analysis diagram explained the influence of audio-visual interactions on psychological responses of young people. The audio-visual context located beside the waterscape with a relatively higher level of acoustic and visual comfort was the most cheerful (2.60), relaxed (2.45), and energetic (2.05), while the audio-visual context close to an urban built environment tended to be both acoustically and visually uncomfortable, and the psychological state was decreased to the most depressed (−0.25), anxious (−0.75), fatigued (−1.13) and distracted (−1.13).

Keywords: audio-visual interaction; audio-visual walk; young people's psychological response; orthogonal analysis; urban parks

1. Introduction

Psychological health issues of specific populations, especially young people, have developed into a major concern. People face a series of economic, academic, social, and life pressures that (without the possibility of recovery) result in vulnerability to stress, and ignoring psychological stress can lead to increased depression [1], diabetes [2], and cardiovascular and neurological illnesses [3]. On the other hand, urban green spaces are recognized as a context that can improve the psychological health of people because the environment in urban green spaces helps to reduce stress and assists with psychological recovery. Therefore, the context of urban green spaces is of importance.

Two theories, namely stress recovery theory (SRT) [4], which focuses on the recovery from stress due to attention to the contact with nature, and attention restoration theory (ART) [5], which focuses on recovery from mental fatigue using the natural environment, have been frequently used to explore the psychological restoration effects of the natural environment. Some previous studies employing SRT and ART explained the psychological restoration effects on the visual aspect perspective. Because watching "green nature" can lower the heartbeat and blood pressure and stimulate the parasympathetic nervous system, it calmed the sympathetic nervous system and increased the user's tendency to relax and experience enjoyment and energy [6]. Much literature has described the application of different visual stimuli using visual stimulations from different open spaces (e.g., urban environment, parks, gardens, and forests) to compare psychological restoration effects in experimental research [7,8] or field studies [9–11]. Some other studies have quantified the visual landscape to explore the extent to which the visual landscape in green spaces can influence psychological responses. For example, a study by Grahn and Stigsdotter carried out in nine Swedish cities claimed that space openness and richness in the resident species, which was described by perceived sensory dimensions (PSDs), were significant factors that influenced the level of stress [12]. Han reported the results from studies in which the objective visual green rate was collected by a camera and analyzed with Photoshop and AutoCAD software. The results showed a significant correlation with fatigue nervousness and confusion reflected by a Profile of Mood State (POMS) in a natural environment on a university campus ($p < 0.05$) [11].

In recent years, some studies have assessed the psychological recovery potential of soundscapes [8,13–15]. They focused on the relationship between the acoustic environment and psychological responses [16,17] and they identified the sound sources that promoted positive emotions (stress recovery) [13,18]. According to a study by Daniel Shepherd et al., the mean scores of psychological well-being described by the WHO's short-form quality of life instrument (WHOQOL-BREF) perceived by residents in quiet areas were higher than in noisy areas [19]. Based on the records of 180 subjects, Goel et al. showed that an auditory stimulus (birdsong enhanced with a classical music background at 60 dB) significantly reduced depression and anger reflected by a POMS after 15 min of exposure [20].

Accumulating evidence has shown that green space can reduce traffic-related annoyance via psychological mechanisms, including visual screening of the noise source and increased restorative quality of the residential environment [21,22]. Yang concluded, based on EEG-recordings, that visually-presented landscape vegetation can "provide excess noise attenuating effects through the subjects' emotional processing" [23]. Thus, when exploring the effects of contextual factors on psychological responses, neither acoustic variables nor visual factors should be neglected, in particular, in green spaces. The importance of acoustic-visual interactions on both mental health and well-being was realized in a few studies [24]. For example, in two studies in the UK, Payne considered both visual and acoustic environments and they proposed that an urban soundscape was perceived as lower in restorative potential than an urban park soundscape, which was perceived as lower than that in rural areas [8]. Shu and Ma compared the effects of an urban park and classroom with 32 visual and auditory stimulation combinations (2 visual × 16 stimuli) on attention recovery of children using the Perceived Restorative Sounds Scale (PRSS) [25].

However, even though the relationship between audio-visual environment and psychological response has been studied in a qualitative way in many previous studies, the mechanism of audio-visual environment and audio-visual perception on the psychological response of users in urban parks still requires further improvement. In addition, the sound environment in an urban green space is complicated, because the green space contains multiple sound sources. However, many studies have focused on the effect of a single sound source. The visual variables analyzed in an audio-visual environment have also been too simplistic. Additionally, whether these psychological benefits could be generalized to young people has not been studied systematically since previous research primarily focused on adults [26,27], children [25,28] and the aged [29]. Urban parks in Europe have been seen as quiet areas that not only protect against noise but also reveal positive sounds [30]. Urban parks in Asia, however, especially in high-density cities in China, are impacted by high-level traffic noise. Thus, a study in urban parks in China is significant.

Two research questions were studied:

RQ1: Do audio-visual contexts and experiences in urban parks influence psychological responses of young people?

RQ2: How do audio-visual interactions determine psychological responses of young people in urban parks?

2. Methods

2.1. Survey Sites

Two typical urban parks, namely Cloves Park and Music Park located in Harbin, China, were selected as survey sites. The reasons why these two urban parks were selected were the following: First, they are frequently visited by residents and tourists and are not far away from an urban center. Second, there are various kinds of landscapes (plants, mountains and lakes) and soundscapes (traffic sound, natural sounds, human activities sound, music and so forth) that enriched the sample. Third, the compositions of sound sources in these two parks may result in differences in psychological responses. In Cloves Park, traffic sounds, construction sounds, animal sounds (birdsong and insect songs), and activity sounds are dominant sounds that were investigated in a preliminary study. Traffic sounds, music, and activity sounds make up the main ingredients, while animal sounds can be heard in less 10% of the areas investigated in a preliminary survey in Music Park.

Previous studies adopted soundwalk methodologies for investigating the visual, acoustic or audio-visual environments on participants' experience, especially acoustic perception in soundscape field [31,32]. Nevertheless, in this study, a new method named audio-visual walk (AV-walk) was used to obtain data on audio-visual contexts, audio-visual experiences, and psychological responses to explore the influence of audio-visual interactions on psychological responses of participants. In a preliminary study, a group (4 persons) that majored in Architecture Landscape was asked to visit these two parks and then mark the stopping locations that impressed them in terms of landscape and soundscape for formal research in each park. The choice of stopping locations is similar to soundwalk the method of Jeon et al. [31]. Then, according to the preference weight (>80%) of the stopping locations, we determined the final 30 survey points. In a formal study, participants were asked to walk on a pre-set path and when they visited one of 30 points in each park, they were asked to perceive the intensity of each sound source for 2–3 min [33], and to report the audio-visual experience and the psychological responses. At the same time, acoustic instruments and a camera were used to obtain data on the sound environment and visual environment, respectively.

The study was conducted in accordance with the Declaration of Helsinki, and the protocol was approved by the Research Ethics Committee of School of Architecture of Harbin Institute of Technology, China. In addition, all participants gave their informed consent for inclusion before the experiment of the audio-visual walk originally started.

2.2. Participants

A total of 36 graduate students (male: 16; female: 20) with self-reported normal vision and hearing [34,35] asserted that they can easily distinguish a certain sound in a complex sound environment, sense the strength of the sound, and recognize different colors from the School of Architecture, Harbin Institute of Technology, volunteered to join the AV-walk survey. The age of the participants ranged from 22–33 years old [36]. Before the formal survey, participants were asked have good sleep on the day before the survey and to study and work for 2–4 h on the survey day to reduce errors of psychological responses. In addition, when the formal survey began, to avoid disturbances among them during perceiving the audio-visual context, they were prohibited from communicating, eating, and walking. Participants were also required to provide their demographic characteristics, such as gender, age (22–25, 25–28, or 28–33 years old), and educational background (bachelor's degree and master's degree, and those reading for a master's or doctoral degree) before the formal investigation.

2.3. Procedure

The survey was performed in the afternoon (from 1:30–3:30) with clear weather from September 20–October 20, 2018, which is the most vigorous season for vegetation growth and bird and insect activity. The range of the average air temperature, wind strength, and air quality indexes (PM 2.5 index [37]) during the experimental procedure was 18–21 °C, 3–4 degrees and 35–75 μg/m^3, respectively. The formal survey consisted of two parts, including audio-visual context measurements and the audio-visual perception questionnaire.

Regarding the audio-visual context, the sound pressure level was recorded with a sound pressure level meter (type: BSWA801, BSWA TECH, Beijing, China) at every survey point. The sound pressure level meter was set to a slow-mode and A-weight, and a reading for instantaneous data was taken every 1 s. The probe of the sound-level meter was positioned more than 1.0 m away from any reflectors and more than 1.2 m off the ground [38]. A total of 3 min of data were obtained at each measurement position, and the corresponding A-weight equivalent sound pressure level (LAeq) was derived. To measure the psychoacoustic indicators, an acoustic recorder (type: SQuadriga II, LANDTOP, Beijing, China) was used simultaneously with the BSWA 801. Artemis 12.0 software (LANDTOP, Beijing, China) was used to analyze the psychoacoustic variables; e.g., loudness (sone), roughness (asper) and sharpness (acum) [39]. The assessment of loudness was based on the N5 value rather than the average because it was more suitable for the evaluation of time-varying sounds [40]. In terms of visual context, based on the quantification of visual landscapes in photos, recent works explored the relationship between landscape attributes and landscape preferences [41,42] and showed the effects of landscape elements on aesthetic appreciation that may impact emotions. Thus, in this study, a single lens reflect camera (35-mm lens) was used to take a picture of a normal setting every 90° with a total of 3 pictures [11] covering a 180° view in the horizontal plane at a height of 1.7 m above the ground at each survey point [15]. The picture was used to obtain landscape elements (e.g., plants, sky and paving) identified by a volunteer. Some visual parameters; i.e., visual green rate (%), sky visibility and paving visibility, were used in this study to quantify these landscape elements. The visible greenness rate quantifies the amount of vegetation that is visible in the visual field and it is a more valid approach than the green cover ratio [11], which was processed and calculated with Photoshop 6.0 software (Adobe, San Jose, CA, USA) [9,43] according to the pixel weight in each photograph. The sky visibility and paving visibility were analyzed with the same process.

Audio-visual context measurement and application of the audio-visual perception questionnaire were performed simultaneously, which means when the volunteer collected data on the audio-visual context, participants were asked to perceive the audio-visual context. The audio-visual perception questionnaire included three parts. First, as participants visited each survey point, they were required to perceive the sound sources and then evaluate the intensity of each sound with a five-point Likert scale: 0, not at all; 1, a little; 2, moderately; 3, a lot; and 4, dominates completely [44]. Second, the participants were asked to assess the audio-visual experience at each location, including acoustic comfort and visual comfort using a 9-point bipolar scale that ranged from not at all to extremely (from −4–4). Third, this study assumed that there are always two dimensions of psychological states in urban green spaces, as assessed in previous studies; that is, positive and negative emotions. Eight adjectives, including 4 positive and 4 negative adjectives, were selected with high reliability and validity from the Profile of Mood State (POMS), the Positive and Negative Affect Scale (PANAS) and the Restoration Scale (RS), based on SRT and ART. In this paper, two dimensions, namely emotion and cognition dimensions, in psychological response were reflected by these adjectives. Among them, 4 adjectives—cheerful, depressed, relaxed and anxious—were used to evaluate the emotion dimension of psychological response [11,45], and other adjectives including energetic, fatigued, focused, and distracted were selected to assess the cognition dimension of psychological response [46]. Additionally, many studies have shown that a psychological assessment appears to be bipolar rather than unipolar or simply categorical. Therefore, these 8 adjectives were divided into 4 items, and each item reflected both positive and negative feelings, which were cheerful-depressed (CD), relaxed-anxious (RA), energetic-fatigued (EF), and focused-distracted (FD), respectively. A 9-point bipolar scale was used to evaluate these 4 items with values ranging from −4 (negative) to 4 (positive).

2.4. Data Statistics

SPSS software [47] was used to analyze the normality of samples, correlations, and regression of indicators in the two parks. First, the Kolmogorov-Smirnov test was used to analyze the normality of the collected data. The results showed that all of the p values were more than 0.05 (except for birdsong in Music Park: $p = 0.008$, and paving visibility in Cloves Park and Music Park: $p = 0.014$ and 0.013, respectively), which indicated all samples had statistical significance. This may be because the sample of birdsong was low: The percentage of birdsong was less than 5% in 80% of the survey points. Second, Pearson's correlation was used to calculate the relationship between the audio-visual context and psychological responses, the relationship between the audio-visual experiences and the psychological responses; a T-test at $p < 0.01$ and $p < 0.05$ was used to test for significant differences. Third, a stepwise linear regression was used to establish the regression equations for audio-visual context and psychological responses, audio-visual experiences and the psychological responses. An ANOVA was used to test the significance of regression equations. In addition, the reliability and validity of the questionnaire were also tested. The reliability and validity was measured by Cronbach's Alpha and Kaiser-Meyer-Olkin (KMO) respectively. The values of Cronbach's Alpha were 0.684 and 0.785 and the scores of KMO were 0.803 and 0.788 in Cloves Park and Music Park, respectively, which means that the reliability and validity of the questionnaire were acceptable [48].

The results of Pearson's correlation analysis between the sound sources and psychological responses showed that traffic sounds and construction sounds were negatively correlated with psychological responses, birdsong and insect songs, and activity sounds were positively correlated with psychological responses in Cloves Park. In Music Park, traffic sounds and activity sounds were negatively correlated with psychological responses, and birdsong and music were positively correlated with psychological responses, although there was a weak correlation between music and psychological responses and between birdsong and psychological responses, which may be because the proportion of birdsong and activity sounds was relatively lower than other sounds at each survey point. Thus, traffic sounds, construction sounds, and activity sounds (in Music Park) were classified as negative sounds and birdsong, insect sounds, music activity sounds (in Cloves Park) were classified as positive sounds.

3. Results

3.1. Identification of Audio-Visual Context and Experiences

Pearson's correlation results between the acoustic context and psychological responses, and between visual context and psychological responses in the two parks are shown in Table 1. The results showed that LAeq, loudness (except for CD), and roughness were significantly negatively correlated with psychological responses in Cloves Park, with correlation coefficient R ranging from −0.850 to −0.396. There was no correlation between sharpness and psychological responses according to significance level (Sig.). It is interesting to note that LAeq and psychoacoustic parameters were uncorrelated with psychological responses in Music Park ($p > 0.05$). One possible reason may be that the composition of positive and negative sounds in Music Park is not significantly different; that is, the ratio of positive and negative sounds was close to 1:1 (ranging from 0.9–1.1) at 46.7% survey points in Music Park. Therefore, objective acoustic parameters may not reflect changes in participants' psychological responses. Regarding visual context, there was no relationship between the visual green rate and psychological responses and between sky visibility and psychological responses in two urban parks (except for a weak correlation between sky visibility and RA in Music Park with a correlation coefficient R that was only 0.366).

Table 1 also shows the relationship between audio experiences and psychological responses and between visual experiences and psychological responses in two urban parks. In Cloves Park, it can be seen that acoustic comfort and visual comfort showed a positive strong correlation with psychological responses ($p < 0.01$) with coefficient R ranging from 0.511–0.889. Audio-visual experiences were also positively correlated with psychological responses ($p < 0.05$) with coefficient R ranging from 0.665–0.873 in Music Park. It can be concluded that, with audio-visual comfort increasing, the level of psychological responses, including CD, RA, EF, and FD, also increased, which was consistent with a recent research result in Spain [17].

Table 1. The Pearson correlation results between acoustic and visual environments and psychological responses in two parks.

	Sig.	Psychological Responses in Cloves Park				Psychological Responses in Music Park			
		CD	RA	EF	FD	CD	RA	EF	FD
Acoustic-visual context	LAeq	0.000 **	0.000 **	0.000 **	0.000 **	0.509	0.370	0.916	0.333
	Loudness	−0.071	0.013 *	0.027 *	0.003 **	0.255	0.455	0.179	0.437
	Roughness	0.030 *	0.004 **	0.009 **	0.001 **	0.436	0.272	0.915	0.289
	Sharpness	0.814	0.731	0.407	0.397	0.961	0.691	0.615	0.673
	Visual green rate	0.774	0.789	0.845	0.738	0.197	0.358	0.451	0.382
	Sky visibility	0.206	0.212	0.174	0.130	0.056	0.046 *	0.183	0.104
Acoustic-visual experience	Acoustic comfort	0.000 **	0.000 **	0.000 **	0.000 **	0.000 **	0.000 **	0.000 **	0.000 **
	Visual comfort	0.000 **	0.000 **	0.001 **	0.004 **	0.000 **	0.000 **	0.000 **	0.000 **

* means $p < 0.05$, ** means $p < 0.01$. cheerful-depressed (CD), relaxed-anxious (RA), energetic-fatigued (EF), focused-distracted (FD). Sig.: significance level.

Stepwise regression models (confidence interval 95%) were established to determine the impact intensity of audio-visual contexts on psychological responses in Cloves Park (shown in Table 2). To decrease errors, the variance inflation factor (VIF) was calculated to test the collinearity among predictors (VIF < 10). It can be seen that only the LAeq can be used to examine CD, RA, EF and FD in Cloves Park. There were no objective acoustic and visual parameters that could determine psychological responses (except for sky visibility) in Music Park.

Table 2. Stepwise regression model for audio-visual contexts and psychological responses in Cloves Park.

Model		Collinearity	Unstandardized Coefficients		Standardized Coefficients	Sig. [a]	Sig. [b]
Variable	Predictors	VIF	Regression Coefficient	Std. Error	Beta		
CD: $R^2 = 0.537$	(Constant)		7.415	1.136		0.000 **	0.000 **
R^2 (adj) = 0.521	LAeq	1.000	−0.125	0.022	−0.733	0.000 **	
RA: $R^2 = 0.558$	(Constant)		7.681	1.117		0.000 **	0.000 **
R^2 (adj) = 0.542	LAeq	1.000	−0.129	0.022	−0.747	0.000 **	
EF: $R^2 = 0.533$	(Constant)		7.590	1.231		0.000 **	0.000 **
R^2 (adj) = 0.517	LAeq	1.000	−0.135	0.024	−0.730	0.000 **	
FD: $R^2 = 0.723$	(Constant)		7.095	0.791		0.000 **	0.000 **
R^2 (adj) = 0.713	LAeq	1.000	−0.131	0.015	−0.850	0.000 **	

** means $p < 0.01$; [a] means significance of regression coefficient; [b] means significance of regression equation. VIF: variance inflation factor.

Table 3 describes the final results of the stepwise regression analysis in terms of the impact intensity of audio-visual experiences on psychological responses, including CD, RA, EF and FD in Cloves Park. The results of a stepwise regression analysis suggested that the regression model was significant and four psychological responses named CD, RA, EF and FD were determined by different predictors. In Cloves Park, CD was determined by acoustic and visual comfort, and acoustic comfort was in a dominant position regarding the influence on CD, with a beta weight of 0.660, compared to visual comfort ($p < 0.01$). RA and EF were also determined by acoustic and visual comfort, and the relative contribution of acoustic comfort was 2.37 and 2.64 times higher than visual comfort ($p < 0.01$), respectively, while FD was only explained by acoustic comfort ($p < 0.01$).

Table 3. The stepwise regression model for audio-visual experiences and psychological responses in Cloves Park.

Model		Collinearity	Unstandardized Coefficients		Standardized Coefficients	Sig. [a]	Sig. [b]
Variable	Predictors	VIF	Regression Coefficient	Std. Error	Beta		
CD: $R^2 = 0.870$ R^2 (adj) = 0.860	(Constant)		0.564	0.096		0.000 **	
	Acoustic comfort	1.248	0.400	0.047	0.660	0.000 **	0.000 **
	Visual comfort	1.248	0.372	0.068	0.427	0.000 **	
RA: $R^2 = 0.870$ R^2 (adj) = 0.860	(Constant)		0.779	0.097		0.000 **	
	Acoustic comfort	1.248	0.456	0.047	0.748	0.000 **	0.000 **
	Visual comfort	1.248	0.277	0.068	0.316	0.000 **	
EF: $R^2 = 0.712$ R^2 (adj) = 0.691	(Constant)		0.564	0.095		0.000 **	
	Acoustic comfort	1.001	0.512	0.067	0.783	0.000 **	0.000 **
	Visual comfort	1.001	0.385	0.134	0.297	0.000 **	
FD: $R^2 = 0.666$ R^2 (adj) = 0.654	(Constant)		0.405	0.073		0.000 **	
	Acoustic comfort	1.000	0.445	0.059	0.816	0.000 **	0.000 **

** means $p < 0.01$; [a] means significance of regression coefficient; [b] means significance of regression equation.

In Music Park (Table 4), psychological responses can be examined by both acoustic comfort and visual comfort ($p < 0.05$). The predictor with the highest contribution was acoustic comfort in the model for both CD and RA. The impact intensities of acoustic comfort on CD and RA were 1.68 and 1.64 times higher than that of visual comfort, respectively, while in the model for EF and FD, visual comfort was more significant than acoustic comfort by 1.37 and 1.35 times, respectively.

Table 4. Stepwise regression model for audio-visual experiences and psychological responses in Music Park.

Model		Collinearity	Unstandardized Coefficients		Standardized Coefficients	Sig. [a]	Sig. [b]
Variable	Predictors	VIF	Regression Coefficient	Std. Error	Beta		
CD: $R^2 = 0.862$ R^2 (adj) = 0.852	(Constant)		0.557	0.081		0.000 **	
	Acoustic comfort	1.512	0.381	0.052	0.649	0.000 **	0.000 **
	Visual comfort	1.512	0.362	0.082	0.387	0.000 **	
RA: $R^2 = 0.854$ R^2 (adj) = 0.843	(Constant)		0.478	0.092		0.000 **	
	Acoustic comfort	1.512	0.417	0.059	0.640	0.000 **	0.000 **
	Visual comfort	1.512	0.405	0.094	0.391	0.000 **	
EF: $R^2 = 0.612$ R^2 (adj) = 0.583	(Constant)		−0.167	0.169		0.331	
	Visual comfort	1.512	0.595	0.173	0.507	0.002 **	0.000 **
	Acoustic comfort	1.512	0.273	0.109	0.370	0.018 *	
FD: $R^2 = 0.758$ R^2 (adj) = 0.740	(Constant)		−0.280	0.117		0.024 *	
	Visual comfort	1.512	0.575	0.119	0.561	0.000 **	0.000 **
	Acoustic comfort	1.512	0.268	0.075	0.415	0.001 **	

** means $p < 0.01$; [a] means significance of regression coefficient; [b] means significance of regression equation.

3.2. Influence of Audio-Visual Interactions on Psychological Responses

The above results show the relationship between audio-visual contexts and psychological responses and between audio-visual experiences and psychological responses, and also analyzed the impact level of audio-visual independent variables on psychological responses in two urban parks. The results of multiple logical regressions showed the psychological health of young people in urban parks was determined by audio-visual experiences reflected by acoustic comfort and visual comfort (except for FD in Cloves Park). How audio-visual interactions determine psychological responses of young people in urban parks remains unclear. Thus, to answer this research question, an orthogonal analysis diagram was established to describe the influence of audio-visual interactions on psychological responses, shown in Figures 1 and 2. The orthogonal analysis method was designed and used in this study to analyze the effects of visual and auditory factors that simultaneously affect the psychological changes acquired by participants instead of employing separate analyses. However, the orthogonal analysis model for FD was not established in this paper because FD cannot be examined by visual comfort. As illustrated in Figures 1 and 2, psychological responses of every survey point were represented in a two-dimensional space defined by acoustic comfort and visual comfort. The positions for psychological responses in the two-dimensional space were determined by the values of acoustic comfort and visual comfort and the levels of psychological responses were represented by the color described in Figures 1 and 2. To analyze the effects of audio-visual experiences in a readily comprehensible way, four quadrants were used to represent audio-visual interactions. The areas of quadrants 1, 2, 3, and 4 show the mean acoustic and visual comfortable (AV), acoustic uncomfortable and visual comfortable (UV), acoustic and visual uncomfortable (UU) and acoustic comfortable and visual uncomfortable (AU) results.

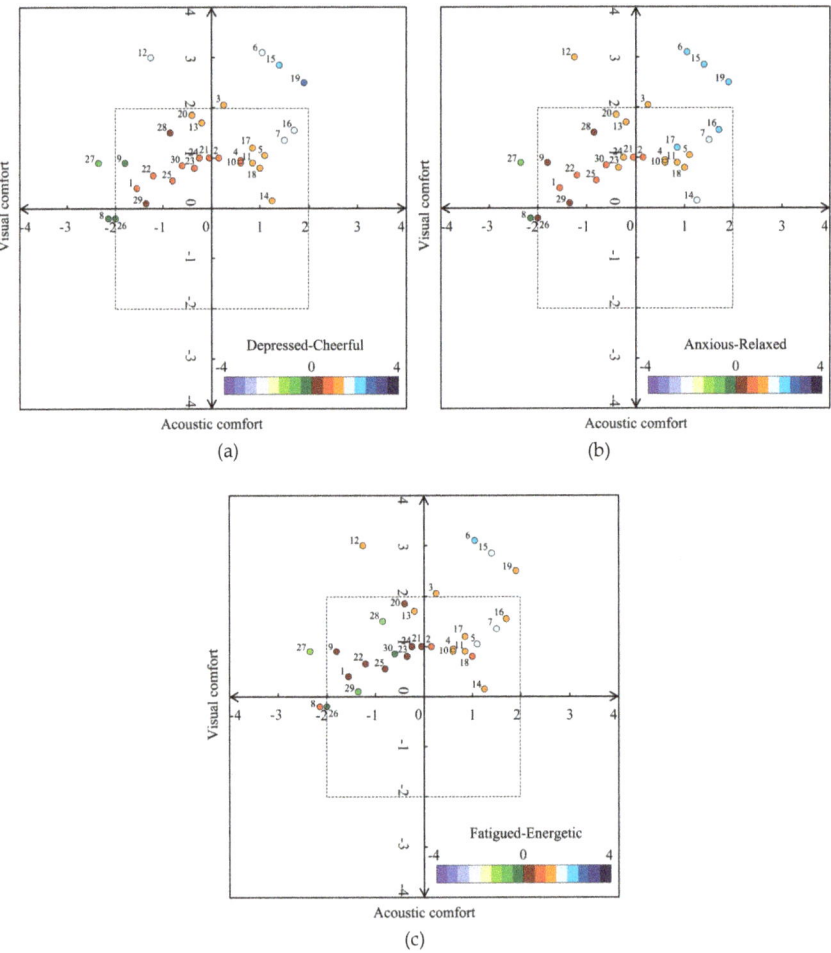

Figure 1. Orthogonal analysis of audio-visual experiences on psychological responses: (**a**) cheerful-depressed (CD); (**b**) relaxed-anxious (RA); (**c**) energetic-fatigued (EF) in Cloves Park.

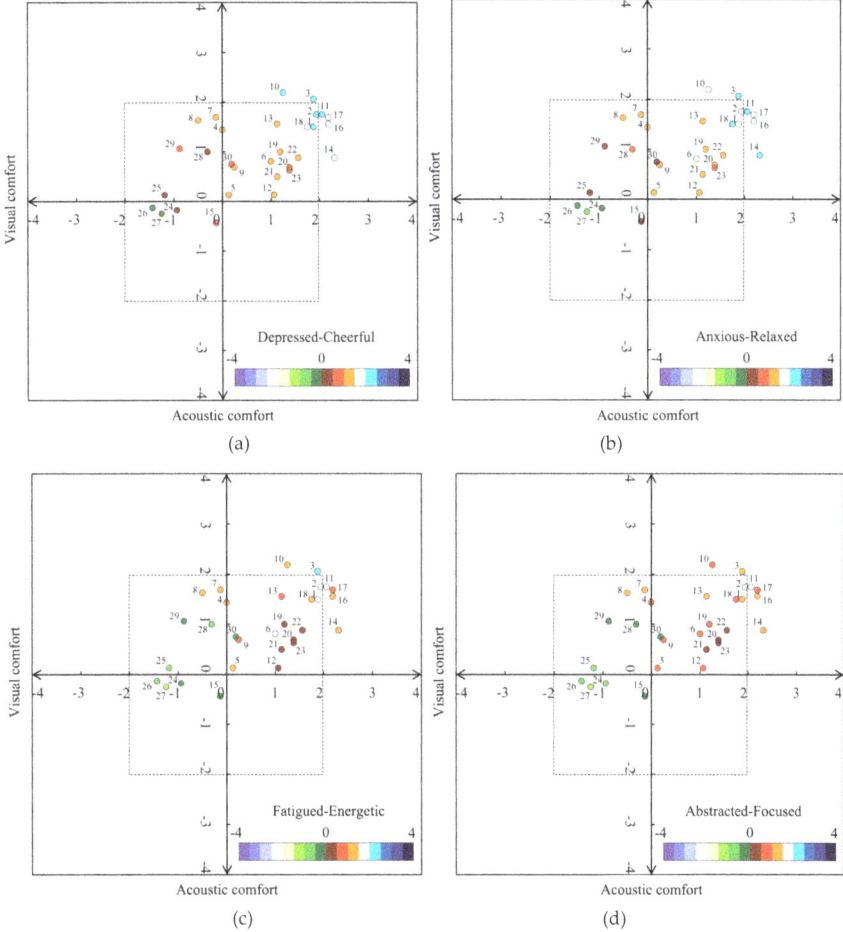

Figure 2. Orthogonal analysis of audio-visual experiences on psychological responses: (**a**) CD; (**b**) RA; (**c**) EF; (**d**) focused-distracted (FD) in Music Park.

In Figure 1, it can be seen that 46.7% of the survey points fell into the AV quadrant, 46.7% of the survey points fell into the UV quadrant, and 6.6% of the survey points fell into the UU quadrant for Cloves Park. Overall, 86.7% of the audio-visual context tended to be cheerful, 93.3% of the context tended to be relaxed, and 83.3% of the context was energetic. In the orthogonal analysis diagram of CD, the values of CD at 78.6% of the survey points were more than 1.00 in the AV quadrant, while the values of CD were more than 1.00 in 14.3% of the survey points in the UV quadrant. In terms of RA, the values of RA in 92.9% of the survey points were more than 1.00 in the AV quadrant, and the values of RA were more than 1.00 in 35.7% of the survey points in the UV quadrant. Regarding EF, the levels of EF in 85.7% of the audio-visual contexts were more than 1.00 in the AV quadrant, while the values of EF were more than 1.00 at 14.3% of the survey points in the UV quadrant.

On the other hand, in the AV quadrant, the audio-visual context at survey point 19 was the most cheerful, with the level of CD at 2.60, compared to point 15 (2.40) and point 6 (1.95). Survey point 19 was also the most relaxed audio-visual context, compared to point 15 (2.35) and point 6 (2.25). In the orthogonal analysis diagram of EF, survey point 6 had the most energetic audio-visual context, with a value of EF at 2.05, compared to point 15 (1.80) and point 7 (1.65), and point 19 was close behind (1.45).

Points 6, 15, and 19 were almost the most cheerful, relaxed and energetic contexts among all points, which is due to three points that were located by the lakeside with better landscapes than others and the percentage of positive sounds in these three points were also higher than others (Figure 3). Points 7 and 16 also had relatively cheerful (1.50, 1.95), relaxed (1.75, 2.10) and energetic (1.65, 1.45) contexts, although they were visually inferior to the above three places. In the UV quadrant, survey point 12 had the most cheerful (1.50) audio-visual context, and the audio-visual context at point 13 was most relaxed (1.30) and energetic (1.35). In fact, both points 12 and 13 had outstanding audio-visual contexts with higher values of CD, RA, and EF than the others, which is likely because they were located on the top of a mountain with unique visual experiences, although the acoustic comfort was negative. The most depressed, anxious and fatigued contexts were at point 27 in the UV quadrant, and the values of CD, RA, and EF at point 27 were even lower than those at points 8 and 26 in the UU quadrant. It can be explained by previous theories; namely, SRT and ART, that the percentages of urban sounds (like traffic noise and construction noise) and urban views were the most salient, and the memory of the daily stress of participants can easily be aroused by these stimuli.

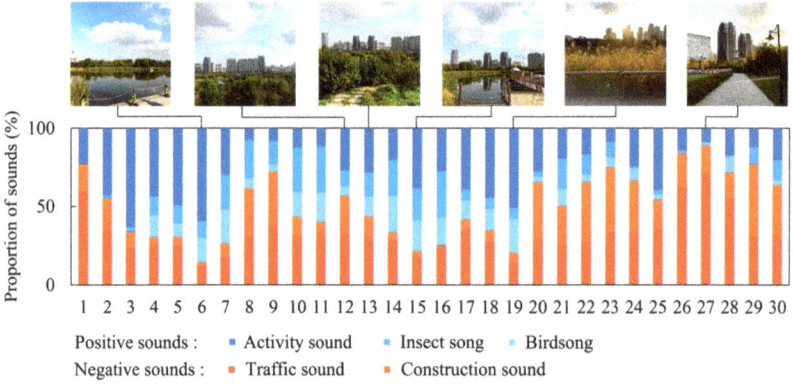

Figure 3. The proportion of sounds in each survey point and photographs in typical survey points in Cloves Park.

In Music Park (Figure 2), it can be seen that 66.7% of the survey points fell into the AV quadrant, 20.0% of the survey points fell into the UV quadrant and 13.3% of the survey points fell into the UU quadrant in Music Park. Overall, 93.3% of the audio-visual context tended to be cheerful, 90.0% of the contexts tended to be relaxed, 73.3% of the contexts were energetic and focused. The values of CD, RA, and EF in 85.0%, 90.0%, and 55.0% of the survey points were more than 1.00 in the AV quadrant, respectively, and the values of CD, RA, and EF were more than 1.00 in only 30.0% of the survey points in the UV quadrant and UU quadrant. However, the value of FD was more than 1.00 in only 23.3% of the survey points in the AV quadrant, the value of FD was less than 0 in 70.0% of the survey points in the UV and UU quadrants. It was interesting to note that, in the model of CD and RA, visual comfort can influence CD and RA to a lower extent than acoustic comfort. For example, the differences in the levels of CD and RA at points 13, 19, 6, 21, and 12 were no more than 0.60, while it reached 1.44 in the model for EF and 1.06 in the model for FD, which testified to the results of stepwise regression models in that acoustic comfort was in a dominant position for CD and RA, and visual comfort was dominant for EF and FD.

On the other hand, in the AV quadrant, audio-visual context at survey point 11 was most cheerful, relaxed and focused, with the levels of CD, RA and FD were 2.25, 2.25, and 1.56, and point 3 had the most energetic audio-visual context with a value of EF at 2.00. In the UV and UU quadrants, point 7 had the most relaxed, energetic, and focused audio-visual context, with the scores of RA, EF and FD at 1.31, 1.19, and 1.13, respectively. Point 8 had scores for RA, EF, and FD of 1.25, 1.13, and 1.00, respectively. The audio-visual context at point 8 was most cheerful, and the score for CD was just 0.06 higher than that of point 7, although the percentage of negative sounds at points 7 and 8 reached 93.2% and 78.5% (Figure 4), respectively. It is interesting to note that, though the proportion of negative sounds at points 24–27 also were at a higher level, ranging from 88.3%–100%, the audio-visual context at these points was almost the most depressed, anxious, fatigued, and distracted, with the level of psychological responses lower than −1.13. The most likely reason may be that participants can be easily influenced by urban views and sounds due to the lack of a masking effect of vegetation.

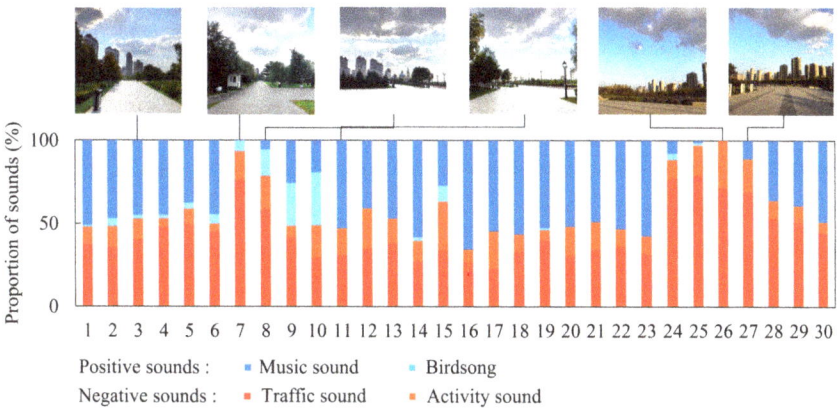

Figure 4. Proportion of sounds in each survey point and photographs in typical survey points in Music Park.

4. Discussion

Previous studies focused on explaining the relationship between green spaces and psychological responses through visual factors or acoustic factors. Although a few studies emphasized the implications of audio-visual interactions on psychological responses, audio-visual interactions were not considered as two-dimensional. Therefore, this study introduced a new method to quantify audio-visual context, audio-visual experiences, and psychological responses in two typical urban parks in China. The relationship between audio-visual context and psychological responses was studied firstly in this paper, and results show that loudness and sharpness were not correlated with psychological responses of the cognition dimension, which was not inconsistent with Shu and Ma's study [25]. One possible reason may be that they took children's psychological responses as a research object. In a recent study in UK, Payne and Bruce reported that relationships between sound levels (subjective and objective) and psychological restoration were not linear, which was also different from this study [16]. It may be because the type of sounds heard and other aspects of the place experience affect the relationships. According to the orthogonal analysis, the psychological responses in audio-visual contexts close to an urban built environment was worse than that in a natural audio-visual context, which was similar to previous related studies [7,8,19].

This study makes a significant contribution to the literature because a new method was designed and executed to specify the audio-visual interactions that affect the psychological responses of young people and how the audio-visual context based on psychological responses relates to the design of soundscapes and landscapes of urban green spaces.

However, there were some limitations to this study. This study employed graduate students as an example of young people, which may have resulted in bias. The psychological state of other young people, such as young workers and officers, was not at the same level as that of graduate students, which may influence the relationship between audio-visual interactions and psychological responses. Therefore, they will be invited to be controlled subjects in future studies. Moreover, a recent work proposed that the differences in seasonal effects may lead to different audio-visual contexts, and psychological responses could consequently be affected [49]. To avoid seasonal influence, this study was carried out only in one season. Furthermore, in the preliminary survey, some participants reported that their emotions could be changed by styles of music in Music Park. To reduce the error, the music in Music Park was set to classical music. The consideration of seasonality, crowd characteristics and types of sounds were important in terms of the creation of audio-visual context in urban green spaces that promotes psychological responses. Thus, in future studies, these factors could also be explained further.

5. Conclusions

Based on a new field method—namely, AV-walk—some interesting results in two typical urban parks are summarized below.

First, on the influence of audio-visual context, there were significant correlations between LAeq and psychological responses and between roughness and psychological responses in Cloves Park ($p < 0.05$), while LAeq and roughness showed no correlation with psychological responses in Music Park.

Second, in terms of the effects of audio-visual experiences, acoustic comfort and visual comfort determined CD, RA, and EF, and only acoustic comfort determined FD in Cloves Park ($p < 0.01$), and the impact intensity of acoustic comfort was 1.55–2.64 times higher than that of visual comfort. In the model for CD and RA (emotion dimension) in Music Park, acoustic comfort was 1.64–1.68 times higher than that of visual comfort, respectively, while in the model for EF and FD (cognition dimension), visual comfort was 1.35–1.37 times than that of acoustic comfort.

In addition, the influence of audio-visual interactions on psychological responses was also analyzed with an orthogonal analysis. The audio-visual context located beside the waterscape with a relatively higher level of acoustic and visual comfort was most cheerful (2.60), relaxed (2.45), and energetic (2.05), and the audio-visual context located on the top of a mountain had better performance; i.e., cheerful (1.50), relaxed (1.30), and energetic (1.35), although the visual context was uncomfortable. The audio-visual context close to an urban built environment, which was both acoustic and visually uncomfortable, was most depressed (−0.25), anxious (−0.75), fatigued (−1.13) and distracted (−1.13).

Author Contributions: Conceptualization: S.Z.; Methodology: S.Z.; Software: S.Z.; Validation: S.Z.; Formal Analysis: S.Z.; Investigation: S.Z.; Data Curation: S.Z.; Writing–original Draft Preparation: S.Z.; Writing–Review and Editing: S.Z.; Visualization: S.Z., Z.Z. and X.Q.; Supervision: X.Z.; Project administration: X.Z.; Funding acquisition: X.Z.

Funding: This work was supported by the National Natural Science Foundation of China (grant numbers 51878206, 51438005).

Acknowledgments: The authors would like to thank graduates from the School of Architecture, Harbin Institute of Technology for their participation in the psychological investigation in Cloves Park. The authors are also grateful to Prof. Hong Jin's group and Associate Qi Meng's group for their help with acoustic software (version: Artemis 12.0) and instrumentation (type: BSWA 801).

Conflicts of Interest: The authors declare no conflict of interest.

References

1. Rachael, D.; Kimberly, R. Freshmen adaptation to university life: Depressive symptoms, stress, and coping. *J. Clin. Psychol.* **2010**, *62*, 1231–1244.
2. Tsiotra, P.C.; Tsigos, C. Stress, the endoplasmic reticulum, and insulin resistance. *Ann. N Y Acad. Sci.* **2010**, *1083*, 63–76. [CrossRef]
3. Nilsson, K.; Sangster, M.; Konijnendijk, C.C. *Forests, Trees and Human Health and Well-being: Introduction*; Springer: Heidelberg, The Netherlands, 2011.
4. Ulrich, R.S.; Simons, R.F.; Losito, B.D.; Fiorito, E.; Miles, M.A.; Zelson, M. Stress recovery during exposure to natural and urban environments. *J. Environ. Psychol.* **1991**, *11*, 201–230. [CrossRef]
5. Kaplan, S. The restorative benefits of nature: Toward an integrative framework. *J. Environ. Psychol.* **1995**, *15*, 169–182. [CrossRef]

6. Maller, C.; Townsend, M.A.; Brown, P.; Leger, S.L. Healthy nature healthy people: 'contact with nature' as an upstream health promotion intervention for populations. *Health Promot. Int.* **2006**, *21*, 45. [CrossRef]
7. Tyrväinen, L.; Ojala, A.; Korpela, K.; Lanki, T.; Tsunetsugu, Y.; Kagawa, T. The influence of urban green environments on stress relief measures: A field experiment. *J. Environ. Psychol.* **2014**, *38*, 1–9. [CrossRef]
8. Payne, S.R. The production of a Perceived Restorativeness Soundscape Scale. *Appl. Acoust.* **2013**, *74*, 255–263. [CrossRef]
9. Kjellgren, A.; Buhrkall, H. A comparison of the restorative effect of a natural environment with that of a simulated natural environment. *J. Environ. Psychol.* **2010**, *30*, 464–472. [CrossRef]
10. Park, B.J.; Tsunetsugu, Y.; Kasetani, T.; Kagawa, T.; Miyazaki, Y. The physiological effects of Shinrin-yoku (taking in the forest atmosphere or forest bathing): Evidence from field experiments in 24 forests across Japan. *Environ. Health Prev. Med.* **2010**, *15*, 18. [CrossRef]
11. Han, K.T. The Effect of Nature and Physical Activity on Emotions and Attention while Engaging in Green Exercise. *Urban For. Urban Green.* **2017**, *24*, 5–13. [CrossRef]
12. Grahn, P.; Stigsdotter, U.K. The relation between perceived sensory dimensions of urban green space and stress restoration. *Lands. Urban Plan.* **2010**, *94*, 264–275. [CrossRef]
13. Alvarsson, J.J.; Wiens, S.; Nilsson, M.E. Stress Recovery during Exposure to Nature Sound and Environmental Noise. *Int. J. Environ. Res. Public Health* **2010**, *7*, 1036–1046. [CrossRef]
14. Aletta, F.; Oberman, T.; Kang, J. Associations between Positive Health-Related Effects and Soundscapes Perceptual Constructs: A Systematic Review. *Int. J. Environ. Res. Public Health* **2018**, *15*, 2392. [CrossRef] [PubMed]
15. Aletta, F.; Kang, J. Towards an Urban Vibrancy Model: A Soundscape Approach. *Int. J. Environ. Res. Public Health* **2018**, *15*, 1712. [CrossRef]
16. Payne, S.R.; Bruce, N. Exploring the Relationship between Urban Quiet Areas and Perceived Restorative Benefits. *Int. J. Environ. Res. Public Health* **2019**, *16*, 1611. [CrossRef] [PubMed]
17. Herranz-Pascual, K.; Aspuru, I.; Iraurgi, I.; Santander, A.; Luis Eguiguren, J.; Garcia, I. Going beyond Quietness: Determining the Emotionally Restorative Effect of Acoustic Environments in Urban Open Public Spaces. *Int. J. Environ. Res. Public Health* **2019**, *16*, 1284. [CrossRef] [PubMed]
18. Hedblom, M.; Gunnarsson, B.; Schaefer, M.; Knez, I.; Thorsson, P.; Lundstrom, J.N. Sounds of Nature in the City: No Evidence of Bird Song Improving Stress Recovery. *Int. J. Environ. Res. Public Health* **2019**, *16*, 1390. [CrossRef]
19. Shepherd, D.; Welch, D.; Dirks, K.N.; Mcbride, D. Do Quiet Areas Afford Greater Health-Related Quality of Life than Noisy Areas? *Int. J. Environ. Res. Public Health* **2013**, *10*, 1284–1303. [CrossRef]
20. Namni, G.; Etwaroo, G.R. Bright light, negative air ions and auditory stimuli produce rapid mood changes in a student population: A placebo-controlled study. *Psychol. Med.* **2006**, *36*, 1253.
21. Renterghem, T.V. Towards explaining the positive effect of vegetation on the perception of environmental noise. *Urban For. Urban Green.* **2019**, *40*, 133–144. [CrossRef]
22. Watts, G.R.; Pheasant, R.J.; Horoshenkov, K.V.; Ragonesi, L. Measurement and Subjective Assessment of Water Generated Sounds. *Acta Acust. United Acust.* **2009**, *95*, 1032–1039. [CrossRef]
23. Yang, F.; Bao, Z.Y.; Zhu, J.Z. An Assessment of Psychological Noise Reduction by Landscape Plants. *Int. J. Environ. Res. Public Health* **2011**, *8*, 1032–1048. [CrossRef]
24. Pheasant, R.J.; Fisher, M.N.; Watts, G.R.; Whitaker, D.J.; Horoshenkov, K.V. The importance of auditory-visual interaction in the construction of 'tranquil space'. *J. Environ. Psychol.* **2010**, *30*, 501–509. [CrossRef]
25. Shu, S.; Ma, H. The restorative environmental sounds perceived by children. *J. Environ. Psychol.* **2018**, *60*, 72–80. [CrossRef]
26. Morita, E.; Fukuda, S.; Nagano, J.; Hamajima, N.; Yamamoto, H.; Iwai, Y.; Nakashima, T.; Ohira, H.; Shirakawa, T. Psychological effects of forest environments on healthy adults: Shinrin-yoku (forest-air bathing, walking) as a possible method of stress reduction. *Public Health* **2007**, *121*, 54–63. [CrossRef]
27. Ming, K. How might contact with nature promote human health? Promising mechanisms and a possible central pathway. *Front. Psychol.* **2015**, *6*, 1093.
28. Bagot, K.L.; Allen, F.C.L.; Toukhasati, S. Perceived restorativeness of children's school playground environments: Nature, playground features and play period experiences. *J. Environ. Psychol.* **2015**, *41*, 1–9. [CrossRef]

29. Artmann, M.; Chen, X.; Iojă, C.; Hof, A.; Onose, D.; Poniży, L.; Lamovšek, A.Z.; Breuste, J. The role of urban green spaces in care facilities for elderly people across European cities. *Urban For. Urban Green.* **2017**, *27*, 203–213. [CrossRef]
30. Cerwén, G.; Mossberg, F. Implementation of Quiet Areas in Sweden. *Int. J. Environ. Res. Public Health* **2019**, *16*, 134. [CrossRef] [PubMed]
31. Jeon, J.Y.; Honga, J.Y.; Lee, P.J. Soundwalk approach to identify urban soundscapes individually. *J. Acoust. Soc. Am.* **2013**, *134*, 803. [CrossRef]
32. Romero, V.P.; Maffei, L.; Brambilla, G.; Ciaburro, G. Acoustic, Visual and Spatial Indicators for the Description of the Soundscape of Waterfront Areas with and without Road Traffic Flow. *Int. J. Environ. Res. Public Health* **2016**, *13*, 934. [CrossRef]
33. Zhang, S.; Meng, Q.; Kang, J. The Influence of Crowd Density on Evaluation of Soundscape in Typical Chinese Restaurant. In Proceedings of the INTER-NOISE 2016—45th International Congress and Exposition on Noise Control Engineering: Towards a Quieter Future, Hamburg, Germany, 21–24 August 2016; German Acoustical Society: Hamburg, Germany, 2016; pp. 6150–6155.
34. Ba, M.; Kang, J. A laboratory study of the sound-odour interaction in urban environments. *Build. Environ.* **2019**, *147*, 314–326. [CrossRef]
35. Shu, S.; Ma, H. Restorative Effects of Classroom Soundscapes on Children's Cognitive Performance. *Int. J. Environ. Res. Public Health* **2019**, *16*, 293. [CrossRef]
36. Chee, G.L.; Wynaden, D.; Heslop, K. Improving metabolic monitoring rate for young people aged 35 and younger taking antipsychotic medications to treat a psychosis: A literature review. *Arch. Psychiatr. Nurs.* **2017**, *31*, 624. [CrossRef]
37. Yang, J.; Zhou, Q.; Liu, X.; Liu, M.; Qu, S.; Bi, J. Biased perception misguided by affect: How does emotional experience lead to incorrect judgments about environmental quality? *Glob. Environ. Chang.* **2018**, *53*, 104–113. [CrossRef]
38. Zhao, X.; Zhang, S.; Meng, Q.; Kang, J. Influence of Contextual Factors on Soundscape in Urban Open Spaces. *Appl. Sci.* **2018**, *8*, 2524. [CrossRef]
39. Fastl, H.; Zwicker, E. *Psychoacoustics—Facts and Models, third Ed.*; Springer: Berlin, Germany, 2007.
40. Tieskens, K.F.; Zanten, B.T.V.; Schulp, C.J.E.; Verburg, P.H. Aesthetic appreciation of the cultural landscape through social media: An analysis of revealed preference in the Dutch river landscape. *Lands. Urban Plann.* **2018**, *177*, 128–137. [CrossRef]
41. Berkel, D.B.V.; Tabrizian, P.; Dorning, M.A.; Smart, L.; Newcomb, D.; Mehaffey, M.; Neale, A.; Meentemeyer, R.K. Quantifying the visual-sensory landscape qualities that contribute to cultural ecosystem services using social media and LiDAR. *Ecosyst. Serv.* **2018**, *31*, 326–335. [CrossRef]
42. Kumar, A.; Yerneni, L. Semi-automated relative quantification of cell culture contamination with mycoplasma by Photoshop-based image analysis on immunofluorescence preparations. *Biologicals* **2009**, *37*, 55–60. [CrossRef]
43. Zhang, X.; Bo, L.; Wang, J.; Zhe, Z.; Shi, K.; Wu, S. Adobe photoshop quantification (PSQ) rather than point-counting: A rapid and precise method for quantifying rock textural data and porosities. *Comput. Geosci.* **2014**, *69*, 62–71. [CrossRef]
44. ISO. Acoustics-Soundscape-Part 2: Data collection and reporting requirements. In *(ISO/TS 12913-2:)*; ISO: Geneva, Switzerland, 2018; pp. 1–29.
45. Thompson, E.R. Development and validation of an internationally reliable short-form of the positive and negative affect schedule (PANAS). *J. Cross Cult. Psychol.* **2007**, *38*, 227–242. [CrossRef]
46. Han, K.-T. A reliable and valid self-rating measure of the restorative quality of natural environments. *Lands. Urban Plann.* **2003**, *64*, 209–232. [CrossRef]
47. Feeney, B.C. *A Simple Guide to IBM SPSS Statistics for Version 20.0.*; Cengage Learning: Boston, MA, USA, 2012.
48. Liu, Q.; Zhang, Y.; Lin, Y.; Wei, Z.; Bosch, C.K.V.D. The relationship between self-rated naturalness of university green space and students' restoration and health. *Urban For. Urban Green.* **2018**, *34*, 259–268. [CrossRef]
49. Brooks, A.M.; Ottley, K.M.; Arbuthnott, K.D.; Sevigny, P. Nature-related mood effects: Season and type of nature contact. *J. Environ. Psychol.* **2017**, *54*, 91–102. [CrossRef]

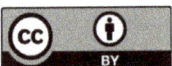

© 2019 by the authors. Licensee MDPI, Basel, Switzerland. This article is an open access article distributed under the terms and conditions of the Creative Commons Attribution (CC BY) license (http://creativecommons.org/licenses/by/4.0/).

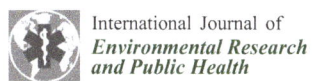

Article

Listening to Japanese Gardens: An Autoethnographic Study on the Soundscape Action Design Tool

Gunnar Cerwén [1,2]

1. Department of Work Science, Business Economics and Environmental Psychology, Swedish University of Agricultural Sciences, Slottsvägen 5, 230 53 Alnarp, Sweden; gunnar.cerwen@slu.se
2. Japanese Society for the Promotion of Science (JSPS) International Research Fellow Programme, School of Cultural and Creative Studies, Aoyama Gakuin University, Shibuya, Tokyo 4-4-25, Japan

Received: 19 June 2019; Accepted: 3 November 2019; Published: 22 November 2019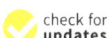

Abstract: Landscape architecture and urban design disciplines could benefit from soundscape thinking in order to enhance experiential qualities in their projects, though the available tools are not yet fully developed nor tested. The present research aims to substantiate one of the available tools, Soundscape Actions, and thereby increase the understanding of soundscape design. The study focuses on the Japanese garden tradition, which is known for high preference ratings, tranquil qualities and consideration for sound and other sensory experiences. An autoethnographic approach was used to conduct field studies in 88 gardens in Japan, the majority of which are located in urban areas with potential noise disturbance. The studies are based on observations in situ, supported by video documentation, field recordings and readings of sound pressure levels (SPL). A total of 19 Soundscape Actions are described and discussed in the paper. They are structured around three main categories: localisation of functions, reduction of unwanted sounds and introduction of wanted sounds. The study provides concrete examples of how the tool can be used to enhance tranquil qualities, particularly focusing on small green spaces in dense urban settings, involving the (simultaneous) reduction of unwanted sounds and enhancement of wanted sounds/effects. The autoethnographic approach allowed for the phenomenological perspective to be brought forward, which contributed new insights regarding the design tool. The findings are discussed in relation to health and soundscape research, focusing on multisensory experiences, masking strategies and potentials for implementation and future developments of the design tool.

Keywords: soundscape design; sonic experience; tranquillity; noise; garden therapy; landscape architecture; Japanese gardens; autoethnography; soundscape actions

---

1. Introduction

Japanese gardens are sources of inspiration for gardeners, landscape architects and designers around the world [1]. Originally inspired by gardens in China, the Japanese garden tradition has a long history with many particular styles, including the dry landscaped garden *karesansui*, the stroll garden *kaiyū-shiki-teien* and the tea garden *cha-niwa* [2,3]. It is a diverse tradition held together by its Japanese sense of aesthetics, characterised by asymmetry, symbolism, geomancy, careful detailing and the use of natural materials (c.f. [4,5]).

Japanese gardens tend to receive high preference ratings compared to other types of gardens and landscapes [6–9], which can partly be explained by their informal character and natural expressions [10]. Rocks, water and vegetation constitute some of the most typical materials, meticulously shaped to represent nature "at its best". For instance, the shape of pruned trees in Japanese gardens have been used as motivation for the "Savannah theory" [11]. Studies have shown that spending time in a Japanese garden can lead to a reduction in heart rate [12] and an improved mood [13]. Some of the most famous gardens are Zen Buddhist gardens, rich with symbolic meaning and spiritual qualities, and sometimes specifically designed to stimulate meditation [3]. Other gardens encourage physical activity and engage the bodily senses [4,14].

The green and natural landscapes of Japanese gardens have constituted an important part of the urban fabric for several hundred years [15]. In contemporary Japan, the gardens still offer a contrast to the restraints of modern life and the highly densified cities that often surround them. Space is a scarce resource in Japan, and gardens are often designed to appear larger than they actually are [16], which makes them interesting as reference objects for pocket parks and other small green spaces.

Today, 55% of the world's population lives in urban areas, with an expected increase to almost 70% in 2050 [17]. It is known that urbanisation and urban lifestyles can lead to stress and negative health effects [18]. Problems relating to stress constitute a major challenge for the global community. While a certain amount of stress is a natural part of human life, extended periods of exposure may lead to negative health effects, such as sleeping problems, depression, cardiovascular disease and chronic fatigue [19].

Research has shown that nature and nature-like environments can alleviate [20] and prevent [21] such negative health effects. Accessibility to green spaces is thus a crucial factor to consider in city planning, albeit one that may be difficult to adhere to, especially as densification proceeds. Gardens and other small green spaces with natural components may prove to be increasingly important in the future, as their spatial requirements are more flexible than parks. Yet, problems with noise from neighbouring urban activities constitute a challenge. This is the case in Japan, as well as in many other countries around the world.

The sound environment influences the quality of gardens and other green spaces [22,23] and has repercussions on health, both positive and negative [24,25]. It is pertinent to ensure that planning and design is optimised to take this into account. However, it has been repeatedly argued that sound is a limited concern within architectural disciplines and that, if sound is considered at all, it is typically with reference to noise issues [26,27].

Soundscape research, on the other hand, adopts a comprehensive understanding of the sound environment, including problems as well as positive experiences. It is a broad and interdisciplinary field, focusing on the contextual and subjective experience of sound environments. Initiated in the late 1960s [28–30], it has gained increased momentum in recent years [31], not least in urban planning and design projects [31–33]. In 2014, soundscape was defined by the International Organization for Standardization (ISO) as an "acoustic environment as perceived or experienced and/or understood by a person or people, in context" [34]. To date, a number of tools and approaches have been developed to aid the design of outdoor environments through use of the soundscape approach [35–39], yet few of these have been tested and validated in situ.

In the present study, one of the available tools called Soundscape Actions [27,36] was applied to study sonic experiences in the Japanese garden tradition. The aim was to substantiate Soundscape Actions as a design tool in landscape architecture and to increase the understanding of the design of tranquil soundscapes. Given their health promoting potential [13] and careful consideration of sonic experiences [4,40–44], Japanese gardens were considered an ideal context to appraise the tool, the idea being that the rich knowledge accumulated in a centuries-old tradition could potentially be used to inform future developments of the tool.

2. Materials and Methods

The present study is based on empirical material that was collected on site in Japan using an autoethnographic approach [45]. The material was collected during 136 visits to 88 renowned Japanese gardens, the majority of which are located in Kyoto (Figure 1). For further details about the selection of gardens, times of visit and other details, see Appendix A and Section 2.2.

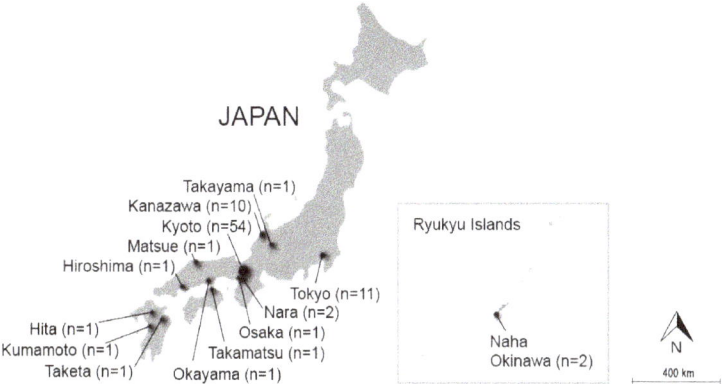

Figure 1. This map illustrates the geographical distribution of the 88 studied Japanese gardens.

Most of the studied gardens have existed for several hundred years, during which time the gardens and their soundscapes may have undergone change to various extents (not least the soundscapes surrounding the gardens). Alas, it should be pointed out that the study does not aim to contribute with historical insights as to how gardens were designed in different periods or regions in Japan. Rather, the tradition is considered as a context from which to draw general understandings regarding soundscape design which can then be applied to other (contemporary) gardens and green areas. It may well be that some of the effects that were experienced in the gardens were not the result of intentional acts by their designer. However, this does not make it any less interesting for the purposes of the study.

Field notes from the gardens were collected in a digital document amounting to a total of about 23,000 words, which served as the main research material. The design tool Soundscape Actions was subsequently applied to analyse and structure the material. The findings are supported by extracts from the field notes as well as photographs, videos, field recordings and sound pressure level (SPL) readings taken in the gardens. For an overview of video and sound material referred to in this paper, see Supplementary Material—List of video files. For further information on data collection, see Section 2.2.

2.1. Using Autoethnography to Substantiate Soundscape Actions

Autoethnography is a qualitative method focusing on the researcher's own experience and reflection of a phenomenon [45]. It has been increasingly applied in architectural disciplines, where it can be used to uncover various aspects of the cultural practice of designing and experiencing landscapes [46–49]. In this study, the autoethnographer has a background as a soundscape researcher and a landscape architect. It is in the intersection of these two fields that sonic experiences in Japanese gardens are notated.

Soundscape research has tended to focus on participants' generalised experiences (e.g., [50–52]), while relatively little attention has been paid to how individual subjects experience a phenomenon in detail. The subjective perspective is emphasised in the ISO definition of soundscape [34] and could potentially lead to a better understanding of how contextual factors influence the experience of sound. Subjectivity could also be an important factor when connecting soundscape research to design disciplines; it has been pointed out that architects often use their own subjective site experiences as a starting point when proposing new design solutions [46]. Autoethnography can be used to bring such experiences to the foreground, allowing for comparisons between practitioners [45]. If experiences are shared as autoethnographic narratives, these may also be studied by other researchers and designers as components of their reference libraries. In the present study autoethnography was used to evaluate a design tool, with the intention of substantiating its usage and making it more accessible to practitioners (c.f. [53]).

The approach is akin to the notion of "skilled listeners" as proposed by Hedfors and Berg [54] which has previously been used to study the relationship between sonic phenomena and landscape architecture [55]. In that study, data from skilled listeners were used to provide intricate understandings regarding the experiential qualities of environmental sounds, which were then formulated as a terminology for practitioners. A related approach has also been used by Amphoux [56], involving trained listeners to map urban soundscapes.

The present study differs from the above by focusing on a single listener's experience, rather than several. As an autoethnographic study it is subjective in nature, and care should be taken when interpreting the results. To ensure validity, efforts have been taken to make subjectivity explicit where it is present [57]. In order to increase generalisability, sonic experiences are discussed in relation to previous research and supported by data collected on site (Section 2.2). In accordance with what has been termed "analytical autoethnography" [58], the findings are used to gain insights on a theoretical framework (Soundscape Actions).

2.2. Data Collection

Most of the research was undertaken during 2018, preceded by some initial surveys in 2015. Following the autoethnographic approach, criteria for site selection were guided by a general intention to learn from the Japanese garden tradition in terms of how soundscapes could be designed (see Sections 2.2.1 and 2.2.2). In total, 88 gardens in multiple locations around Japan were visited (see Figure 1 and Appendix A). The majority of these (n = 54) were located in Kyoto, which is known for its many gardens of high quality. During the spring and autumn of 2018, a total of three months were devoted to field studies in Kyoto. Additionally, a number of gardens in Tokyo (n = 11) and Kanazawa (n = 10) were included in the study, as well as chosen gardens in other locations. The data collection process can roughly be divided into five phases as discussed below. However, it should be noted that the chronology sometimes overlapped. For instance, when a new city was visited, Phases II and III were repeated.

2.2.1. Phase I: Surveying the Field

In the first phase, a survey of previous literature pertaining to Japanese gardens (e.g., [2–5,14,16]) and their soundscapes (e.g., [40–44]) was undertaken. Contact was also established with key researchers in Japan, leading to some valuable recommendations for gardens to study. Based on the literature review and contact with researchers, prospective gardens were continuously plotted using Google Maps.

2.2.2. Phase II: Initial Study Visits in Gardens

This phase was intended to provide an overview of a wide variety of traditional gardens in Japan. Visits in this phase were relatively short (typically 15–45 min), the intention being to identify gardens that would be able to contribute with insights on soundscape design. Each garden was briefly described in a notebook, including the general impression, the context for the visit, notable features, the date, weather and soundscapes. The notes were brief, though could be elaborated if there were particular sonic features. The notes were taken either directly on site or written down later in the evening of the same day. Each garden was photographed, and in case there were notable sonic features, these were recorded.

2.2.3. Phase III: Extended Visits to Gardens

Gardens that had been noted for further investigation in Phase II were revisited once or several times, with the intention to study selected sonic events more thoroughly. Visits in Phase III were longer, typically lasting more than one hour. The extended time allowed for reflective on-site writing and the capturing of video, SPL readings and field recordings (for technical details, see Table 1). In a few gardens that were difficult to access, Phases II and III were combined.

Table 1. Equipment and processes used to notate sonic experiences in the gardens.

Type of Data	Description
Field notes	The most central piece of equipment was a small (analogue) notebook that was used to list garden encounters, focusing on soundscapes and sonic events in relation to landscape architecture. Notes were continuously transcribed digitally in a Microsoft Word document.
Images and video	To capture photos, a Canon EOS 6D DSLR camera was used together with a 35 mm f/2 lens and (during autumn 2018) a Canon EF 28–105 mm f/3.5–4.5 USM lens. In addition, the built-in camera of an IPhone SE was used to capture panorama and HDR images and video. Video was recorded at HD (1080 p, 30 fps).
Field recordings	A Zoom H2n was used to record sound, and in most cases the built-in microphones were used in the XY setting together with a thick wind screen. In cases where a wider spatial effect was deemed necessary, a pair of external Roland CS-10 EM binaural microphones was used. The quality was set to 24 bits at 44 kHz at all times.
Sound Pressure Levels (SPL)	SPLs were measured with an IPhone SE (internal microphone) together with the application NIOSH SLM (Version 1.0.6.24) to obtain approximated instantaneous readings in dBA [1]. Instantaneous readings were taken at approximately 1.5 metres above the ground for a few seconds; care was taken to protect the device from direct wind exposure and hand noise. In cases where a particular source was evaluated, the microphone was directed towards that source.

[1] The setting had been tested prior to the study in an urban environment sheltered from wind (SPL varying between 50–65 dBA). A Norsonic 140 (Class 1) SPL meter was used as control, and the manual setting in NIOSH SLM was calibrated to −2.1 dBA. After the study, the setting was tested again, this time by playing back different types of noises indoors and using a Brüel & Kjaer 2270 (Class 1) SPL meter as control. This test indicated that the setting had been satisfactory for the situations observed in the study (35–65 dBA), where the discrepancy did not exceed ±1.5 dBA. With this being said, it should be noted that SPL readings taken with smartphone applications do not comply with international standards. Studies on smartphone applications for SPL measurements have shown that, even though some of them may be suitable to measure occupational noise [59], the performance varies and limitations in accuracy can be problematic in the wrong context [60]. The SPL readings should be interpreted with this in mind.

2.2.4. Phase IV: Summary of Research Material

Garden visits were continuously noted in a Microsoft Excel spreadsheet (Appendix A). Field notes were collected in a digital document, amounting to a total of 23,000 words. This document served as the main research material. Images, video and sound were organised as a digital library that was used as a reference during the process of analysis. Extracts from this library were used to support the findings in this paper.

2.2.5. Phase V: Control

This phase was carried out in conjunction with data analysis, and entailed revisits to some of the previously studied gardens. The intention for these visits was either to confirm findings, make further comparisons between gardens and/or to collect audio-visual material and SPL readings. Most of the work in Phase V was completed in the autumn of 2018.

2.3. Analysis of Data

The Soundscape Action tool was used as a framework to analyse the research material and present the results. The tool was originally developed in collaboration with practitioners aiming to improve urban areas exposed to noise [27,36,61]. The tool has been described as "a group of acts that can be taken with the intention of designing a soundscape" ([36], p. 509). There are currently 23 Soundscape Actions divided into three main categories: localisation of functions, reduction of unwanted sounds and introduction of wanted sounds (Figure 2).

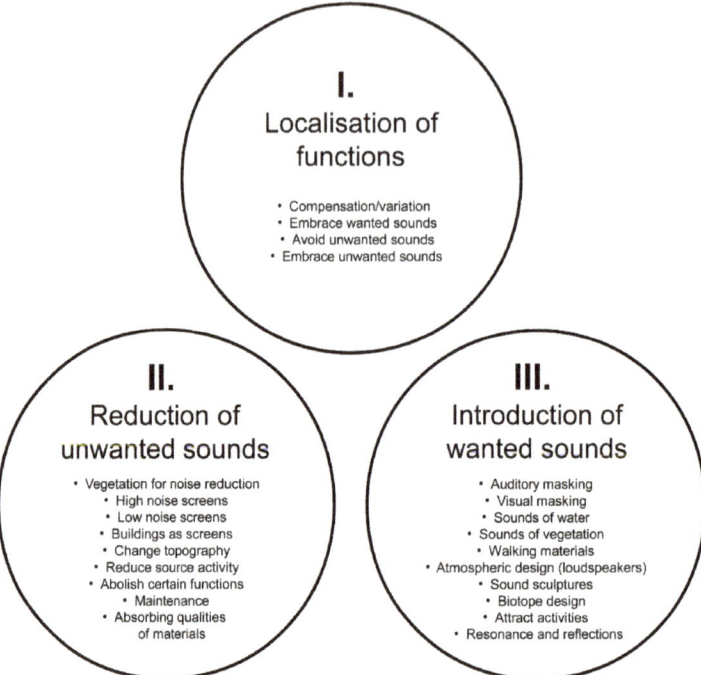

Figure 2. The design tool Soundscape Actions was used as the basis for analysis. In total there are 23 Soundscape Actions divided into three main categories: localisation of functions, reduction of unwanted sounds and introduction of wanted sounds.

The field studies were conducted in 88 gardens around Japan, but the analysis and presentation focuses on gardens located in Kyoto (n = 54). The focus on Kyoto is partly a result of the extensive material collected in this area, and it was also deemed necessary for reasons of clarity. The focus on Kyoto is most evident in Category I (localisation of functions), where other gardens are excluded entirely, so as to allow for comparisons within the city.

Before analysis was initiated, all field notes had been studied and checked for connections to supportive data. In cases where additional data or controls were required, this was noted and carried out (Section 2.2.5). In the analysis, each of the Soundscape Actions was compared with the field notes in order to identify relevant sections in the material; this process was guided by the author's recollection of the visits as well as strategic searches within the notes. Identified passages were copied to a new Microsoft Word document which was used as a base from which to summarise the findings. Supportive data was compared with the Soundscape Actions and, where applicable, links were provided in the new document.

It was found that four of the 23 Soundscape Actions were not applicable to the given context—embrace unwanted sounds, abolish certain functions, low noise screens and atmospheric design (loudspeaker-based)—and have thus been omitted from Section 3, leaving a total of 19 Soundscape Actions. These four are further described and discussed in Section 4.

3. Soundscape Actions in Japanese Gardens: Descriptions and Findings

The results are structured according to the three main categories illustrated in Figure 2. Each of these three categories is first given a brief *Category introduction* including any particular *Prerequisites and delimitations* of importance to the study. The 19 subcategories (Soundscape Actions) are then introduced using the following three headings: *Description*—A brief definition of each Soundscape Action based on previous studies; *Gardens of particular interest*—A list of gardens that were important for the findings presented and; *Findings*—A description of how the Soundscape Action related to the studied Japanese gardens and the findings that were made. Where applicable, connections to previous research are indicated.

3.1. Localisation of Functions

Category introduction: The first main category in the Soundscape Action tool regards the localisation of functions in relation to their surroundings (in the present study: gardens in relation to their urban surroundings). This category typically entails the consideration of noise and the compatibility between functions.

Prerequisites and delimitations: The Soundscape Actions in this category are mainly described based on observations and comparisons between gardens, complemented with the mapping of garden locations, images and SPL readings. For the purposes of clarity, all gardens mentioned in this main category are limited to one city, i.e., Kyoto (Figure 3). While acknowledging the considerable age of many gardens and the complex development of the city over time, the study focuses on how the gardens and their contexts are conceived today.

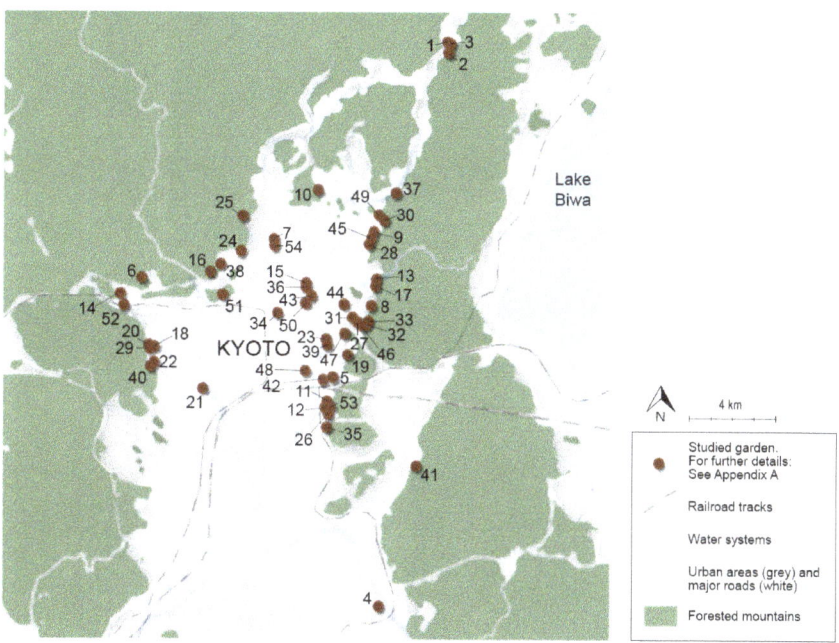

Figure 3. This map illustrates the locations of the 54 gardens that were studied in and around Kyoto. See Appendix A for names and further details of the study visits.

3.1.1. Compensation/Variation

Description: Compensation/Variation acknowledges the differences between neighbouring soundscapes as a potential quality. Gardens are frequently referred to as "safe havens" and "oases", thus implying a relative tranquillity and quietness where it is possible to escape from the hustle of the outside (urban) world. Consequently, busy urban settings surrounding a garden may be regarded as an asset, by offering contrast and juxtaposition (provided that the tranquillity inside the garden can be maintained).

Gardens of particular interest: Ōhashi-ke (35), Konchi-in (27), Murin-an (31).

Findings: The notion of Compensation/Variation was particularly pronounced in lesser known gardens located close to busy tourist routes. For instance, Ōhashi-ke garden in southeast Kyoto is located only two to three hundred metres from the immensely popular Shinto shrine Fushimi-Inari Taisha. In this intense tourist area, the narrow roads are filled with visitors en route to or returning from the shrine, lingering among market stalls and food shops (Figure 4a). In the study, the overwhelming intensity around Fushimi-Inari Taisha was found to influence the experience inside Ōhashi-ke by making the garden seem calm and quiet in comparison. Hence, the experience of the garden's soundscape depended not only on sounds experienced inside the garden, but also on previous encounters in the surrounding area. This polarity was captured in a comparative recording between the two sites (Video S1, https://vimeo.com/350108144).

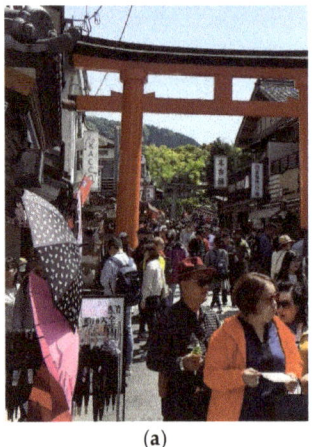 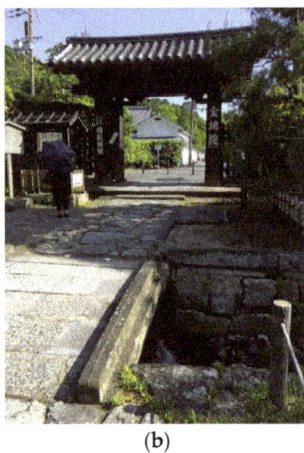

(a) (b)

Figure 4. Intense soundscapes may work as a contrast to enhance tranquillity in nearby gardens. (a) A busy tourist street at Fushimi Inari-Taisha in Kyoto. (b) The entrance to Konchi-in temple leads the visitor across a loud water stream.

A similar effect of contrast can be experienced about 5 km north, in Konchi-in garden, where the effect is articulated through the sound of water (in addition to the proximity of a tourist route). In order to reach the garden, the visitor needs to cross a loud water stream (Figure 4b). On the bridge across the water, the SPL temporarily reaches over 60 decibels (62 dBA; 21 April 2018), but drops rapidly as the main gate is approached on the other side. Inside the garden itself, the SPL is about 20 decibels lower (38–43 dBA, as observed in different parts of the garden; 21 April 2018). This example illustrates how the addition of sound could be intentionally used to temporarily raise the SPL in order to produce a relative tranquillity at the offset. The effect could arguably be further enhanced if it were combined with screens to increase the contrast. Such a combination can be experienced in another garden in the vicinity, Murin-an, though only occasionally, as the channel that produces the sound is dependent on rainfall to reach sufficient water flow.

3.1.2. Embrace Wanted Sounds

Description: To embrace wanted sounds is to make use of pre-existing sounds as a quality when selecting the locations of new functions. For instance, by selecting a location next to a forest, this may add the sound of twittering birds and rustling vegetation, among other experiences.

Gardens of particular interest: Nanzen-in (32), Sanbō-in (41), Entsū-ji (10), Shisen-dō (45), Sanzen-in (2), Ruriko-in (37).

Findings: Kyoto is surrounded by wooded mountain ranges on three sides: Higashiyama to the east, Kitayama to the north and Nishiyama to the west. A substantial amount of the most well-known gardens in Kyoto are located on the fringes of the city (c.f. Figure 3), often bordering the foothills of the mountain ranges directly. Not only is this a scenic setting which offers good views, but the proximity to nature also creates good prerequisites for a rich soundscape, inviting the sound of rustling leaves, purling water streams and the twittering of birds to be "borrowed" from the surrounding mountains:

> *Nanzen-in is an exquisitely designed small pond garden, parts of which date back to the 13th century. Lush mountainous woodlands surround the garden and add to the atmosphere through fragrance and sound. In the southeastern corner of the garden, a waterfall supplies fresh mountain water to the ponds.*
>
> Nanzen-in garden; 14 May 2018 (Figure 5)

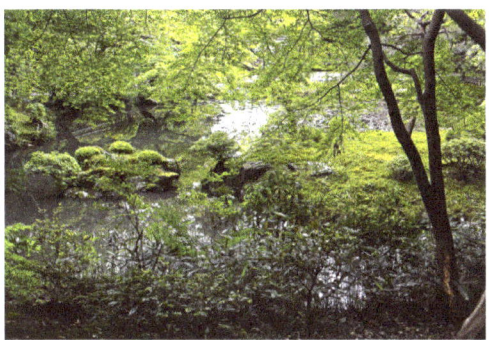

Figure 5. Nanzen-in, a sub-temple to the Nanzen-ji complex, has a small pond garden that borders mountainous woodlands attractive to birds and other animals.

In the Japanese garden discourse, *shakkei* is an important concept used to describe a technique whereby scenic features from the surrounding landscapes are "borrowed" and incorporated as part of the garden design. A typical example is when a distant mountain is framed to become part of the garden, articulated by carefully pruned vegetation. The notion of *shakkei* has mostly been discussed as a visual concept [62], however it is also fruitful to consider it as referring to sound and the other senses (c.f. [42]). This is exemplified in Nanzen-in above, as well as in other gardens like Sanbō-in (Video S2, https://vimeo.com/312665806), Entsū-ji, Shisen-dō, Sanzen-in and Ruriko-in.

3.1.3. Avoid Unwanted Sounds

Description: Avoiding unwanted sound is about considering existing sound sources that could potentially be disturbing and to make sure to locate new functions in areas shielded from such sources by providing sufficient distance and/or using shelter from buildings, mounds and other existing features.

Gardens of particular interest: Enkō-ji (9), Rurikoin (37), Shisen-dō (45), Konpuku-ji (28), Giou-ji (14), Saihoji (40), Shōsei-en (48).

Findings: Studying several gardens in the same city made it possible to make comparisons between different locations. While the majority of studied gardens were located on the fringes of the city, others had more urban locations, and thus provided an important reference. Almost all gardens located on the fringes of the city were perceived as quiet. Enkō-ji is an example of one such garden, where the background ambience was found to be around 40 dBA (12 May 2018). In that example, most of the ambience consisted of subtle natural sounds from the garden and the surrounding forest. It was striking how the low SPL made it possible to hear "further away":

I measure the background ambience at the veranda to be around 40 dBA. The ambience consists of a stream, distant birds and the occasional wind in the trees. In a way, it is so quiet that it seems I can hear further away.

Enkō-ji; 12 May 2018 (Figure 6)

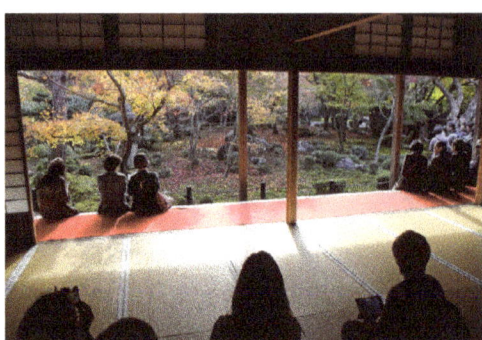

Figure 6. Autumn in Enkō-ji temple. The sliding doors to the main hall have been opened, thus allowing the sounds and sights from the garden to enter into the building.

Needless to say, gardens in central locations tended to be more exposed to noise, inevitably leading to reduced dynamics and a shorter "acoustic horizon" [30]. Gardens in urban locations could still be experienced as surprisingly tranquil, partly owing to the extensive use of water streams with masking capabilities (see further in Section 3.3.1. Auditory Masking). Other important factors for reducing noise include distance to major roads, use of vegetation and screens (garden walls and other structures).

The most problematic of the gardens studied in Kyoto was Shōsei-en, located close to the central station. Shōsei-en is a large garden, and the disturbances varied quite extensively inside the garden (45–60 dBA, as observed on different locations in the central parts of the garden; 29 April 2018). Such local variations constitute important prerequisites when functions within a garden are planned, as some features are more sensitive to noise than others.

3.2. Reduction of Unwanted Sounds

Category introduction: Soundscape Actions in this main category concern the reduction of unwanted sounds, most typically sounds from urban settlements and related activities like traffic. In contrast to the previous category, these Soundscape Actions are performed after the relative locations of functions have been decided upon.

Prerequisites and delimitations: Descriptions in this category are mainly based on observations. It was not deemed fruitful to use SPL to assess noise reduction in most cases, the reason being that this would have required comparisons that could not be obtained due to practical reasons (such as observing SPL with and without a garden wall). Instead, the studies focused on how various features in the gardens were designed, and discussed this in relation to previous research. The focus remains on gardens in Kyoto, though other examples are included as well.

3.2.1. Vegetation for Noise Reduction

Description: Vegetation is commonly used to reduce the impact of noise; one of the most typical applications is vegetation belts along roads. However, the actual effect of vegetation for reducing SPL is debated [63], most likely because the effect varies extensively depending on a number of factors such as vegetation type/s, distribution pattern, and the absorbing qualities of the ground cover [63–65]. Psychological factors are also important, in particular source visibility [66] (see further in Section 3.3.2.

Visual Masking). Moreover, the sound of vegetation can have a positive masking effect that shifts focus from noise (see also Section 3.3.1. Auditory Masking and Section 3.3.4. Sounds of Vegetation).

Gardens of particular interest: Saihoji (40), Murin-an (31), Shin'en (44), Chishaku-in (5).

Findings: Woodlands constitute a recurring feature in Japanese gardens, often found together with moss as in the famous Saihoji: the moss temple (Figure 7). Woodlands' effect on noise reduction is multifaceted. The trees themselves have some effect, depending on species composition, stem thickness, stand density and other factors [63–65], though there are several indirect factors that need to be taken into consideration, such as interference from wind. Wind is known to carry noise, hence woodlands can limit noise propagation in some situations [64]. For gardens, the wind reduction is particularly important along garden walls where there is otherwise a risk of micro-metrological turbulence that can have extensive negative effects.

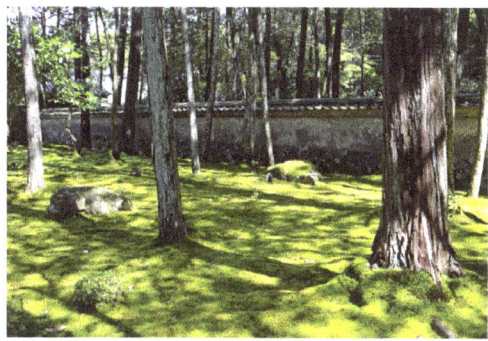

Figure 7. Moss and a garden wall in the woodland of Saihoji in Kyoto.

Almost all Japanese gardens in the study had garden walls, and these were often combined with vegetation. The combined effect of vegetation and wall is beneficial, not only for its enhanced noise reduction [64], but also as a means of articulating the garden space and delimiting it from the outside world (Video S3, https://vimeo.com/311434655, see further in Section 3.3.2. Visual Masking). Moreover, wind causes trees to rustle and this sound (together with birds and sounds from other animals attracted to the forest) can have the effect of masking noise (see further in Section 3.3.1. Auditory Masking and Section 3.3.7. Biotope Design).

Another aspect of woodlands is the effect that trees have on the ground cover. For instance, moss is one of the most characteristic features in Japanese gardens and it seems to thrive particularly well in moist woodlands, where it is shaded by the tree canopy (see further in Section 3.2.7. Absorbing Qualities of Materials). Moss is interesting for present purposes as it has a good ability to absorb ambient noise, an ability it shares with organic soil, grass and other soft ground covers (c.f. [67]).

3.2.2. High noise Screens

Description: A screen or wall with the approximate height of 1.8 metres or above is a high noise screen. Like all screens, they should be located as close to the source as possible [68]. High noise screens make it difficult for most people to see to the other side of the screen (unless the screen is transparent).

Gardens of particular interest: Murin-an (31), Shin'en (44), Saihoji (40).

Findings: Garden walls constitute a characteristic feature in the Japanese garden. Traditionally, the walls are made from clay, resting on a foundation of rocks and with a tile roofing (Figure 7), yet there are also examples of constructions based on other materials such as wood and stone. The height of garden walls vary; most are tall enough to offer visual seclusion, and some are three metres or higher, thus suggesting that screening of noise might have been an important consideration in addition to visual/spatial seclusion. Walls can be used to define the edges of a garden as well as having an effect on noise reduction from the outside. The actual noise reducing effect varies depending on several factors, and the reduction is most effective when the screen is located close to the source (or alternatively close to the receiver) [68]. As previously discussed, vegetation can improve the effect [64].

3.2.3. Buildings as Screens

Description: This Soundscape Action acknowledges the potential of strategically located buildings to reduce unwanted sound. Buildings can be effective noise screens, especially if they are tall and made of solid material [38]. They may also be combined with traditional noise screens.

Gardens of particular interest: Enkō-ji (9), Shisen-dō (45), Rurikoin (37).

Findings: Most buildings in and around the studied gardens were built in traditional style. One characteristic feature of traditional Japanese buildings is that they are made of light materials. In fact, some parts are even made of paper, including the *Shōji*, sliding doors. Moreover, the buildings are regularly opened up to the garden (c.f. Figure 6). In this respect, traditional buildings are not ideal when it comes to noise reduction, and the lower frequencies particularly are able to pass through buildings easily. However, these limitations with traditional buildings were seldom experienced as problematic in the study. One reason could be that the buildings tended to be located inside the boundaries of the garden walls and/or that they were located with sufficient distance from the noise.

There is an opposite and positive effect associated with the traditional buildings' ability to carry sound. The light construction can be said to "invite" sounds from the garden such that these may be experienced from inside the building, making it possible to listen to water, birds, the chanting of monks, the occasional bell, the murmur of other visitors or any other sound in the vicinity. Japanese buildings are known for their ability to blur the borders between inside and outside [14], and sound plays an important part in this.

3.2.4. Change Topography

Description: Land masses can be shaped to form strategic topographical patterns like mounds and/or valleys, which can be used to screen noise. The effect varies depending on factors such as height, width, detailed shape as well as planted vegetation (if any) [64].

Gardens of particular interest: Katsura Rikyū (21), Kōrakuen (76), Koishikawa-Kōrakuen (59) Suizen-ji Joju-en (77), Rikugi-en (64), Adachi Museum garden (79), Goten (Ninna-ji) (16).

Findings: Topographical features constitute a recurring design feature in the Japanese garden. In Katsura Rikyū in Kyoto, for instance, a pond was dug out and the soil was used to create an artificial mound, *tsukiyama* [4], where a tea house is located. Topographical features offer good views over the landscape, but they can also be visually striking in their own right, such as the characteristically shaped hills in Kōrakuen in Okayama and Koishikawa-Kōrakuen in Tokyo. Mounds are often designed to represent famous and/or sacred mountains, in which case they have a symbolic value [2,3]. The almost perfectly shaped grass cone in Suizen-ji Joju-en, Kumamoto, made to look like Mount Fuji, is a good example.

Topographical features constitute a useful means to reduce noise, if strategically located [64]. However, neither of the features mentioned above seem to have been built with the deliberate purpose of screening noise from the outside, as they are typically located in the central parts of the gardens where the effect should be limited, given the distance to the source [68].

On the other hand, it has been suggested that topographical features in some Japanese gardens are used with the intention of reducing the sonic impact of waterfalls inside the gardens [4]. The idea is that by "muffling" the sound of a waterfall in this way, it may seem to be further away than it actually is, hence making the garden appear larger (c.f. *shakkei* in Section 3.1.2). This effect was encountered in three gardens: Rikugi-en in Tokyo (Video S4, https://vimeo.com/312519101), Adachi Museum garden outside Matsue and Goten (Ninna-ji) in Kyoto.

3.2.5. Reduce Source Activity

Description: This Soundscape Action is concerned with everyday activities in the environment. It focuses on how unwanted sound from such activities can be reduced by decisions made in planning and design, such as enforcement of speed limits on roads or restrictions on social behaviour.

Gardens of particular interest: Tenryū-ji (52), Daisen-in (7), Shisen-dō (45), Goten (16).

Findings: Many Japanese gardens are popular attractions, and it is common to experience sounds from other visitors. These sounds can be quite intense, particularly in famous gardens with high accessibility, like the UNESCO World Heritage Site Tenryū-ji, which attracts many tourists. Taking photographs is a popular activity inside the gardens, and one which generates a lot of sound including discussions, shutter sounds and so on. Some gardens, like Daisen-in, do not allow photography, and this seems to have a positive effect on the soundscape as well as corresponding better with the "mindful" spirit of zen in that temple. In some gardens, like Shisen-dō and Goten, there are signs encouraging people to be respectful in their visits (Figure 8).

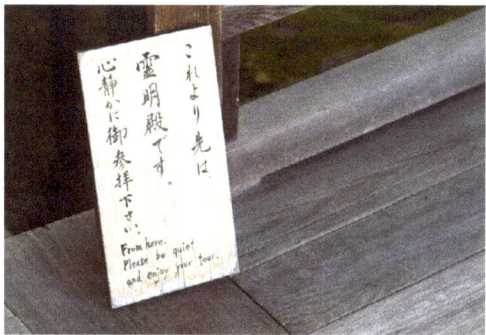

Figure 8. A sign in Goten, Kyoto, encouraging people to be quiet during their visit: "From here. Please be quiet and enjoy your tour.".

3.2.6. Maintenance

Description: Maintenance can generate a lot of noise, particularly when combustion engines are used. On the other hand, the use of hand-driven equipment and/or animals can potentially add a quality to the soundscape. Maintenance can be controlled in maintenance plans, but it is also influenced by design solutions. For instance, a lawn requires constant mowing, while a free-growing meadow is less intensive.

Gardens of particular interest: Ginkaku-ji (13), Rurikoin (37), Konchi-in (27), Shūgaku-in Rikyū (49).

Findings: Generally speaking, Japanese gardens are intensive when it comes to maintenance. Fallen leaves and other litter are removed meticulously, as are weeds. Moreover, the characteristic shape of trees and shrubs requires extensive pruning to be maintained and the gravelled areas of the dry gardens, *karesansui*, are raked every morning. On the other hand, the widespread use of moss rather than grass reduces the need for lawn mowing. Despite the intensive care required, as well as the fact that a lot of maintenance is carried out during opening hours, the work was rarely perceived as disturbing during the study. To a great extent, this might be ascribed to the fact that most tasks are performed by hand. The soft clipping of secateurs or the sweeping of a broom are sounds that add a layer to the experience, rather than disturb it (Figure 9a,b and Video S2, https://vimeo.com/312665806).

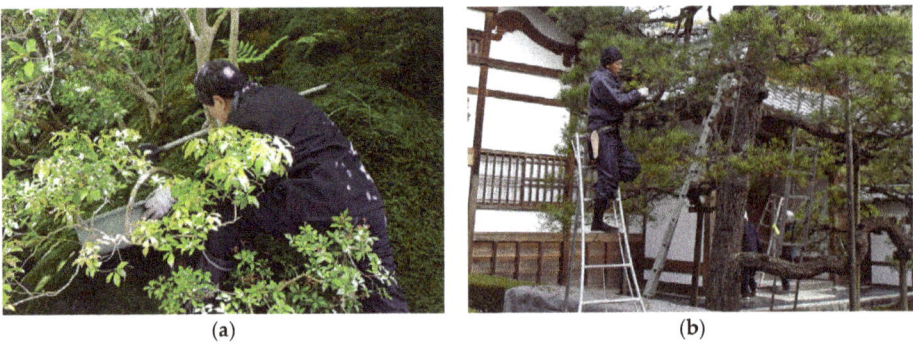

Figure 9. (**a**) A garden worker sweeping the moss in Rurikoin, Kyoto. (**b**) A garden worker pruning a pine tree in Ginkaku-ji, Kyoto.

Modern equipment is unusual, but was noted on a few occasions when it became quite disturbing. For example, in a garden normally perceived as a quiet gem, Konchi-in, a leaf blower was encountered on one visit, raising the SPL from 41 dBA to 65 dBA (15–20 m from the machine, 14 May 2018). Leaf blowers were also noted on two visits to Shūgaku-in Rikyū, though the garden workers there waited until the visitors had passed before using the machines (visits to Shūgaku-in Rikyū are organised in groups with a guide).

3.2.7. Absorbing Qualities of Materials

Description: This Soundscape Action regards the strategic application of materials with absorbing qualities, such as vegetation soil and moss, to reduce noise impact.

Gardens of particular interest: Saihoji (40), Rurikoin (37), Enkō-ji (9), Sanzen-in (2).

Findings: The prerequisites for moss are good in Japan, as the proximity to the ocean creates a humid climate which helps the moss to thrive. The timeless expression and subtle atmospheric appeal of moss corresponds with the Japanese aesthetics known as *wabi-sabi* [69] and many gardens cultivate moss intentionally. Moss can have a positive effect on the sound environment, as it grows to create a soft and absorbing surface on the ground (c.f. [64,67]). The famous moss temple Saihoji, for instance (Figure 7), was found to be one of the most quiet gardens in the field studies. The ambience at the entrance to the pond section of the garden was noted at 35 dBA (18 November 2018). As speculated during an earlier visit to the garden, moss could be one of several explanations for the quietness:

> *I attribute the silence partly to the fact that the garden is situated in the outskirts of Kyoto, making it less likely to be affected by city noise. However, the silence can also in part be attributed to the extensive coverage of moss, which is known to absorb sound. Moreover, the garden is surrounded by walls on the one side, and hills on the other, to offer a shelter from the surroundings.*
>
> Saihoji; 15 May 2018 (Figure 7)

3.3. Introduction of Wanted Sounds

Category introduction: Soundscape Actions in this category can be used to introduce, stimulate or enhance sounds that are considered wanted in a particular situation. Needless to say, wanted sounds vary depending on context and individual preferences along with a number of other cues [51,52,70,71], yet sounds from nature, like water, birds and rustling vegetation, are typically considered to be wanted sources [50].

Prerequisites and delimitations: Descriptions of Soundscape Actions in this category are based on subjective observations supported by field recordings, images and SPL readings. The focus remains on gardens in Kyoto, but other examples are included as well.

3.3.1. Auditory Masking

Description: Auditory masking is an effect where one sound (masker) is used to reduce the impact of another sound (target). Auditory masking has been used in a number of urban design projects, typically involving water features to reduce the impact of traffic noise [72]. Essentially, there are two types of auditory masking: energetic masking and informational masking [73]. In energetic masking the masker sound literally covers the target sound, rendering it inaudible. It has been found that, in the case of urban water features, an increase of about 8–10 dBA is required to achieve this effect [74]. In informational masking on the other hand, both sounds are audible, yet the focus shifts from the target to the masker.

Gardens of particular interest: Eikan-dō (8), Murin-an (31), Shōsei-en (48), Koishikawa-Kōrakuen (59), Nezu museum garden (63), Kenroku-en (68).

Findings: The ample use of water features in Japanese gardens constitutes an ideal setting to study auditory masking. The notion of energetic masking was conceived to be relatively straightforward. It would typically be experienced in the proximity of loud water features, where all surrounding sounds were effectively covered. Informational masking, on the other hand, was found to be much more complex, involving several cues including the physical characteristics of the inherent sound sources and their relative locations in space. The studies also indicate that informational masking could be affected by visual information (c.f. Section 3.3.2. Visual Masking), as well as the notion of gestalt psychology (c.f. [30,75]), as the following experience from Eikan-dō illustrates:

> A loud stream and two waterfalls border the garden on its southern side. In a way, the powerful sound seems to be reinforcing the edge of the garden, which is also marked by a fence. Behind the fence, there is a high school and a kindergarten. This creates an interesting and potentially disturbing situation, as the sound of the children playing can collide with the activities in the temple, activities that presumably are best performed in a tranquil and quiet environment. The sound of children playing is loud, but it is partly masked by the powerful sound of the water. It can still be heard through the water, but in a way, it is as though it becomes located on a different spatial layer, or to use gestalt psychology, in the background. Without the water, the sound of children would probably have been much more intrusive.
>
> Eikan-dō; 18 April 2018 (Figure 10a)

Sound level is an important factor to consider in relation to masking strategies. It has been argued that if the SPL reaches above 65–70 dBA, all sounds start to become disturbing, in which case masking strategies are not fruitful [39]. To achieve tranquil qualities, much lower levels than this are needed. It has been shown that good soundscape quality in suburban green areas and city parks typically require a level below 50 dBA [76] and that informational masking is more efficient at levels below 52.5 dBA (traffic noise) [77]. In Eikan-dō, the SPL was 58 dBA (29 November 2018) at the point where the above description was noted, a few metres from the stream that borders the garden's edge.

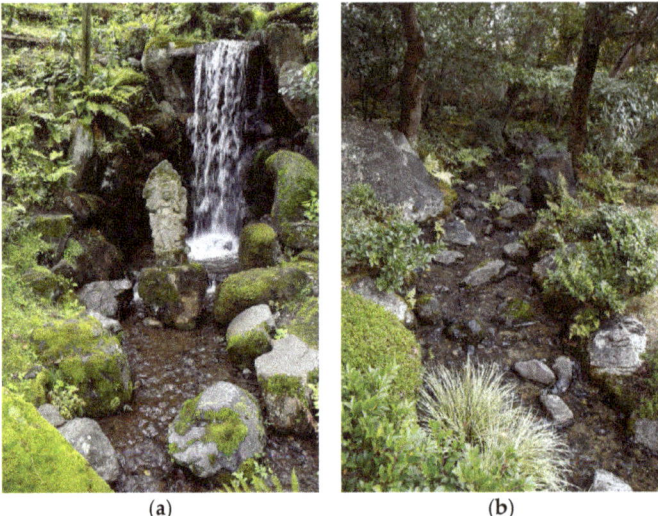

Figure 10. Loud water features can be used to mask outside noise. (**a**) A waterfall in Eikan-dō, Kyoto. (**b**) A stream in Murin-an garden, Kyoto.

3.3.2. Visual Masking

Description: The idea behind visual masking is that if the source of a noise is hidden from view it is less likely to attract attention and cause disturbance. It has been argued that visual masking can be a fruitful strategy as long as the noise that is being hidden is not too prominent [66,78]. This strategy has also been referred to as source (in)visibility [66] and is related to the notion of acousmatics [79].

Gardens of particular interest: Murin-an (31), Shin'en (44), Chishaku-in (5), Eikan-dō (8), Shōsei-en (48).

Findings: As previously discussed, Japanese gardens make extensive use of garden walls combined with vegetation to mark the edges of the premises. The clearly defined visual spaces keep the visitor's attention within the garden, presumably making noise from the outside world less likely to be noticed (Video S3, https://vimeo.com/311434655). In a similar manner as auditory masking discussed above, visual masking seems to entail a kind of layering of experiences in terms of background and foreground. In fact, it was found that these two masking effects may work together, as the following example from Murin-an garden in Kyoto illustrates:

> *It seems the garden wall manages to shield the sound from the street well; the combined effect of screening and lack of visual contact makes me feel as though the cars belong to another world. Moreover, I think it helps that the sound of cars mixes nicely with the rustling of vegetation above the wall, as it is a windy day when I visit. In fact, the vegetation follows the exact same stretch as the road, but because only the vegetation is visible from where I sit, it is easy to partly ascribe the sound of the traffic to the vegetation. Suddenly, a bus passes by, I can clearly see its white roof above the wall, and the illusion is broken for an instance. The sound seems disturbing now, partly I think because I can see the bus, and partly because the sound is louder; I can even feel the vibration from where I am sitting. As the bus passes away, it becomes quiet again.*
>
> Main building, Murin-an; 6 May 2018 (Figure 10b)

The ambience in the example (without passing cars) was noted at around 46 dBA (6 May 2018). The rather high wall surrounding the main building shields noise effectively, and the SPL was only raised by a couple of decibels when cars were passing by, thus helping to keep the noise "not prominent" [66]. As a reference, outside the wall on the sidewalk, the ambience was noted at around 54 dBA, which was increased by more than 10 dBA as a car passed by (14 May 2018).

3.3.3. Sounds of Water

Description: Water has the potential to create a vast amount of sonic effects, ranging from the powerful broadband noise of a waterfall through to the subtle tickling of a single drop. Water can be made to vary in tone, rhythm and strength [80,81]. It is generally perceived as a pleasant sound, though can be annoying depending on the character [82]. Water features have repeatedly been used to produce masking effects from urban noise in strategic locations [32,72,74].

Gardens of particular interest: Tsujike teien (75), Kenroku-en (68), Murin-an (31), Eikan-dō (8), Shin'en (44), Ginkaku-ji (13), Funda-in (12), Rurikoin (37), Chishaku-in (5), Tenryū-ji (52).

Findings: The ample rainfall and mountainous geography of Japan supplies many gardens with direct access to natural water with a high flow rate. As a general trait, water features in Japanese gardens tend to echo expressions that can be found in nature (Figure 10a,b and Figure 11a,b). For instance, Japanese gardens make frequent use of ponds, natural streams and waterfalls, while formalistic expressions like fountains are less frequent.

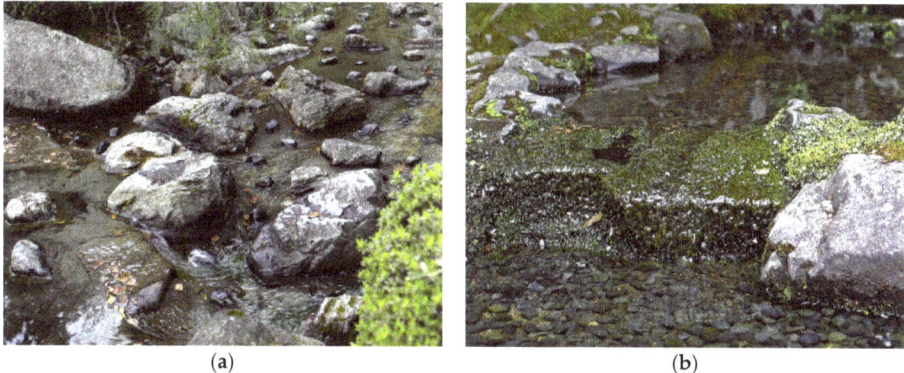

(a)   (b)

Figure 11. Two strategies to articulate water sound in Japanese gardens. (**a**) Stones are strategically laid out to enhance the sound of a water stream in Shin'en garden (Heian Jingu Shrine), Kyoto (Video S5). (**b**) A barely audible miniature waterfall in Ginkaku-ji, Kyoto (Video S6b).

Streams and waterfalls with loud and roaring sounds can be found in Tsujike Teien and Kenroku-en in Kanazawa, as well as Murin-an and Eikan-dō in Kyoto. Such loud water features are particularly useful to mask out urban noise through energetic masking (c.f. Section 3.3.1. Auditory Masking). In some gardens, stones are used to deliberately enhance the sound of streams. In Shin'en garden in Kyoto, a stream that connects the eastern and northern ponds is narrowed by the use of boulders, which increases the speed and directs the flow (Figure 11a and Video S5, https://vimeo.com/311170428). As the water descends towards the next level, rocks are strategically located to break the flow. This makes the stream full of life and produces a stronger and more interesting sound than would otherwise have been the case. This technique can be traced back to at least the 11th century in Japan, where it is mentioned in the classic novel *The Tale of Genji*: "The stream above the waterfall was cleared out and deepened to a considerable distance; and that the noise of the cascade might carry further, he set great boulders in mid-stream, against which the current crashed and broke" ([83], p. 428).

If some water features are created in a way that enhances their sound, it is also common to find opposite and more delicate approaches where extremely low sound levels are emphasised. In some cases, such kinds of subtle water features are in fact just above the audibility threshold. They are often found in zen gardens, which could suggest that they are used to support meditation practices (c.f. [3]). The expressions vary from the tranquil dripping of water in a small washing basin, *chozubachi*, as experienced in Funda-in in Kyoto, through to what could essentially be described as miniature waterfalls, found in gardens like Rurikoin, Chishaku-in (Video S6a, https://vimeo.com/311182675) and Ginkaku-ji (Figure 11b and Video S6b, https://vimeo.com/311079936) in Kyoto. Another expression of this kind of aesthetics can be found in the "dry waterfall", *karetaki*, (e.g., Tenryū-ji in Kyoto), where stones are arranged to look like a waterfall but intentionally kept dry, thus only suggesting the sound [43].

3.3.4. Sounds of Vegetation

Description: Vegetation sound is perhaps most commonly associated with leaves that rustle in the wind. The character of the rustle varies depending on several factors, including species composition, spatial layout and wind [27]. Tree branches can produce crackling sounds if they are swaying in the wind, and large leaves can enhance the sound of rain as raindrops fall on them [84]. Some species are known as good rustlers, including the poplar genus (aspen) and bamboo [84,85].

Gardens of particular interest: Funda-in (12), Chishaku-in (5), Rikugi-en (64), Rentaroh Taki's Memorial garden (81).

Findings: The sound of rustling leaves could be experienced in most gardens, the character varying from a tranquil and subtle atmosphere to strong gusts. On windy days, when the effect was most pronounced, the leaves could take over and drown out other sounds (c.f. Section 3.3.1. Auditory Masking and Section 3.3.2. Visual Masking). Observations in this study indicate that the sound could be enhanced if the trees are surrounded by open land or planted as an avenue to allow the wind better access to the leaves, however no SPL readings could be taken to confirm this. In some gardens, like Funda-in, Chishaku-in, and Rikugi-en, it was apparent that trees planted on mounds had a strategic position to catch the wind. This was particularly evident in Funda-in and Chishaku-in, where the bamboo was planted on mounds:

> *A few moments of tense silence before a gust of wind starts to build up in the distance. At first, I can hear how the tall bamboo trees in the left back side of the garden start to move. They are strategically located on a high position which exposes them to more wind. The wind gust gradually approaches the garden, and I can now hear the rustle of the vegetation on the top of the hill, where a variety of species adds to the composition. Eventually, I can feel the wind passing the veranda and hear how the shoji doors behind me shake slightly as a response, before it quiets down again.*
>
> Chishaku-in; 21 May 2018 (Video S6a)

Bamboo has previously been acknowledged for its ability to invite sound into a garden, in China [84] as well as in Japan [44]. When describing the soundscape design in Rentaroh Taki's Memorial garden in Taketa, Torigoe mentions how bamboo makes "sound when blowing in the wind, rustling its leaves and squeaking its stems" [44] (p. 112).

3.3.5. Walking Materials

Description: Materials like gravel and wood are known to generate ample sonic responses when walked upon, while other materials like asphalt and stone are quieter. Furthermore, different materials can contribute with different connotations which have bearing on preference [86]. The sound of other people walking may be experienced as a pleasant atmosphere, or in some cases, as a warning [85].

Gardens of particular interest: Rentaroh Taki's memorial garden (81), Nomura-ke samurai teien (70), Ryōan-ji (38), Shoren-in (47), Nijō-jō (34).

Findings: One of the most typical materials used to produce walking paths in Japanese gardens is no doubt stone. Stones are used in different ways: sometimes to create wide, cohesive and formal paths and sometimes as informal stepping stones carefully laid out in the ground, *tobi-ishi* or in water, *sawatari*. Stone paths do not produce so much sound today, though when they were originally conceived, traditional wooden shoes known as *geta* would have created a characteristic clonking sound [43,44]. This effect can still be experienced in Rentaroh Taki's Memorial garden where such shoes are offered to visitors.

Another noteworthy feature is the extensive use of wooden floors. They are typically found in the verandas known as *engawa* (Figure 12). Some gardens, including the famous Ryōan-ji, are designed to be experienced from the *engawa*, where the thumping sound of wood becomes a characteristic *soundmark* [30]. It is quite common for the wooden verandas to extend into the garden as a system of roofed walkways that connect various buildings on the premises. Such walkways offer shade on hot days and shelter from precipitation, while the sound of thumping and squeaking floorboards constitute a potentially pleasant accompaniment, as the following example from Shoren-in illustrates:

> *The wooden walkways make for a nice stroll through the garden, as the roof provides shade in the sunshine. The floor is made from thick wooden floorboards; it has a nice, raw tactility to it. Each floorboard is slightly different in character; the thickness varies. Some floorboards make a heavy thumping sound when walked upon.*
>
> Shoren-in; 28 April 2018

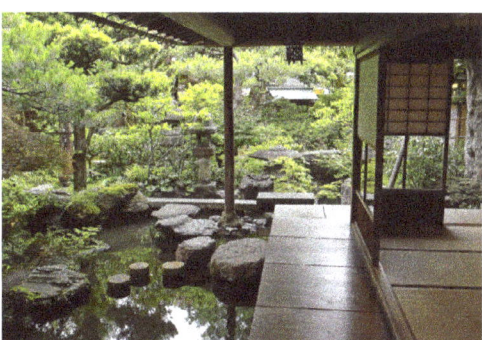

Figure 12. Nomura-ke Samurai teien in Kanazawa. View from the east overlooking the upper pond.

The sound of the verandas' wooden floors differs between gardens depending on the construction. One particularly noteworthy effect is the squeaking sound which has come to be called *uguisubari*, or nightingale floor, after the Japanese bush warbler, *uguisu* (*Horornis diphone*), whose sound it supposedly resembles (Video S7, https://vimeo.com/311380259). Legend has it that the sound of the *uguisubari* was used to warn inhabitants of assassins and other unwelcome guests. This particular function may have played out its role today, yet there may be related applications in other contexts. For instance, in a study reporting on the role of soundscape in a rehabilitation garden, it was found that a patient who wanted to experience "social quietness" used the sound of a gravel path as a warning system from the potential approach of other patients in the garden [85]. Gravel paths can also be found in Japanese gardens, though the extensive use of stone and wood makes it less of a characteristic feature.

3.3.6. Sound Sculptures

Description: A sound sculpture is a multisensory embellishment where sound plays an important part. There are many types of sound sculptures, and they can be driven by sources such as wind, water or electricity (speakers). The sound is usually accompanied by some sort of visual container that is typically designed to be a part of the expression.

Gardens of particular interest: Ōhashi-ke (35), Enkō-ji (9), Taizō-in (51), Giou-ji (14), Shisen-dō (45).

Findings: Two kinds of garden features that qualify as sound sculptures were studied: *suikinkutsu* and *sōzu (shishi-odoshi)*.

Suikinkutsu is a simple but elegant design element that can be found in conjunction with some washing places, *tsukubai* (Figure 13a). The sound is created as excess water from the water basin, *chozubashi*, is led to drop into a hidden cavity below ground. The cavity essentially consists of a pot which is turned upside down and buried in the ground. The sound is generated at the bottom of the cavity where the drops break a water surface. The sound can be described as metallic and vibrant, fresh and melodic. The sound of *suikinkutsu* was experienced and documented in four gardens (Video S8a–e, https://vimeo.com/showcase/5683754). As a sound sculpture, *suikinkutsu* is unusual, as part of it is hidden beneath ground.

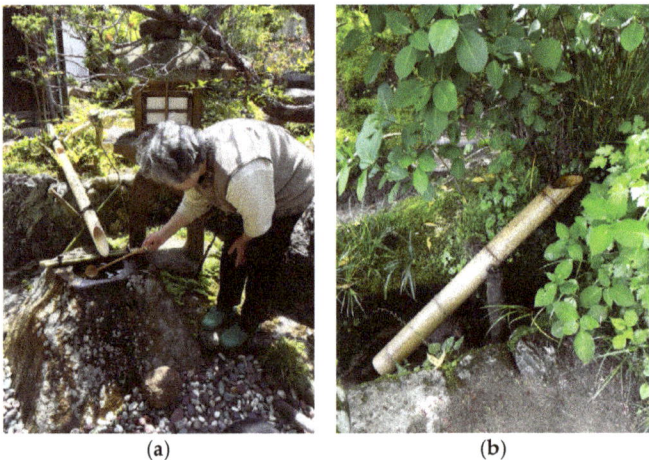

Figure 13. Two typical sound sculptures found in Japanese gardens. (**a**) A suikinkutsu in Ōhashi-ke, Kyoto (Video S8b,). (**b**) A *sōzu*, also known as *shishi-odoshi* in Shisen-dō, Kyoto (Video S9a).

A *sōzu* is a contraption originally developed by farmers to keep deer, boars and other wild animals away from their fields (Figure 13b). It was subsequently incorporated as a design element in gardens [43]. It consists of a bamboo tube, which is opened up on one side to allow water to flow inside. The tube is mounted on a rack that works as a hinge so that the tube can move freely around the axes. The open end of the tube is located beneath a water supply. As the tube fills up, its center of gravity gradually shifts until it passes the hinge, causing the contraption to fall over, emptying its water and then making a distinct sound as it falls back to its resting position (Video S9a,b, https://vimeo.com/showcase/5683758). The *sōzu* is often called a *shishi-odoshi*, in which case a more overarching reference is inferred; both terms are generally translated as deer scarer.

3.3.7. Biotope Design

Description: Biotopes and natural ecosystems can have positive effects on the soundscape, including the presence of song birds and other animals [87]. Song birds are generally attracted by basic features like access to water, shelter and food (most typically insects, seeds and berries) [88,89]. A general guideline is that birds prefer vegetation that is multi-layered, dense and variated.

Gardens of particular interest: Rurikoin (37), Shisen-dō (45), Sanbō-in (41), Shin'en (44) Rurikoin (37), Nanzen-in (32), Shisen-dō (45), Rentaroh Taki's memorial garden (81).

Findings: Many of the studies of Japanese gardens were conducted during April and May, which provided ample opportunities to experience birds and other animals, particularly in gardens that bordered forests, such as Rurikoin, Shisen-dō and Sanbō-in, or gardens that included woodlands, such as Shin'en (Heian Jingu Shrine). Some species, like heron, seemed to enjoy sitting on stones laid out in ponds. It has previously been suggested that such stones were deliberately laid out in shallow water with the purpose of attracting birds [43]. Prerequisites for birds may also be increased by the use of vegetation, particularly fruit-bearing plants [44].

Spring is also the mating season for frogs, and the sometimes intense croaking could be experienced in pond gardens like Rurikoin, Nanzen-in and Shisen-dō. The effect was particularly breathtaking on May 15th 2018 in Nanzen-in, where the whole system of ponds seemed to be "illuminated" by croaking frogs, creating an intense spatial presence (Video S10, https://vimeo.com/270885125). Frogs may in fact have been actively placed in Nanzen-in when the garden was created in the late Kamakura period, as indicated by 15th century sources accessible to Ueyakato Landscape, that manages the garden today [90].

Two other animals are commonly placed in Japanese gardens: turtles and carp fish (Figure 14). Almost all ponds encountered in the study had carp fish, while turtles were less common. In some gardens, for example Konchi-in, carp and turtles live side by side, creating spectacular sightings and the occasional splash. Both carp fish and turtles can make rather loud splashes, an effect that amuses visitors and possibly stimulates a heightened and active "listening" to the environment (as compared to a passive "hearing") [91].

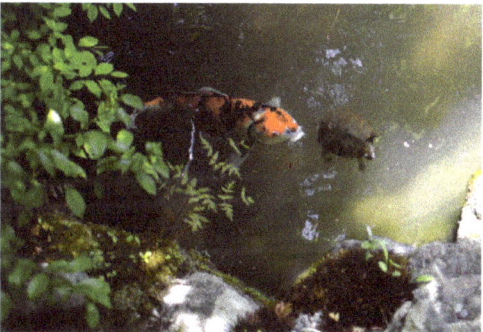

Figure 14. A turtle and a carp fish in Konchi-in temple garden, Kyoto.

3.3.8. Attract Activities

Description: This Soundscape Action acknowledges the relationship between landscape functions and sound by emphasising the fact that the introduction of new functions may generate activities that benefit the soundscape. A typical example of such a function is a café, the atmosphere of which can also be a quality for people passing by.

Gardens of particular interest: Chishaku-in (5), Daisen-in (7), Konchi-in (27), Nanzen-ji (33), Rurikoin (37), Tenryū-ji (52), Suizen-ji Joju-en (77).

Findings: Ticket sales, souvenir shops and cafés constitute some examples of recurring activities noted in the study. Religious activities could be experienced in gardens located in (or in the vicinity of) Buddhist temples and Shinto shrines. Even if secluded, the sound of religious activities would easily travel through the thin walls of the traditional buildings, making it customary to hear monks' chanting or the distant ringing of a gong as a faint, mystical atmosphere. For the visitor, these atmospheric tints may constitute a reminder of the sacred context in which the gardens are located. The act of praying is ritualised in Shinto shrines as well as in Buddhist temples. In both cases, praying involves throwing a coin into an offering box, *saisen-bako*: an event which can create a rather loud sound if the box has resonating qualities.

A *temizuya* is a kind of water basin, where visitors go to purify themselves before a visit. The purification is carried out with the aid of a wooden ladle which is used to pour water on one's hands and mouth. The *temizuya* generates a rather specific soundscape typically involving the murmur of people, the sound of water splashing on the ground and the distinct wooden clonks as the ladles are put down. The *temizuya* are typically associated with Shinto shrines though can also be found in Buddhist temples.

To sum up, the sound of activities signals the presence of other people and may be charged with symbolic meaning and atmospheric qualities. In design situations, such aspects should be given consideration in relation to the intended purpose. Social activities may be regarded as a quality in many contexts, yet may also be problematic in some situations. This is the case in gardens intended for recovery from stress-related illnesses, where seclusion from some forms of social activities is required [85,92].

3.3.9. Resonance/Reflection

Description: Resonance/Reflection is concerned with how acoustically hard materials can be used to enhance wanted sound sources. For instance, if a concrete wall is strategically located behind a water feature, the sound of water can be enhanced by the reflections the wall creates.

Gardens of particular interest: Sanbō-in (41), Konchi-in (27), Shoren-in (47), Murin-an (31).

Findings: These kinds of acoustical effects were mainly found in and around water features, typically enforced by stones enhancing and directing the sound of water in gardens like Sanbō-in, Konchi-in and Shoren-in. The design intentions underlying these cavities could be several, and resonance may not have been the main one. Some of these cavities also worked to direct the sound, as the following notation from Konchi-in in Kyoto indicates:

> *The use of the grotto has other advantages as well. Not only is the sound amplified through the resonance it creates, but the grotto also seems to have a parabolic shape leading the sound across the pond towards the entrance.*

Konchi-in; 21 April 2018

This way of directing sound opens up for a wide range of creative possibilities and experiential effects. In the above example, the sound of the waterfall is best experienced from the opposite (northern) side of the pond, yet because it cannot be seen from that point, an anticipation is created that encourages further exploration of the garden in search for the source. It has previously been described how the sound of hidden water features can be used to create a "spatial appeal" that invites a visitor to go from a "here" to search for a "there" [41]. Such kind of explorations seem to be related to the notion of "soft fascination" as described by Kaplan and Kaplan, as part of their attention restoration theory (c.f. [48,85,93]).

4. Discussion

4.1. Soundscape Actions as a Design Tool

The Soundscape Actions presented in the study constitute a collection of examples, illustrating how landscape architects and other professionals could think about soundscape design in their work [27,36]. Covering a total of 23 Soundscape Actions divided in three categories, it is an extensive framework. This emerged as beneficial in the study, as it provided a variety of entry points from which to understand the soundscapes of Japanese gardens. In this way, aspects that would not necessarily have been noted otherwise could be highlighted.

In the study, 19 of the 23 Soundscape Actions were applicable. The other four (Embrace unwanted sounds, Abolish certain functions, Low noise screens and Atmospheric design) were excluded because no concrete examples were encountered. This is partly owing to the particular character of Japanese gardens, where certain expressions are not likely to be found, such as urban vibrancy (Embrace unwanted sounds) or artificial speaker installations (Atmospheric design). In future developments of the tool, it might be possible to take this into consideration by designing a system in which Soundscape Actions are tagged based on their appropriate application (for instance urban vibrancy, traffic planning and parks/gardens). The other two excluded actions seem relevant for Japanese gardens, yet could not be registered in the study. "Abolish certain functions" (such as roads, factories or air conditioners) should be a fruitful strategy to enhance garden experiences, however no clear examples were identified (in part, owing to language difficulties). "Low noise screens" is a novel solution for traffic noise reduction and only a limited number of practical applications are known worldwide.

Some sonic experiences that were noted in the study did not correspond directly to any of the 23 Soundscape Actions. These experiences could generally be described to be of a phenomenological nature, including effects related to movement, orientation, behaviour and subjective contemplation. This discrepancy may partly be regarded as a consequence of the autoethnographic approach, in which such experiences should be expected to be brought forward; it might also be taken to indicate specificities associated with the context being studied, i.e., Japanese gardens. The encountered effects were referred to in the study in conjunction with related Soundscape Actions (for example subtle water features in Section 3.3.3 and interactive walking materials in Section 3.3.5). There seems to be scope to formulate new Soundscape Actions. This potential will be further examined in upcoming publications.

4.2. Implementation and Usage

The Soundscape Actions constitute a set of strategies with the potential to improve experiential qualities in gardens and other urban (green) spaces. However, it should be noted that, because each situation is unique, the effect of Soundscape Actions will vary, and all of them will not necessarily lead to an improvement every time. One of the challenges of soundscape design is to understand complex relationships and the degree to which various factors effect a situation. The tool brings together a collection of central aspects as a framework that can be used to build an experience base. In future work, this base could be further developed by applying the tool in other contexts and with other participants. The material thus generated could be collected and presented online for accessibility. A digital platform suitable for this purpose already exists (https://soundscapedesign.info). Practitioners should be involved in future developments so as to safeguard compatibility with established working patterns. One way forward could be to evaluate the tool in design workshops and/or use it to build an intervention (which could subsequently be evaluated). Future work could also explore the possibility of integrating the tool with computer aided calculations, known as auralisation. This would potentially allow for real time comparisons between Soundscape Actions in different scenarios.

The study focused on tranquil soundscapes in Japanese gardens, taking into consideration the potential for negative as well as positive health effects [24,25]. The study did not assess health effects per se, but rather used existing research to envisage the effects. As discussed above, there is a strong body of research showing that exposure to noise increases stress and leads to a number of severe negative health effects [24]. This should be taken in account when designing outdoor spaces. Problems with noise have primarily been addressed by engineers and acousticians, yet much can also be achieved by urban planners and designers [27,28,32,94,95]. Increased collaboration across disciplines could further enhance prerequisites for health promoting environments. In terms of positive health effects, there is an increasing number of studies indicating that exposure to nature sounds have beneficial effects on health [25]. This should also be given consideration in design situations so that such sounds are afforded the best possible prerequisites. The present study provided several examples of how this could be accomplished.

5. Conclusions

This study has focused on the Japanese garden tradition in order to gain insights on the design tool Soundscape Actions, and how it can be used to improve soundscapes in gardens and other green spaces. Field studies were conducted in 88 Japanese gardens, and notated experiences from (in total) 136 visits to those gardens were used as empirical material. Most of the analysis and presentation centred on gardens located in Kyoto (n = 54), as this allowed for comparisons within the city.

The research was designed using an autoethnographic approach [45]. This made it possible to obtain detailed understandings on the intersection between landscape architecture and soundscape research. Autoethnography emphasises subjectivity and therefore allows for embodied experiences to be brought forward. This enables the researcher to go into detail and consider the interplay between senses and various site-specific factors. It should be pointed out that the subjective nature of the method could limit the applicability of the findings in other contexts. To increase generalisability, supportive data was collected in situ, including SPL readings, images, videos and field recordings. This material has been made available in the paper, and should mitigate interpretation. Where applicable, findings were compared and discussed in relation to previous research. Yet, caution should be taken when interpreting the results, and future studies involving more participants are recommended to validate the findings.

Sound constitutes one of several aspects of the environmental experience, and it should be stressed that the interplay between the senses is of importance, even when focusing on a particular sense [85]. The study highlights the role of such relationships when discussing masking and other complex mechanisms. Masking is based on the assumption that sounds experienced as positive can be used to reduce the annoyance caused by traffic and other (unwanted) technological sources [72,74,82]. The benefits of masking have been debated, partly because the underlying mechanisms are not fully understood. This study indicated that spatial context and multisensory impressions play an important role, and that such factors should be given increased consideration in future research. The subjective experience of individuals seems to be essential if these effects are to be uncovered further. Subjectivity is emphasised in the ISO definition of soundscape [34], yet has been given surprisingly little attention in research thus far.

Much effort has been invested to analyse and uncover the knowledge existing in the Japanese garden tradition, though most previous publications have tended to prioritise visual aspects. The present study illustrates how Japanese gardens can also be informative regarding sound. The findings presented here follow the Soundscape Action design tool and cover a wide array of perspectives. The study illustrates multiple strategies to avoid noise, such as the use of remote locations, garden walls and absorbent moss. Reduction of noise allows for other and more delicate experiences to come forward, like sounds of nature. Sounds of nature constitute an essential element in Japanese gardens and they can be articulated and enhanced in design solutions. This is highlighted in the study through the way that rustling trees are used, how animals are attracted and how the sound of water is orchestrated to produce loud masking sounds. Taken together, the soundscapes of Japanese gardens are surprisingly tranquil considering the modern and densified cities that often surround them.

Supplementary Materials: The following are available online at http://www.mdpi.com/1660-4601/16/23/4648/s1, Video S1: Compensation/Variation in Ōhashi-ke; Video S2: Spring in Sanbō-in; Video S3: Screening and Masking in Murin-an; Video S4: Muffled Waterfall in Rikgui-en; Video S5: Enhanced Water Stream in Shin'en; Video S6a: Water and Wind in Chishaku-in; Video S6b: Subtle Water Drops in Ginkaku-ji; Video S7: Nightingale Floors; Video S8a: Suikinkutsu in Ōhashi-ke, 1/2; Video S8b: Suikinkutsu in Ōhashi-ke, 2/2; Video S8c: Suikinkutsu in Enkō-ji; Video S8d: Suikinkutsu in Taizō-in; Video S8e: Suikinkutsu in Giou-ji; Video S9a: Shishi-odoshi in Shisen-dō; Video S9b: Shishi-odoshi in Taizō-in; Video S10: Frogs in Nanzen-in.

Funding: This research was funded by the Japanese Society for the Promotion of Science, JSPS, through an International Research Fellow programme (Postdoctoral short term).

Acknowledgments: The author wishes to thank Keiko Torigoe, Kozo Hiramatsu, Ann Bergsjö, Yoshio Tsuchida, Haruyoshi Sowa, Masafumi Komatsu, Jitka Svensson, Catherine Szanto, Sanae Kumakura and Isami Kinoshita for recommendations on soundscapes and gardens in Japan. Moreover, the author wishes to thank Martin Tunbjörk and Gábor Felcsuti at SWECO Acoustics in Malmö, Sweden, for evaluating the equipment used for sound pressure level measurements. Finally, the author wishes to thank three anonymous reviewers as well as Ida Isaksson for valuable comments on the manuscript.

Conflicts of Interest: The author declares no conflict of interest.

Appendix A

This appendix of Japanese gardens provides detailed information about all study visits that were carried out (Table A1).

Table A1. An overview indicating the numbers, names and locations of the studied gardens, as well as number of visits, dates for visits and total time spent in each garden.

Nr	Garden's Name	Location	Number of Visits	Date/s for Visits	Total Time Spent (min)
1	Hōsen-in	Ohara, Kyoto	1	10 April 2018	110
2	Sanzen-in	Ohara, Kyoto	1	10 April 2018	40
3	Shorin-in	Ohara, Kyoto	1	10 April 2018	40
4	Byōdō-in	Uji, Kyoto	1	12 December 2018	60
5	Chishaku-in	Kyoto	3	21 April 2018, 21 May 2018, 29 November 2018	240
6	Daikaku-ji	Kyoto	1	02 December 2018	70
7	Daisen-in	Kyoto	2	06 April 2018, 06 December 2018	60
8	Eikan-dō	Kyoto	2	18 April 2018, 29 November 2018	120
9	Enkō-ji	Kyoto	3	08 April 2018, 12 May 2018, 27 November 2018	315
10	Entsū-ji	Kyoto	1	19 April 2018	40
11	Fumon-in	Kyoto	2	24 April 2015, 30 April 2018	30
12	Funda-in	Kyoto	1	30 April 2018	100
13	Ginkaku-ji	Kyoto	3	23 April 2015, 04 April 2018, 20 December 2018	130
14	Giou-ji	Kyoto	1	02 December 2018	60
15	Gonaitei (Imperial palace)	Kyoto	1	01 December 2018	45
16	Goten (Ninna-ji)	Kyoto	1	02 December 2018	75
17	Hōnen-in	Kyoto	1	12 April 2018	30
18	Horai-no-niwa (Matsuno'o Taisha)	Kyoto	1	13 December 2018	40
19	Jōjuin	Kyoto	1	29 November 2018	45
20	Jōkō-no-niwa (Matsuno'o Taisha)	Kyoto	1	13 December 2018	40
21	Katsura Rikyū	Kyoto	2	24 April 2015, 04 April 2018	120
22	Kegon-ji	Kyoto	1	15 April 2018	30
23	Kennin-ji	Kyoto	1	16 April 2018	80
24	Kinkaku-ji	Kyoto	2	22 April 2015, 01 December 2018	60
25	Koetsu-ji	Kyoto	1	01 December 2018	20
26	Kōmyō-in	Kyoto	1	13 April 2018	30
27	Konchi-in	Kyoto	2	21 April 2018, 14 May 2018	150
28	Konpuku-ji	Kyoto	1	26 April 2018	30
29	Kyokusui-no-niwa (Matsuno'o Taisha)	Kyoto	1	13 December 2018	40
30	Manshu-in	Kyoto	1	27 November 2018	60
31	Murin-an	Kyoto	7	23 April 2015, 25 April 2015, 06 May 2018, 14 May 2018, 20 May 2018, 20 November 2018, 08 December 2018	365
32	Nanzen-in	Kyoto	2	18 April 2018, 14 May 2018	60
33	Nanzen-ji	Kyoto	2	23 April 2015, 05 April 2018	60
34	Nijō-jō	Kyoto	1	07 April 2018	80
35	Ōhashi-ke	Kyoto	1	13 April 2018	50
36	Oikeniwa (Imperial palace)	Kyoto	1	01 December 2018	20
37	Rurikoin	Kyoto	2	19 April 2018, 19 November 2018	270
38	Ryōan-ji	Kyoto	3	22 April 2015, 06 April 2018, 02 December 2018	160
39	Ryosoku-in	Kyoto	1	30 May 2018	20
40	Saihoji (Kokedera)	Kyoto	2	15 April 2018, 18 November 2018	270
41	Sanbō-in	Kyoto	1	23 April 2018	60
42	Sanjūsangendō	Kyoto	1	26 November 2018	15
43	Sentō Imperial Palace	Kyoto	2	18 April 2018, 05 December 2018	120
44	Shin'en (Heian Jingu)	Kyoto	2	09 April 2018, 05 May 2018	180
45	Shisen-dō	Kyoto	5	06 April 2018, 10 April 2018, 26 April 2018, 15 May 2018, 27 November 2018	240
46	Shōinan	Kyoto	1	23 April 2015	15
47	Shoren-in	Kyoto	2	23 April 2015, 28 April 2018	285
48	Shōsei-en	Kyoto	3	29 April 2018, 21 May 2018, 26 November 2018	210

Table A1. Cont.

Nr	Garden's Name	Location	Number of Visits	Date/s for Visits	Total Time Spent (min)
49	Shūgaku-in Rikyū	Kyoto	2	19 April 2018, 06 December 2018	180
50	Shūsui-tei	Kyoto	2	16 March 2018, 05 December 2018	30
51	Taizō-in	Kyoto	1	18 December 2018	90
52	Tenryū-ji	Kyoto	2	20 April 2018, 18 November 2018	95
53	Tōfuku-ji	Kyoto	3	24 April 2015, 07 April 2018, 20 November 2018	145
54	Zuihō-in	Kyoto	1	06 December 2018	60
55	Denbo-in Teien	Tokyo	1	14 March 2015	15
56	Hama-rikyu	Tokyo	1	20 October 2018	60
57	Kakuuntei	Tokyo	1	31 August 2018	30
58	Kiyosumi Teien	Tokyo	1	19 January 2019	45
59	Koishikawa-Kōrakuen	Tokyo	2	02 August 2015, 03 June 2018	80
60	Kyū-Furukawa Teien	Tokyo	1	19 August 2018	30
61	Kyu-Shiba-rikyu	Tokyo	1	20 October 2018	85
62	Mukōjima-Hyakkaen	Tokyo	1	19 January 2019	15
63	Nezu museum garden	Tokyo	1	08 September 2018	60
64	Rikugi-en	Tokyo	5	02 August 2015, 31 March 2018, 19 August 2018, 19 October 2018, 20 January 2019	320
65	Shinjuku Gyoen	Tokyo	2	09 April 2015, 30 March 2018	150
66	Gyokusen-en teien	Kanazawa	1	14 June 2018	40
67	Gyokusen-in-maru	Kanazawa	1	14 June 2018	10
68	Kenroku-en	Kanazawa	2	14 June 2018, 18 June 2018	120
69	Kurando Terashima teien	Kanazawa	1	18 June 2018	40
70	Nomura-ke Samurai teien	Kanazawa	2	14 June 2018, 15 June 2018	80
71	Oyama shrine pond garden	Kanazawa	1	14 June 2018	10
72	Seisonkaku	Kanazawa	1	14 June 2018	40
73	Shofukaku	Kanazawa	1	15 June 2018	40
74	Takada family home garden	Kanazawa	1	15 June 2018	10
75	Tsujike teien	Kanazawa	1	14 June 2018	30
76	Kōrakuen	Okayama	1	24 April 2018	60
77	Suizen-ji Joju-en	Kumamoto	1	21 February 2019	90
78	Kusano Honke	Hita	1	19 February 2019	15
79	Adachi Museum Garden	Matsue	1	22 February 2019	240
80	Ritsurin Kōen	Takamatsu	1	24 February 2019	170
81	Rentaroh Taki's Memorial garden	Taketa	2	20 February 2019, 21 February 2019	70
82	Isui-en	Nara	2	26 August 2015, 21 December 2018	100
83	Yoshiki-en	Nara	1	21 December 2018	50
84	Keitakuen	Osaka	1	15 December 2018	60
85	Takayama Jin'ya	Takayama	1	16 June 2018	30
86	Shukkeien	Hiroshima	1	15 July 2015	20
87	Shiki-naen	Naha	1	24 June 2018	100
88	Shuri-jo	Naha	1	24 June 2018	45
	Total: 88 gardens		Total: 136 visits		Total: 7750 min (= 129 h)

References

1. Stauskis, G. Japanese gardens outside of Japan: From the export of art to the art of export. *Town Plan. Archit.* **2011**, *35*, 212–221. [CrossRef]
2. Itō, T. *The Japanese Garden; An Approach to Nature*; Yale University Press: New Haven, CT, USA, 1972.
3. Nitschke, G. *Japanese Gardens: Right Angle and Natural Form*; Taschen: Köln, Germany, 1999.
4. Slawson, D.A. *Secret Teachings in the Art of Japanese Gardens: Design Principles, Aesthetic Values*; Kodansha International: Tokyo, Japan, 1987.
5. Takei, J.; Keane, M.P. *Sakuteiki: Visions of the Japanese Garden*; Tuttle Publishing: Tokyo, Japan, 2011.
6. Byoung, E.; Kaplan, R. The perception of landscape style: A cross-cultural comparison. *Landsc. Urban Plan.* **1990**, *19*, 251–262. [CrossRef]
7. Goto, S. Visual preference for garden design: Appreciation of the Japanese garden. *J. Ther. Hortic.* **2012**, *22*, 24–37.
8. Yang, B.-E.; Brown, T.J. A cross-cultural comparison of preferences for landscape styles and landscape elements. *Environ. Behav.* **1992**, *24*, 471–507. [CrossRef]
9. Elsadek, M.; Sun, M.; Sugiyama, R.; Fujii, E. Cross-cultural comparison of physiological and psychological responses to different garden styles. *Urban For. Urban Green.* **2019**, *38*, 74–83. [CrossRef]

10. Twedt, E.; Rainey, R.M.; Proffitt, D.R. Designed natural spaces: Informal gardens are perceived to be more restorative than formal gardens. *Front. Psychol.* **2016**, *7*, 88. [CrossRef] [PubMed]
11. Orians, G.H. An ecological and evolutionary approach to landscape aesthetics. In *Landscape Meanings and Values*; Penning-Rowsell, E.C., Lowenthal, D., Eds.; Allen & Unwin: London, UK, 1986.
12. Goto, S.; Gianfagia, T.J.; Munafo, J.P.; Fujii, E.; Shen, X.; Sun, M.; Shi, B.E.; Liu, C.; Hamano, H.; Herrup, K. The power of traditional design techniques: The effects of viewing a Japanese garden on individuals with cognitive impairment. *HERD* **2017**, *10*, 74–86. [CrossRef]
13. Goto, S.; Park, B.-J.; Tsunetsugu, Y.; Herrup, K.; Miyazaki, Y. The effect of garden designs on mood and heart output in older adults residing in an assisted living facility. *HERD* **2013**, *6*, 27–42. [CrossRef]
14. Fridh, K. *Japanska Rum: Om Tomhet och Föränderlighet i Traditionell och Nutida Japansk Arkitektur [Japanese Space: On Emptiness and Temporality in Traditional and Contemporary Japanese Architecture]*; Svensk byggtjänst: Stockholm, Sweden, 2004.
15. Senoglu, B.; Oktay, E.; Kinoshita, I. Visitors' perception of high-rise building effect on the scenery of traditional gardens: A case study in Hama-Rikyu gardens, Tokyo. *Civil Eng. Archit.* **2018**, *6*, 136–148. [CrossRef]
16. Itō, T. *Space and Illusion in the Japanese Garden*; Weatherhill: New York, NY, USA, 1973.
17. UN. *World Urbanization Prospects: The 2018 Revision*; Department of Economic and Social Affairs, United Nations: San Francisco, CA, USA, 2018.
18. Godfrey, R.; Julien, M. Urbanisation and health. *Clin. Med.* **2005**, *5*, 137–141. [CrossRef]
19. Danielsson, M.; Heimerson, I.; Lundberg, U.; Perski, A.; Stefansson, C.-G.; Åkerstedt, T. Psychosocial stress and health problems: Health in Sweden: The national public health report 2012. Chapter 6. *Scand. J. Public Health* **2012**, *40*, 121–134. [CrossRef] [PubMed]
20. Pálsdóttir, A.M.; Sempik, J.; Bird, W.; Van den Bosch, M. Using Nature as A Treatment Option. In *Oxford Textbook of Nature and Public Health: The Role of Nature in Improving the Health of a Population*; van den Bosch, M., Bird, W., Eds.; Oxford University Press: Oxford, UK, 2018.
21. Song, C.; Ikei, H.; Miyazaki, Y. Physiological effects of nature therapy: A review of the research in Japan. *Int. J. Environ. Res. Public Health* **2016**, *13*, 781. [CrossRef] [PubMed]
22. Pheasant, R.; Horoshenkov, K.; Watts, G.; Barrett, B. The acoustic and visual factors influencing the construction of tranquil space in urban and rural environments tranquil spaces-quiet places? *J. Acoust. Soc. Am.* **2008**, *123*, 1446–1457. [CrossRef] [PubMed]
23. Wang, R.; Zhao, J. A good sound in the right place: Exploring the effects of auditory-visual combinations on aesthetic preference. *Urban For. Urban Green.* **2019**, *43*, 126356. [CrossRef]
24. WHO. *Environmental Noise Guidelines for the European Region*; World Health Organization Regional Office for Europe: Copenhagen, Denmark, 2018.
25. Aletta, F.; Oberman, T.; Kang, J. Associations between positive health-related effects and soundscapes perceptual constructs: A systematic review. *Int. J. Environ. Res. Public Health* **2018**, *15*, 2392. [CrossRef] [PubMed]
26. Steele, D. Bridging the Gap from Soundscape Research to Urban Planning and Design Practice: How do Professionals Conceptualize, Work with, and Seek Information about Sound? Ph.D. Thesis, McGill University, Montreal, QC, Canada, 2018.
27. Cerwén, G. Sound in Landscape Architecture: A Soundscape Approach to Noise. Ph.D. Thesis, Swedish University of Agricultural Sciences, Alnarp, Sweden, 2017.
28. Southworth, M. The sonic environment of cities. *Environ. Behav.* **1969**, *1*, 49–70.
29. Truax, B. Soundscape studies: An introduction to the World Soundscape Project. *Numus-West* **1974**, *5*, 36–39.
30. Schafer, R.M. *The Soundscape: Our Sonic Environment and the Tuning of the World*; Destiny Books: Rochester, VT, USA, 1994 [1977].
31. Kang, J.; Aletta, F. The impact and outreach of soundscape research. *Environments* **2018**, *5*, 58. [CrossRef]
32. Kang, J.; Aletta, F.; Gjestland, T.T.; Brown, L.A.; Botteldooren, D.; Schulte-Fortkamp, B.; Lercher, P.; van Kamp, I.; Genuit, K.; Fiebig, A.; et al. Ten questions on the soundscapes of the built environment. *Build. Environ.* **2016**, *108*, 284–294. [CrossRef]
33. Axelsson, Ö. Designing Soundscape for Sustainable Urban Development. In Proceedings of the Environment and Health Administration, Stockholm, Sweden, 30 September–1 October 2010.
34. ISO. *ISO 12913-1:2014 Acoustics-Soundscape—Part 1: Definition and Conceptual Framework*; ISO: Geneva, Switzerland, 2014.

35. Brown, A.L.; Muhar, A. An approach to the acoustic design of outdoor space. *J. Environ. Plan. Manag.* **2004**, *47*, 827–842. [CrossRef]
36. Cerwén, G.; Kreutzfeldt, J.; Wingren, C. Soundscape actions: A tool for noise treatment based on three workshops in landscape architecture. *Front. Archit. Res.* **2017**, *6*, 504–518. [CrossRef]
37. Lacey, J. *Sonic Rupture: A Practice-led Approach to Urban Soundscape Design*; Bloomsbury: New York, NY, USA, 2016.
38. Hellström, B.; Torehammar, C.; Malm, P.; Grundfelt, G. *Stadens Ljud—Akustisk Design & Hållbar Stadsutveckling [City Sounds—Acoustic Design and Sustainable Development]*; Exploateringskontoret: Stockholm, Sweden, 2013.
39. Zhang, M.; Kang, J. Towards the evaluation, description, and creation of soundscapes in urban open spaces. *Environ. Plan. B Plan. Des.* **2007**, *34*, 68–86. [CrossRef]
40. Sowa, H. The Study on the Soundscape of Three Japanese Gardens. In Proceedings of the 2nd International Conference, Archi-Cultural Translations through the Silk Road, Nishinomiya, Japan, 14–16 July 2012; Mukogawa Women's University: Nishinomiya, Japan.
41. Szanto, C. The Polysensory Dynamics of Ambiance. Exemple of a Japanese Garden (Murin-An). In Proceedings of the Ambiances, tomorrow, 3rd Conference on Ambiances, Volos, Greece, 21–24 September 2016; Rémy, N., Tixier, N., Eds.; University of Thessaly: Volos, Greece, 2016; pp. 683–688.
42. Fowler, M.D. Sound as a considered design parameter in the Japanese garden. *Stud. Hist. Gard. Des. Landsc. An Int. Q.* **2015**, *35*, 312–327. [CrossRef]
43. Fowler, M.D. *Sound Worlds of Japanese Gardens: An Interdisciplinary Approach to Spatial Thinking*; Transcript Verlag: Wetzlar, Germany, 2014.
44. Torigoe, K. A Soniferous Garden of Rentaroh. In *Hearing Places: Sound, Place, Time and Culture*; Bandt, R., Duffy, M., MacKinnon, D., Eds.; Cambridge Scholars Publishing: Newcastle Upon Tyne, UK, 2007.
45. Ellis, C.; Adams, T.; Bochner, A.P. Autoethnography: An overview. *Forum Qual. Soc. Res.* **2011**, *12*. [CrossRef]
46. Lawaczeck Körner, K. *Walking Along Wandering off and Going Astray: A Critical Normativity Approach to Walking as a Situated Architectural Experience*; Department of Architecture and Built Environment, Lund University: Lund, Sweden, 2016.
47. Philips, C. Experiencing Constructed Landscapes: The Use of Autoethnography in the Practice of Architectural History. In Proceedings of the AUDIENCE: The 28th Annual SAHANZ Conference, Brisbane, Australia, 7–10 July 2011; Moulis, A., van der Plaat, D., Eds.; Sahanz: Brisbane, Australia, 2011; pp. 1–17.
48. Dahlin, F.; Berglind, L. Ljudupplevelser: En Vidgad Förståelse för Urbana Ljud som Kvalitet. [Sonic Experiences: An Expanded Understanding for Urban Sounds as Quality]. Master Thesis, Swedish University of Agricultural Sciences, Alnarp, Sweden, 2018.
49. Wingren, C. En Landskapsarkitekts Konstnärliga Praktik: Kunskapsutveckling via en Självbiografisk Studie. [The Artistic Practice of a Landscape Architect: Knowledge Development through an Autobiographical Study]. Ph.D. Thesis, Department of Landscape Architecture, Swedish University of Agricultural Sciences, Alnarp, Sweden, 2009.
50. Axelsson, Ö.; Nilsson, M.E.; Berglund, B. A principal components model of soundscape perception. *J. Acoust. Soc. Am.* **2010**, *128*, 2836–2846. [CrossRef]
51. Yang, W.; Kang, J. Acoustic comfort evaluation in urban open public spaces. *Appl. Acoust.* **2005**, *66*, 211–229. [CrossRef]
52. Hong, J.Y.; Jeon, J.Y. Influence of urban contexts on soundscape perceptions: A structural equation modeling approach. *Landsc. Urban Plan.* **2015**, *141*, 78–87. [CrossRef]
53. Cross, N. Designerly ways of knowing: Design discipline versus design science. *Des. Issues* **2001**, *17*, 49–55. [CrossRef]
54. Hedfors, P.; Berg, P.G. Site Interpretation by Skilled Listeners—Methods for Communicating Soundscapes in Landscape Architecture and Planning. In *Soundscape Studies and Methods*; Järviluoma, H., Wagstaff, G., Eds.; Finnish Society for Ethnomusicology: Helsinki, Finland, 2002.
55. Hedfors, P.; Berg, P.G. The sounds of two landscape settings: Auditory concepts for physical planning and design. *Landsc. Res.* **2003**, *28*, 245–263. [CrossRef]
56. Amphoux, P. *L'identité Sonore des Villes Européennes: Guide Méthodologique. [The Sonic Identity of European Cities: Methodological Guide]*; CRESSON: Grenoble, France, 1993.
57. Le Roux, C.S. Exploring rigour in autoethnographic research. *Int. J. Soc. Res. Methodol.* **2017**, *20*, 195–207. [CrossRef]

58. Anderson, L. Analytic autoethnography. *J. Contemp. Ethnogr.* **2006**, *35*, 373–395. [CrossRef]
59. Kardous, C.A.; Shaw, P.B. Evaluation of smartphone sound measurement applications. *J. Acoust. Soc. Am.* **2014**, *135*, EL186–EL192. [CrossRef] [PubMed]
60. Murphy, E.; King, E.A. Testing the accuracy of smartphones and sound level meter applications for measuring environmental noise. *Appl. Acoust.* **2016**, *106*, 16–22. [CrossRef]
61. Cerwén, G.; Wingren, C.; Qviström, M. Evaluating soundscape intentions in landscape architecture: A study of competition entries for a new cemetery in Järva, Stockholm. *J. Environ. Plan. Manag.* **2017**, *60*, 1253–1275. [CrossRef]
62. Kuitert, W. *Themes in the History of Japanese Garden Art*; University of Hawaii Press: Honolulu, HI, USA, 2002.
63. Van Renterghem, T.; Attenborough, K.; Jean, P. Designing Vegetation and Tree Belts along Roads. In *Environmental Methods for Transport Noise Reduction*; Nilsson, M., Bengtsson, J., Klæboe, R., Eds.; CRC Press (Imprint of Taylor & Francis): Boca Raton, FL, USA, 2015.
64. HOSANNA. *Novel Solutions for Quieter and Greener Cities*; EU FP7: Bandhagen, Sweden, 2013.
65. Bucur, V. *Urban Forest Acoustics*; Springer: Berlin, Germany, 2006.
66. Van Renterghem, T. Towards explaining the positive effect of vegetation on the perception of environmental noise. *Urban For. Urban Green.* **2019**, *40*, 133–144. [CrossRef]
67. Attenborough, K.; Taherzadeh, S.; Bashir, I.; Forssén, J.; Van der Aa, B.; Männel, M. Porous Ground, Crops, and Buried Resonators. In *Environmental Methods for Transport Noise Reduction*; Nilsson, M., Bengtsson, J., Klæboe, R., Eds.; CRC Press (Imprint of Taylor & Francis): Boca Raton, FL, USA, 2015.
68. Forssén, J.; Kropp, W.; Kihlman, T. Introduction to Traffic Noise Abatement. In *Environmental Methods for Transport Noise Reduction*; Nilsson, M., Bengtsson, J., Klæboe, R., Eds.; CRC Press (Imprint of Taylor & Francis): Boca Raton, FL, USA, 2015.
69. Nordström, U. *Moss*; Penguin Books, Ltd., Michael Joseph: London, UK, 2019.
70. Ratcliffe, E.; Gatersleben, B.; Sowden, P.T. Bird sounds and their contributions to perceived attention restoration and stress recovery. *J. Environ. Psychol.* **2013**, *36*, 221–228. [CrossRef]
71. Yu, L.; Kang, J. Factors influencing the sound preference in urban open spaces. *Appl. Acoust.* **2010**, *71*, 622–633. [CrossRef]
72. Galbrun, L.; Ali, T.T. Acoustical and perceptual assessment of water sounds and their use over road traffic noise. *J. Acoust. Soc. Am.* **2013**, *133*, 227–237. [CrossRef]
73. Moore, B.C.J. *An Introduction to the Psychology of Hearing*; Emerald: Bingley, UK, 2012.
74. Brown, A.L.; Rutherford, S. Using the sound of water in the city. *Landsc. Aust.* **1994**, *2*, 103–107.
75. Hedfors, P. Site Soundscapes: Landscape Architecture in the Light of Sound. Ph.D. Thesis, Swedish University of Agricultural Sciences, Uppsala, Sweden, 2003.
76. Nilsson, M.E.; Berglund, B. Soundscape quality in suburban green areas and city parks. *Acta Acust. United Acust.* **2006**, *92*, 903–911.
77. Hao, Y.; Kang, J.; Wortche, H. Assessment of the masking effects of birdsong on the road traffic noise environment. *J. Acoust. Soc. Am.* **2016**, *140*, 978. [CrossRef] [PubMed]
78. Botteldooren, D.; Andringa, T.C.; Aspuru, I.; Brown, A.L.; Dubois, D.; Guastavino, C.; Kang, J.; Lavandier, C.; Nilsson, M.E.; Preis, A.; et al. From Sonic Environment to Soundscape. In *Soundscape and the Built Environment*; Kang, J., Schulte-Fortkamp, B., Eds.; Taylor & Francis Group: Boca Raton, FL, USA, 2016; pp. 1–16.
79. Schaeffer, P. *Traité des Objets Musicaux: Essai Interdisciplines [Treatise on Musical Objects: An Essay across Disciplines]*; Seuil: Paris, France, 1966.
80. Nikolajew, M. At Læse Vandet: Et Redskab til Analyse af Vandkunst og Fontæner [Reading the Water: An Approach to the Analysis of Water Art and Fountains]. Ph.D. Thesis, The Royal Danish Academy of Fine Arts, København, Denmark, 2003.
81. Halprin, L. *Cities*; MIT Press: Cambridge, MA, USA, 1973.
82. Rådsten Ekman, M. Unwanted Wanted Sounds: Perception of Sounds from Water Structures in Urban Soundscapes. Ph.D. Thesis, Stockholm University, Stockholm, Sweden, 2015.
83. Shikibu, M. *Tale of Genji*; Tuttle Publishing: North Clarendon, Vermont, 2011.
84. Yang, S.; Xie, H.; Mao, H.; Xia, T.; Cheng, Y.; Li, H. A summary of the spatial construction of soundscape in chinese gardens. In Proceedings of the 22nd International Congress on Acoustics, ICA 2016, Buenos Aires, Argentina, 5–9 September 2016.

85. Cerwén, G.; Pedersen, E.; Pálsdóttir, A.M. The role of soundscape in nature-based rehabilitation: A patient perspective. *Int. J. Environ. Res. Public Health* **2016**, *13*, 1229. [CrossRef] [PubMed]
86. Aletta, F.; Kang, J.; Astolfi, A.; Fuda, S. Differences in soundscape appreciation of walking sounds from different footpath materials in urban parks. *Sustain. Cities Soc.* **2016**, *27*, 367–376. [CrossRef]
87. Dawson, K.J. Flight, fancy, and the garden's song. *Landsc. J.* **1988**, *7*, 170–175. [CrossRef]
88. DeGraaf, R.M. *Trees, Shrubs, and Vines for Attracting Birds*; University Press of New England: Hanover, Germany, 2002.
89. Forman, R.T.T. *Urban Ecology: Science of Cities*; Cambridge University Press: Cambridge, UK, 2014.
90. Ueyakato Landscape: Nanzen-in Temple. Available online: https://ueyakato.jp/en/gardens/nanzenin/ (accessed on 18 October 2018).
91. Truax, B. *Acoustic Communication*; Ablex Publishing: Westport, CT, USA, 2001.
92. Pálsdóttir, A.M.; Persson, D.; Persson, B.; Grahn, P. The journey of recovery and empowerment embraced by nature—Clients' perspectives on nature-based rehabilitation in relation to the role of the natural environment. *Int. J. Environ. Res. Public Health* **2014**, *11*, 7094–7115. [CrossRef]
93. Kaplan, R.; Kaplan, S. *The Experience of Nature: A Psychological Perspective*; Cambridge University Press: Cambridge, UK, 1989.
94. Bild, E.; Coler, M.; Pfeffer, K.; Bertolini, L. Considering sound in planning and designing public spaces. *J. Plan. Lit.* **2016**, *31*, 419–434. [CrossRef]
95. Brown, A.L. Soundscapes and environmental noise management. *Noise Control Eng. J.* **2010**, *58*, 493–500. [CrossRef]

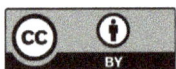

© 2019 by the author. Licensee MDPI, Basel, Switzerland. This article is an open access article distributed under the terms and conditions of the Creative Commons Attribution (CC BY) license (http://creativecommons.org/licenses/by/4.0/).

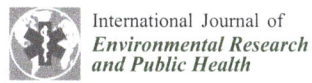

Article

Implementation of Quiet Areas in Sweden

Gunnar Cerwén [1,*,†] and **Frans Mossberg [2]**

1. Department of Landscape Architecture, Planning and Management, Swedish University of Agricultural Sciences, 230 53 Alnarp, Sweden
2. Sound Environment Center, Lund University, 222 10 Lund, Sweden; frans.mossberg@kultur.lu.se
* Correspondence: gunnar.cerwen@slu.se
† Parts of this work have been presented previously at the 2018 Euronoise in Crete, Greece, and the 2018 AESOP Congress in Gothenburg, Sweden. The study has also been described in a research report entitled "Tysta områden i Sverige" from the Sound Environment Center at Lund University, Sweden.

Received: 26 November 2018; Accepted: 20 December 2018; Published: 7 January 2019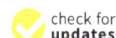

Abstract: The notion of quiet areas has received increasing attention within the EU in recent years. The EU Environmental Noise Directive (END) of 2002 stipulates that member states should map existing quiet areas and formulate strategies to keep these quiet. Quiet areas could play an important role in balancing densified urban development by ensuring access to relative quietness and associated health benefits. This paper reports on a recent study investigating how the notion of quiet areas has been implemented in Sweden. The study, initiated by the Sound Environment Center in 2017, was carried out in two phases. In phase one, an overview of the current situation was obtained by scrutinizing regional and municipal mapping initiatives, aided by a short digital questionnaire sent out to all 290 municipalities in Sweden. This provided a general understanding and highlighted initiatives for further study in phase two. The results revealed that 41% (n = 118) of Sweden's municipalities include quiet areas in their general plans, but that significantly fewer of these have sophisticated strategies for implementation (n = 16; 6%). Moreover, the interest in quiet areas in municipalities does not seem to be directly related to the END, but is instead inspired by previous regional initiatives in Sweden. The study highlights a number of considerations and examples of how quiet areas are approached in Sweden today. In general, Sweden has come a long way in terms of identifying and mapping quiet areas, but more progress is needed in developing strategies to protect, maintain, and publicize quiet areas.

Keywords: quiet areas; environmental noise; noise abatement; soundscape design; landscape planning; urban planning; general plan; sustainability

1. Introduction

In the EU's Environmental Noise Directive (END) of 2002 (2002/49/EC) [1], member states are asked to make an inventory of existing quiet areas and devise strategies for their protection. The whole concept of quiet areas could be regarded as a way to turn the question of sound environment around, to focus on potential positive qualities of the sound environment and not only on noise and disturbances. The concept connects to tendencies in cultural and general environmental movements of the time with roots back in the soundscape movement [2] and acknowledges the fact that sound may have positive health effects [3].

Sweden is known as one of the countries in Europe working more actively with quiet areas, including several initiatives on regional and municipal level. This could be related to Sweden's early implementation of the soundscape perspective in research on environmental noise, not least through the Mistra project "Soundscape for better health" [4], carried out between 2000 and 2007, in which the notion of "quiet façade" was introduced.

Recent exposure data from the European Environment Agency (EEA) demonstrate that more than 100 million European citizens are negatively affected by high noise levels, impacting human health [5]. The World Health Organization estimates that one million healthy life-years in Western Europe are lost annually as a result of exposure to traffic noise [6]. Noise has been shown to have severe negative effects on health, including hearing damage, sleep disturbance, hypertension, and cardiovascular disease [7,8].

The situation in Sweden concerning exposure to traffic noise, and to airborne particles, in the immediate vicinity of permanent dwellings has become increasingly problematic since the introduction of more relaxed noise regulations by the Swedish government in 2015 [9], in response to political pressure [10]. In sharp contrast to the scientific advice from the research community on health and the environment, more noise is now permitted close to people's dwellings than was the case before the updates to the legislation. This proved to be politically acceptable because of an urgent need for housing, but also because of building industry and business interests. The higher threshold levels now in place mean that, in principle, unlimited noise is permitted on the noisiest side of dwellings in noise-exposed urban areas [9,11].

The recently published Environmental Noise Guidelines for the European Region [7] define the aim of these guiding principles as reducing noise while conserving quiet areas. Based on previous research [12–14], the report states that "people appreciate quiet areas as beneficial for their health and well-being, especially in urban areas" [7]. A growing number of studies indicate that exposure to natural sounds may have positive health effects by reducing stress [3]. Thus quiet areas not only protect against noise, but also reveal positive sounds that would otherwise be masked by noise.

Urban areas around the world are currently facing new challenges, as there is increasing demand for densification related to sustainability. In order to safeguard the quality of parks and other recreational spaces in the future, quiet areas are likely to become even more important, not only in cities, but also in the vicinity of cities and in open country.

There are good reasons to build on the notion of quiet areas, as postulated in the END [1]. The present study investigated how the concept has been implemented in regional and municipal contexts in Sweden. The results may be useful as reference for further implementation of the concept in Sweden and other countries, as well as informing future strategies and guidelines on EU level.

2. Materials and Methods

The study comprised two phases: a quantitative phase providing an overview of the situation in Sweden and a qualitative phase in which chosen examples were studied further.

In phase one, an overview was made and background information on quiet areas in Sweden was obtained by studying government documents and reports dealing with quiet areas. The internet was searched extensively and key individuals were contacted. The outcomes are described in Section 3 of this paper.

Based on the findings, a subdivision was made into regional and municipal initiatives when selecting examples for further studies. The regional initiatives were studied manually, by going through reports and other documents describing these. A total of 10 initiatives were identified and are described in Section 4. In order to study municipal initiatives, an email was sent out to the registrar of all 290 municipal authorities in Sweden. The email included a short description of the project and a digital questionnaire containing three introductory questions on how the municipality works with quiet areas, which the registrar was asked to redirect to the appropriate department. These questions were intended to provide an overview of the extent to which the concept of quiet areas appears in the municipalities' general plans (Question 2) and to identify initiatives for further study (Questions 1 and 2). Question 3 was included to obtain contact details. For Questions 1 and 2, a set of pre-given options was provided, plus a box for comments:

1. Is there any area in your municipality that has been designated a quiet area, a noise-free area or anything corresponding to this? 1a) Yes, in an urban setting. 1b) Yes, in a rural setting. 1c) No, not at all. 1d) Other (comment box).
2. Is "quiet areas" included as a question to be dealt with in your municipality's general plan? 2a) Yes, elaborated. 2b) Yes, briefly. 2c) No, our municipality does not have a need for quiet areas. 2d) No, but we have discussed implementation in our future plan. 2e) No, and it has not been up for discussion. 2f) Other (comment box).
3. Is there anyone at the municipality we can contact for follow-up questions? (please supply email address/es).

Within one month, during which two reminders were sent out, 208 of the municipalities had answered (response rate 71.7%).

In order to provide a full overview for question 2, the remaining 82 municipalities were investigated manually by means of a digital search in their respective general plans. The search words used were "quiet" (Swedish: tyst) and "noise-free" (bullerfri). In this way, it was determined whether each of these municipalities deals with quiet areas or not. Moreover, if it was found that the municipality mentioned quiet areas, it was determined whether this mention was brief or comprehensive (corresponding to the alternatives in Question 2). Any other trends or noteworthy issues were entered in an Excel spreadsheet.

A total of 47 municipalities were identified in phase one as interesting for further study. This selection was based on answers given to the questions and information obtained in the manual search of general plans. Moreover, some initiatives were added to this group based on searches on the internet and tips from the public (the project generated media attention that encouraged some people to make contact).

In phase two of the study, the 47 chosen initiatives were investigated further to obtain more information about how quiet areas are treated in Sweden. Furthermore, efforts were made to identify municipalities that had taken action and to explain why others had not taken any action at all. We also sought to identify and discuss general tendencies, challenges, and future possibilities.

Data were collected in phase two through different methods. Initially, a more detailed questionnaire was sent out to municipalities selected for further study. This questionnaire was sent out digitally to email addresses obtained in response to Question 3 in the first digital questionnaire. The detailed questionnaire consisted of 23 questions that dealt with how the municipality had gained inspiration for its work on quiet areas, if there were any measures to protect the quiet areas, and if these areas were used in marketing and tourism, as well as general questions about the level of knowledge and potential for improvement. After one month and one reminder, 25 out of 47 questionnaires were returned (53.2% response rate). Further correspondence followed in some cases.

Results from both research phases are reported below, starting with an overview of how the notion of quiet areas has developed in Sweden and the EU, and important initiatives and definitions (Section 3). We then go on to describe how the concept is used in Sweden, on regional level (Section 4) and municipal level (Section 5). This is followed by a discussion of general trends and challenges identified (Section 6) and conclusions (Section 7).

3. Quiet Areas: Background and Definitions

In Sweden, the notion of quiet areas can be traced to the late 1990s, when the Swedish Road Administration initiated a pilot project in which two municipalities in Jönköping County were mapped for relative quietness [15]. Within a few years, similar mapping initiatives had been undertaken in two other counties [16,17] and in major urban regions [18,19]. Several of these initiatives were connected to a collaborative project officially launched in 2002 with the purpose of developing a method for inventory of quiet areas [20]. The collaboration involved influential stakeholders, such as the Road Administration, the Rail Administration, the National Board of Housing, the Civil Aviation Administration, the Environmental Protection Agency, and two major county councils. The project finished in 2005 [21], and the outcomes were made accessible in an influential report entitled "A Good Sound Environment—More than Merely Absence of Noise" published by the Swedish Environmental Protection Agency [22].

The method used in the collaborative project was based on the assumption that disturbances vary depending on context, and it considers areas divided into five different noise classes (A–E). Noise class A has the highest demands; it corresponds to areas completely free from community noise, such as remote areas in the mountains, forests, and national parks. The benchmark for noise class A is set at 25 dBA (A-weighted instantaneous sound pressure level), whereas the class with the next-highest demand, noise-class B, has a benchmark of 35 dBA. Noise classes C and D are intended for forests and recreation areas in proximity to urban developments and are both based on a benchmark of 45 dBA (instantaneous), but what is called the "exceeding time" differs. The lowest demands are found in noise class E, where the benchmark is set to 45–50 dBA (equivalent), or 10–20 dBA lower than the surrounding sound pressure level. Noise class E is intended to be applied in urban areas such as parks.

In the EU, the development of quiet areas can be traced back to 1996 and the document "Green Paper on Future Noise Policy" [23], where it is mentioned how noise mapping could be used to identify quiet areas. The thoughts raised in this green paper are enforced in the END [1]. However, the instructions in the END are relatively vague, which has resulted in different interpretations and implementations.

In 2014, "The Good Practice Guide on Quiet Areas" [24] followed up on the END by mapping how the question had been dealt with, through examining existing examples and initiatives. The report provided a good overview of existing initiatives in Europe. No specific recommendations were given, but it was suggested that the review could be used as inspiration and reference was made to "competent authorities" for further guidance.

In 2016, the report "Quiet Areas in Europe: The Environment Unaffected by Noise Pollution" [25] introduced a method called Quietness Suitability Index (QSI) for identifying quiet areas in rural contexts. The QSI approach makes use of existing noise mapping data combined with land use data to identify areas that are potentially quiet. No applications of the method have been made yet in Sweden.

The END [1] distinguishes between two different kinds of quiet areas, "open country" and "agglomerations", which are defined as follows:

"A quiet area in open country' shall mean an area, delimited by the competent authority, that is undisturbed by noise from traffic, industry or recreational activities."

"A quiet area in an agglomeration' shall mean an area, delimited by the competent authority, for instance which is not exposed to a value of Lden or of another appropriate noise indicator greater than a certain value set by the Member State, from any noise source."

In both definitions, the END refers to the "competent authority" of the member state. In Sweden, the competent authority can be said to correspond to the collaboration group mentioned above and the noise classes it proposed [22]. Thus in Sweden, the END definition for rural settings can be said to correspond to noise classes A and B, while the END definition for urban settings corresponds to noise class E. Noise classes C and D, are intermediate, suggesting that there is scope for a third type of quiet area, i.e., those in 'proximity to urban areas'.

The collaboration group's noise classes have been influential for assessing and mapping quiet areas in Sweden. Many of the municipalities in Sweden refer to the benchmarks suggested in the method. However, there are other values that do not relate to this framework. For instance, two benchmarks, 30 dBA and 40dBA, which are still used relatively frequently, derive from early regional initiatives in Sweden undertaken by the Road Administration [16,17] and an earlier version of the collaboration group's method [20].

Moreover, it is common for the benchmarks to be adjusted, depending on the context in which the noise classes are applied and the data available. In most of the initiatives studied here, only one or two of the classes were used. Non-acoustic factors were influential when quiet areas were defined, including accessibility, natural qualities, and cultural qualities.

More recently, two new methods have been proposed in Sweden [26,27], as well as the QSI on EU level [25], but it is too soon to assess how they are being applied in Sweden.

4. Regional Initiatives in Sweden

On regional level, a total of 10 initiatives, together covering 121 municipalities, were recorded (see Figure 1a). As can be seen from the map, some of these regional initiatives overlap each other. These areas, indicated with darker color on the map, correspond to some of the most densely populated areas in Sweden, which could be a result of more extensive noise problems in these areas. Moreover, it is interesting to note that, of the 15 municipalities found to have carried out more far-reaching work on quiet areas (see Section 5.1 and Figure 1b), all except one had been preceded by a regional initiative. This suggests that regional initiatives are an important catalyst for implementation of quiet areas.

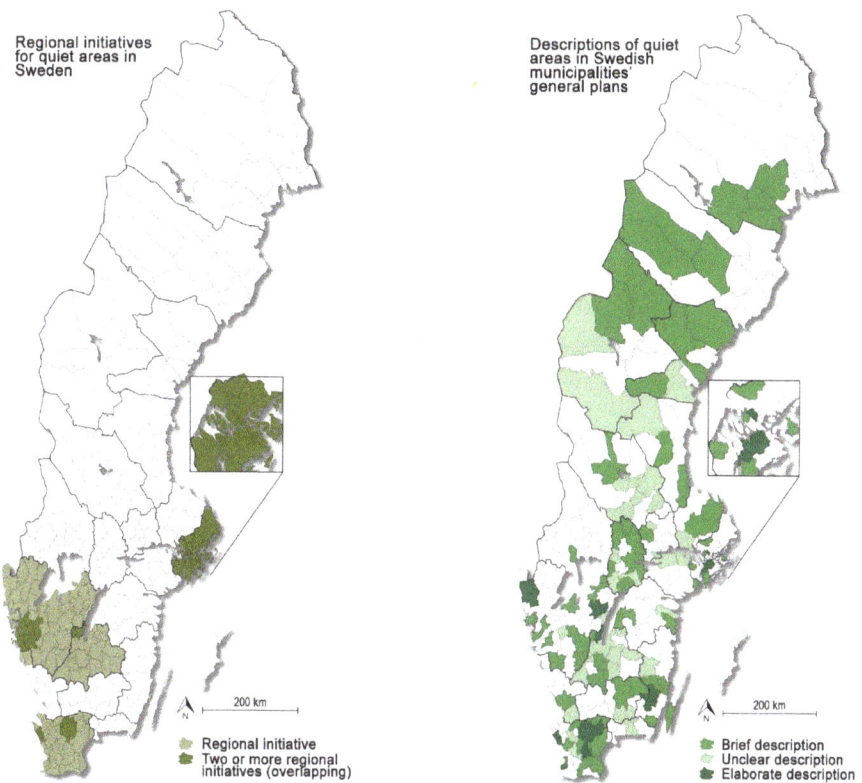

Figure 1. (a) Location of regional initiatives for quiet areas in Sweden. Overlapping initiatives are marked with darker color. (b) Location of municipalities that describe quiet areas in their general plans, with these descriptions divided into three categories: brief, unclear, and elaborate.

A short summary of the regional initiatives is presented below, following the chronological order of introduction within the respective region (see Table 1 for an overview).

The first regional initiative was that in Jönköping County by the Swedish Road Administration, in 1998 [15]. Starting from a 30 dBA level equivalent for the noise sources mapped (road, industry, rail, and recreational activities), four quiet areas were identified. Seventeen years later, Jönköping County Council conducted mapping for the whole county on the methodological basis of GIS data [26]. The method was presented as potentially useful for other areas in Sweden as a cost-effective method for modeling larger areas, including vegetation data. By including vegetation data, it was found that it was possible to increase the number of quiet areas. The mapping took account not only of human wellbeing, but also of wildlife. Five categories were introduced, described with words rather than decibel levels. The mapping revealed that 22% of the area of Jönköping County fell within the strictest category, i.e., free from noise.

Table 1. Overview of regional 'quiet area' initiatives in Sweden.

Region:	Year:	Term Used:	Type of Setting:	Benchmark:	Identified Area/s:
Jönköping County [15]	1998	Quiet areas	Rural	30 dBA (equivalent)	4 areas
Jönköping County [26]	2015	Undisturbed areas	Rural/Urban proximity	Undisturbed (approximately 40 dBA)	Illustrated coverage (22% of county area)
Västra Götaland County [17]	2001	Quiet areas	Rural	30 dBA (equivalent)	Illustrated coverage (at least half of county area)
Gothenburg region [28]	2014	Quiet areas	Rural/Urban proximity	45 dBA (max and equivalent), stricter for some events	9 areas
Scania County [16]	2003	Noise free areas	Rural/Urban proximity	30 dBA and 40 dBA (equivalent)	Illustrated coverage in maps
Scania County [29]	2004	Noise free areas	Rural/Urban	40 dBA (equivalent)	7 areas (4 urban and 3 rural)
Stockholm region [19]	2000	Quiet areas	Urban proximity	45 dBA (equivalent, year)	Quiet areas in green wedges
Stockholm region [30]	2005	Quiet areas	Urban proximity	45 dBA (instantaneous)	5 areas studied
Stockholm region [31]	2010	Quiet areas	Urban proximity	45 dBA (equivalent)	Illustrated coverage in maps
Stockholm County [27]	2016	Noise free areas	Rural/Urban/Urban proximity	Four noise classes (20–40 dBA equivalent day/evening)	Proposed methodology for mapping

Västra Götaland County in Western Sweden mapped its quiet areas in 2001 [17]. A benchmark of 30 dBA (equivalent, year) was used and, despite this relatively strict value, it was found that more than half of the area in the county qualified. In that case, the mapping of noise data was coordinated with land use, and quiet areas with experiential potential for nature and recreation were illustrated in maps in a final report. In another initiative in the same county, the municipalities around the Gothenburg region conducted mapping that was published in 2014 [28]. This mapping was based on noise emanating from outside the agglomeration, i.e., roads, rail, air traffic, wind power, industry, and noisy recreational activities. It concerned noise class C (45 dBA instantaneous), as proposed by the collaboration project [22] described in Section 3, but the demands set were higher for some noise sources (large industry, harbor activity, wind power, quarries, dumps, and crushing plants) and equivalent levels were combined with maximum levels as indicators. In all, nine major quiet areas were identified in the region and presented on an illustrated map.

In Scania County, at the southern tip of Sweden, broad mapping was conducted in 2003 based on two benchmarks, 30 dBA and 40 dBA (equivalent levels) [16]. The outcomes were correlated with areas judged to have natural, cultural, and recreational qualities, and these were illustrated in maps. The mapping showed that noise-free areas were rare in Scania County, especially in western parts. Based on this finding, the final report suggested that quiet areas should be valued more highly, particularly if they lie in proximity to urban areas, have connections to other quiet areas, or have high accessibility. For instance, it was found that areas below 30 dBA were generally far away from urban agglomerations, whereas access to areas between 30 dBA and 40 dBA was better. The regional mapping in Scania county was followed up in the next year, when the outcomes were applied in two municipalities, one characterized by an urban setting (Helsingborg) and one characterized by a rural setting (Hässleholm) [29]. In the urban setting, the benchmark 40 dBA was used to identify four areas. In the rural setting, the benchmarks 30 dBA and 40 dBA (equivalent levels) were overlapped with other factors to identify three areas. The municipality found that it was possible to co-locate noisy activities and to use quiet areas to promote the region. In both municipalities, topographical variations were identified as an important factor to consider.

In the Stockholm area, a number of mappings have been conducted on various regional levels since the turn of the millennium [19,27,30,31]. In the first of these carried out in 2000 [19], the benchmark 45 dBA (equivalent) was used to identify quiet areas in relation to green structures. A few years later, another initiative was taken in which five areas were chosen on the basis that they should both be quiet and have other recreational qualities [30]. Data were extracted through a combination of calculations, measurements, and user interviews. The benchmark 45 dBA (instantaneous) was identified as a threshold for experienced quietness, with a certain exceeding time that varied depending on context. This initiative was linked to the collaboration project mentioned in Section 3 [21]. Another initiative taken at county level proposes a new method for mapping of quiet areas in the region [27]. In addition to these initiatives, the region has a shared development plan in which the notion of quiet areas is emphasized, particularly in relation to green structure [31], and Stockholm County Board has presented a map of quiet areas in the region.

5. Initiatives on the Municipality Level

The following presentation of municipal initiatives is divided into three parts. The first part provides a quantitative overview of how the notion of quiet areas has been dealt with in Swedish municipalities' general plans. In the second part, experiences from six municipalities that have progressed further in this work are described. The third part deals with municipalities that have not been working with the concept of quiet areas and looks at the different reasons for this.

5.1. Quiet Areas in the General Plans

It was found that 118 of Sweden's 290 municipalities (41%) mention the concept as part of their strategies in their general plans. Based on how extensive the initiatives were, the municipalities were divided into three categories; brief, unclear, and elaborate descriptions (see Figure 1b and Table 2). These categories are further described below. As indicated in Table 2, the majority of these municipalities focus on rural rather than urban settings. Even though several of these rural initiatives are located in proximity to agglomerations, the lack of focus on urban settings suggest that there is scope to elaborate on quiet areas within such contexts in Sweden.

Table 2. Overview of municipal initiatives in Sweden, highlighting the context focused upon in the initiative (urban and/or rural).

Type of Initiative:	Urban Setting:	Rural Setting:	Urban and Rural Setting:	Setting not Known or not Applicable:	Total:
Brief description:	0	33	0	37	70
Unclear description:	0	20	0	12	32
Elaborated description:	1	10	5	0	16
Total:	1 (1%)	63 (53%)	5 (4%)	49 (42%)	118 (100%)

"Brief descriptions" (n = 70; 24%) generally contained a short description and a positive attitude to the notion of quiet areas. Reference was sometimes made to a regional initiative and it was sometimes stated that this issue will be dealt with in future work. Brief descriptions sometimes lacked a definition of how to classify quiet areas and, in most cases, no particular areas were set aside or mapped.

The descriptions of quiet areas provided by 32 of the municipalities (11%) were categorized as "unclear". In these cases, the term 'quiet areas' was confused with other established planning concepts, such as "large unaffected areas" (stora opåverkade områden), "nature reserves" (naturreservat), and "radiation-free areas" (strålningsfria områden).

The descriptions of quiet areas provided by 16 municipalities (6%) in their general plans were categorized as "elaborate". These descriptions generally included definitions of what a quiet area is, as well as maps of designated areas. In some cases, designated areas were protected and descriptions were provided of how they should be maintained. The 16 municipalities with elaborate descriptions were: Botkyrka, Habo, Helsingborg, Huddinge, Hässleholm, Hörby, Malmö, Munkedal, Nybro, Skövde, Sollentuna, Stockholm, Sundbyberg, Tanum, Tibro, and Östra Göinge. As previously mentioned, 15 of these 16 initiatives (94%) were preceded by a regional initiative (see Figure 1b). In contrast, for the other two categories, brief and unclear descriptions, the corresponding values were 43% ($n = 30$) and 31% ($n = 10$) respectively (Table 3).

Table 3. Number and percentage of municipal initiatives that were preceded by a regional initiative.

Type of Initiative:	Number of Municipalities:	Number (and Proportion) Preceded by a Regional Initiative:
Brief description:	70	30 (43%)
Unclear description:	32	10 (31%)
Elaborated description:	16	15 (94%)
Total:	118	55 (47%)

This suggests that the regional initiatives were important in inspiring initiatives on municipal level. This was confirmed to some extent by responses to the more detailed questionnaire, where municipalities that had progressed in their work were asked to explain their sources of inspiration. The responses revealed that inspiration from regional mappings accounted for 28% ($n = 7$), while inspiration from neighboring municipalities accounted for 12% ($n = 3$). Local motiving forces emerged as the most important source of inspiration, for 60% ($n = 15$) of the initiatives. Interestingly, only 4% of responding municipalities ($n = 1$) said that the END had been an important factor, suggesting that there is scope for further promotion and/or enforcement of the directive.

5.2. Examples of Municipal Initiatives

Initiatives on municipal level were selected for further study with the ambition to focus on examples that could be inspiring for future work, including initiatives that applied more unusual ways of tackling the subject.

Starting in rural locations, the municipality of Munkedal, north of Gothenburg, was covered by regional mapping in 2001 [17]. In the municipality's general plan, Munkedal ÖP 14 [32], the question is treated on a more detailed level and two quiet areas are designated, both of which border on a wildlife area designated "large unaffected area" (Figure 2). In the plan, the municipality distinguishes between "unaffected" and "quiet areas", but acknowledges overlapping so that certain parts of larger unaffected areas may include quiet areas. This was not the case in some other municipalities, where instead it was assumed that "large unaffected areas" were also quiet areas by definition. The same problem was found in relation to "nature reserves" and other recreational areas.

Nybro, another small municipality in a rural setting, included an addition about quiet areas to its general plan in 2015 [33]. All known sources for noise were mapped. Based on the noise classes proposed by the collaboration group [22], two benchmarks were introduced (35 dBA and 45 dBA, instantaneous). The idea was that by using two different definitions, the various preconditions in the region could be accounted for. After taking account of non-acoustic factors, four areas were proclaimed as free from noise and it was stated that they should remain so. According to the municipality, the designation of quiet areas has already prevented exploitation of wind power in some of these areas. The municipality also says that the areas are maintained through reviewing permits and by supervision, but that more could be done in terms of publicizing them and making them accessible.

In the municipality of Hörby, the initiative to designate quiet areas in the region arose out of activities by the citizens themselves, which were met with positive attitudes by the town council's planning department. In the current general plan adopted in 2016 [34], parts in the east and north of the municipality are designated free from noise and protected (Figure 3). The definition is based on a previous regional mapping that utilized the benchmark 30 dBA [16]. The general plan includes a detailed account of how the quiet areas are to be protected. For instance, wind farms, shooting ranges, sawmills, and similar activities are to be avoided.

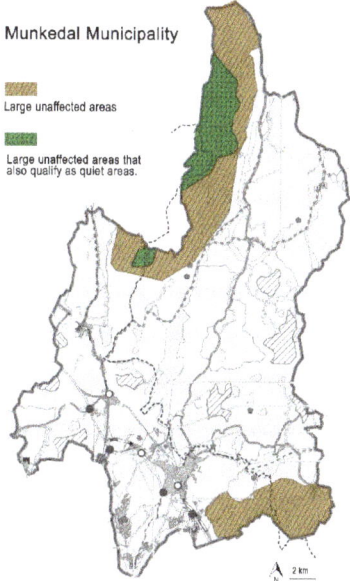

Figure 2. Map of Munkedal municipality, where "quiet areas" overlap with "large unaffected areas". Adapted and translated from Munkedal's general plan ÖP14 [32].

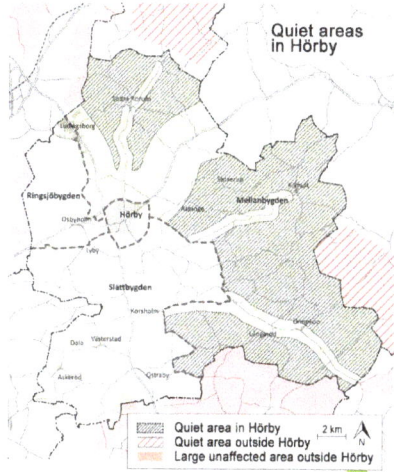

Figure 3. Map of quiet areas in the municipality of Hörby and neighboring municipalities. Adjusted and translated from [34].

In Stockholm, as previously mentioned, several noise mappings on regional level have been made from the turn of the millennium onwards. In 2013, the concept "Guide to Silence" was introduced in the region, and so far it has been tested in the three municipalities: Sollentuna, Sundbyberg, and Stockholm [35]. The "Guide to Silence" distinguishes itself as the most outgoing of the initiatives found in Sweden. Accessibility is an important aspect and the concept includes publicizing quiet areas on the internet and in illustrated brochures. Signs with maps and symbols have been erected at the sites. According to questionnaire responses from one of the municipalities, Sundbyberg, the concept has been used in marketing the municipality and has received a good response from residents.

The City of Malmö was early to acknowledge quiet areas. Noise measurements of designated areas have been made four times since 1998 [36] and the development can be followed by residents on the City's website [37]. The results have been quite disappointing since, even though these areas were chosen for their relative quietness, there are extensive problems with noise. An alternative way of working with quiet areas was tested in 2011, when an artificial quiet space was constructed in an urban square (Figure 4). Noise screens covered with ivy were used to form a small and secluded arbor next to a noise-exposed road. It was found that the arbor improved the soundscape compared with outside the arbor, and that this effect was further enhanced when sounds of nature were played inside the space to mask traffic noise [38]. The results illustrated that it is fruitful to combine noise reduction with introduction of masking sounds, thus confirming the fact that it is not only sound pressure levels which are important when discussing quiet areas, but also the quality of the sound.

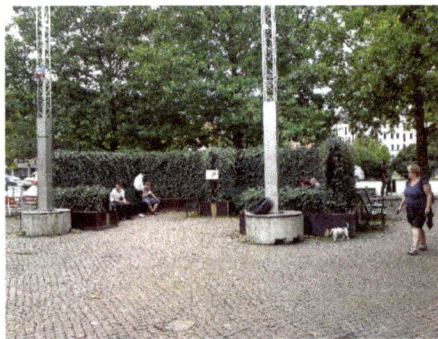

Figure 4. City of Malmö. A small arbor constructed from noise screens covered with ivy. Sounds of nature were added using concealed speakers and visitors' experiences were evaluated [38]. Photo: Gunnar Cerwén.

Helsingborg was one of the municipalities that participated in the early initiative undertaken by the Swedish Road Administration in the region [29]. In the municipality's current general plan, the notion of quiet areas is mentioned briefly, but it is further discussed in the action plan for noise [39]. A benchmark of 40 dBA (equivalent level) is used for rural areas. For parks inside the city, another benchmark is used, incorporating accessibility as a factor. It is thus stated that residents should have a maximum of 300 m to a green area where at least half the area is below 50 dBA. Based on noise data from the City's parks, accessibility is illustrated in a map (Figure 5). This approach was included here as it illustrates how the notion of quiet areas could be used to ensure variation in a city soundscape. While some urban sounds can be a quality, it is also important to ensure relative quietness [38,40], as this allows residents to choose an environment based on preference, mood, and other factors.

5.3. Reasons Why Some Municipalities Are Not Working with Quiet Areas

This section discusses the main reason why some Swedish municipalities do not include quiet areas in their planning. Municipalities that answered no in the questionnaire were given the chance to explain why by ticking boxes. A total of 117 such answers were collected. Among the reasons for lack of activity listed in the questionnaire, "No, our municipality does not have a need for quiet areas" (option 2c) was ticked by 22 municipalities. These municipalities were typically located in remote areas with relatively little human activity and hence good access to quiet areas already. Another 59 municipalities ticked the option "No, and it has not been up for discussion" (option 2e). It was found that the reasons varied, as some municipalities stated that their knowledge was insufficient or that it was an ambiguous term. There were also examples of municipalities, like Salem, which thought that it was useless to work with quiet areas due to the high noise exposure in the region. Another 36 municipalities stated that they had started working on the concept, ticking the option "No, but we have discussed implementation in our future plan" (option 2d), but added that it was not yet implemented in the general plan or that they were about to start work on it soon.

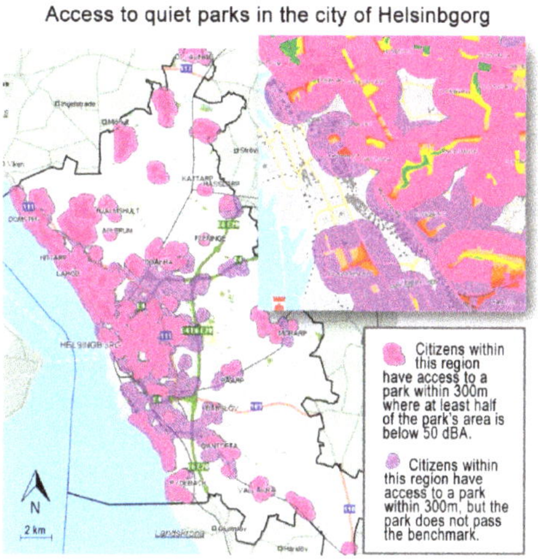

Figure 5. Map showing accessibility of parks and quiet parks in the City of Helsingborg. Adjusted and translated from the City's action plan against noise [39].

6. General Trends, Challenges, and Future Prospects

The final part of the study focused on tendencies and challenges, especially in light of future development, legislation, and implementation.

6.1. Confusion Surrounding the Concepts

There is some confusion about the concept of quiet areas as such, as a few different terms are used interchangeably in the Swedish planning community. The terms "quiet areas" (tysta områden) and "noise-free areas" (bullerfria områden) are the most well-established, but there are also other terms, such as "undisturbed areas" (ostörda områden), "carefulness areas" (varsamhetsområden), and "tranquil areas" (lugna områden), that are used more or less synonymously.

There are several other closely related terms in the planning discourse, including "large unaffected areas" (stora opåverkade områden), "radiation-free areas" (strålningsfria områden), "consideration areas" (hänsynsområden), "nature reserves" (naturreservat), "green structure" (grönstruktur) and "areas for recreation" (rekreationsområden). As described previously (see Sections 5.1 and 5.2), some of these concepts were confused with quiet areas in the survey responses. This was particularly noteworthy for "large unaffected areas", where it was assumed that these areas were also quiet. For instance, the municipality of Halmstad reported that it had not focused specifically on quiet areas, but that "in the concept of large unaffected areas, the sound environment is naturally included". However, as the municipality went on to state, in two of the areas identified as "unaffected", it was evident that only one would qualify as "quiet". The municipality of Åre, similarly, argues that because a large part of the municipality is protected as a nature reserve, it is probably quiet.

Assumptions such as these could be problematic and confirm the need for a term like "quiet areas" or "noise-free areas" that focuses specifically on the sonic aspects. Some of the other terms, such as "undisturbed areas" and "tranquil areas", do not specifically focus on sound and the use of such concepts may increase the confusion further.

It was found that the notion of "quiet areas" can be overlapped with other planning concepts to provide a more nuanced understanding, as illustrated by the municipality Munkedal [32] and its use of the concept (see Section 5.2).

6.2. Definitions and Identification of Quiet Areas

Definitions of quiet areas vary widely in Sweden. Most definitions include a reference to a benchmarked sound pressure level, which is derived either from a regional initiative and/or from five different classes of noise exposure developed by a number of influential stakeholders [22]. In Sweden, the noise classes can be said to correspond to what the EU END [1] describes as a "competent authority".

The END distinguishes between two main types of quiet areas, i.e., in "open country" and in "agglomerations". This division was used as a starting point in the present study. It was found that it was significantly more common for Swedish municipalities to work with the concept in open country, suggesting that there is scope to further develop strategies for agglomerations. Such focused initiatives have been undertaken in other parts of Europe [41–44]. Moreover, the findings suggest that it would be feasible to extend the division to three types of quiet areas (urban, urban proximity, and rural), in order to account for areas that are in close proximity to agglomerations. Such a division would allow for a more nuanced and contextual use of quiet areas, as exemplified in the five noise classes discussed in the study [22].

This study confirms what has already been noted in Europe [24], i.e., that approaches and definitions vary extensively. This is not necessarily a problem given that various contexts set different demands. However, the ambiguities surrounding the concept were reported as being problematic by some municipalities, resulting in a need for clarification. An overview of approaches has previously been published on EU level [24], and the present paper contributes a Swedish perspective. It provides an overview of current methods and approaches in use in Sweden, and this can hopefully provide some guidance for future work. However, an independent evaluation of the many methods that are currently being used would be useful for future research.

The overview on EU level [24] describes four main types of methods to identify quiet areas; noise calculations, noise measurements, evaluations by experts, and evaluations by users (e.g., interviews and surveys). No specific recommendations are presented, except that a combination of these four methods should be used. All four methods were found in Sweden and at least two of the methods were simultaneously put into practice in most cases. Most typically, benchmarks of sound pressure levels were combined with expert evaluations. The experts typically contributed knowledge about aspects such as land use, accessibility, and natural and recreational qualities. Of the four methods, user participation emerged as least commonly applied, although there were examples of its use, e.g., in Upplands Väsby, where interviews were used to identify quiet areas. In future implementations, it is possible that users could be involved in a more cost-effective manner through use of digital tools like smart phone applications (see Section 6.4).

6.3. Maintenance and Enforcement

While there are many approaches for identifying and mapping quiet areas, there are fewer examples in Sweden of active maintenance and enforcement of quiet areas. In many cases where mapping of quiet areas had been performed, it has been used mainly as an inventory, possibly with a recommendation to avoid further exploitation in the areas identified, if possible. For instance, the municipality of Växjö reported that it had been 15 years since it performed its inventory and that it had not made any follow-up since then. Sävsjö reported similar experiences, stating that "quiet areas have been mapped, but other than that, it is not something that has come to concrete usage when we make our detailed planning".

There were some examples in which quiet areas are explicitly protected in the municipality's general plans, sometimes with clear instructions on the types of activities and exploitation that should be avoided. One such municipality is Nybro [33], which reported that the designation of quiet areas had been used to limit wind power installations.

The conflict between economic interests, on the one hand, and quietness, on the other, was a recurring theme. In particular, wind power was a question that seemed to upset people, as several such conflicts were noted in the study. The conflicts sometimes extended across regional borders, e.g., the municipality of Grums reported that it had designated an area as quiet, yet experienced disturbance from the neighboring municipality: "One area has been designated (as quiet), but on the other side of the municipal border, that municipality and the county have decided to locate a wind power park (12 mills), because it is in the outskirts and few people are disturbed there."

Another recurring theme, particularly in Northern Sweden, was regulation of snow scooter traffic. Such enforcements were noted in three northern municipalities: Arjeplog, Dorotea, and Kiruna. The municipality of Umeå reported that it had a ban on motor boats but, apart from this, there were few reports of these kinds of restrictions for private citizens in the study.

A related concept to quiet areas, called "consideration areas", was developed rather recently in a collaboration between three Swedish counties [45]. Consideration areas are used in designated archipelagos, where visitors are encouraged to be careful and not make noise. Boats are encouraged to drive more slowly and to avoid noisy activities. The concept does not have legal support, but is based on common will and collaboration. The experiences to date are reported to be good [45].

Another related initiative should be mentioned in this context; quiet sections in trains. Originally introduced in the early 2000s, quiet sections are now established and used extensively in public transportation around Sweden. A quiet section is usually a separate compartment, secluded from the rest of the train. Potentially disturbing activities such as conversations and mobile phones are prohibited inside the compartment, which allows travelers to work, read, or relax.

To conclude, even though there are some interesting examples in Sweden in terms of maintenance and enforcement of quiet areas in Sweden, there is much scope for further improvement as most of the examples are from other contexts. Maintenance was noted in the questionnaire by 20% of the municipalities as being one of the greatest future challenges. Some related ideas and concepts from other contexts that are described here could possibly be used to promote future development.

6.4. Accessibility and Marketing

This section is related to the Section 6.3 (Maintenance and Enforcement), as both deal with outward activities aimed at the end users. As mentioned, it was found that there was scope for improving accessibility and marketing quiet areas. Mappings of quiet areas described in general plans and other planning documents may be difficult for the end user to access, and it is therefore noteworthy that few municipalities have focused on outward activities. Even municipalities that have come far in their mapping of quiet areas, such as Nybro, reported that there is more to be done in terms of publicizing these areas and making them accessible to the public.

There was a demand for good examples as inspiration in the municipalities' own work. Relatively few such good examples were identified in the study, with the exception of the "Guide to Silence" in the Stockholm region (see Section 5.2). A related initiative has been developed in the UK and is called "Tranquility Trails" [44].

The internet can be an effective way to reach residents, via channels already established by the municipalities and via marketing on independent websites. No dedicated apps for smartphones were reported to have been developed in Sweden, but an application, Hush City, in the EU allows users to measure sound pressure levels, document favorite places, and inform other users about their favorite quiet areas [41]. It is also possible to plot quiet trails in Google maps.

Signs are another way to raise awareness about quiet areas. This is used in the "Guide to Silence" (Figure 6), where each trail's starting point is marked with a large sign containing a map and a short description of the concept [35]. Moreover, a dedicated symbol is placed at strategic locations. Signs are also used in the related concept of "consideration areas" [45].

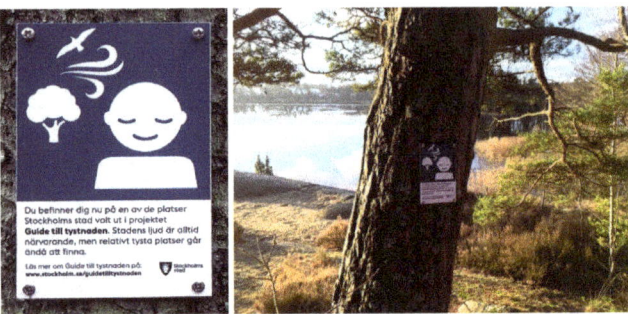

Figure 6. In the "Guide to Silence" concept, quiet areas are marked by signs. This one reads: "You are now in one of the places chosen by the City of Stockholm for the project "Guide to Silence". The sounds of the city are always present, but relative quietness can be found." Photo and illustration: Ulf Bohman.

The spatial distribution of quiet areas is an important factor for accessibility and one that can be controlled in planning. In Sweden, it is generally suggested that urban dwellers should be at most 300 m (about 5 min' walking distance) from the nearest green area or park [46]. This recommendation has been discussed as a possible benchmark for quiet areas in urban regions [40,47] and has been applied in the City of Helsingborg (see Section 5.2) [39]. Spatial distribution is a factor that could be given more attention, in particular as it lends itself to quantification. However, for rural regions, no corresponding recommendations were encountered. It can be assumed that the quieter an area is, the farther people are willing to travel to get there. Thus, quiet areas in urban regions compensate for the relative noise exposure by proximity, while quiet areas in open country do the opposite. In formulation of future recommendations, it is possible that multifractal modeling could be used as inspiration [48], i.e., that the distribution could be varied depending on type of quiet area and relationships between different types of quiet areas.

Designation of quiet areas is sometimes associated with economic conflicts, as activities like wind power and other industries cannot exist in the proximity of quiet areas. However, there is also the possibility of positive repercussions for the economy if quiet areas are used in marketing. For instance, in the City of Malmö it is clear that the income levels of residents in different neighborhoods correlate with freedom from noise disturbance [49]. Quietness thus appears to be an experiential quality that can be valued economically. There is potential to use quiet areas to create added value by attracting inhabitants and tourists.

A survey conducted at EU level [25] using the Quietness Suitability Index (QSI) has shown that the Nordic region has relatively good access to quiet environments (see Figure 7). The access to quietness could thus be used as a potential tool in tourism-related marketing. However, only a few examples were found where quietness was marketed in this way, suggesting that there is scope for development in this respect. This could result in economic benefits and also serve as a way to highlight and value quiet areas further, thus providing a means by which to protect them in the future.

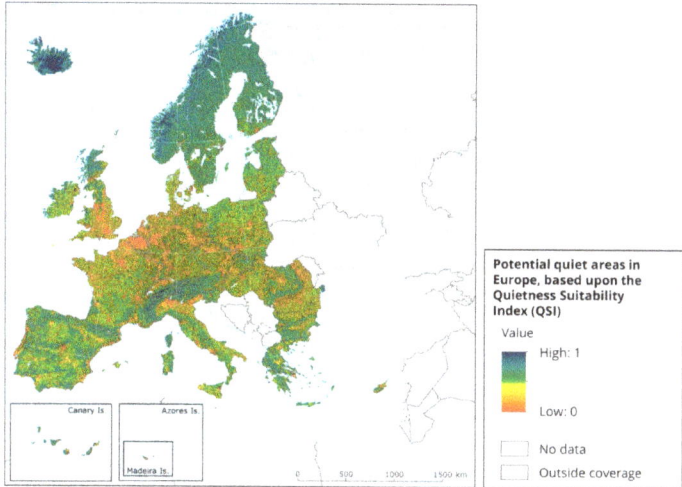

Figure 7. Map of Europe created using the Quietness Suitability Index (QSI), where the potential for quiet areas is based on noise data and land use. Map previously published by the European Environmental Agency [25].

7. Conclusions

Although quiet areas are becoming rare in some urban regions in Sweden, it can be concluded that there is growing interest in preserving existing quiet areas. It was found that the concept is well-known in the Swedish planning community, but that few municipalities have been dealing with it in a comprehensive manner. This seems to be due to ambiguities surrounding the concept and lack of good examples. Continuous revision and development of strategies for working with quiet areas is suggested. The study identified a total of 16 municipalities in Sweden that have come further in their work than others and experiences from some of these are described.

The results do not indicate that the EU's Environmental Noise Directive (END) has had a significant impact on the development of quiet areas on municipal level. A more important factor in Sweden seems to be various regional initiatives undertaken in recent decades. The municipality's own driving force and inspiration from neighboring municipalities also appear to be important factors.

A number of challenges to future work on quiet areas, in Sweden and at EU level, were identified. In Sweden, many initiatives have focused on mapping and identification of quiet areas, but less has been done regarding maintenance and enforcement. If the principles stated in the recent World Health Organization guidelines on reducing noise while conserving quiet areas are to be followed, more attention definitely needs to be given to such aspects. Some activities are more problematic than others as regards noise emissions, such as snow scooter use in open country, motorsports, and wind farms. In a few cases, activities like these were specifically described in the environmental strategies of some Swedish municipalities as unwanted and undesirable. However, examples of limitations such as these affecting individual activities were fairly rare in the survey data.

There were significant differences in how municipalities work with quiet areas. Such differences are not necessarily problematic per se, as the prerequisites for quiet areas vary depending on context, but it was found that further clarification and guidelines could benefit applicability. In particular, there is a need for an independent evaluation of the methods and definitions available. In the END, a distinction between two types of quiet areas is proposed (agglomerations and open country), but our results indicate that this could be extended to three types: urban areas (agglomerations), areas in urban proximity, and rural areas (open country).

There were very few examples of public communications and marketing of quiet areas by Swedish municipalities, although quiet areas can be beneficial for residents and for tourism, i.e., they are beneficial for health, quality of life, and the local economy. Many parts of Northern Europe, including Sweden, provide rich access to quiet areas and this could play a more prominent role in marketing the country. In addition to economic benefits from tourism, this could also be a way to raise the value and awareness of quiet recreational areas so that they are protected and maintained in the future.

Author Contributions: G.C. and F.M. collaborated throughout the project, where G.C. had a more active role. G.C. collected the data and analyzed the results, guided by continuous discussions with F.M. Both authors contributed to writing the paper, G.C. provided the majority of the writing.

Funding: This research was funded by The Sound Environment Center at Lund University, through the project "Quiet Areas in Sweden" (Tysta områden i Sverige).

Acknowledgments: The authors wish to thank Eja Pedersen and Magnus Lindqvist for valuable comments during the project. Moreover, the authors thank all municipalities that participated in the study, particularly those that took part in the follow-up study and those that granted the use of images.

Conflicts of Interest: The authors declare no conflict of interest.

References

1. EU. Directive 2002/49/EC of the European Parliament and of the Council Relating to the Assessment and Management of Environmental Noise. European Union, Official Journal of the European Communities: L 189, 2002. Available online: https://eur-lex.europa.eu/legal-content/EN/TXT/?uri=celex:32002L0049 (accessed on 23 November 2018).
2. Schafer, R.M. *The Soundscape: Our Sonic Environment and the Tuning of the World*; Destiny Books: Rochester, VT, USA, 1994.
3. Aletta, F.; Oberman, T.; Kang, J. Associations between positive health-related effects and soundscapes perceptual constructs: A systematic review. *Int. J. Environ. Res. Public Health* **2018**, *15*, 2392. [CrossRef] [PubMed]
4. Gidlöf-Gunnarsson, A.; Öhrström, E.; Berglund, B.; Kropp, W.; Kihlman, T.; Nilsson, M.; Forssén, J. *Ljudlandskap för Bättre Hälsa: Resultat och Slutsatser från ett Multidisciplinärt Forskningsprogram. Soundscape Support to Health (Final Report)*; Arbets-Och Miljömedicin, Sahlgrenska Akademin, Göteborgs Universitet: Gothenburg, Sweden, 2008.
5. EEA. *Population Exposure to Environmental Noise*; Report nr: IND-233-en; European Environmental Agency: Luxembourg, 2018.
6. WHO. *Burden of Disease from Environmental Noise—Quantification of Healthy Life Years Lost in Europe*; World Health Organization, Regional Office for Europe: Copenhagen, Denmark, 2011.
7. WHO. *Environmental Noise Guidelines for the European Region*; World Health Organization, Regional Office for Europe: Copenhagen, Denmark, 2018.
8. Basner, M.; Babisch, W.; Davis, A.; Brink, M.; Clark, C.; Janssen, S.; Stansfeld, S. Auditory and non-auditory effects of noise on health. *Lancet* **2014**, *383*, 1325–1332. [CrossRef]
9. Ministry of Enterprise and Innovation. *Förordning om Riktvärden för Trafikbuller vid Bostadsbyggnader Regulation for Traffic Noise Close to Housing*; Regeringskansliet 2015, SFS nr: 2015:16. Available online: https://www.riksdagen.se/sv/dokument-lagar/dokument/svensk-forfattningssamling/forordning-2015216-om-trafikbuller-vid_sfs-2015-216 (accessed on 23 November 2018).
10. Kristersson, U.; Billström, T.; Thalén Finné, E.; Enström, K.; Waltersson Grönvall, C.; Svantesson, E.; Wallmark, H.; Avsan, A.; Finstorp, L.; Magnusson, C. *Ökat Byggande och fler Bostäder. Increased Building and More Housing*; Motion nr: 2017/18:3570; Riksdagen, Moderaterna, Motion to parliament: Stockholm, Sweden, 2017.
11. Ministry of Enterprise and Innovation. Nya Riktvärden för Trafikbuller. New Guidelines for Traffic Noise. Regeringskansliet, 2017. Available online: https://www.regeringen.se/pressmeddelanden/2017/05/nya-riktvarden-for-trafikbuller/ (accessed on 23 November 2018).
12. Shepherd, D.; Welch, D.; Dirks, K.N.; McBride, D. Do quiet areas afford greater health-related quality of life than noisy areas? *Int. J. Environ. Res. Public Health* **2013**, *10*, 1284–1303. [CrossRef] [PubMed]

13. Gidlöf-Gunnarsson, A.; Öhrström, E. Noise and well-being in urban residential environments: The potential role of perceived availability to nearby green areas. *Landsc. Urban Plan* **2007**, *83*, 115–126. [CrossRef]
14. Öhrström, E.; Skånberg, A.; Svensson, H.; Gidlöf-Gunnarsson, A. Effects of road traffic noise and the benefit of access to quietness. *J. Sound Vib.* **2006**, *295*, 40–59. [CrossRef]
15. Ingemansson. *Kartläggning av Bullerkällor i Mullsjö och Habo. Mapping of Noise Sources in Mullsjö and Habo Municipalities*; Report nr: B-1280-B 1998-03-20; Vägverket: Borlänge, Sweden, 1998.
16. Scania County. *Bullerfria Områden i Skåne. Noise-Free Areas in Scania*; Report nr: 1010; Länsstyrelsen i Skåne och Vägverket: Malmö, Sweden, 2003.
17. Västra Götaland County. *Tysta Områden i Västra Götalands län. Quiet Areas in the County of Västra Götaland*; Report nr: 2001:18; Länsstyrelsen i Västra Götalands Län: Göteborg, Sweden, 2001.
18. Ingemansson. *Malmö Stad: Kartläggning av Ljudmiljön i "Tysta Områden". City of Malmö: Mapping of the Sound Environment in "Quiet Areas"*; Report nr: M-2744-r-A; Miljöförvaltningen i Malmö stad: Malmö, Sweden, 1999.
19. Regional plan office in Stockholm. *Tysta Områden, en Kartläggning av Buller i Regionens Grönstruktur. Quiet Areas, a Mapping of Noise in the Region's Green Structure*; Promemoria nr: 5; Regionplanekontoret: Stockholm, Sweden, 2000.
20. Collaboration Group on Quiet Areas. *Ljudkvalitet i Natur- och Kulturmiljöer—Förslag till Mått, Mätetal och Inventeringsmetod. Sound Quality in Natural and Cultural Environments—Proposing Measurements and Methods*; Report nr: 2002-12-18; Naturvårdsverket: Bromma, Sweden, 2002.
21. Collaboration Group on Quiet Areas. *Utvärdering och Utveckling av Mått, Mätetal och Inventeringsmetod: Slutrapport i ett Samarbetsprojekt. Evaluation and Development of Measurements and Methods: Final Report in a Collaboration Project*; Report nr: 5440; Naturvårdsverket: Bromma, Sweden, 2005.
22. Collaboration Group on Quiet Areas. *God ljudmiljö … … Mer Än bara Frihet Från Buller: Ljudkvalitet i Natur- och Kulturmiljöer. A Good Sound Environment … … More Than Merely Absence from Noise: Sound Quality in Natural and Cultural Environments*; Report nr: 5709; Naturvårdsverket: Bromma, Sweden, 2007.
23. EUC. *Future Noise Policy. European Commission Green Paper*; Commission of the European Communities: Brussels, Belgium, 1996.
24. EEA. *Good Practice Guide on Quiet Areas*; Report no 4; European Environment Agency/Publications Office of the European Union: Luxembourg, 2014.
25. EEA. *Quiet Areas in Europe: The Environment Unaffected by Noise Pollution*; Report No 14; European Environment Agency/Publications Office of the European Union: Luxembourg, 2016.
26. Jönköping County. *Ostörda Områden var Finns de? En GIS-Modell för Identifiering av Bullerfria Områden. Undisturbed Areas Where Are They? A GIS-Model for Identification of Noise-Free Areas*; Report nr: 2015:01; Länsstyrelsen i Jönköpings län: Jönköping, Sweden, 2015.
27. Stockholm County. *Kartläggning av Bullerfria Områden. Metodbeskrivning för Stockholms län. Mapping of Quiet Areas: Method Description for Stockholm County*; Report nr: 2016:04; Centrum för Arbetsmedicin vid Stockholms läns landsting: Stockholm, Sweden, 2016.
28. Gothenburg Region. *Tysta Områden Inom GR: Kartläggning av Bullerpåverkan i Natur och Grönområden. Quiet Areas in the Gothenburg Region: Mapping of Noise in Nature and Green Areas*; Report nr: 590711; Göteborgsregionen och Länsstyrelsen Västra Götaland: Göteborg, Sweden, 2014.
29. Scania County. *Bullerfria Områden i Skåne del 2: Redovisning av Pilotprojekt i Helsingborgs stad och Hässleholms Kommun. Noise Free Areas in the Municipality of Skåne Part 2: Presentation of a Pilot Project in Helsingborg and Hässleholm*; Report 2004:186; Helsingborg, Hässleholm, Vägverket och Länsstyrelsen i Skåne län: Malmö, Sweden, 2004.
30. Environmental Protection Agency in Sweden. *Stockholms Tysta, Gröna Områden—Ljudnivåer och Inventering; Quiet Areas of Stockholm—Sound Pressure Levels and Inventory*; Report nr: 5441; Naturvårdsverket: Bromma, Sweden, 2005.
31. Regional Plan Office in Stockholm. *Regional Utvecklingsplan för Stockholmsregionen RUFS. Regional Development Plan for the Stockholm area RUFS*; Regionplanekontoret: Stockholm, Sweden, 2010.
32. Munkedal municipality. *Framtidsplan: ÖP14 Munkedal. General Plan in Munkedal Municipality, ÖP14*; Munkedals Kommun: Munkedal, Sweden, 2014.

33. Nybro municipality. *Bullerfria Områden i Nybro Kommun: Tematiskt Tillägg till Översiktsplanen. Noise free areas in Nybro: Amendment to the General Plan*; Teknik- och Samhällsbyggnadsnämnden: Nybro Kommun, Sweden, 2015.
34. Hörby municipality. *Översiktsplan 2030. General Plan 20130*; Hörby Kommun: Hörby, Sweden, 2016.
35. Ulf Bohman. Guide till Tystnaden Guide to Silence (Homepage). Available online: http://www.guidetosilence.org/ (accessed on 14 November 2018).
36. Tyréns. *Malmö Stad: Uppföljande Ljudmätning av Ljudmiljön i "Tysta Områden". City of Malmö: A Follow Up on Noise Measurements in "Quiet Areas"*; Report nr: 248329; Malmö stad: Malmö, Sweden, 2016.
37. City of Malmö. Ljudnivå i Tysta Stadsmiljöer. Sound Pressure Levels in Quiet Urban Areas. Available online: http://miljobarometern.malmo.se/buller/tysta-omraden/ljudniva-i-tysta-stadsmiljoer/ (accessed on 23 November 2018).
38. Cerwén, G. Urban soundscapes: A quasi-experiment in landscape architecture. *Landsc. Res.* **2016**, *41*, 481–494. [CrossRef]
39. Helsingborg municipality. *Buller: Åtgärdsprogram Buller 2014–2018. Noise: Action Plan against Noise 2014–2018*; Stadsbyggnadsförvaltningen, Helsingborgs Kommun: Helsingborg, Sweden, 2014.
40. Cerwén, G. Sound in Landscape Architecture: A Soundscape Approach to Noise. Ph.D. Thesis, SLU, Alnarp, Sweden, 2017.
41. Radicchi, A. From crowdsourced data to open source planning: The implementation of the hush city app in Berlin. In Proceedings of the Internoise 2018, Chicago, IL, USA, 26–29 August 2018.
42. Tsaligopoulos, A.; Economou, C.; Matsinos, Y. Identification, prioritization and assessment of urban quiet areas. In *Handbook of Research on Perception-Driven Approaches to Urban Assessment and Design*; Aletta, F., Xiao, J., Eds.; IGI Global: Hershey, PA, USA, 2018; pp. 150–180.
43. Booi, H.; van den Berg, F. Quiet areas and the need for quietness in Amsterdam. *Int. J. Envron. Res. Public Health* **2012**, *9*, 1030–1050. [CrossRef] [PubMed]
44. Watts, G. Tranquillity trails for urban areas. *Urban For. Urban Green.* **2018**, *29*, 154–161. [CrossRef]
45. Coast State Provincial Offices. *Arbetet med Hänsynsområden i Kust och Skärgård: Kustlänsstyrelsernas Gemensamma Rapportering av Regeringsuppdrag 51d Enligt Regleringsbrev 2007*; Document nr: (Lst Stockholm) 501-2007-102617; Länsstyrelserna: Stockholm, Sweden, 2009.
46. National Board of Housing, Building and Planning. *Bostadsnära Natur—Inspiration & Vägledning Nature and Housing—Guidelines & Inspiration*; Boverket: Karlskrona, Sweden, 2007.
47. Hedfors, P. Site Soundscapes: Landscape Architecture in the Light of Sound. Ph.D. Thesis, SLU, Uppsala, Sweden, 2003.
48. Frankhauser, P.; Tannier, C.; Vuidel, G.; Houot, H. An integrated multifractal modelling to urban and regional planning. *Comput. Environ. Urban Syst.* **2018**, *67*, 132–146. [CrossRef]
49. Skärbäck, E.; Grahn, P. Rofylldhet: En Planfaktor att Beakta. Tranquility: A Parameter to Consider in Planning. *Plan* **2015**, *5*, 14–19.

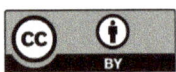

© 2019 by the authors. Licensee MDPI, Basel, Switzerland. This article is an open access article distributed under the terms and conditions of the Creative Commons Attribution (CC BY) license (http://creativecommons.org/licenses/by/4.0/).

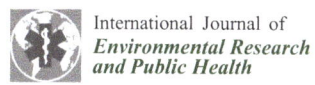

Article

Going beyond Quietness: Determining the Emotionally Restorative Effect of Acoustic Environments in Urban Open Public Spaces

Karmele Herranz-Pascual [1], Itziar Aspuru [1,*], Ioseba Iraurgi [2], Álvaro Santander [1], Jose Luis Eguiguren [1] and Igone García [1]

[1] TECNALIA Research and Innovation, Parque Tecnológico de Bizkaia, Calle Geldo, Edificio 700, 48160 Derio, Bizkaia, Spain; karmele.herranz@tecnalia.com (K.H.-P.); alvaro.santander@tecnalia.com (Á.S.); jluis.eguiguren@tecnalia.com (J.L.E.); igone.garcia@tecnalia.com (I.G.)

[2] DeustoPsych, University of Deusto, Unibertsitate Etorb. 24, 48007 Bilbao, Bizkaia, Spain; ioseba.iraurgi@deusto.es

* Correspondence: igone.garcia@tecnalia.com; Tel.: +34-902-760-004

Received: 15 February 2019; Accepted: 7 April 2019; Published: 10 April 2019

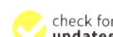

Abstract: The capacity of natural settings to promote psychological restoration has attracted increasing research attention, especially with regards to the visual dimension. However, there is a need to extend these studies to urban settings, such as squares, parks or gardens, due to the global trend towards urbanisation, and to integrate the dimension of sound into landscape. Such was the main aim of this study, in which 53 participants assessed four public spaces in Vitoria-Gasteiz (Spain) as part of the CITI-SENSE Project (137 observations were used for analysis). A smartphone application was used to simultaneously collect objective and subjective data. The results show that at the end of the urban environmental experience, there was a statistically significant reduction in negative emotions and perceived stress, and a slight increase in positive emotions. Emotional restoration was mainly associated with prior emotional states, but also with global environmental comfort and acoustic comfort. The soundscape characteristics that contributed to greater emotional restoration and a reduction in perceived stress were pleasantness, calm, fun and naturalness. Therefore, in agreement with previous research, the findings of the present study indicate that besides contributing to the quietness of the urban environment, the urban soundscape can promote psychological restoration in users of these spaces.

Keywords: quietness; soundscape; psychological restoration; emotions; acoustic environment; urban open public spaces; urban design

1. Introduction

Restorative environments enhance or facilitate psychological restoration, and thus contribute to human health and well-being. The most influential theories on this topic are attention restoration theory (ART) developed by Kaplan and Kaplan [1] and the stress recovery theory (SRT), postulated by Ulrich [2–4].

ART states that natural environments can restore the cognitive resources that people use in their daily activities (e.g., work, studies, responsibilities). In ART theory, the restorative potential of environments, known as restorativeness, is defined by four fundamental dimensions: (a) "being away", which refers to a series of perceived characteristics that allow individuals to distance themselves physically or psychologically from that which requires their directed attention; (b) "extent", which refers to the environmental qualities that invite exploration beyond what is immediately perceived; (c) "fascination", the perceived characteristics that attract people's attention (this refers to involuntary attention, which does not require excessive mental exertion); and (d) "compatibility", which refers to the perception that the environment is consonant with the goals of the person experiencing it [1].

Meanwhile, Ulrich's theory postulates that despite its adaptive value, the stress response elicited by some life events drains psychological energy and leads to the emergence of a negative emotional state. Thus, a positive affective response to open natural settings enables the individual to recover from fatigue and its negative emotional outcomes.

In recent decades, the study of psychological restoration has attracted considerable research interest in environmental psychology and beyond, although most studies have focused primarily on natural settings (outside urban areas) such as parks and forests. It has been found that exposure to green or blue natural environments (with vegetation and water, respectively) can provide a more effective restorative experience than exposure to artificial urban areas [1–10]. However, this restorative experience does not occur solely in natural settings, although it is enhanced by them [6,10–12], and not all such environments contribute to restoration [13]. In connection with the latter, research conducted by Ojala et al. [14] is particularly noteworthy. It assesses how differences in orientation towards built vs. natural environments as well as noise sensibility affect psychological and physiological restoration in three different urban places.

Very few recent studies have explored the restorative capacity of urban settings, since these are generally approached from a negative point of view, considering cities as settings which may give rise to psychological ill health and social disruption as a result of social, economic, environmental and spatial factors [6–17]. Urban settings are consequently seen as more stressful and less attractive than natural ones, and in some way responsible for negative effects that can only be palliated through contact with nature.

There is thus a need to extend research on restorative environments to urban settings in order to determine whether these may also be considered restorative, as some recent studies would seem to suggest [18]. The results of one recent study revealed that participants' psychological state improved after spending half an hour in one of two selected urban squares [19,20]. Visitors to both squares showed better cognitive performance, reduced negative affect variables (tension-anxiety, anger-hostility, fatigue and stress) and reported an increase in happiness. Consequently, applying the restorative environment approach to cities may be an effective way of ameliorating urban life and contributing to people's health and well-being.

The United Nations Department of Economic and Social Affairs has reported that the urban population has increased exponentially—from 751 million in 1950 to 4200 million in 2018—and that this trend will continue [21]: currently, 55% of world's population lives in cities and this number is expected to rise to 68% by 2050. In this context, research on restorative environments could help to improve the health and well-being of people living in an urban world, where the workload (or lack thereof) is so stressful.

Another important aspect of previous research on restorative environments is that it has focused primarily on the visual dimension of nature, as reflected in the terms used to describe them (e.g., contemplation, scene, views, green elements), as well as the dimensions that define them (e.g., extent, being away, fascination). These terms are difficult to apply to senses other than sight; however, perception is a holistic process that integrates information from various senses, including sight and hearing. While it is an important environmental element, with social and aesthetic attributes, the quality of soundscape is one of the key factors for environmental perception in urban public open spaces [22–24].

In addition, there is a prevailing tendency to consider the urban acoustic environment solely from the perspective of noise pollution. As a result, studies in this field have focused on its harmful effects on people. In its recent publication "Environmental Noise Guidelines for the European Region" [25], the World Health Organization (WHO) regional office for Europe reported that sufficient scientific evidence was available to quantify the health effects of noise for cardiovascular disease

(CVD), which includes ischaemic heart disease (IHD) and hypertension (HT), sleep disturbance (SD), annoyance (HA), hearing loss and tinnitus (HL/T) and cognitive impairment (CI). Noise also exerts an adverse effect on newborns, metabolic function, quality of life, mental health and well-being.

Recent years have witnessed an increase in studies analysing the acoustic environment from a positive perspective, focusing attention on its beneficial effects on people [26,27]. In the city of Rotterdam, where 16 urban parks were assessed, restorative levels were mainly due to the park size and the average noise level [28]. For its part, in Milan it was confirmed that the perceived environmental quality of five urban parks was dependent on the type of soundscape [29,30].

Studies also started to explore the impact of soundscape on restoration [10]. A survey conducted in the city of Sheffield showed that the soundscape of urban parks played a significant role in their restorative experience [31].

This current trend includes the study of restorative aspects linked to the soundscape and new surveys on quiet areas [32]. In fact, the restoration theory has very rarely been addressed as a reference in soundscape studies, apart from Payne et al. [33,34], who included two adjectives in their soundscape scale, grouped in the "pleasantness" dimension, which refer to the known positive perception of "nature" and to the restorative capacity of the soundscape. In other laboratory research, Zhang, et al. [35] reported how the typical urban soundscapes with natural elements in densely populated Chinese cities had significant effects on individuals' restorative experiences; natural sounds will boost the restoration of the individual's attention, whereas traffic and machine sounds will have a negative effect [10].

Other projects have assessed the sound environment from the point of view of acoustic comfort [36–39], thus falling within the field of research on environmental comfort. A "comfortable place" is understood as one that can create a pleasant environmental experience for the people and the communities that use it, carrying out individual or social activities [40].

The acoustic dimension of environmental comfort can be assessed using the concept of soundscape. This concept has been developed within the framework of several European actions and projects (many of which formed part of the COST-Action on "Soundscape of European Cities and Landscapes") aimed at collecting people's perceptions of the acoustic environment (i.e., the soundscape) and analysing the sound environment from a positive perspective that transcends the restrictive pollution-related approach.

The key principles of soundscape are defined in international standard ISO 12913, in which the notion of soundscape is viewed as an acoustic analogy of landscape. ISO 12913:1:2014 provides the definition of a conceptual framework for the term soundscape [41], while ISO/TS 12913-2:2018 supplementary materials about data collection regarding soundscape studies [42]. According to this standard, soundscape is "the acoustic environment as perceived or experienced and/or understood by a person or people in context".

But what are the beneficial effects of restorative environments on human health? According to Kaplan and Kaplan's [1] and Ulrich's [2–4] theories, natural settings reduce stress and alleviate negative emotional states, but there are few references to their impact on positive emotional states. Hence, San Juan et al. [19] have argued that urban design can also significantly contribute to improving people's well-being and quality of life, reducing their stress and restoring their psychological state. Other studies on the soundscape have highlighted the benefits of sound environments for well-being, mainly focusing on natural [43] or human sounds [44]. Thus, several studies have tried to provide scientific evidence of the benefits of the "soundscape approach" for public engagement, health and well-being [45,46]. Consequently, the soundscape should be considered part of urban design [47,48], incorporating specific urban furniture [49] to improve people's perceptions of urban places and their environmental experiences.

According to the WHO, "health is a state of complete physical, mental and social well-being rather than the absence of illness or discomfort" [50]. Hence, any analysis of restorative environments should consider both their capacity to mitigate negative health states (e.g., negative emotions, stress) and their benefits for positive health states (e.g., comfort, calm, happiness).

The literature shows that psychological restoration in natural settings has received considerable research attention in recent years, but such studies have focused mainly on the visual dimension. However, due to the global trend towards urbanisation, there is a need to extend these studies to urban settings, to integrate the dimension of sound into landscape, and to study the benefits for positive health states.

Therefore, the main objective of the present study was to determine the influence in urban open public spaces of the sound environment and its perception (soundscape) on users' health. To this end, the effects on positive and negative emotional states and perceived stress were measured. A further aim was to identify the characteristics of the soundscape that enhance emotional restoration and reduce perceived stress.

Within the scope of this article, the authors consider urban open public spaces "as the total surface of the built-up areas of cities devoted to streets and boulevards—including walkways, sidewalks, and bicycle lanes—and the areas devoted to public parks, squares, recreational green areas, public playgrounds and open areas of public facilities" [51]. The present study focused on open public urban spaces whose primary function was to provide a leisure area, such as squares, parks or gardens.

The study hypothesis was that comfortable urban places with a pleasant soundscape are restorative in terms of their effect on emotions, complementing other studies on other restorative aspects, such as the physiological effects or considering their effect on attention, and should therefore be associated with an increase in positive emotions and a reduction in negative emotions such as perceived stress.

2. Materials and Methods

The present study was conducted using a toolkit developed as part of the CITI-SENSE EU Project [52,53] (for more information, visit the project web site www.citi-sense.eu.) which allowed a simultaneous assessment of the acoustic environment and its perception (soundscape) on site. This toolkit [37] is an adapted smartphone and app designed to facilitate observations of open spaces (see Figure 1).

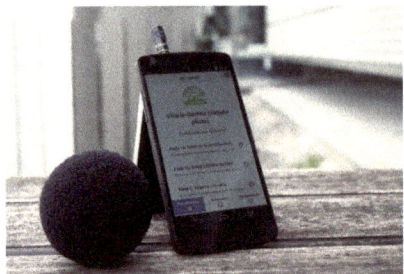

Figure 1. CITI-SENSE observation toolkit.

It comprises five elements: (a) a smartphone, which can be used to post-process acoustic signals; (b) an external microphone for measuring acoustic levels; (c) a user-friendly smartphone app that enables people to provide an assessment and collects data on their perceptions of the area via an embedded questionnaire; (d) a procedure for measuring the acoustic environment and soundscape, based on the state-of-the-art; and (e) a protocol for conducting observations that includes clear instructions for participants.

As explained above, the present study focused on open public urban spaces whose primary function was to provide a leisure area, such as squares, parks or gardens. These places were selected because people visit them to rest, relax or socialise, activities that are closely associated with restorative environments and which also define the functions of urban open public spaces. Hence, if these types of urban places are pleasant, they are more likely to have a restorative capacity because people will spend more time enjoying them. The combination of the characteristics of these places and people's perceptions and enjoyment of them determines environmental and acoustic comfort. The public spaces analysed in this study will henceforth be referred to as "urban places".

Other types of urban public space, such as streets, stations or enclosed spaces, were not included in the study because the main function of the first is to provide a place of transit, while the latter two usually offer very little contact with natural elements related to vegetation (green) or water (blue).

2.1. Case Studies

Four urban places in the city of Vitoria-Gasteiz (Spain) were selected to carry out the study. Selection was conducted with the aim of obtaining a sample of places with diverse characteristics in terms of the presence of natural elements (green and blue) and their function in the city (frequently used and located in the city centre or more sporadically used and located in a peri-urban environment). The places selected were (Figure 2):

- Los Herrán (Figure 2a). Stretch of the Los Herrán street in which the city's central bus station was previously located. The place analysed in this street is the central area with leisure use (boulevard), which is surrounded by high traffic flow roads and is close to a school.
- Constitución (Figure 2b). Constitución square is situated next to the northern entrance to the city. To the left of the square, there is a relatively quiet green street.
- Salinillas (Figure 2c). Salinillas de Buradón park is situated in a new urban area and sits on a small hill close to the city's green belt. The park has very few trees.
- Olarizu (Figure 2d). Olarizu park is part of the city's green belt and home to the Environmental Research Centre (CEA), which receives thousands of visitors throughout the year. Some of these spend the day in the surrounding area.

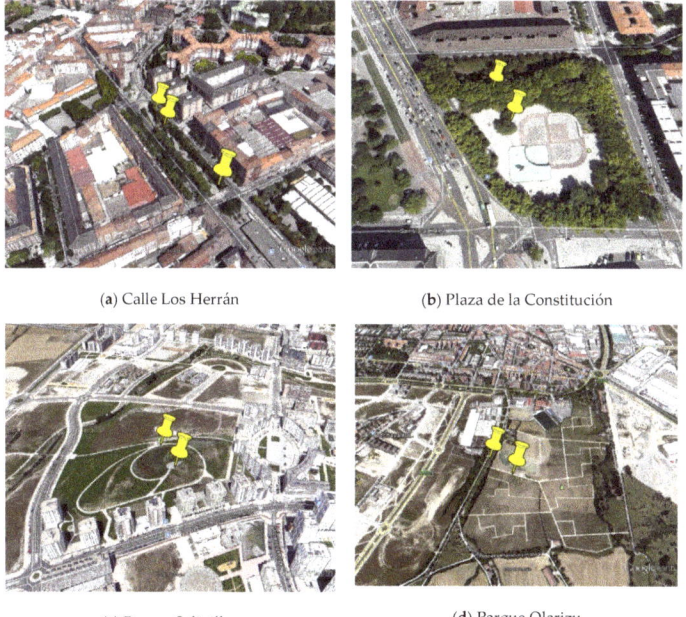

(a) Calle Los Herrán (b) Plaza de la Constitución

(c) Parque Salinillas (d) Parque Olarizu

Figure 2. Pictures of the four urban places, indicating the evaluation points. Source: Google Earth.

The method proposed to characterise each urban place comprised an assessment of a set of objective variables related to the quality of services and the diversity of each place, the presence of green (green), cultural (landmarks and heritage) and water (blue) elements, the level of artificiality (grey) and the proportion of openness (% sky) [37].

The maintenance, safety, presence of businesses (shops), traffic, facilities and tall vegetation (trees) were also evaluated. These were assessed on a scale of 0–3 (0 not applicable; 1 low; 2 medium; 3 high). In addition, water, landmarks and heritage were assessed on a scale of 0–2 (0 not present; 1 yes, it can be seen from the study area; 2 yes, it is part of the study area). These evaluations were based on the ratings of three project technicians and are the result of a consensus process (Delphi Method). More detailed information on this evaluation methodology is available in QUADMAP guidelines [54].

Table 1 provides a description of the four urban places analysed in relation to their physical and landscape features.

Table 1. Description of the four urban places selected.

Evaluation (1)	Los Herrán	Constitución	Salinillas	Olarizu
Maintenance	3	3	2	3
Safety	2	3	1	2
Shops	2	1	0	1
Traffic	3	1	1	1
Facilities	2	2	0	1
Trees	2	2	1	2
Presence (2)	**Los Herrán**	**Constitución**	**Salinillas**	**Olarizu**
Water	0	2	0	2
Landmarks	0	0	0	1
Heritage	0	1	0	0
Percentage	**Los Herrán**	**Constitución**	**Salinillas**	**Olarizu**
% green	25	40	90	80
% blue	0	25	0	25
% sky	35	30	100	80
% grey	85	60	10	10

(1) Evaluation: 1 low; 2 medium; 3 high; 0 not applicable. (2) Presence: 0 no; 1 yes, it can be seen from the study area; 2 yes, it is part of the study area.

The four places displayed a great deal of homogeneity in terms of maintenance, which was generally high, the presence of water, landmarks and heritage. In contrast, they differed widely in terms of safety, facilities, traffic, economic activity, trees and green areas. These differences were also reflected in characterisation of the places in terms of greenness (% green), water (% blue), artificiality (% grey) and openness (% sky).

When the places were ranked according to the results of this analysis, a dichotomous dimension emerged: grey versus green (or artificiality versus naturalness). Grey was defined by building elements and artificiality, such as the presence of shops, traffic and facilities (urbanisation), whereas green was defined by the presence of vegetation, greenness and water (naturalness). The four places analysed in the study were ranked as follows according to this dimension: Los Herrán, the greyest place; Constitución, a grey place; Salinillas, a green place with sparse vegetation; and Olarizu, the greenest place with water.

2.2. Procedure and Data Collection

A protocol was established to define how participants should conduct their acoustic observations of the urban places. Since the observational procedure was both crucial and complex, participants were accompanied by a member of the team who guided them in order to ensure that it was applied correctly during the exercise. At the beginning, participants spent five minutes observing the location to gain experience of the urban place (urban environmental experience), as they were expected to make conscious observations and assessments. Sound events could occur at any time during the observation, and each time one was detected, a pop-up message was displayed on the smartphone screen. The message prompted users to identify their perception (i.e., pleasant or unpleasant) and the type of acoustic source for the event. Participants identified the main acoustic sources noticed, but without identifying the potential keynote sounds of each urban place. As soon as the evaluation was completed, data were post-processed, providing observers with easily interpretable feedback on their evaluation.

The observations were conducted from the 17th to the 30th of April, 2015. It was important for this study that the weather facilitated enjoyment of the urban places analysed; consequently, data collection was conducted on sunny spring days when it was neither very cold nor very hot and participants were available. Experiences were usually collected at times when the spaces were most crowded (10am–1pm and 5–8pm). The mean duration of experiences was 12.45 min (SD = 6.76), with no significant differences between places.

The acoustic indicators were measured for the duration of the observer's experience in these places.

Data protection legislation and participants' rights and obligations with respect to the data they collected were observed at all times. To fulfil the legal requirements of the European Directive 95/46/EC, 24th October 1995 on the protection of individuals with regard to the processing of personal data and on the free movement of such data, and Spanish Law 15/1999, 13rd December, of Protection of Personal Data) a privacy policy document was drafted. It described the type of data to be collected, its intended use (e.g., for research and scientific publications), data storage and protection. All these details were gathered in two documents signed by users/participants (i.e., the Privacy Policy and the User Agreement) [55].

2.3. Sample

Participation was voluntary, and subjects were recruited from among residents of the city of Vitoria-Gasteiz, through civic associations. The criteria for selecting participants were established by the Iritziak Batuz team, and the process is described in deliverable D3.4 of the CITI-SENSE project [56]. A total of 53 people conducted field observations in the four urban places. They produced a total of 137 observations that were used for analysis, and each participant evaluated at least two sites in the same or in different urban places. In this regard, the unit of analysis for this study was each of these 137 observations.

2.4. Assessment of Sound Environment

Preliminary tests under environmental conditions indicated that the smartphone's built-in microphone was highly sensitive to wind (contribution higher than 5 dB with wind intensity above 1.5 m/s), which would have affected outdoor measurements. Therefore, an external microphone with a standard protective windscreen was added to the measurement protocol. After analysis and a search for a low-cost microphone, the Edutige EIM-003 was chosen. The improvement in accuracy was tested in an anechoic chamber, and it was found that the average deviations of 6.7 dB (obtained using the smartphone with an internal microphone) were reduced to 1 dB (obtained using the smartphone with an external microphone), compared using a class 1 sound level meter.

The toolkit was designed to measure global $LAeq,1s$ levels, as other acoustic indicators can be constructed from this parameter: $LAeq,T$, minimum $LAeq,1s$ as $LAmin$ and maximum $LAeq,1s$ as $LAmax$. As part of the measurement, the time history is registered and displayed on the smartphone screen, as is the global mean $LAeq,T$ level and the maximum and minimum $LAeq,1s$ levels during the measurement period. In addition, the toolkit detects sound events by applying a dynamic threshold principle, and when an event is detected, the participant is prompted to provide an assessment (e.g., pleasantness and type of sound source).

This method is based on a comparison of the instantaneous LAeq,1s level with the energy means of the LAeq,5s, downstream (5 s earlier) and LAeq,5s, upstream (5 s later). Thus, a sound event is detected when the acoustic level variation indicates a difference with both downstream and upstream means that exceeds the threshold (6.5 dBA fixed value). The fixed threshold value was defined using expertise to identify events in noisy or quiet urban environments alike.

2.5. CITI-SENSE Questionnaire: Emotions, Soundscape and Other Issues

Although the CITI-SENSE toolkit allows a simultaneous assessment of the sound environment and collection of environmental perceptions on site, participants' responses to the questionnaire were independent of sound or acoustic environment measurements. The questionnaire was only interrupted when an event was detected during the two minutes that the acoustic environment was being measured, to ask participants what kind of event it was and whether or not they found it pleasant.

The CITI-SENSE questionnaire, which can be consulted in the Supplementary Materials, collected information on participants' emotional states, the soundscape and other variables that might also influence emotional state.

Emotional impact was evaluated using an emotions scale that included four basic emotions, two of which were positive; happiness (high arousal) and calm (low arousal), and two negatives; anger (high arousal) and sadness (low arousal). The five-point scale also included an item to measure perceived stress. These five items were assessed at two different times, once at the beginning of the questionnaire (referring to emotional states in the preceding days), and subsequently at the end of the questionnaire (referring to present emotional state after urban environmental experience). Differences in the scale between these two moments indicated the emotional impact of urban environmental experiences in the places analysed.

Soundscape (SSC) was evaluated by means of an ad hoc questionnaire, using a semantic differential (SD) scale that contained 13 pairs of bipolar adjectives such as unpleasant-pleasant, noisy-calm, stressful-relaxing, artificial-natural, monotonous-lively (vibrant), informative-uninformative and inappropriate-appropriate to surroundings, rated using a five-point ordinal scale. The data collection method corresponded to that described in ISO/TS 12913:2 on soundscape [42].

A semantic differential five-point scale was also used for landscape (LSC), with 3 items related to unpleasant-pleasantness, noisy-quietness and artificial-naturalness. These items did not specifically include visual aspects.

In addition, other aspects were considered that might influence the relationship between soundscape and its emotional impact. These included sociodemographic variables, residential factors, general self-perceptions of health and acoustic and environmental comfort.

Acoustic and environmental comfort were evaluated by means of two specific items measured on a 5-point ordinal scale (where 1 = very uncomfortable and 5 = very comfortable). The scale also included assessments of thermal, lighting and visual comfort, which were not specifically analysed in the present study.

2.6. Data AnalysisStrategy

To describe the data, the mean and standard deviation (M± SD) were calculated in the case of continuous variables, and the frequency and percentage (n, %) in the case of nominal variables. The contrast of proportions was performed through the Chi-Square test (χ^2) or the equivalent Fisher's exact test in the case of expected frequencies less than five. For the contrast of mean differences, the analysis of variance test (ANOVA) was used, and in the case of non-compliance with the homoscedasticity assumption, the Brown-Forsythe robust test was applied. Normal distribution was also checked prior to contrast analysis using the Kolmogorov-Smirnov test. The degree of association between variables was estimated using Pearson's (r) product-moment correlation coefficient. Likewise, multiple linear regression models were used to determine the predictors of the emotional response, with an estimation of the validity of the model (ANOVA test), the level of variance explained by the retained factors (R^2) and an estimation of the standardised coefficient (β) of each of them. For all analyses, the level of significance considered was $\alpha = 0.05$.

3. Results

The results obtained for the proposed solution as regards the research objectives are presented below and include: (1) characterisation of study participants; (2) characterisation of the urban places: acoustic levels and soundscape; (3) emotional effect of the urban environmental experience (henceforth urban experience); (4) explanation of the emotional effect of urban environmental experiences (UEE).

3.1. Characterisation of Study Participants

Women accounted for 54% of the study sample and men, 46%. The mean age of participants was 42.3 years (SD = 14.18 years, min = 19; max = 75). In addition, 46.4% had a university and 39.0% a secondary education, and 40.4% were employed while 16.9% were unemployed.

As shown in Table 2, in general, there were no significant social or demographic differences between the observers in each of the urban places. The only significant difference concerned place of residence ($\chi^2 = 28.263$; df = 15; $p < 0.05$), whereby residents of Vitoria-Gasteiz accounted for all (100%) of the participants who assessed Olarizu but only 80.7% of those who assessed Constitución square.

Table 2. Participant characteristics by urban places in Vitoria-Gasteiz (total), and significance (p) of Chi-square analysis.

No. of Observations	Los Herrán 42	Constitución 31	Salinillas 34	Olarizu 30	% GLOBAL 137	N	p
Gender (women)	52.4%	51.6%	61.8%	50.0%	54.0%	74	0.769
Residence (Vitoria-Gasteiz)	92.9%	80.7%	94.1%	100.0%	92.0%	126	0.020
University education	43.9%	45.2%	50.0%	46.7%	46.3%	63	
Secondary education	46.3%	32.3%	35.3%	40.0%	39.0%	53	0.885
Primary education	4.9%	12.9%	8.8%	10.0%	8.8%	12	
Other	4.9%	9.7%	5.9%	3.3%	5.9%	8	
Employed	36.6%	45.2%	41.2%	40.0%	40.4%	55	
Unemployed	14.6%	6.5%	20.6%	26.7%	16.9%	23	
Students	29.3%	12.9%	8.8%	0.0%	14.0%	19	0.069
Retirees	7.3%	16.1%	5.9%	10.0%	9.6%	13	
Other	12.2%	19.4%	23.5%	23.3%	19.1%	26	
Perceived health: good and very good	76.1%	71.0%	82.4%	83.4%	78.1%	107	
P. Health: fair	23.9%	29.0%	17.6%	16.6%	21.9%	30	0.605
P. Health: bad	0.0%	0.0%	0.0%	0.0%	0.0%	0	

N: frequency of response by category; p (probability of χ2): * $p < 0.05$; ns: not significant.

Neither was a statistically significant difference between urban places and participants' perceived health status, which was generally good (51.1%) or very good (27%). No participants perceived their health status to be bad.

These results indicate that composition of the participant group did not affect the results of the analysis.

3.2. Characterisation of the Urban Places: Sound Environment and Soundscape

The urban places with the highest acoustic levels were Los Herrán and Constitución, at 60.9 and 60.5 dBA LAeq, mean, respectively (Table 3). Los Herrán was also where the highest maximum level was recorded (79.3 dBA maximum-LAeq,1s), whereas the highest minimum level was recorded at Constitución (51.9 dBA minimum-LAeq,1s). Acoustic events were barely detected at these places.

Participants were asked to identify the most characteristic sound sources in the urban places and the pleasantness of their sound environments. The most common source of sound was traffic (64.3%) at Los Herrán, natural sounds (29.0%) and traffic (25.8%) at Constitución and sounds associated with nature at the greener places, Olarizu and Salinillas (93.3% and 55.0%, respectively) ($\chi^2 = 89.81$; df = 18; $p < 0.001$). Thus, the main sound source at Los Herrán, the most artificial place, was considered unpleasant (85.7%), while at Olarizu, the greenest place, it was considered pleasant (93.3%), and these differences were statistically significant ($\chi^2 = 78.26$; df = 12; $p < 0.001$). In relation to the above, it can be seen that the number of acoustic events (mostly positive) was higher in the greener than in the greyer place.

Table 3. Characterisation of the urban places analysed (mean scores ± standard deviation), by sound environment, landscape, environmental comfort and soundscape, and significance (p) of ANOVA analysis.

N	Los Herrán 42	Constitución 31	Salinillas 34	Olarizu 30	Global 137	p
dB LAeq,mean	60.9 ± 4.21	60.5 ± 10.38	52.9 ± 16.63	55.9 ± 8.92	57.7 ± 9.78	0.001
dB max LAeq,1s	79.3 ± 6.09	74.7 ± 10.65	76.3 ± 15.54	74.7 ± 9.46	76.4 ± 10.83	0.261
dB minLAeq,1s	47.6 ± 3.36	51.9 ± 6.21	43.8 ± 11.81	43.4 ± 6.83	46.7 ± 8.13	<0.001
No. total events	1.41 ± 1.97	1.10 ± 9.80	7.98 ± 1.19	8.23 ± 7.02	4.49 ± 6.87	<0.001
No. positive events	0.53 ± 0.88	0.77 ± 5.57	4.91 ± 1.07	5.31 ± 4.92	2.73 ± 4.33	<0.001
No. negative events	0.80 ± 1.19	0.29 ± 3.60	1.94 ± 0.59	2.57 ± 4.47	1.36 ± 2.95	0.007
LSC_pleasant	2.71 ± 1.07	3.74 ± 0.77	3.76 ± 0.99	4.53 ± 0.73	3.61 ± 1.13	<0.001
LSC_quiet	1.98 ± 1.07	3.32 ± 1.19	4.03 ± 0.87	4.20 ± 0.71	3.28 ± 1.34	<0.001
LSC_natural	2.36 ± 1.01	2.61 ± 0.99	3.32 ± 1.12	4.53 ± 0.63	3.13 ± 1.26	<0.001
Environmental comfort	2.60 ± 0.80	3.32 ± 0.96	3.56 ± 0.75	4.10 ± 0.66	3.33 ± 0.97	<0.001
Acoustic comfort	2.24 ± 0.82	2.90 ± 0.84	3.79 ± 0.83	4.03 ± 0.72	3.17 ± 1.09	<0.001
SSC_pleasant	1.90 ± 0.88	2.97 ± 0.93	3.53 ± 1.05	4.10 ± 0.66	3.03 ± 1.22	<0.001
SSC_calm	1.69 ± 0.84	2.90 ± 0.99	3.62 ± 1.04	3.97 ± 0.76	2.94 ± 1.28	<0.001
SSC_relaxing	2.24 ± 0,91	3.23 ± 0.83	3.82 ± 0.76	4.10 ± 0.71	3.26 ± 1.10	<0.001
SSC_uninterrupted	3.79 ± 0.95	3.48 ± 0.86	3.47 ± 0.89	3.67 ± 1.03	3.61 ± 0.93	0.407
SSC_familiar	4.02 ± 0.90	4.03 ± 1.08	3.50 ± 0.84	4.10 ± 0.80	3.91 ± 0.94	0.029
SSC_facilitates conversation	2.48 ± 0.83	3.23 ± 0.88	3.88 ± 0.76	4.33 ± 0.66	3.40 ± 1.07	<0.001
SSC_informative	2.48 ± 0.89	2.87 ± 0.74	3.24 ± 0.76	3.23 ± 1.10	2.92 ± 0.93	0.001
SSC_clear	2.57 ± 1.15	3.19 ± 0.73	3.79 ± 0.86	4.03 ± 0.81	3.34 ± 1.09	<0.001
SC_characteristic	2.36 ± 1.32	2.90 ± 0.94	3.29 ± 1.16	3.90 ± 0.96	3.05 ± 1.25	<0.001
SSC_lively (vibrant)	2.60 ± 1.15	2.77 ± 0.98	3.21 ± 0.88	3.17 ± 0.99	2.91 ± 1.04	0.028
SSC_fun	2.43 ± 1.08	2.71 ± 1.03	3.09 ± 0.97	3.67 ± 0.92	2.93 ± 1.03	<0.001
SSC_natural	1.90 ± 0.96	2.58 ± 1.32	3.32 ± 1.12	4.40 ± 0.67	2.96 ± 1.39	<0.001
SSC_appropriate-surroundings	3.10 ± 1.14	3.58 ± 1.13	3.62 ± 0.81	4.20 ± 0.66	3.58 ± 1.05	<0.001

SSC: soundscape; LSC: landscape; SSC, LSC and comfort: 5-point scales; p: probability.

Acoustic and environmental comfort (assessed using a 5-point ordinal scale) was high in Olarizu (4.0 and 4.1, respectively), medium-high in Salinillas (3.8 and 3.6), average in Constitución (2.9 and 3.3) and low (2.2) or medium-low (2.6) in Los Herrán, and all of these differences were statistically significant ($F(3,133) = 37.92$; $p < 0.001$ and $F(3,133) = 21.78$; $p < 0.001$).

The results for soundscape (SSC) characterisation were similar to those for comfort, as can be seen in Table 3. A semantic differential five-point scale with bipolar adjectives was used to assess the soundscape; however, the table only gives the right-hand adjective of each pair, which corresponds to the highest value (5) for the response options.

Soundscapes at Olarizu were generally associated with positive scores (mean values around 4, on a scale of 1–5), with the exception of the score for lively, which was neutral (3.2). Overall, the Olarizu soundscape was characterised by naturalness (4.5) and capacity to facilitate conversation (4.3).

The Salinillas soundscapes were associated with scores between neutral and positive (values between 3 and 4). Meanwhile, at Constitución, they were associated with neutral scores (around 3), scoring higher for familiarity (4.0), appropriacy to the environment (3.6) and uninterrupted (3.5).

The soundscapes at Los Herrán obtained the lowest scores, especially for lack of calm (1.7), naturalness or pleasantness (1.9). As with Constitución, its soundscapes were also familiar (4.0) and uninterrupted (3.8).

Perceptions of the degree of naturalness of the landscape in each urban place confirmed the previous ranking of these according to the dimension of grey versus green. Thus, Olarizu, the urban place ranked as the most natural because it contained the most green and blue elements (Table 1), was the one that participants perceived as the most natural (mean 4.53 in LSC-natural: Table 3), whereas Los Herrán, the most artificial place (85% grey in Table 1) with the least green elements (25%) was perceived as the most artificial (mean 2.36 in LSC_natural: Table 3).

3.3. Emotional Effect of the Urban Environmental Experience

Environmental experiences in the four urban places analysed in Vitoria-Gasteiz gave rise to emotional changes, as can be seen in Figure 3, which gives the mean scores of the total number of observations, for each of the four basic emotions considered and perceived stress at the beginning (T01) and end (T02) of the urban experiences.

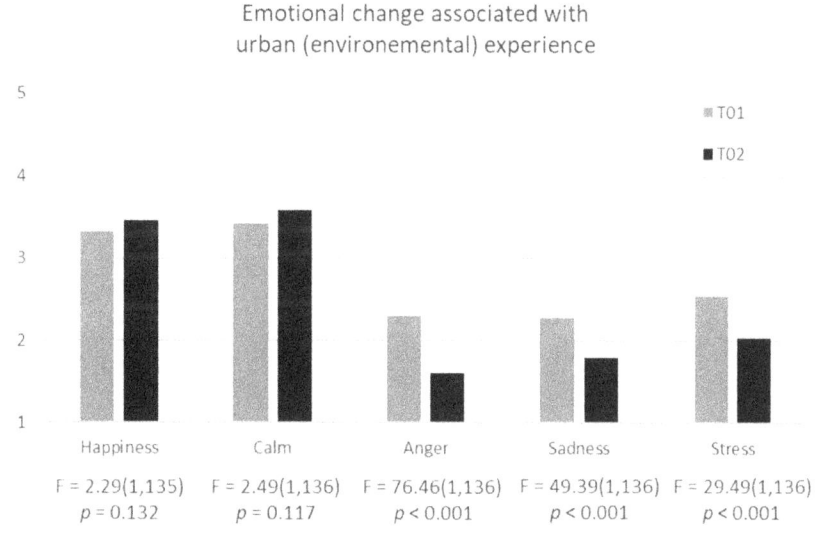

Figure 3. Effect of the urban experience on the four basic emotions and perceived stress, before (T01) and after (T02) renovation of the urban places (ANOVA test).

The changes indicate that after the urban environmental experience, even if this had been of a short duration, positive emotions increased slightly, and negative emotions and perceived stress were reduced. A repeated measure analysis revealed that differences in the positive emotions of happiness and calm were not statistically significant. In contrast, reductions in negative emotions and perceived stress were statistically significant. Anger dropped by 0.69 points (30%) ($F(1,136) = 76.493$; $p < 0.001$), sadness by 0.49 (21.55%) ($F(1,136) = 49.386$; $p < 0.001$) and perceived stress by 0.50 (19.7%) ($F(1,136) = 29.493$; $p < 0.001$). The effect size (partial Eta squared: η^2) was large in all three cases (0.360 for anger, 0.266 for sadness and 0.178 for perceived stress).

Table 4 presents the mean scores for emotional states before and after the urban experiences, and the difference between both, for the total number of observations and for the places analysed.

As can be seen in the table, apparent differences emerged between the urban places, although these did not reach statistical significance.

Table 4. Characterisation of emotional states at the beginning (T01) and end (T02) of the urban experience, and the difference between both (mean scores ± standard deviation) in the four urban places, and significance (p) of ANOVA analysis.

N	Los Herrán	Constitución	Salinillas	Olarizu	Global	p
	42	31	34	30	137	
Happiness_T01	3.29 ± 1.04	3.35 ± 1.07	3.21 ± 1.14	3.47 ± 0.90	3.32 ± 1.04	0.782
Happiness_T02	3.29 ± 0.74	3.48 ± 0.97	3.45 ± 0.81	3.70 ± 0.75	3.46 ± 0.82	0.218
Happiness_Dif	0.00 ± 0.91	0.13 ± 1.15	0.24 ± 1.35	0.23 ± 0.90	0.14 ± 1.08	0.748
Calm_T01	3.40 ± 1.25	3.74 ± 1.03	3.09 ± 1.18	3.47 ± 0.97	3.42 ± 1.14	0.141
Calm_T02	3.40 ± 0.89	3.74 ± 0.96	3.59 ± 1.00	3.67 ± 0.92	3.58 ± 0.94	0.452
Calm_Dif	0.00 ± 1.14	0.00 ± 1.21	0.50 ± 1.35	0.20 ± 1.27	0.16 ± 1.25	0.291
Anger_T01	2.31 ± 0.95	2.16 ± 1.16	2.41 ± 1.00	2.30 ± 1.02	2.30 ± 1.02	0.810
Anger_T02	1.71 ± 0.94	1.45 ± 0.88	1.68 ± 0.89	1.53 ± 0.82	1.61 ± 0.89	0.580
Anger_Dif	−0.60 ± 0.77	−0.71 ± 0.94	−0.73 ± 0.90	−0.77 ± 1.17	−0.69 ± 0.93	0.868
Sadness_T01	2.40 ± 0.94	2.32 ± 0.92	2.24 ± 0.98	2.13 ± 0.90	2.28 ± 0.93	0.655
Sadness_T02	1.95 ± 0.94	1.71 ± 0.76	1.71 ± 0.97	1.77 ± 0.74	1.80 ± 0.89	0.593
Sadness_Dif	−0.45 ± 0.67	−0.61 ± 0.95	−0.53 ± 0.71	−0.36 ± 0.96	−0.48 ± 0.81	0.672
Stress_T01	2.71 ± 0.97	2.35 ± 1.11	2.56 ± 1.02	2.47 ± 1.04	2.54 ± 1.03	0.503
Stress_T02	2.31 ± 1.00	1.77 ± 0.76	2.03 ± 0.96	1.93 ± 0.74	2.04 ± 0.89	0.071
Stress_Dif	−0.40 ± 1.19	−0.58 ± 1.09	−0.53 ± 0.86	−0.54 ± 1.20	−0.50 ± 1.09	0.911

T01: initial emotional stages; T02: final emotional stages; Dif: T02-T01; p: probability.

These differences (Table 4) suggest that at Los Herrán, the least green place, the urban experiences did not change positive emotions. However, they reduced negative ones and perceived stress, although to a lesser extent than in the other urban places. In Los Herrán, perceived stress was greater at the end of the urban experience, presenting tendential differences to the other urban places ($F(3,133) = 2.40$; $p = 0.07$).

Urban experiences in the second least green place, Constitución, were not associated with changes in positive emotions either, but again, they did reduce negative ones and perceived stress, even to a slightly greater extent than experiences in the parks of Salinillas and Olarizu, the greener places. Urban experiences in these latter were associated with a slight increase in positive emotions and a reduction in negative emotions, mainly anger, and perceived stress (Table 4).

Table 5 shows the relationships (Pearson correlation) between the dimensions of environmental and acoustic comfort and emotional states at the end of the urban experience. As can be seen, comfort was inversely associated with negative emotional states (as the former increased, the latter decreased), whereas it presented a direct relationship with positive emotional states (as the former increased, so did the latter).

Table 5. Pearson correlations (r) for the four basic emotions and perceived stress at the end of the urban experience (T02), and comfort and soundscape variables.

T2	Happiness	Calm	Anger	Sadness	Stress
Environmental comfort	0.38 ***	0.21 **	−0.28 **	−0.20 **	−0.42 ***
Acoustic comfort	0.32 ***	0.25 **	−0.25 **	−0.19 *	−0.36 ***
SSC_pleasant	0.37 ***	0.24 **	−0.21 **	−0.28 **	−0.35 ***
SSC_calm	0.40 ***	0.24 **	- - -	- - -	−0.24 **
SSC_fun	0.3 ***	0.23 **	- - -	- - -	−0.23 **
SSC_lively	- - -	- - -	- - -	−0.18 *	- - -
SSC_natural	0.32 ***	0.25 **	- - -	−0.20 *	−0.19 *

*** $p < 0.001$; ** $p < 0.01$; * $p < 0.05$.

Thus, happiness in the urban settings was directly related to perceptions that the soundscape was calm and pleasant and to the environmental comfort of the urban environmental experience (UEE) ($r \approx 0.40$). It was also associated—albeit less strongly—with acoustic comfort and the fun and naturalness of the soundscape ($r \approx 0.40$). Calm at the end of the urban experience was also related to environmental and acoustic comfort and to perceptions of pleasantness, calm, fun and naturalness of the soundscape ($r \approx 0.25$. As with happiness, perceived stress also presented a strong association with environmental and acoustic comfort and with pleasantness of the soundscape, but this time inversely ($r \approx -0.40$).

Similarly, the negative emotions of anger and sadness were inversely associated with environmental and acoustic comfort and the pleasantness of the soundscape (correlations between −0.2 and −0.3). Sadness was also inversely related to the liveliness or vibrancy and naturalness of soundscapes; thus, the livelier and more natural the soundscape, the lower the sadness at the end of the urban experiences.

3.4. Explaining the Emotional Effect Of Urban Environmental Experiences

To determine the explanatory power of the factors considered, mainly those related to the soundscape and the sound environment, for emotional effect and perceived stress, multiple regression models were constructed.

Having selected four basic emotions (happiness, calm, anger and sadness) and perceived stress as outcome variables, five regression models were constructed using the same set of independent variables: sociodemographic variables (e.g., age, sex and educational level), the parameters used to characterise the acoustic environment of the urban places analysed (LAeq,mean, min-LAeq,1s, max-LAeq,1s, no. of positive, negative and total events, and pleasantness of the two main sound sources), acoustic and environmental comfort of the places and soundscape (13 dimensions considered in the semantic differential scale). To control for the effect of participants' emotional state when commencing the experience, baseline measurements of the five emotional variables were included in the regression model. Each model was constructed using a stepwise strategy whereby those factors that did not significantly explain the emotion assessed were gradually discarded.

Table 6 shows the five regression models, one per column, together with the predictive variables that were statistically significant in one of the models. The predictive model for the emotion of calm was the most modest, explaining 22.5% of the variance ($R^2 = 0.225$) and identifying three predictors, whereas the predictive model for stress was the most robust ($R^2 = 0.519$).

Table 6. Effect (standardised Beta) of the urban environmental experience (UEE) on the four basic emotions and perceived stress.

Independent Vatriables	Happiness (T02)	Calm (T02)	Anger (T02)	Sadness (T02)	Stress (T02)
Calm (T01)	0.251				
Anger (T01)	−0.204		0.454	0.204	0.332
Sadness (T01)			0.281	0.473	0.229
Stress (T01)	−0.203	−0.380			0.192
Age			−0.240		
Education					−0.211
dB LAeq,mean		0.164		−0.170	
Environmental comfort	0.277		−0.259		−0.338
Acoustic comfort		0.270			
SSC_fun			0.324		
SSC_lively					0.295
F	18.96	13.94	19.14	31.56	25.11
d.f.	4129	3131	5129	3131	6128
p	<0.001	<0.001	<0.001	<0.001	<0.001
R^2 adjusted	0.351	0.225	0.404	0.406	0.519

T01: scores at the start of the EEU; T02: scores at the end of the EEU; SSC: soundscape.

It should be noted that in the social sciences, the average value of associations between variables is around 0.21 [56]; therefore, the correlation value obtained in the present study was close to this average and even a little above.

An analysis of the data presented in the table for stress indicated that this model was statistically significant (F = 25.11; $p < 0.001$) and identified six predictors of stress: experiencing low environmental comfort ($\beta = -0.34$), the presence of high baseline anger ($\beta = 0.33$), perceptions of the soundscape as lively or vibrant ($\beta = 0.29$), the presence of baseline sadness ($\beta = 0.23$), a lower educational level ($\beta = -0.21$) and a high baseline level of stress ($\beta = 0.19$).

Focusing on the factors involved in the expression of emotional states, the results can be assessed by analysing how many of the emotions presented a given explanatory factor. In this regard, for example, a baseline emotion of anger was associated with four of the emotional states: negatively with happiness ($\beta = -0.20$) and positively with anger ($\beta = 0.45$), stress ($\beta = 0.33$) and sadness ($\beta = 0.20$). Meanwhile, environmental comfort was associated with greater happiness ($\beta = 0.27$) and less stress ($\beta = -0.34$) or anger ($\beta = -0.26$).

These results indicate that emotional states after the urban experience were generally associated with previous emotional states, but primarily with negative emotions and perceived stress.

For the acoustic environment, only the LAeq, mean was significantly associated with the emotional states of calm and sadness after the urban experience. Higher sound levels were associated with emotional states of greater calm and less sadness.

The environmental experiences in more comfortable urban places were associated with greater happiness and less anger or perceived stress.

With regard to the soundscape, differences were observed according to the emotion considered. Calm was associated with acoustic comfort, while in contrast, the negative emotion of anger was positively associated with the soundscape's capacity for fun: the more fun a soundscape was considered, the more anger the observer felt at the end of the experience. Similarly, the more lively or vibrant the sound environment was perceived to be, the more stressed the observer felt at the end of the urban experience.

4. Discussion

In agreement with other studies [6,10,11,14,19,20], the results reported here confirm the initial study hypothesis that some urban places exert a positive impact on people's well–being and quality of life. Thus, the present study has demonstrated a positive effect that reflects the emotionally restorative capacity of the urban places analysed, whereby environmental experiences in these places yielded a statistically significant reduction in perceived stress and the negative emotions of sadness and anger, and a trend towards an increase in the positive emotions of happiness and calm.

In this study, the effect on positive emotions did not reach statistical significance. This may be because these emotional states are more resistant to change and require visits of a longer duration to reflect these benefits; recall that the duration of the urban environmental experiences in this study was short. A further possibility is that the beneficial effect on positive emotions is more strongly associated with the naturalness of places [1–5] and it is therefore more difficult to find this effect in urban environments. Another possible explanation may be the paradox whereby it is difficult to improve situations that are already close to their maximum. In general, when people are asked about positive emotional states, health, life satisfaction or residential surroundings, they tend to respond positively and close to the maximum, leaving little room for improvement. As with all horizontal asymptotes, the value of "y" will never be equal, and it can always be improved and brought closer to the maximum; however, in practice, the difference is imperceptible and sometimes even irrelevant. It might therefore be more difficult to improve positive emotions than negative ones. The same occurs in other areas such as athletic performance or life expectancy, which evidence increasingly smaller improvements.

The results presented here also indicate that the emotionally restorative capacity of the urban places was influenced by the environmental comfort experienced by the participants. Evidently, emotional states, especially negative ones, at the end of the urban environmental experiences were to a large extent determined by prior emotional states. However, besides these, the other aspect that exerted the most influence on participants' emotional states at the end of the experience was environmental comfort, conceived holistically (globally). These results highlight the need for a holistic vision of experiences of places in urban environments, in order to integrate information from all the senses.

Besides global environmental comfort, acoustic comfort was also associated with a reduction in negative and an increase in positive emotional states. This result is in agreement with recent studies analysing the relationship between soundscape and health [57] and the restorative capacity of the soundscape in urban settings e.g., [33,34]. In this respect, this work complements other studies aimed at improving physiological and attention restoration [1,2,10,14]. This study found that the soundscape characteristics which contributed to greater emotional restoration and a reduction in perceived stress were pleasantness, calm, fun and naturalness. It therefore contributes to analyses of the soundscape characteristics that can exert positive health-related effects. A recently published systematic review of associations between positive soundscapes (e.g., pleasant, calm, less annoying) and health (e.g., increased restoration, reduced stress-inducing mechanisms) found that positive soundscapes are associated with faster stress recovery processes in laboratory experiments and better self-reported health in large-scale surveys [46]. Hence, the present study adds to the above-mentioned research by providing results obtained using a method applied in real urban environments.

Although this study was conducted on site, the method applied made it possible to collect objective and subjective data simultaneously; consequently, the objective acoustic environment indicators referred specifically to the period of time in which each participant's urban environmental experience took place. In this respect, the present study supports the use of the new technologies, a smartphone application in this case, to conduct soundscape research based on subjective data reported directly by users of the places. However, the application of this method proved somewhat complex and might present limitations compared to laboratory studies, as might the study sample size and the low diversity of urban spaces have considered. It is also possible that the experiment itself or the attention the participants received contributed to the effect on emotional restoration. Nevertheless, the method applied has proved interesting, and the study findings, while not conclusive, are consistent with the results obtained in earlier studies employing other research methods.

In addition, in this study, environmental comfort (both global and acoustic) presented an increase associated with the dichotomous dimension of artificiality (% grey elements) versus naturalness (% green and blue), as shown in Figure 4. The greener the places, the more environmentally and acoustically comfortable they were.

The analysis of acoustic environments and their perception (soundscape) indicates that besides naturalness, sound diversity was associated with greater pleasantness and comfort. Acoustic environments in more artificial places were characterised by higher acoustic levels, meaning that fewer sound events were detected. In contrast, the acoustic environment of spaces with a high presence of natural elements presented lower acoustic levels and a higher number of events, which tended to be perceived positively. In addition, the most characteristic sound sources in these environments, usually human or natural, were considered pleasant. Participants were not asked to identify potential keynote sounds, and therefore it was not possible to analyse whether these contributed to the acoustic comfort or restorative capacity of urban open public spaces.

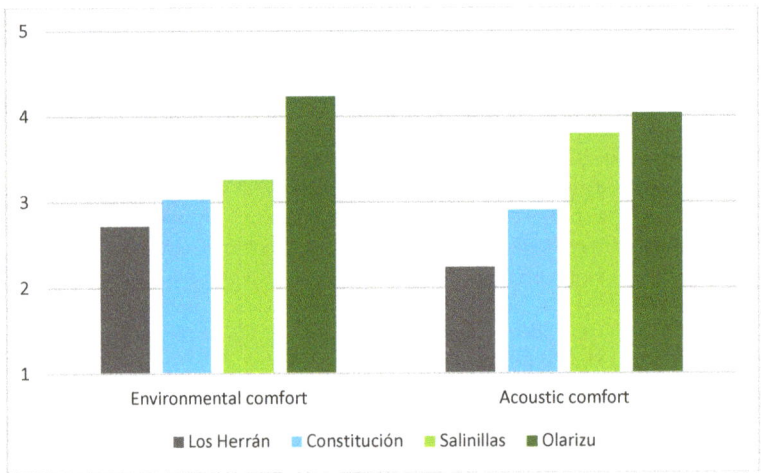

Figure 4. Mean scores for environmental and acoustic comfort in relation to the artificial-natural continuum.

The classical theories of attention restoration—ART [1] and stress recovery, SRT [2–4]—state that there is a direct link between naturalness and restorative capacity. Consequently, and given the relationship between comfort and naturalness detected in the present study, it would seem logical to conclude that naturalness influences emotional restoration. However, no evidence of a direct association between the two was obtained in the present study, since no significant differences were observed between the urban places for any of the emotions analysed. This would seem to indicate an indirect relationship mediated by the environmental comfort experienced by users in the place.

The results evidence some limitations since it has not been possible to provide very strong evidence of the restorative capacity of urban open public spaces or to quantify the relationship between restorative capacity and the presence of natural elements in urban places. Nevertheless, the study has provided indications in the expected direction. This suggests the need to continue to conduct research in this area, which encompasses two topics for which previous studies have reported firm evidence, namely the restorative capacity of some urban settings and the contribution of the soundscape to this positive effect on health and well-being.

This work complements other studies [10], as it is focused on small urban public spaces. In future research, it would be interesting to extend the diversity of urban open public spaces in order to further elucidate the contribution of different elements: green (e.g., grass, shrubs, trees), blue (e.g., fountains, rivers, lakes, seas), and grey (e.g., types of material, design). It would also be interesting in future research to consider cultural diversity (mainly related to cultural heritage and signs of identity), social diversity (related to users) and animal biodiversity (the activity of which could contribute to increase the richness of the associated soundscape).

The findings of this study, although not conclusive, give evidence of the potential use of this method to analyse the restorative effect of the quality of urban public spaces, and their soundscape, on emotions. In combination with ICT technologies, it can enable studies where citizens can take part as users of the spaces, reducing their participation effort. As an example of this, the observation time necessary in this survey was around 20 minutes, lower than that needed in other studies [10,14,19,20]. Consequently, the completion of field studies was much easier and the outcomes showed that emotional restorative effects could be noticed with short periods of environmental experience. Nonetheless, the influence of the length of time of the test should be investigated in greater depth, considering the target restorative effect to be assessed (physiological, attention, emotions or other). As other authors have noted, it is "necessary to plan and conducive to the soundscape and health research within the

5. Conclusions

The main conclusion that can be drawn from this study is that the capacity for psychological restoration is not unique to natural settings outside cities, but may also be a characteristic of some urban spaces, since it was found that even for short periods of time, the use of urban places was associated with a significant decrease in negative emotions and perceived stress, as well as a slight increase in positive emotions.

Another important aspect is that restorative capacity is associated with global environmental comfort and acoustic comfort in particular. Thus, the higher the comfort, the better the emotional state detected. Consequently, acoustically comfortable urban places with a pleasant soundscape can be considered restorative environments.

Since the urban soundscape can promote the psychological restoration of users, it should clearly form part of planning and architectural design [47,58], incorporating specific urban furniture [49] to improve the perception of urban places. In this respect, collaboration from the initial stages of project development between those responsible for urban design and acoustics experts represents a crucial element in urban renovation processes [59]. The human and social sciences should also play a key role in holistic soundscape studies because soundscape is a construct of human perception.

This study identified the soundscape characteristics that contributed to greater positive health-related effects, namely pleasantness and calm, as well as the attributes of fun and naturalness. These findings confirm the known benefits of enhancing the natural component of urban places and increasing their acoustic diversity, for example by encouraging insects and birds, facilitating the interaction between wind and plants, or introducing the sound of water. In addition, designing and creating other positive acoustic events and sound sources would also contribute to improving environmental experiences in these urban places.

Supplementary Materials: It is available online at http://www.mdpi.com/1660-4601/16/7/1284/s1.

Author Contributions: Conceptualisation, K.H.-P. and I.A.; data collection, K.H.-P., I.I. and Á.S.; data analysis, K.H.-P. and I.I.; funding acquisition, I.A.; research, K.H.-P., I.I., I.G. Á.S. and J.L.E.; methodology, K.H.-P., I.A. and I.I.; project administration, I.A. and I.G.; resources, I.G.; software, Á.S.; supervision, K.H.-P., J.L.E. and I.A.; validation, K.H.-P.; visualisation, K.H.-P. and Á.S.; writing –original draft, K.H.-P., I.A., I.I., J.L.E. and Á.S.; Writing –review & editing, K.H.-P., J.L.E. and I.G.

Funding: This research formed part of the CITI-SENSE project funded under the European Union Seventh Framework Programme for research, technological development and demonstration, grant agreement no 308524.

Conflicts of Interest: The authors declare no conflict of interest.

References

1. Kaplan, R.; Kaplan, S. *The Experience of Nature. A Psychological Perspective*; Cambridge University Press: New York, NY, USA, 1989.
2. Ulrich, R.S. Natural versus urban scenes. Some psychophysiological effects. *Environ. Behav.* **1981**, *13*, 523–556. [CrossRef]
3. Ulrich, R.S. View through a window may influence recovery. *Science* **1984**, *224*, 420–421. [CrossRef]
4. Ulrich, R.S.; Simons, R.F.; Losito, B.D.; Fiorito, E.; Miles, M.A.; Zelson, M. Stress recovery during exposure to natural and urban environments. *J. Environ. Psychol.* **1991**, *11*, 201–230. [CrossRef]
5. Hernández, B.; Hidalgo, M.C. Effect of urban vegetation on psychological restorativeness. *Psychol. Rep.* **2005**, *96*, 1025–1028. [CrossRef] [PubMed]
6. Hartig, T.; Mang, M.; Evans, G. Restorative Effects of Natural Environment Experiences. *Environ. Behav.* **1991**, *23*, 3–26. [CrossRef]
7. Tennessen, C.H.; Cimprich, B. Views to nature: Effects on attention. *J. Environ. Psychol.* **1995**, *15*, 77–85. [CrossRef]

8. Kaplan, R. The nature of the view from home-psychological benefits. *Environ. Behav.* **2001**, *3*, 507–542. [CrossRef]
9. Herzog, T.R.; Black, A.M.; Fountaine, K.A.; Knotts, D.J. Reflection and attentional recovery as distinctive benefits of restorative environments. *J. Environ. Psychol.* **1997**, *17*, 165–170. [CrossRef]
10. Zhang, Y.; Kang, J.; Kang, J. Effects of Soundscape on the Environmental Restoration in Urban Natural Environments. *Noise Health* **2017**, *19*, 65–72.
11. Stigsdotter, U.K.; Corazon, S.S.; Sidenius, U.; Kristiansen, J.; Grahn, P. It is not all bad for the grey city—A crossover study on physiological and psychological restoration in a forest and an urban environment. *Health Place* **2017**, *46*, 145–154. [CrossRef]
12. Keniger, L.E.; Gaston, K.J.; Irvine, K.N.; Fuller, R.A. What are the benefits of interacting with nature? *Int. J. Environ. Res. Public Health* **2013**, *10*, 913–935. [CrossRef]
13. Van den Berg, A.; Hartig, A.; Staats, H. Preference for nature in urbanized societies: Stress, restoration and the pursuit of sustainability. *J. Soc. Issues* **2007**, *63*, 79–96. [CrossRef]
14. Ojala, A.; Korpela, K.; Tyrväinen, L.; Tiittanen, P.; Lankic, P. Restorative effects of urban green environments and the role of urban-nature orientedness and noise sensitivity: A field experiment. *Health Place* **2019**, *55*, 59–70. [CrossRef]
15. Milgram, S. The experience of living in cities. *Science* **1970**, *167*, 1461–1468. [CrossRef]
16. Marsella, A.J. Urbanization, mental health, and social deviancy. A review of issues and research. *Am. Psychol.* **1998**, *53*, 624–634. [CrossRef]
17. Nelson, A.L.; Schwirian, K.P.; Schwirian, P.M. Social and economic distress in large cities, 1970–1990: A test of the urban crisis thesis. *Soc. Sci. Res.* **1998**, *27*, 410–431. [CrossRef]
18. Staats, H.; Jahncke, H.; Herzog, T.R.; Hartig, T. Urban options for psychological restoration: Common strategies in everyday situations. *PLoS ONE* **2016**, *11*, e0146213. [CrossRef]
19. San Juan, C.; Subiza-Pérez, M.; Vozmediano, L. Restoration and the City: The Role of Public Urban Squares. *Front. Psychol.* **2017**. [CrossRef]
20. Subiza-Pérez, M.; Vozmediano, L.; San Juan, C. Restoration in urban settings: Pilot adaptation and psychometric properties of two psychological restoration and place bonding scales/Restauración en contextos urbanos: Adaptación piloto y propiedades psicométricas de dos escalas de restauración psicológica y vinculación con el espacio. *Psyecology* **2017**, *8*, 234–255. [CrossRef]
21. ONU. Las Ciudades Seguirán Creciendo, Sobre Todo en los Países en Desarrollo. Available online: https://www.un.org/development/desa/es/news/population/2018-world-urbanization-prospects.html (accessed on 23 January 2019).
22. Kang, J. *Urban Sound Environment*; Taylor & Francis Incorporating Spon: London, UK, 2006.
23. Brown, A.L.; Muhar, A. An approach to the acoustic design of outdoor space. *J. Environ. Plan. Manag.* **2004**, *47*, 827–842. [CrossRef]
24. Jeon, J.Y.; Lee, J.P.; Hong, J.Y. Non-auditory factors affecting urban soundscape evaluation. *J. Acoust. Soc. Am.* **2011**, *130*, 3761–3770. [CrossRef]
25. WHO. Environmental Noise Guidelines for the European Region. Available online: http://www.euro.who.int/en/health-topics/environment-and-health/noise/publications/2018/environmental-noise-guidelines-for-the-european-region-2018 (accessed on 4 April 2019).
26. Cain, R.; Jennings, P.; Poxon, J. The development and application of the emotional dimensions of a soundscape. *Appl. Acoust.* **2013**, *74*, 232–239. [CrossRef]
27. Brown, A.L.; Gjestland, T.; Dubois, D. Acoustic Environments and Soundscapes. In *Soundscape and the Built Environment*; Kang, J., Schulte-Fortkamp, B., Eds.; CRC Press, Taylor & Francis Group: Boca Raton, FL, USA, 2016; pp. 1–16.
28. Jabben, J.; Weber, M.; Verheijen, E. A framework for rating environmental value of urban parks. *Sci. Total Environ.* **2013**, *508*, 395–401. [CrossRef]
29. Yu, C.J.; Kang, J. Effects of cultural factors on the evaluation of acoustic quality in residential areas. In Proceedings of the 20th International Congress on Acoustics, ICA 2010, Sydney, Australia, 23–27 August 2010.
30. Brambilla, G.; Gallo, V.; Zambon, G. The soundscape quality in some urban parks in Milan, Italy. *Int. J. Environ. Res. Public Health* **2013**, *10*, 2348–2369.

31. Payne, S.R. Are perceived soundscape within urban parks restorative. *J. Acoust. Soc. Am.* **2008**, *123*, 3809. [CrossRef]
32. QUADMAP Project. Quiet Areas Definition and Management in Action Plans, Final Report. Covering the Project Activities from 01/09/2011 to 31/03/2015. 2016. Available online: http://www.quadmap.eu/wp-content/uploads/2016/01/Final-Report_QUADMAP_technical.pdf (accessed on 2 November 2016).
33. Payne, S.R. The production of a Perceived Restorativeness Soundscape Scale. *Appl. Acoust.* **2013**, *74*, 255–263.
34. Payne, S.R.; Guastavino, C. Exploring the Validity of the Perceived Restorativeness Soundscape Scale: A Psycholinguistic Approach. *Front. Psychol.* **2018**, *9*. [CrossRef]
35. Zhang, Y. Research on soundscape restorative benefits of urban open space and promotion strategy of the acoustic environment quality. *New Arch.* **2014**, *165*, 18–22.
36. Yang, W.; Kang, J. Acoustic comfort evaluation in urban open public spaces. *Appl. Acoust.* **2005**, *66*, 211–229. [CrossRef]
37. Herranz-Pascual, K.; García, I.; Aspuru, I.; Díez, I.; Santander, A. Progress in the understanding of soundscape: Objective variables and objectifiable criteria that predict acoustic comfort in urban places. *Noise Mapp.* **2016**, *3*, 247–263. [CrossRef]
38. Cassina, L.; Fredianelli, L.; Menichini, I.; Chiari, C.; Licitra, G. Audio-visual preferences and tranquillity ratings in urban areas. *Environments* **2018**, *5*, 1. [CrossRef]
39. Garcia, I.; Herranz-Pascual, K.; Aspuru, I.; Gutierrez, L.; Acero, J.A.; Santander, S. Indicators of Environmental Comfort Sensitive to Human Perception (Chapter 22). In *Handbook of Research on Perception-Driven Approaches to Urban Assessment and Design*; Aletta, F., Xiao, J., Eds.; IGI Global: Hershey, PA, USA, 2018; pp. 508–533.
40. Herranz-Pascual, K.; Gutiérrez, L.; Acero, J.A.; García, I.; Santander, A.; Aspuru, I. Environmental comfort as criteria for designing urban places. In Proceedings of the Architecture, Education and Society, Barcelona, Spain, 4–6 June 2014.
41. ISO 12913:1. *Acoustics—Soundscape—Part 1: Definition and Conceptual Framework*; International Association for Standardization: Geneva, Switzerland, 2014.
42. ISO/TS 12913:2. *Acoustics—Soundscape—Part 2: Data Collection and Reporting Requirements*; International Association for Standardization: Geneva, Switzerland, 2018.
43. Allou, C.; Pearson, A.; Rzotkiewicz, A.; Buxton, R. Positive Effects of Natural Sounds on Human Health and Well-Being: a Systematic Review. Available online: http://www.crd.york.ac.uk/PROSPERO/display_record.php?ID=CRD42018095537 (accessed on 22 October 2018).
44. Aletta, F.; Kang, J. Towards an Urban Vibrancy Model: A Soundscape Approach. *Int. J. Environ. Res. Public Health* **2018**, *15*, 1712. [CrossRef]
45. Lercher, P.; van Kamp, I.; von Lindern, E.; Botteldooren, D. Perceived Soundscapes and Health-Related Quality of Life, Context, Restoration, and Personal Characteristics. In *Soundscape and the Built Environment*; Kang, J., Schulte-Fortkamp, B., Eds.; CRC Press: Boca Raton, FL, USA, 2015.
46. Aletta, F.; Oberman, T.; Kang, J. Associations between Positive Health-Related Effects and Soundscapes Perceptual Constructs: A Systematic Review. *Int. J. Environ. Res. Public Health* **2018**, *15*, 2392. [CrossRef]
47. Cerwén, G. Urban soundscapes: A quasi-experiment in landscape architecture. *Landscape Res.* **2016**, *41*, 481–494. [CrossRef]
48. Echevarria-Sanchez, G.M.; Alves, S.; Botteldooren, D. Urban Sound Planning: An Essential Component in Urbanism and Landscape Architecture (Chapter 1). In *Handbook of Research on Perception-Driven Approaches to Urban Assessment and Design*; Aletta, F., Xiao, J., Eds.; IGI Global: Hershey, PA, USA, 2018; pp. 1–22.
49. Fusaro, G.; D'Alessandro, F.; Baldinelli, G.; Kang, J. Design of urban furniture to enhance the soundscape: A case study. *Build. Acoust.* **2018**, *25*, 61–75. [CrossRef]
50. WHO. Preamble to the Constitution of the World Health Organization as Adopted by the International Health Conference. In Proceedings of the International Health Conference, New York, NY, USA, 19–22 June 1946.
51. UN-Habitat. Streets as Public Spaces and Drivers of Urban Prosperity. Available online: http://unhabitat.org/books/streets-as-public-spaces-and-drivers-of-urban-prosperity/ (accessed on 4 April 2019).
52. CITISENSE. Global Citizen Observatory—The Role of Individuals in Observing and Understanding Our Changing World (European Environment Agency, 2009). Available online: http://www.eea.europa.eu/pressroom/speeches/global-citizen-observatory-the-roleof-individuals-in-observing-and-understanding-our-changingworld (accessed on 4 April 2019).

53. Aspuru, I.; García, I.; Herranz-Pascual, K.; Santander, A. CITI-SENSE: Methods and tools for empowering citizens to observe acoustic comfort in outdoor public spaces. *Noise Mapp.* **2016**, *3*, 37–48. [CrossRef]
54. QUADMAP. Guidelines for the Identification, Selection, Analysis and Management of Quiet Urban Areas (ver.2.0). QUADMAP Project: QUiet Areas Definition & Management in Action Plans. LIFE10 ENV/IT/000407. March 2015. Available online: http://www.quadmap.eu/wp-content/uploads/2012/01/Guidelines_QUADMAP_ver2.0.pdf (accessed on 4 April 2019).
55. Aspuru, I.; García, I.; Rubio, A.; Bartonova, A. Evaluation of the performance of the user cases: Public Places. Deliverable D3.4 of CITI-SENSE Project Development of Sensor-Based Citizens' Observatory Community for Improving Quality of Life in Cities (Grant Agreement No: 308524). 2016. Available online: https://social.citi-sense.eu/Portals/1/Deliverables/WP3-Public%20places_FINAL.pdf?ver=2016-12-23-103731-863 (accessed on 4 February 2019).
56. Richard, F.D.; Bond, C.F., Jr.; Stokes-Zoota, J.J. One Hundred Years of Social Psychology Quantitatively Described. *Rev. Gen. Psychol.* **2003**, *7*, 331–363. [CrossRef]
57. Van Kamp, B.; Klæboe, R.; Brown, L.; Lercher, P. Soundscapes, Human Restoration, and Quality of Life. In *Soundscape and the Built Environment*; Kang, J., Schulte-Fortkamp, B., Eds.; CRC Press, Taylor & Francis Group: Boca Raton, FL, USA, 2016; pp. 43–68.
58. Elmqvist, T. Designing the Urban Soundscape. Available online: https://www.thenatureofcities.com/2013/08/25/designing-the-urban-soundscape/ (accessed on 14 February 2019).
59. Herranz-Pascual, K.; Garcia, I.; Aspuru, I.; Iraurgi, I.; Eguiguren, J.L.; Santander, S. Incorporating the acoustic dimension into urban design: Making progress in the quietness of public spaces and their users' emotional health. *J. Urbna Des.* **2019**. in revision.

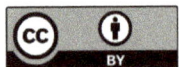

© 2019 by the authors. Licensee MDPI, Basel, Switzerland. This article is an open access article distributed under the terms and conditions of the Creative Commons Attribution (CC BY) license (http://creativecommons.org/licenses/by/4.0/).

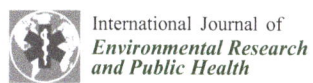

Article

Towards an Urban Vibrancy Model: A Soundscape Approach

Francesco Aletta and Jian Kang *

UCL Institute for Environmental Design and Engineering, The Bartlett, University College London (UCL), Central House, 14 Upper Woburn Place, London WC1H 0NN, UK; f.aletta@ucl.ac.uk
* Correspondence: j.kang@ucl.ac.uk; Tel.: +44-(0)20-3108-7338

Received: 12 July 2018; Accepted: 8 August 2018; Published: 10 August 2018

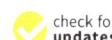

Abstract: Soundscape research needs to develop predictive tools for environmental design. A number of descriptor-indicator(s) models have been proposed so far, particularly for the "tranquility" dimension to manage "quiet areas" in urban contexts. However, there is a current lack of models addressing environments offering actively engaging soundscapes, i.e., the "vibrancy" dimension. The main aim of this study was to establish a predictive model for a vibrancy descriptor based on physical parameters, which could be used by designers and practitioners. A group interview was carried out to formulate a hypothesis on what elements would be influential for vibrancy perception. Afterwards, data on vibrancy perception were collected for different locations in the UK and China through a laboratory experiment and their physical parameters were used as indicators to establish a predictive model. Such indicators included both aural and visual parameters. The model, based on Roughness, Presence of People, Fluctuation Strength, Loudness and Presence of Music as predictors, explained 76% of the variance in the mean individual vibrancy scores. A statistically significant correlation was found between vibrancy scores and eventfulness scores, but not between vibrancy scores and pleasantness scores. Overall results showed that vibrancy is contextual and depends both on the soundscape and on the visual scenery.

Keywords: soundscape; environmental sounds; quietness; vibrancy; acoustic environments; urban sound planning

---

1. Introduction

The quality of the acoustic environments of modern cities is becoming a growing concern at a global scale. When such quality is poor because of (among other issues) high exposures to unwanted sounds, there will likely be noise pollution, which has been recognised as an element "affecting quality of life and well-being and (. . .) as an important public health issue" [1]. At different levels, noise issues are the object of attention of several groups with potentially competing interests towards the acoustic environment, including citizens, companies, policy-makers, local authorities, and planning and design professionals. The policy framework for this topic in the Member States of the European Union is provided by the so-called "Environmental Noise Directive (END)" [2], which brings guidance on the "assessment and management of environmental noise". It is now generally acknowledged that the management of the urban acoustic environments can no longer rely on a mere noise control or acoustic retrofitting approach [3–6] and it should extend to a broader concept of "urban sound planning" [7]. A number of local authorities around Europe embraced this cause and tried to implement several actions into their policies, aimed at enhancing the environmental sound quality in a "proactive", rather than a "reactive", way (e.g., [8–10]).

This shift towards a quality paradigm calls for further attention on how acoustic environments are perceived. Within this framework, the soundscape philosophy plays a key role. Soundscape is the perceptual construct deriving from the human experience and understanding of any acoustic environment, in context [11]. Ever since its appearance as a research field, soundscape soon became a relevant topic for planners and designers questioning the "sonic identity" of cities and how this would match their "visible" reality [12,13].

In recent years, soundscape research has been going through rapid expansion, with international experts and research groups aiming at standardizing definitions, methods and analysis procedures [11,14–16]. This is possibly due to the scientific community's will to provide policy-makers and practitioners with operative tools (i.e., predictive models). There is a current lack of soundscape descriptors and indicators, which has been previously identified as a gap to fill, in order to introduce the soundscape approach into the urban realm's management (e.g., [17–19]).

Aletta et al. [20] recently reviewed the main soundscape descriptors and indicators, where "descriptors" are meant as "measures of how people perceive the acoustic environment" and "indicators" are "measures used to predict the value of a soundscape descriptor". The review showed that overall descriptors referred either to single dimensions of soundscape appreciation (e.g., calmness), or to soundscape holistically (e.g., soundscape quality). It also pointed out that many descriptors have a focus on calmness or similar constructs (e.g., tranquillity, quietness). A possible explanation for this is that the Environmental Noise Directive explicitly urged the Member States to identify and preserve quiet areas but provided little guidance on the criteria to consider. Thus, a lot of research efforts went in that direction (e.g., [21–27]). Consequently, the European Environmental Agency (EEA) released a good practice guide on quiet areas, where the soundscape methodology is officially endorsed for the first time at an international policy level [6]. The EEA review also includes the tranquillity rating tool, developed by Watts and his colleagues, which considers the ratio of greenery features in a scene and sound pressure level as main predictors (i.e., indicators) for the tranquillity descriptor.

Nonetheless, it is worth noticing that a soundscape descriptor related to a single dimension should be relevant for the investigated context. Would it make sense to use a tranquillity descriptor to assess the soundscape quality of Piccadilly Circus in London? Possibly not. But this doesn't necessarily mean that such a place is not able to elicit positive soundscapes. Local authorities and planners may need to work out the soundscape quality of places where "the quieter, the better" strategy might not be the best option [28,29].

Models for soundscape characterisation have been proposed by Axelsson et al. [30] and Cain et al. [31]. These seem to converge towards two-dimensional models of perceived affective quality and provide for the most comprehensive information about soundscape appreciation [20]. Axelsson et al.'s model is defined by two orthogonal factors "Pleasantness" and "Eventfulness", which are located at a 45° degrees rotation from the second set of orthogonal factors "Calmness" and "Excitement". According to this model, a soundscape that is both pleasant and eventful will be "exciting", whilst a soundscape that is both pleasant and uneventful will be "calm". Likewise, the model by Cain et al. includes two orthogonal factors, i.e., "Calmness" and "Vibrancy" (instead of "Excitement"). Figure 1 summarises the two models and shows how they seem to agree on the fact that, for a soundscape to be positive (i.e., pleasant), this should either be calm or vibrant, and these two factors are not straightforwardly related to sound levels [31]. The first factor relates to the possibility of achieving quiet and restorative soundscapes (i.e., the calm construct); the latter is more oriented to the potential of offering actively engaging soundscapes (i.e., the vibrant construct). Both models point out one aspect of soundscape, namely the "vibrancy" or "excitement", which has not been previously covered by descriptor-indicator(s) models [20]. Within the framework of this research we will refer to the term "vibrancy". This is ultimately the descriptor that is being sought in order to characterise (and eventually plan and design) in a more relevant way the soundscape quality of pleasant and eventful places (like Piccadilly Circus, for instance). Thus, this work acknowledges the need to develop a predictive model for vibrancy based on a set of corresponding physical indicators, as a tool to be used by planners and designers, in contexts where such a descriptor is likely to be relevant.

It is worth pointing out at this stage that the soundscape (or rather, the acoustic environment) of a place should not be treated in isolation or designed independently of other factors of an urban environment. From a planning and design point of view, measuring the vibrancy of an acoustic environment as an independent factor would be a pointless exercise, since in the real world it does not seem likely that a place (as a whole) would be vibrant while its soundscape (alone) would be not. The research on tranquillity of Watts and colleagues [22–25] faced a similar issue, where they did not assess the tranquillity of a place as a separate dimension from its soundscape, but rather investigated the tranquillity of the place as a whole, including both visual and acoustic aspects. Such methodological approach is typical in soundscape studies, as soundscape research aims at considering several environmental components and their interactions in contest in a holistic way, rather than treating them as unrelated parts of the built environment.

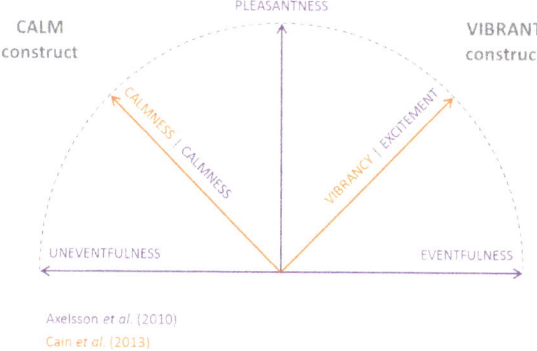

Figure 1. Schematic representation of the models for soundscape characterisation. Figure adapted from Axelsson et al. [30] and Cain et al. [31].

The main aims of this study are: (1) to investigate how the vibrancy construct is overall understood and how it could be relevant for soundscape research; (2) to establish a predictive model (i.e., identifying indicators) for a "vibrancy" descriptor; and (3) to further explore the relationships between the vibrant, eventful and pleasant constructs in soundscape. In order to address the first aim, a group interview was carried out with acousticians and designers to explore the vibrancy construct so to formulate a hypothesis on what elements would be influential for vibrancy perception. For the second aim, a laboratory experiment was carried out to collect soundscape data on vibrancy perception and to establish a predictive model using indicators derived from the group interview stage. While both the descriptors and indicators considered in this study might be already known in soundscape literature, it was considered useful to perform the group interview and use data derived from it to inform the second part of the study (laboratory experiment). To some extent, this helps to limit a potential "experimenter's bias", which could have occurred if the indicators were selected on a totally arbitrary basis.

2. Materials and Methods

Despite sounding like a relatively familiar concept, little is known about how "vibrancy" is defined or understood, under a planning and design perspective. Hence, the first stage of the work aimed to establish a framework that would inform the group interview stage, which was in turn supposed to provide information about what elements people perceive to be relevant for the vibrant construct. Having extrapolated the likely vibrancy influential elements from the group interview, it was possible to make a hypothesis on potential physical metrics (i.e., indicators) that could be proxy for the abovementioned elements. For the experimental stage, these metrics would then be computed for the collected recordings and used as predictors of the vibrancy descriptor in a statistical model. Figure 2 shows the methodological approach adopted in the current research. The flowchart reflects that, since a number of assumptions needed to be made, the workflow did not follow a linear development. Boxes correspond to sub-sections of the paper, as addressed in the main sections, namely Methods and Results.

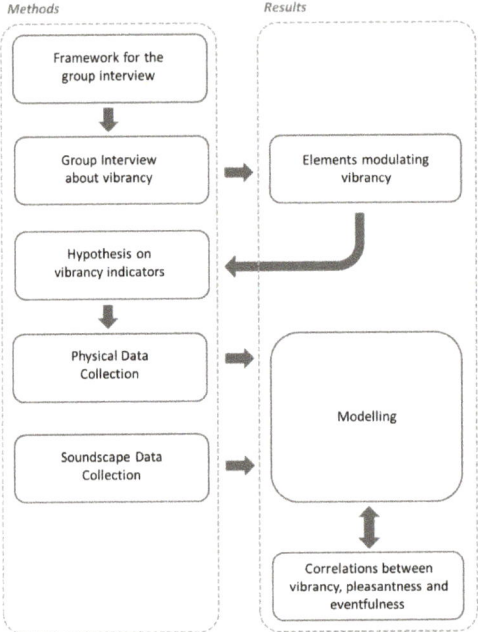

Figure 2. Schematic representation of the methodological workflow considered within the current research.

This study was granted ethical approval by the Research Ethics Committee of the School of Architecture of the University of Sheffield, UK (former institution of the authors; this is where the study originally started), with approval letter ref. 007015 (01.12.2015). All participants, both for the group interview and the audio-visual experiment presented below, provided informed consent.

2.1. Framework for the Group Interview

As a preparatory work for the group interview stage, the vibrancy concept was explored in urban studies and soundscape literature so to prepare a framework to inform questions and aspects to ask people about, when it comes to their perception and understanding of vibrancy.

The attribute "vibrant" is usually referred to something that is "full of energy and life" [32]. In urban studies, it is not a new concept and is conventionally associated with downtowns and cities (e.g., [33,34]), and environments that "facilitate non-motorized transportation, connect activities in space, promote health and equity, emphasizes diverse land uses, preserve environmental resources, and encourage social exchange in the public realm." (ref. [35], as cited in [36]). Braun and Malizia [36] developed a composite vibrancy index to describe the vibrancy of 48 downtown areas, taking into account urban compactness, density, regional and local connectivity, destination accessibility, land use, and social diversity. They found that vibrancy is associated with more favourable population-level health and safety outcomes in central urban environments. Such findings might be particularly relevant under an urban design perspective, and support the cities' efforts at a policy level to generate "more vibrant centres in support of innovation and economic development".

In soundscape studies, the vibrancy concept has been addressed in several studies (e.g., [30,31,37]) and there it has been suggested that the vibrant construct is positively associated to the pleasantness dimension of soundscapes (e.g., [38]). Davies et al. [37] concluded that soundscape vibrancy is related to two auditory aspects: organisation of sounds and changes over time. These two aspects can be in turn described by two qualitative dimensions, namely: cacophony-hubbub and constant-temporal, which can elicit a vibrancy response in the listener.

However, Hall et al. [38] showed that the association between vibrancy responses and conventional psycho-acoustic metrics (e.g., loudness, roughness, fluctuation strength and sharpness, or metrics based on averaged spectral shape) is not straightforward. In their experimental study, even though some psycho-acoustic metrics significantly correlated with vibrancy responses, the final model only explained 3% of the overall variance in the data. This suggests that when it comes to perceived soundscape vibrancy, people might be affected by other non-acoustic factors. Thus, it seems fair to investigate further what indicators are likely to be relevant for such a descriptor.

2.2. Group Inteview about the Vibrancy Concept

Given the sociological nature of soundscape research, semi-structured interview techniques, like group interviews and focus groups, are often considered as a suitable method for collecting data about the perception of sound environments or some of their components (e.g., [39,40]). Within the framework of this research, there was a need to investigate how the concept of vibrancy of a place is overall understood, so to consider what factors could be relevant to provide a "vibrant urban environment" to people. For this purpose, a group interview was organised. Seven postgraduate students, doctoral students and researchers in architecture, acoustics and planning were invited to take part. The rationale for participants' selection was having a group with a relatively common background, but not necessarily the same attitude towards a topic [41], as well as participants who were likely to provide useful insights into the vibrancy perceptual attribute, under a planning and design perspective.

The session took place in a meeting room of the School of Architecture of the University of Sheffield. Two experimenters coordinated the discussion asking open questions, and participants had the opportunity to express their views, exchange ideas and agree on a number of points. The session lasted approximately 45 min and it was audio-recorded for further semantic analysis (consent had been previously collected from participants for this purpose). The questions were: "What does vibrancy mean for you?", "Overall, is vibrancy something good for you?"; "What would the opposite of vibrant be?"; "What elements contribute to make a vibrant urban environment for you?"; "Can you give me an example of an urban environment that is/is not very vibrant?"; "How would a vibrant urban environment sound like?"; "How would a vibrant urban environment look like?". It is important to highlight that the concept of vibrancy, in general, might be understood differently across different cultures or simply personal backgrounds. While the aim of this study was establishing a preliminary vibrancy model, more studies targeting specific cultures and countries might be useful.

2.3. Hypothesis on Vibrancy Indicators

The results of the group interview stage will be discussed in Section 3.1, but for the sake of clarity they are briefly anticipated here, as they serve as basis for the hypothesis on the vibrancy indicators. Overall, people agreed that the elements modulating the vibrancy perception are related both to the aural (i.e., loudness, variability, human voices, and music) and the visual (i.e., people and activity) domain.

In order to establish a vibrancy model, a hypothesis was made about what physical indicators (i.e., measurable quantities) could potentially be effective predictors of the perceptual elements derived from the group interview [20]. This resulted in the following parameters: Loudness (N), Loudness

Variability (N_{10}–N_{90}), Roughness (R), Fluctuation Strength (Fls), Presence of Music (MUSIC) and Presence of People (PEOPLE). The rationale for the parameters' selection was finding the best physical proxy for the perceptual descriptors. Since soundscape is a complex and multi-layered construct, it was assumed that different indicators might refer to the same perceptual elements; likewise, a single perceptual element might well be represented by different indicators, as schematised in Figure 3. The metrics are briefly described below.

The loudness of a sound reflects the intensity sensation of the energy content of sound on the human hearing. In perceptual studies it is usually preferred to other metrics like sound pressure level, as it is considered to better represent how the human ear perceives sounds [42]. There are several methods for calculating the loudness. This study will refer to Loudness (N) as defined in Fastl and Zwicker [43] and its values are expressed in *sones*. In order to account for Loudness changes over time, statistical levels of Loudness (i.e., levels exceeded for an N_x percentage of time, with respect to the reference period) will be considered. Thus, the Loudness Variability over time (N_{10}–N_{90}) can be represented by the difference between the Loudness peak values (N_{10}) and the Loudness background values (N_{90}).

Roughness (R) is a metric related to the perceptual effect of fast amplitude modulation of a sound (15–300 Hz) and it is measured in *aspers* [43]. Likewise, Fluctuation Strength (Fls) is a metric related to slower (up to 20 Hz) amplitude modulation of a sound and it is measured in *vacils* [43]. Both these metrics are usually considered to be representative of a sound's temporal variation [44].

For the purposes of this study, Presence of People (PEOPLE) was defined as a numerical variable and computed for a site by summing the persons represented in a scene; thus it is expressed in integers. On the other hand, Presence of Music (MUSIC) was defined as a binary variable, considering whether music can (1) or cannot (0) be heard at any moment during a reference auditory stimulus.

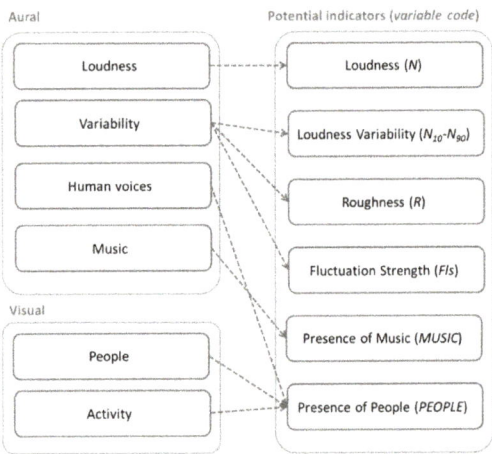

Figure 3. Schematisation of variables hypothesised for the elements of the group interview.

2.4. Physical Data Collection

Audio-visual data were collected from 46 locations across England and China using a Canon EOS 500D camera to record the visual information and a binaural headset (in-ear 1/8" DPA microphones) connected to an Edirol R44 portable recorder to capture the auditory and acoustic data [45]. The locations chosen for the study were selected from the city centre of Sheffield and Doncaster (UK), and Beijing and Tangshan (China). The reasons for this were: (1) to provide a wide range of urban environments with different activities (e.g., commercial, residential, service areas);

(2) to sample stimuli from the entire two-dimensional soundscape model so that, for instance, also calm or chaotic or monotonous environments are considered (and not only vibrant ones); (3) to provide different cultural and social backgrounds between European and Asian contexts; and (4) to consider cities that could be representative of different urban sizes (compared to the corresponding countries). Table 1 reports the selected locations for data collection and the corresponding main urban activities as noted during the on-site campaign.

At each location, for visual data, an operator swept clockwise taking a picture on a normal setting every 45° (with approximately one-second intervals) so to have eight contiguous pictures covering a 360° view in the horizontal plane, at a height of 1.70 m [25]. Immediately after that, the operator performed a 30-s audio-recording with the binaural headset, with a steady head orientation. The audio-visual recording procedure is summarised in Figure 4.

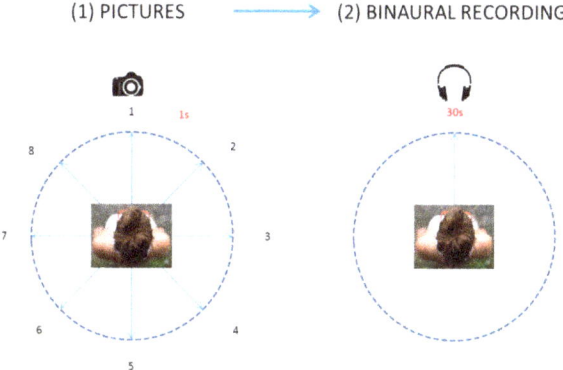

Figure 4. Scheme representing the procedure for audio-visual data collection.

Table 1. Locations selected for data collection and main urban activity taking place there.

ID	City	Reference	Coordinates	Main Urban Activity
UK1		Students' Union	53°22′52.09″ N, 1°29′14.57″ E	Tertiary
UK2		West Street	53°22′49.68″ N, 1°28′39.10″ E	Entertainment
UK3		Division Street	53°22′46.65″ N, 1°28′35.98″ E	Entertainment
UK4		Barker's Pool	53°22′49.42″ N, 1°28′18.58″ E	Commercial
UK5		Leopold Square	53°22′54.21″ N, 1°28′18.52″ E	Entertainment
UK6		Orchard Square	53°22′54.23″ N, 1°28′13.77″ E	Commercial
UK7		Fargate	53°22′52.47″ N, 1°28′10.48″ E	Entertainment
UK8		Peace Gardens	53°22′47.57″ N, 1°28′11.02″ E	Green areas
UK9		The Moor	53°22′32.29″ N, 1°28′26.55″ E	Commercial
UK10		Crookes Valley Park	53°23′1.85″ N, 1°29′37.39″ E	Green areas
UK11		Elmore & Marlborough Road	53°22′52.27″ N, 1°29′51.07″ E	Residential
UK12	Sheffield	Botanical Gardens	53°22′21.44″ N, 1°29′55.31″ E	Green areas
UK13		Fargate cross Black Swan Walk	53°22′56.29″ N, 1°28′6.46″ E	Commercial
UK14		Castle Square	53°22′58.85″ N, 1°27′58.19″ E	Commercial
UK15		Howard Street	53°22′41.21″ N, 1°27′54.38″ E	Tertiary
UK16		St Georges' Church	53°22′54.61″ N, 1°28′48.26″ E	Tertiary
UK17		Weston Park	53°22′56.17″ N, 1°29′22.82″ E	Green areas
UK18		Headford Gardens	53°22′40.17″ N, 1°28′53.76″ E	Residential
UK19		Bolton Street	53°22′41.50″ N, 1°28′55.72″ E	Residential
UK20		Broomspring Close	53°22′39.47″ N, 1°28′58.42″ E	Residential
UK21		Broomhall Place	53°22′29.85″ N, 1°29′8.33″ E	Residential
UK22		Victoria Road	53°22′28.73″ N, 1°29′12.11″ E	Residential
UK23		Ecclesall Road	53°22′16.06″ N, 1°29′23.37″ E	Commercial
UK24		St Sepulchre Gate	53°31′21.73″ N, 1°8′11.23″ E	Commercial
UK25	Doncaster	High Street	53°31′25.46″ N, 1°8′7.67″ E	Commercial
UK26		Market Place	53°31′28.66″ N, 1°8′2.00″ E	Entertainment

Table 1. Cont.

ID	City	Reference	Coordinates	Main Urban Activity
CH1		Community activity area	39°44'6.29" N, 118°41'31.11" E	Residential
CH2		Community North Gate	39°44'10.03" N, 118°41'25.61" E	Residential
CH3		Shopping centre parking lot	39°44'9.65" N, 118°41'51.36" E	Commercial
CH4		South entrance of the square	39°44'12.27" N, 118°41'50.92" E	Commercial
CH5		Leisure area near North entrance	39°44'17.32" N, 118°41'51.14" E	Entertainment
CH6		North entrance of the square	39°44'19.20" N, 118°41'50.92" E	Entertainment
CH7	Tangshan	South entrance of the pedestrian street	39°44'23.94" N, 118°41'55.59" E	Commercial
CH8		Middle area of the pedestrian street	39°44'32.12" N, 118°41'55.30" E	Commercial
CH9		Middle area of the pedestrian street	39°44'31.83" N, 118°41'48.95" E	Commercial
CH10		Middle area of the pedestrian street	39°44'26.27" N, 118°41'49.67" E	Commercial
CH11		Market	39°43'53.83" N, 118°42'24.18" E	Commercial
CH12		Market	39°43'53.21" N, 118°42'24.20" E	Commercial
CH13		Market	39°43'53.86" N, 118°42'25.41" E	Commercial
CH14		East entrance of the Beijing Old street	39°56'22.49" N, 116°24'8.96" E	Commercial
CH15		Bus stop of a street in Beijing	39°56'22.53" N, 116°24'14.87" E	Commercial
CH16		Beijing Dongcheng District First Library	39°56'22.85" N, 116°24'23.41" E	Tertiary
CH17	Beijing	Middle island in front of the Orient Plaza	39°54'28.54" N, 116°24'23.98" E	Tertiary
CH18		Entrance of Orient Plaza office building	39°54'26.52" N, 116°24'21.93" E	Tertiary
CH19		Entrance to Orient Plaza Shopping Mall	39°54'28.61" N, 116°24'19.88" E	Commercial
CH20		Wangfujing Avenue	39°54'35.41" N, 116°24'18.57" E	Commercial

With the purpose of providing input data for the modelling stage, the indicators described in Section 2.3 were calculated for each of the 46 sample locations. Table 2 reports the values of the different variables for each of the 46 locations considered in the study. The psychoacoustic indicators were computed using the software Artemis v.11 [46], while the other variables where computed manually through audio-visual inspections, and cross-validated by two research students.

Table 2. Computed indicators for the selected locations of the experiment.

Location ID	N	$N_{10}-N_{90}$	R	FIs	PEOPLE	MUSIC
UK1	19.85	7.35	2.37	0.0301	80	0
UK2	16.40	10.69	2.13	0.0244	24	0
UK3	15.30	5.47	2.27	0.0153	15	0
UK4	16.75	4.90	2.10	0.0171	60	1
UK5	19.85	4.80	2.45	0.0168	6	0
UK6	15.10	4.03	2.06	0.0125	27	0
UK7	33.75	11.20	2.48	0.0599	117	1
UK8	26.25	3.00	2.62	0.0121	98	0
UK9	23.60	8.05	2.44	0.0456	80	1
UK10	5.96	2.23	1.25	0.0093	4	0
UK11	5.78	3.03	1.16	0.0117	4	0
UK12	6.08	1.10	1.26	0.0066	7	0
UK13	17.80	6.00	2.16	0.0178	117	0
UK14	22.50	4.75	2.51	0.0122	130	0
UK15	16.25	6.35	2.12	0.0209	51	0
UK16	13.60	4.92	2.01	0.0172	28	0
UK17	9.60	1.96	1.64	0.0189	17	0
UK18	7.97	2.01	1.44	0.0067	0	0
UK19	12.65	8.36	2.07	0.0315	34	0
UK20	9.15	4.48	1.56	0.0090	3	0
UK21	10.06	3.75	1.82	0.0105	15	0
UK22	7.87	4.75	1.50	0.0107	15	0
UK23	30.10	18.75	2.93	0.0119	15	0
UK24	18.45	5.15	2.33	0.0195	127	0
UK25	24.50	6.70	2.47	0.0277	126	1
UK26	17.55	7.35	2.22	0.0430	122	0
CH1	6.39	4.33	1.21	0.0211	3	0
CH2	14.25	8.25	2.00	0.0142	14	0
CH3	20.40	8.85	2.13	0.0611	26	0
CH4	19.80	11.60	2.41	0.0571	23	0
CH5	11.85	6.33	1.77	0.0427	42	0
CH6	16.55	18.85	0.79	0.0273	37	0
CH7	23.70	9.85	1.30	0.0329	51	0
CH8	16.80	6.20	0.56	0.0244	57	0

Table 2. Cont.

Location ID	N	N_{10}–N_{90}	R	Fls	PEOPLE	MUSIC
CH9	14.30	4.45	1.87	0.0155	22	0
CH10	16.30	18.88	2.11	0.0159	6	0
CH11	18.70	9.60	2.01	0.0344	54	0
CH12	24.75	11.90	2.45	0.0385	48	0
CH13	16.50	6.65	1.80	0.0342	73	0
CH14	19.60	7.75	2.38	0.0224	34	0
CH15	17.55	16.60	2.27	0.0170	25	0
CH16	17.45	12.00	2.15	0.0174	9	0
CH17	10.19	3.21	1.38	0.0147	11	0
CH18	14.40	6.40	1.92	0.0171	23	0
CH19	18.25	7.30	2.25	0.0270	85	0
CH20	20.70	7.95	2.29	0.0234	142	0

2.5. Soundscape Data Collection

According to the conceptual framework for the development of soundscape predictive models proposed in Aletta et al. [20], after the physical characterisation of the acoustic (or visual) environment, it is necessary to gather individual data about perception. For this purpose, a laboratory experiment was carried out to collect responses on the perceived vibrancy of the investigated urban environments. Axelsson et al. [30] define vibrant (or exciting) the soundscape that is both pleasant and eventful. Thus, individual responses were collected also for the latter attributes, in order to further validate the perceptual information.

Thirty-five undergraduates and postgraduates and staff members at the University of Sheffield, 18 to 46 years old, took part in the experiment (19 women, 16 men; M_{age} = 26.5 years, SD = 5.8). Participants were selected from a group of 200+ persons who completed an online survey circulated via the established email list for research volunteers at the University of Sheffield. The online survey was designed to achieve a varied sample of participants in terms of gender, age and ethnic origin. The 35 participants who completed the experiment received 5 GBP as a token of appreciation for volunteering in the experiment.

Forty-six videos (30 s) were used for this experiment, corresponding to the 46 locations where physical data were collected. The auditory part of the video consisted of the 30-s binaural recordings, as collected on site. The visual part consisted of a transition of the eight pictures, (from picture 1 to picture 8, as shown in Figure 4), for 3.75 s each [22]. The equipment used for the experiment consisted of a 16" laptop (HP EliteBook 850, Hewlett-Packard, Palo Alto, CA, USA), and a pair of open, circum-aural headphones (HD 558, Sennheiser, Wedemark, Germany). The audio part of the video was played back at the original sound-pressure level as recorded on site (Type 4231 calibrator, Brüel & Kjær, Nærum, Denmark).

The experiments were carried out in a silent meeting room (background noise <25 dBA) at the School of Architecture of the University of Sheffield. Participants took part individually. Upon arriving, they were asked to sign the informed consent and report if they had a normal or corrected to normal hearing and vision. Some demographic information was collected for descriptive purposes. Sitting at a desk with the laptop, participants were given the headphones and the experiment started. The stimuli were presented via an online platform in a randomised sequence for each participant, so to limit potential order effects. Participants were only allowed to listen to the recordings once. The experimental sessions lasted between 30 and 40 min.

After each scenario, participants were asked to answer three questions on a ten-point scale ranging from "not at all" (0) to "extremely" (10): (a) "Overall, how vibrant was the sound environment that you have just experienced?"; (b) "Overall, how eventful was the sound environment that you have just experienced?"; (c) "Overall, how pleasant was the sound environment that you have just experienced?". Since "eventful" and "vibrant" are attributes that are likely to generate ambiguity, participants were previously instructed to consider eventful a sound environment that "is related to the presence of significant events that characterize the sound environment, defining it as a non-flat context", and to consider vibrant a sound environment relating to "excitement, creating a soundscape that is 'full of life' and activating". While participants were tutored to consider the vibrancy of the place "holistically" (i.e., both aurally and visually), the questions explicitly mentioned the "sound environment" so that the sample would pay particular attention to the soundscape construct, which in such complex audio-visual stimuli could be possibly disregarded in favour of vision.

Since the meaning attributed to "vibrant" was crucial for the experiment, particular attention was given to this concept to avoid that it could be confused with the abovementioned "eventful". When the meaning was not clear, participants were offered synonyms for vibrant, such as "exciting" or "lively". This is a common practice in behavioural science, where multiple attributes are typically used to define an index for the underlying construct, since this increases the quality of the data, and the likelihood of valid results [47].

3. Results

Results are divided in three sub-sections. Section 3.1 reports the output of the group interview about vibrancy, which has been already referred in Section 2.3 to state the hypothesis about the potential vibrancy indicators. Section 3.2 establishes the predictive model for the vibrancy descriptor, based on the perceptual and physical data. Section 3.3 eventually explores further associations between vibrancy and its underpinning dimensions (i.e., eventfulness and pleasantness).

3.1. Elements Modulating Vibrancy

The transcription of the group interview was coded using general concepts that could help to define how vibrancy is understood in the urban realm [48]. This thematic analysis refers to the "grounded theory", which is becoming an increasingly important methodological approach in soundscape studies [40,49]. According to this method, the investigation should start with a (set of) question(s) and collection of qualitative data (the transcription of the group interview, in this case). Recurring concepts are then tagged with "codes" in an iterative process; codes are then grouped into concepts, and then into categories. The final categories are those likely to become the basis for a new framework/theory.

Overall, the group agreed that vibrancy is related to a pleasantness dimension (e.g., "To me, [vibrancy] implies positive feelings, so if an area is vibrant it implies that it makes you feel good and gets yourself in a state of excitement"), which is consistent with previous literature [30,48], and it might be affected by people's preconceptions or background about a specific urban context (e.g., "I think your preconceptions as well can influence. If you have heard an area is exciting, I think you bring your own biases and preconceptions about the area as well and get yourself in that mood" or "... you might hear from some friend that this area is very cool, a lot of bars etc., you should go ... and this might influence your perception of vibrancy").

Regarding the elements that contribute to a vibrant perception of an urban context, the thematic analysis of the group interview transcription revealed that there are a number of core elements (codes), which can be in turn sorted into two main categories, namely: aural factors and visual factors. Table 3 reports the main factors that emerged from the group interview, that participants considered being relevant for the vibrancy of an urban environment.

Table 3. Main elements contributing to the vibrancy of an urban environment, as coded in the group interview.

Factors (Categories)	Elements (Codes)	Examples of Excerpts from the Group Interview
Aural	Human Voices	"It sort of implies to me human voices; you can hear some sort of hubbub going on"
	Variability	"It is vibrant, it is not stable, it is changing"
	Loudness	"It is loud, not quiet", "You are closer to every sound", "You feel the vibes ... "
	Music	"It is like when you have festivals, or funfairs or concerts in the street"
Visual	People	"I think vibrancy to me implies people, social context"
	Activity	"The railway station is vibrant: many people are walking and going and I think that this helps defining vibrancy with a sort of rhythm"

3.2. Modeling Vibrancy

A stepwise linear regression analysis was conducted, using the vibrancy scores (individual values averaged across the 35 participants, for each site) as dependent variables and the set of six parameters as independent variables (SPSS 22 for Windows, IBM Corporation, Armonk, NY, USA). The model explained 75.9% of the variance in the dependent variable. The strongest predictors of vibrancy were R ($t = 6.314$, $p < 0.001$), PEOPLE ($t = 4.447$, $p < 0.001$), Fls ($t = 4.163$, $p < 0.001$), N ($t = -4.358$, $p < 0.001$), and MUSIC ($t = 3.123$, $p = 0.003$); ($F_{5, 40} = 25.21$, $p < 0.001$, $R^2 = 0.76$). The sixth variable (N_{10}–N_{90}) was excluded by the regression algorithms: this is further discussed in Section 4.1.

Table 4 shows that R explained 39.4% of the variance in vibrancy. When controlling for this variable, PEOPLE explained an additional 14.6% of the variance. Likewise, Fls, N, and MUSIC explained an additional 6.7%, 9.3% and 5.9% of the variance, accordingly. Overall, the positive relationship between vibrancy and R shows that there was more rapid amplitude modulation associated with the acoustic environments interpreted as vibrant. For the visual aspects, the more people in the scene, the more vibrant the environment was perceived. Figure 5 shows the strength of the relationship between the average vibrancy scores collected during the listening experiment, and those predicted by the vibrancy model proposed above.

Table 4. Linear regression model for vibrancy.

Predictor	R^2 Change	Coefficient (β)
R	0.39	0.682
PEOPLE	0.15	0.436
Fls	0.07	0.383
N	0.09	−0.579
MUSIC	0.06	0.272

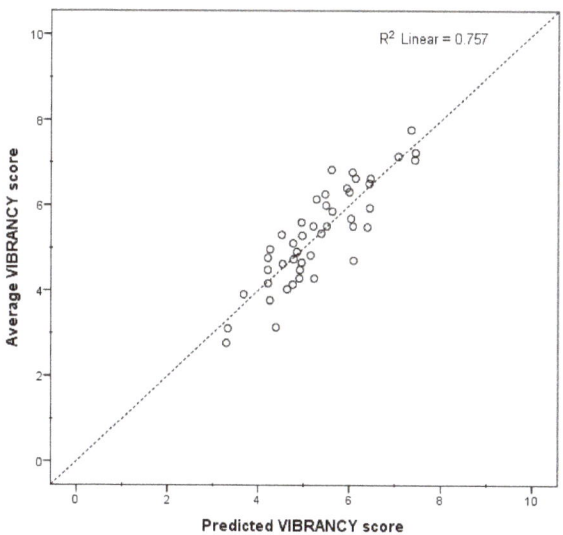

Figure 5. Predicted vibrancy scores vs. actual vibrancy scores (average across all participants).

Strong collinearity between variables was dismissed after checking for the variance inflation factor (VIF) of the predictors used for the vibrancy model (VIF values: R, 1.936; PEOPLE, 1.594; Fls, 1.402; N, 2.934; MUSIC, 1.260).

As a further check on the reliability of the model, a filter variable was created in the original database to randomly select a subset of approximately 75% of the sample. This subset and the other covering the remaining 25% of the dataset were used to calibrate the model. The linear regression algorithm was run again using 75% of the dataset and achieved an explained variance of approximately 73%, compared to the 76% of the full dataset. Afterwards, a bivariate correlation analysis between the vibrancy scores and the predicted vibrancy values of the models from the two subsets was performed. The Pearson's product-moment correlation coefficients for the two subsets were similar: $r(34) = 0.847$, $p < 0.001$ for the subset of the 75% of the sample and $r(12) = 0.889$, $p < 0.001$ for the subset of the remaining 25% of the sample. Thus, severe issues of overfitting were deemed to be negligible.

3.3. Correlation between Vibrancy, Pleasantness and Eventfulness

In order to provide further insights into vibrancy perception, two Pearson product-moment correlation coefficients were computed to assess the relationships between the mean vibrancy scores and the mean pleasantness scores, and the mean vibrancy scores and the mean eventfulness scores. There was a strong positive correlation between vibrancy and eventfulness, $r(46) = 0.926$, $p < 0.001$. However, no statistically significant correlation was observed between vibrancy and pleasantness: $r(46) = 0.079$, $p = 0.604$. Figure 6 summarises these results.

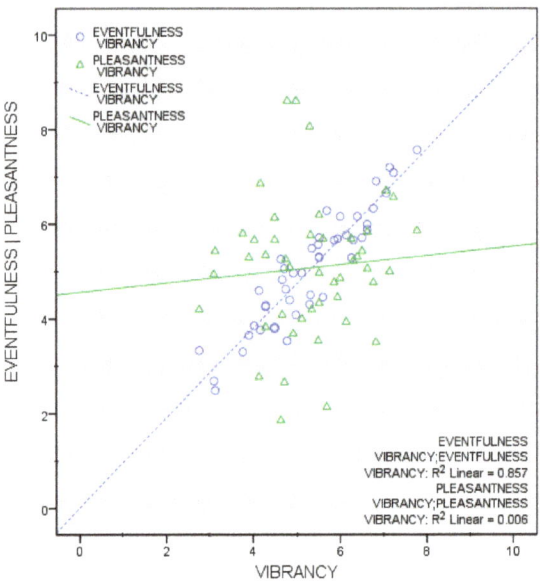

Figure 6. Scatterplots for mean vibrancy scores vs. mean eventfulness scores and mean vibrancy scores vs. mean pleasantness scores.

Such lack of correlation was further explored, while controlling for the "main urban activity" (as per in Table 1) variable. No statistically significant correlation between vibrancy and pleasantness emerged in this case either, for most of the urban activity categories: tertiary, $r(6) = -0.417$, $p = 0.411$; entertainment, $r(7) = 0.614$, $p = 0.143$; commercial, $r(21) = 0.405$, $p = .069$; residential, $r(8) = -0.228$, $p = 0.588$. The only exception was the strong and statistically significant negative correlation between vibrancy and pleasantness for the urban activity category green areas: $r(4) = -0.985$, $p = 0.015$. This was somewhat expected since green areas, when eliciting pleasantness, are most likely assessed as calm (and not vibrant) [22–25].

This suggests that while the association between vibrancy and eventfulness coming from previous studies [30] is perceptually appreciated in this experiment, pleasantness might be more affected by the contextual information (e.g., visual factors). To support this hypothesis, a one-way between subjects ANOVA was conducted to compare the effect of the main urban activity (as reported in Table 1) taking place in each of the 46 locations of this study (as a proxy for context) on the mean pleasantness scores. There was a general significant effect of the context on pleasantness scores, $F(4, 41) = 8.597$, $p < 0.001$. A post hoc Bonferroni test indeed revealed that, for the pleasantness scores, "green" locations (e.g., urban parks) significantly differed from all other contexts: "tertiary" ($p = 0.024$); "entertainment" ($p = 0.002$); "commercial" ($p < 0.001$); and "residential" ($p = 0.027$). Figure 7 reports the mean scores for the three variables considered in the laboratory experiments, where such differences can be observed.

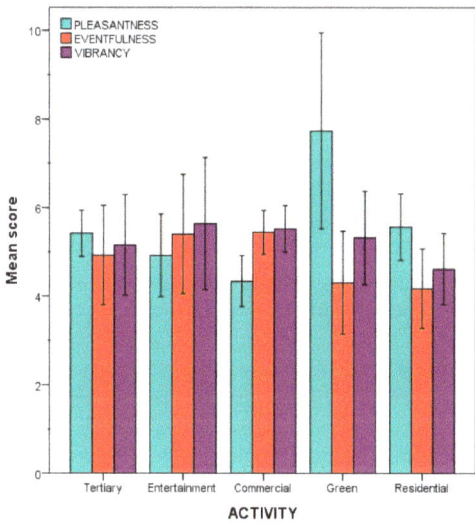

Figure 7. Mean scores for pleasantness, eventfulness and vibrancy (Error bars: 95% CI).

Furthermore, a set of independent-sample *t*-tests was run to determine if there were differences in pleasantness, eventfulness or vibrancy between UK (Sheffield and Doncaster) and Chinese (Tangshan and Beijing) sites. No statistically significant differences emerged, for any of the three variables; pleasantness: UK ($M = 5.50$, $SD = 1.19$), China ($M = 4.84$, $SD = 1.04$), $p = 0.059$; eventfulness: UK ($M = 5.49$, $SD = 1.17$), China ($M = 4.82$, $SD = 1.04$), $p = 0.052$; vibrancy: UK ($M = 5.56$, $SD = 1.19$), China ($M = 4.99$, $SD = 1.07$), $p = 0.102$. This suggests that, at least for this experiment, the sample was not particularly influenced by the "cultural" content of the stimuli, either aurally (e.g., language of the voices heard, type of music, etc.) or visually (e.g., language of the shops' windows, ethnicity of the people in the scene, etc.).

4. Discussion

The construct of vibrancy has been showed to be multi-dimensional and to rely on different sensory elements. While the physical characteristics and information content of the acoustic environment are certainly important, the group interview conducted in this study pointed out that other visual aspects might contribute to modulate vibrancy perception, which is in line with the holistic approach underpinning the soundscape theory [11]. Particularly, the presence of people, as both aural (i.e., human voices) and visual (i.e., groups or individuals within sight) sources, was regarded as a key component of the vibrancy experience. The presence of people is indeed likely to provide a social dimension that seems to be at the core of vibrancy perception, and previous studies reported that even the aural presence of humans alone can enhance the perceived safety of a place [50].

4.1. The Vibrancy Model

In a previous study based on a listening laboratory experiment, Hall et al. [38] proposed a predictive model for soundscape vibrancy, but they found that even though some acoustical and psycho-acoustical factors were significantly correlated with vibrancy scores, it was not possible to explain more than 3% of the model variance. The authors attributed this issue to individual differences in the listeners' approach to soundscape rating or other non-acoustic factors. The point raised in this study is that also visual elements are crucial in vibrancy appreciation and when the auditory stimuli are presented together with the visual context, the listeners integrate the information coming from the aural and visual domain and report assessments that are better predicted by the physical indicators.

Roughness and Fluctuation Strength together accounted for more than 45% of the variance in vibrancy scores. To some extent this was expected, considering that these parameters are often related to the "impression" of a sound's temporal variation [44], which is one of the elements emerged from the group interview. Interestingly, Roughness has usually been considered as a negative feature for "soundscape quality", i.e., the rougher the acoustic environment, the poorer the soundscape quality [51]. Thus, this finding suggests that the same indicator might perform differently at predicting a single soundscape dimension, like vibrancy, rather than soundscape "holistically" (i.e., whether a soundscape is "good" or "bad") [20,39,42].

The loudness variability (N_{10}–N_{90}) indicator was excluded from the model by the stepwise linear regression algorithm. When plotting the mean vibrancy scores versus the N_{10}–N_{90} values for the 46 investigated locations, it appears clearly that such a relationship is not linear, as reported in Figure 8. However, a quadratic fit for the loudness variability was found to explain 25% of the variance in vibrancy. Particularly, low and high loudness variability levels corresponded to low vibrancy, while moderate loudness variability increased vibrancy. A possible explanation for this is that, for a soundscape to be vibrant, loudness changes in time are relevant, but if these become overwhelming (e.g., like for acoustic environments dominated by traffic noise), the vibrant construct evolves into something different (possibly, chaotic, according to Axelsson et al. [30]).

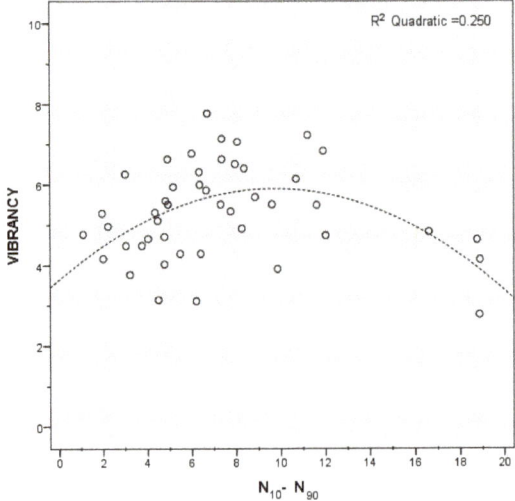

Figure 8. Scatter plot of the loudness variability (N_{10}–N_{90}) values vs. the mean vibrancy scores.

Regarding the *PEOPLE* and *MUSIC* factors, it could be argued that they are oversimplified representations for a complex urban environment. However, there was a deliberate attempt for keeping these variables simple, so that the predictive model could potentially be implemented in future automatic monitoring systems, with limited computational resources.

4.2. Vibrancy, Pleasantness and Eventfulness

According to soundscape literature, vibrancy should be correlated with both eventfulness and pleasantness, and the latter two variables should be independent. The measurements of vibrancy gathered in this study correlated with eventfulness and not with pleasantness, seemingly suggesting that an eventfulness measurement was collected. However, as mentioned in Section 2.5, the participants of the audio-visual experiment were clear about the meaning of vibrant and eventful. The rationale for seeking correlations between vibrancy and eventfulness, and vibrancy and pleasantness, was indeed testing the theory developed by Axelsson et al. [30], stating that an "exciting" (or else, vibrant) soundscape is both eventful and pleasant. This was also confirmed by the information gathered during the group interview stage of this study. On the other hand, Hall et al. [38] in their study on psychoacoustic properties of urban soundscapes found no evidence for a relationship between the vibrant and pleasant constructs and concluded that these attributes are referred to independent dimensions. Nevertheless, the abovementioned studies [30,38] relied on audio-only laboratory experiments, and the group interview of this study addressed (soundscape) vibrancy perception "in theory", while the participants of the audio-visual experiment looked at (vibrant) environments as a whole. That is, the visual information could not be disregarded. The results of the present study are somewhat in line with the findings of Hall et al. [38], as no correlation was found between vibrancy and pleasantness, but this should be considered in the broader understanding that the vibrancy construct is maybe too complex to be captured by auditory factors alone, and it could be highly affected by the contextual (e.g., visual) situation [52]. In order to confirm this outcome, it could be useful to perform further experiments including control conditions (e.g., audio-only or video-only stimuli) to gain a better understanding of the corresponding weights of the auditory and visual domains in the vibrancy construct. However, this was out of the scope of the present work, the primary aim of which was testing a predictive model.

It could still be meaningful to assess soundscape vibrancy in isolation from the context as some have done in the past, for mapping and assessment purposes, although this is less relevant if the purpose is to plan and design a (vibrant) place. Then, the soundscape cannot be treated separately, but must be approached as an integrated part of the place as a whole.

5. Conclusions

This paper aimed to provide further insights into the perceptual construct of vibrancy in soundscape studies and to provide a predictive model for the vibrancy descriptor using physical indicators. For this purpose a two-stage data collection was organised through a group interview and a laboratory experiment. Overall, the main conclusions of this study are:

- Vibrancy perception depends on both aural and visual cues, and the presence of people is relevant for both sensory domains.
- A vibrancy model based on Roughness, Presence of People, Fluctuation Strength, Loudness and Presence of Music as predictors, can explain up to 76% of the variance in the mean individual vibrancy scores.
- Within this audio-visual laboratory experiment, mean vibrancy scores resulted strongly correlated with mean eventfulness scores, but not correlated with mean pleasantness scores.

From a holistic perspective, this study suggests that the pleasantness dimension is contextual and highly dependent on the visual scenery. Taken together, the findings of this study show that there is room for the implementation of predictive models for new soundscape descriptors and these can be useful operative design tools within a broader urban sound planning framework.

Author Contributions: Conceptualization, F.A. and J.K.; Methodology, F.A. and J.K.; Software, F.A.; Validation, F.A. and J.K.; Formal Analysis, F.A.; Investigation, F.A. and J.K.; Resources, J.K.; Data Curation, F.A.; Writing-Original Draft Preparation, F.A.; Writing-Review & Editing, F.A. and J.K.; Visualization, F.A.; Supervision, J.K.; Project Administration, J.K.; Funding Acquisition, J.K.

Funding: This research was funded through the People Programme (Marie Curie Actions) of the European Union's 7th Framework Programme FP7/2007-2013 under REA grant agreement no. 290110, SONORUS "Urban Sound Planner" and through the European Research Council (ERC) Advanced Grant (no. 740696) on "Soundscape Indices" (SSID).

Acknowledgments: The authors are also grateful to Federica Lepore and Eirini Kostara-Konstantinou for their support during data collection.

Conflicts of Interest: The authors declare no conflict of interest. The funders had no role in the design of the study; in the collection, analyses, or interpretation of data; in the writing of the manuscript, and in the decision to publish the results.

References

1. European Environment Agency. *Noise in Europe 2014*; Publications Office of the European Union: Luxembourg, 2014.
2. European Parliament and Council. *Directive 2002/49/EC Relating to the Assessment and Management of Environmental Noise*; Publications Office of the European Union: Brussels, Belgium, 2002.
3. Kang, J. *Urban Sound Environment*; Taylor & Francis incorporating Spon: London, UK, 2007.
4. Andringa, T.C.; Weber, M.; Payne, S.R.; Krijnders, J.D.; Dixon, M.N.; van der Linden, R.; de Kock, E.G.; Lanser, J.J. Positioning soundscape research and management. *J. Acoust. Soc. Am.* **2013**, *134*, 2739–2747. [CrossRef] [PubMed]
5. Maffei, L.; Di Gabriele, M.; Masullo, M.; Aletta, F. On the perception of Limited Traffic Zones as urban noise mitigation action. *Noise Mapp.* **2014**, *1*, 50–58. [CrossRef]
6. European Environment Agency. *Good Practice Guide on Quiet Areas*; Publications Office of the European Union: Luxembourg, 2014.
7. Alves, S.; Altreuther, B.; Scheuren, J. Holistic Concept for Urban Sound Planning Applied to Real Sites. In Proceedings of the Forum Acusticum 2014 Conference, Krakow, Poland, 7–12 September 2014.
8. Lavia, L.; Easteal, M.; Close, D.; Witchel, H.J.; Axelsson, Ö. Sounding Brighton: Practical approaches towards better Soundscapes. In Proceedings of the Internoise 2012 Conference, New York, NY, USA, 19–22 August 2012.
9. Easteal, M.; Bannister, S.; Kang, J.; Aletta, F.; Lavia, L.; Witchel, H. Urban Sound Planning in Brighton and Hove. In Proceedings of the Forum Acusticum 2014 Conference, Krakow, Poland, 7–12 September 2014.
10. Alves, S.; Estévez-Mauriz, L.; Aletta, F.; Echevarria-Sanchez, G.M.; Puyana Romero, V. Towards the integration of urban sound planning in urban development processes: The study of four test sites within the SONORUS project. *Noise Mapp.* **2015**, *2*, 57–85.
11. International Organization for Standardization. *ISO 12913-1:2014 Acoustics—Soundscape—Part 1: Definition and Conceptual Framework*; ISO: Geneva, Switzerland, 2014.
12. Schafer, R.M. *The Tuning of the World*; Knopf: New York, NY, USA, 1977.
13. Southworth, M. The sonic environment of cities. *Environ. Behav.* **1969**, *1*, 49–70.
14. Axelsson, Ö.; Nilsson, M.E.; Berglund, B. A Swedish instrument for measuring soundscape quality. In Proceedings of the Euronoise 2009 Conference, Edinburgh, UK, 26–28 October 2009.
15. Axelsson, Ö. The ISO 12913 series on soundscape. In Proceedings of the Forum Acusticum 2011 Conference, Aalborg, Denmark, 27 June–1 July 2011.
16. Brown, A.L.; Kang, J.; Gjestland, T. Towards standardization in soundscape preference assessment. *Appl. Acoust.* **2011**, *72*, 387–392. [CrossRef]
17. Payne, S.R.; Davies, W.J.; Adams, M.D. *Research into the Practical and Policy Applications of Soundscape Concepts and Techniques in Urban Areas (NANR 200)*; Department for Environment Food and Rural Affairs: London, UK, 2009.

18. Van Kempen, E.; Devilee, J.; Swart, W.; van Kamp, I. Characterizing urban areas with good sound quality: Development of a research protocol. *Noise Health* **2014**, *16*, 380–387. [CrossRef] [PubMed]
19. Aletta, F.; Axelsson, Ö.; Kang, J. Towards acoustic indicators for soundscape design. In Proceedings of the Forum Acusticum 2014 Conference, Krakow, Poland, 7–12 September 2014.
20. Aletta, F.; Kang, J.; Axelsson, Ö. Soundscape descriptors and a conceptual framework for developing predictive soundscape models. *Landsc. Urban Plan.* **2016**, *149*, 65–74. [CrossRef]
21. Brambilla, G.; Maffei, L. Responses to noise in urban parks and in rural quiet areas. *Acta Acust. United Acust.* **2006**, *92*, 881–886.
22. Pheasant, R.J.; Horoshenkov, K.; Watts, G.; Barret, B.T. The acoustic and visual factors influencing the construction of tranquil space in urban andrural environments tranquil spaces-quiet places? *J. Acoust. Soc. Am.* **2008**, *123*, 1446–1457. [CrossRef] [PubMed]
23. Pheasant, R.J.; Horoshenkov, K.V.; Watts, G.R. The role of audio-visual interaction on the perception of tranquility. In Proceedings of the Euronoise Conference, Edinburgh, UK, 26–28 October 2009.
24. Pheasant, R.J.; Fisher, M.N.; Watts, G.R.; Whitaker, D.J.; Horoshenkov, K.V. The importance of auditory-visual interaction in the construction of 'tranquil space'. *J. Environ. Psychol.* **2010**, *30*, 501–509. [CrossRef]
25. Watts, G.R.; Pheasant, R.J.; Horoshenkov, K.V. Predicting perceived tranquillity in urban parks and open spaces. *Environ. Plan. B* **2011**, *38*, 585–594. [CrossRef]
26. García, I.; Aspuru, I.; Herranz, K.; Bustamante, M.T. Application of the methodology to assess quiet urban areas in Bilbao: Case pilot of QUADMAP. In Proceedings of the Internoise 2013 Conference, Innsbruck, Austria, 15–18 September 2013.
27. Wolfert, H. QUADMAP, three pilots and a methodology. In Proceedings of the Internoise 2014 Conference, Melbourne, Australia, 16–19 November 2014.
28. Aletta, F.; Kang, J. Soundscape approach integrating noise mapping techniques: A case study in Brighton, UK. *Noise Mapp.* **2015**, *2*, 1–12. [CrossRef]
29. Aletta, F.; Margaritis, E.; Filipan, K.; Puyana Romero, V.; Axelsson, Ö.; Kang, J. Characterization of the soundscape in Valley Gardens, Brighton, by a soundwalk prior to an urban design intervention. In Proceedings of the Euronoise 2015 Conference, Maastricht, The Netherland, 31 May–3 June 2015.
30. Axelsson, Ö.; Nilsson, M.; Berglund, B. A principal components model of soundscape perception. *J. Acoust. Soc. Am.* **2010**, *128*, 2836–2846. [CrossRef] [PubMed]
31. Cain, R.; Jennings, P.; Poxon, J. The development and application of the emotional dimensions of a soundscape. *Appl. Acoust.* **2013**, *74*, 232–239. [CrossRef]
32. Oxford Dictionaries. *Oxford Dictionary of English*; Oxford University Press: Oxford, UK, 2010.
33. Jackson, L.E. The relationship of urban design to human health and condition. *Landsc. Urban Plan.* **2003**, *64*, 191–200. [CrossRef]
34. Samadi, Z.; Yunus, R.M.; Omar, D.; Bakri, A.F. Experiencing urban through on-street activity. *Procedia Soc. Behav. Sci.* **2015**, *170*, 653–658. [CrossRef]
35. Talen, E. *City Rules: How Regulations Affect Urban Form*; Island Press: Washington, DC, USA, 2012.
36. Braun, L.M.; Malizia, E. Downtown vibrancy influences public health and safety outcomes in urban counties. *J. Transp. Health* **2015**, *2*, 540–548. [CrossRef]
37. Davies, W.J.; Adams, M.D.; Bruce, N.S.; Cain, R.; Carlyle, A.; Cusack, P.; Hall, D.A.; Hume, K.I.; Irwin, A.; Jennings, P. Perception of soundscapes: An interdisciplinary approach. *Appl. Acoust.* **2013**, *74*, 224–231. [CrossRef]
38. Hall, D.A.; Irwin, A.; Edmondson-Jones, M.; Philips, S.; Poxon, J.E. An exploratory evaluation of perceptual, psychoacoustic and acoustical properties of urban soundscapes. *Appl. Acoust.* **2013**, *74*, 248–254. [CrossRef]
39. Fiebig, A.; Schulte-Fortkamp, B. Soundscapes and their influence on inhabitants—New findings with the help of a grounded theory approach. *J. Acoust. Soc. Am.* **2004**, *115*, 2496. [CrossRef]
40. Liu, F.; Kang, J. A grounded theory approach to the subjective understanding of urban soundscape in Sheffield. *Cities* **2016**, *50*, 28–39. [CrossRef]
41. Barbour, R. *Doing Focus Groups*; SAGE Publications Ltd.: London, UK, 2007.
42. Genuit, K.; Fiebig, A. Psychoacoustics and its Benefits for the Soundscape Approach. *Acta Acust. United Acust.* **2006**, *92*, 1–7.
43. Fastl, H.; Zwicker, E. *Psychoacoustics—Facts and Models*; Springer: Berlin, Germany, 1990.

44. Rychtáriková, M.; Vermeir, G. Soundscape categorization on the basis of objective acoustical parameters. *Appl. Acoust.* **2013**, 240–247. [CrossRef]
45. Pheasant, R.J.; Watts, G.R. Towards predicting wildness in the United Kingdom. *Landsc. Urban Plan.* **2015**, *133*, 87–97. [CrossRef]
46. HEAD Acoustics. Artemis. 2011. Available online: http://www.head-acoustics.de/eng/nvh_artemis.htm (accessed on 30 July 2017).
47. Van den Bosch, K.A. *Safe and Sound: Soundscape Research in Special Needs Care*; University of Groningen: Groningen, The Netherland, 2015.
48. Axelsson, Ö. How to measure soundscape quality. In Proceedings of the Euronoise 2015 Conference, Maastricht, The Netherland, 31 May–3 June 2015; pp. 1477–1481.
49. Yilmazer, S.; Acun, V. A grounded theory approach to assess indoor soundscape in historic religious spaces of Anatolian culture: A case study on Hacı Bayram Mosque. *Build. Acoust.* **2018**, *25*, 137–150. [CrossRef]
50. Sayin, E.; Krishna, A.; Ardelet, C.; Briand Decré, G.; Goudey, A. "Sound and safe": The effect of ambient sound on the perceived safety of public spaces. *Int. J. Res. Mark.* **2015**, *32*, 343–353. [CrossRef]
51. Aletta, F.; Kang, J.; Astolfi, A.; Fuda, S. Differences in soundscape appreciation of walking sounds from different footpath materials in urban parks. *Sustain. Cities Soc.* **2016**, *27*, 367–376. [CrossRef]
52. Hong, J.Y.; Jeon, J.Y. Influence of urban contexts on soundscape perceptions: A structural equation modeling approach. *Landsc. Urban Plan.* **2015**, *141*, 78–87. [CrossRef]

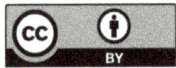

© 2018 by the authors. Licensee MDPI, Basel, Switzerland. This article is an open access article distributed under the terms and conditions of the Creative Commons Attribution (CC BY) license (http://creativecommons.org/licenses/by/4.0/).

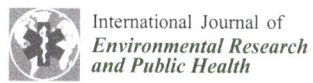

Article

Soundtracking the Public Space: Outcomes of the Musikiosk Soundscape Intervention

Daniel Steele [1,*], Edda Bild [2], Cynthia Tarlao [1] and Catherine Guastavino [1]

[1] School of Information Studies and CIRMMT, McGill University, Montreal, QC H3A 0G4, Canada; cynthia.tarlao@mail.mcgill.ca (C.T.); catherine.guastavino@mcgill.ca (C.G.)
[2] Department of Geography, Planning and International Development, University of Amsterdam, 1018WV Amsterdam, The Netherlands; A.E.Bild@uva.nl
* Correspondence: daniel.steele@mail.mcgill.ca

Received: 1 April 2019; Accepted: 12 May 2019; Published: 27 May 2019

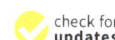

Abstract: Decades of research support the idea that striving for lower sound levels is the cornerstone of protecting urban public health. Growing insight on urban soundscapes, however, highlights a more complex role of sound in public spaces, mediated by context, and the potential of soundscape interventions to contribute to the urban experience. We discuss Musikiosk, an unsupervised installation allowing users to play audio content from their own devices over publicly provided speakers. Deployed in the gazebo of a pocket park in Montreal (Parc du Portugal), in the summer of 2015, its effects over the quality of the public urban experience of park users were researched using a mixed methods approach, combining questionnaires, interviews, behavioral observations, and acoustic monitoring, as well as public outreach activities. An integrated analysis of results revealed positive outcomes both at the individual level (in terms of soundscape evaluations and mood benefits) and at the social level (in terms of increased interaction and lingering behaviors). The park was perceived as more pleasant and convivial for both users and non-users, and the perceived soundscape calmness and appropriateness were not affected. Musikiosk animated an underused section of the park without displacing existing users while promoting increased interaction and sharing, particularly of music. It also led to a strategy for interacting with both residents and city decision-makers on matters related to urban sound.

Keywords: Musikiosk; soundscape; sound perception; soundscape intervention; democratic soundscape installation; quality of the urban public experience; mixed methods study; pocket park; urban sound planning

---

1. Introduction

The deleterious effects of noise on everyday life (particularly in urban settings) is well established. Organizations at national, international, and supranational levels have (rightfully) emphasized the negative effects of noise on public health and have emphasized the "cost of noise pollution" (See e.g. Ireland: http://www.askaboutireland.ie/enfo/irelands-environment/noise/cost-of-noise-pollution/). While the field of noise abatement has achieved dramatic reductions in the presence of sounds in urban spaces that exceed harmful sound levels or cause excessive annoyance, it remains impossible, as well as undesirable, to conceive of a city that makes no sound. Today's approaches, heavily reliant on the measurement of sound level (and its subsequent reduction) offer little guidance on identifying what sounds belong in the city once the harmful sources have been mitigated. We suppose that sounds are a reflection of public life [1], playing a complex role in our urban experience. In the sound-oriented research community, there is a growing understanding that exclusive reliance on physical measurements, and particularly sound levels, fails to capture the complexity of the human experience (e.g., [2–5]), providing limited guidance to planners and designers on identifying or designing better sounding cities.

Conversely, an extensive and ever-growing body of research on soundscape (defined as the acoustic environment as perceived, experienced, and/or understood by people or society, in context [6]) offers a new approach for urban sound management, centered on the idea of sound as an urban resource [2,7–11]. Studies embedded in this tradition are based on the experience of the city user and on a complex understanding of the urban auditory experience, repeatedly demonstrating that urban soundscape strongly influences overall health but not always in a negative way (see Aletta et al. [7] for a review of positive outcomes, including stress recovery [12,13]). Despite this knowledge collected in the research community, urban sound management remains driven by noise abatement strategies, on both the city-maker side (i.e., planners, politicians) [14] and the city-user side (i.e., communities, stakeholders) [15].

To investigate the role of sound in urban experience, we deployed a soundscape intervention in the gazebo of a Montreal public park. Musikiosk provided free, unsupervised access to an audio jack and speakers. It allowed people to play whatever audio content they wished in the public space. A stakeholder-based approach as well as rules set forth, described in the Methods section, started in advance of the intervention were intended to minimize risks to the project, as described in the Results section. This study addresses the following research question: "How does a soundscape installation like Musikiosk affect the quality of the urban public experience for users of a public space?".

To this end, we introduce the hybrid concept of "quality of the urban public experience" (QUPE) as a bridge between public health and the present topic of this special issue, soundscape. The QUPE concept comprises themes that are both operationalizable and measurable, providing the opportunity to empirically research the effects of a democratic soundscape installation on the users of a pocket park in Montreal.

Musikiosk was developed based on ideas of sound as a resource and of providing park users with the opportunity (and responsibility) of sonically appropriating their space. We bring into the conversation insights from a number of social and human domains of science (including sociology, psychology, acoustics, soundscape research, and public space research) to define QUPE. To date, the positive link between the conceptualization of "sound as a resource" [4] and public health has been posed as an obvious one, yet there are no available models to utilize.

QUPE thus serves as a catch-all, multidisciplinary concept into which we can integrate the complexity of the psychological, behavioral, and other social aspects of urban space use, with a focus on the quality, including sound quality, of the interaction between city users and their urban public spaces. QUPE (see Figure 1) is operationalized along three axes (which for the purposes of this paper are most elaborated in the sonic dimension): (1) sound-related evaluation (does Musikiosk change the evaluation of soundscapes and specific sounds?), (2) public space engagement (does Musikiosk impact how users engage in the space and interact with others?), and (3) psychological outcomes (does Musikiosk affect users' behaviors and feelings?). Within each of these three dimensions, themes related to the presence of Musikiosk emerge and are elaborated in this manuscript.

We situate the study of the aforementioned effects in a specific spatial context i.e., an urban pocket park, with its own physical, social, and acoustic idiosyncrasies, as well as a politico-technological context, referring to the implications of developing and engaging with an installation that encourages a novel, democratic appropriation of public spaces through sound (particularly music).

We report on the results of a mixed-methods study centered on the Musikiosk intervention and highlighting only results that could be elaborated across multiple methods. The QUPE model links the axes of soundscape and public space evaluations to concepts in the public health literature. The Review section steps through this QUPE model, including a necessary background on soundscape evaluations, and other relevant contexts of the study. The Methods section outlines seven different qualitative and quantitative methods, outlining their integration. The Results section elaborates on findings about Musikiosk across multiple methods, organized by the three QUPE axes. The Discussion section situates these results in the context of the QUPE model and other literature while the Conclusions explain theoretical and practical contributions of the study.

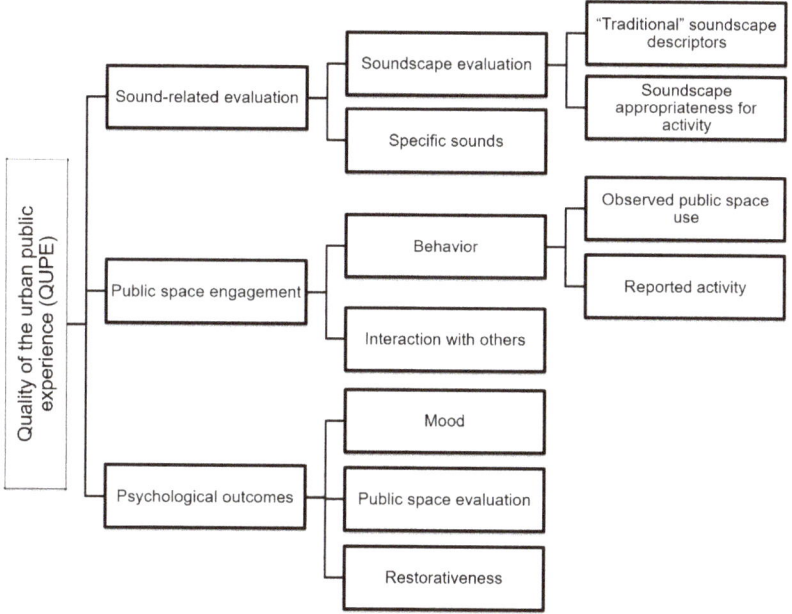

Figure 1. The QUPE (quality of the urban public experience) model. Three axes are elaborated and inform the structure of the present study.

2. Literature Review

As Musikiosk is primarily an intervention with an effect on the sound of the urban environment, it is important to focus on research that both highlights the ways people evaluate soundscape and soundscape interventions, but also the relationship of soundscape (interventions) to broader aspects of the quality of the public experience, for example, the restorative capabilities of soundscapes. The literature review steps through the axes of the quality of urban public experience (QUPE) outlined in the introduction. This is followed by a review of work on the contexts (i.e., spatial and politico-technological) relevant to Musikiosk.

2.1. Sound-Related Evaluation

The first axis of QUPE deals specifically with the evaluation of sound(s) and the sound environment itself.

2.1.1. Soundscape Evaluation

We first review evaluations of the soundscape as a whole, followed by literature on the way people describe specific sounds within the urban sound environment.

"Traditional" Soundscape Descriptors

Soundscape descriptors have been proposed to help explain or predict users' evaluations [16,17] (see [7] for a review). Among these efforts, the Swedish Soundscape-Quality Protocol (SSQP) has stood out as a useful tool to both characterize and compare soundscapes and their perceived affective quality. The scale is composed of a composite of a holistic scale (Good–Bad) [18] paired with a set of eight Likert scales related to *pleasantness, unpleasantness, eventfulness, uneventfulness, vibrancy, monotony, calmness*, and *chaoticness* [19,20]. While originally developed in Swedish, SSQP has been translated in a number of languages, including English, Korean. The in-house French translation, used in this research [21] faced a number of challenges, including the validation of the translation, which led to the *uneventful* rating being dropped.

Recent laboratory and on-site soundscape studies, attempting to further refine soundscape evaluation, have shown the need to add a measurement of the appropriateness of soundscape for a location [7,22,23] and *appropriate* has thus been suggested as a complement to the SSQP ratings [18].

Soundscape Appropriateness for Activity

While the role of users' activities has been suggested almost 20 years ago [3,24] and has also been discussed in relation to the acoustic design of outdoor spaces [25], the integration of activity in models attempting to characterize urban soundscapes is still in its exploratory phase [26–31]. Empirical studies offer some evidence on the importance of activities in both laboratory study tasks (e.g., [32,33]) and in-situ soundscape evaluations [34]. However, most such research projects arise from more practice-oriented questions, either dealing with specific soundscape interventions with some form of behavioral control in mind (see [23,26]) or investigating the effect soundscapes play on relaxation or rehabilitation activities or in relation to aspects of indoor and outdoor auditory comfort [35–38].

In Guastavino's [32] free sorting tasks of recorded sound environments, participants spontaneously grouped soundscapes in terms of activities, describing them in terms of the actions performed (e.g., "do the groceries", "take a walk", "have a drink") in relation to the type of locations ("market," "café", "restaurant," "park") and specific sound sources ("vendors," "music," "birds"), indicative of the activities. Davies et al. [33], using soundwalks, laboratory studies, and focus groups, found consistently that "soundscapes that are compatible for one's own purposes and support one's own behaviors are [...] evaluated as positive". Nielbo et al. [39] further observed that various recorded "soundscapes" were evaluated as being more or less appropriate for different imagined activities by participants in a listening experiment.

Furthermore, recent studies suggest that the level of social interaction of users' activities also influences how public space users evaluate their soundscapes [31,40]). Therefore, in this paper we understand appropriateness of soundscapes not in relation to a location, but rather to one's potential or actual activities in the context of outdoor, public space settings [31].

2.1.2. Specific Sounds

In an urban outdoor setting, added sound has been proven to be an efficient masker for other (potentially unpleasant) sounds, and this approach has been used both for purposeful acoustic design, e.g., by installing fountains in parks to reduce annoyance [25,41] or using curated (added) sound art [37,42–44]. Added sound has also been used in the context of noise pollution management to, for example, reduce annoyance to mechanical sound [45] or to highway noise [46]. A study on auditory comfort in public spaces showed that introducing sounds that were considered pleasant (such as music and water), even rather loud ones, produced a considerable improvement in evaluations acoustic comfort [47]. Worth noting, is that all of these added sounds were chosen and "composed" by sound designers in a top-down approach. None of the interventions allowed space users to have any control over levels or content. Through the democratic nature of Musikiosk, we are addressing this gap specifically by not predefining what is played, leaving content and even levels (to an extent) up to users.

Music, as another type of added sound, stands out as a sound with an "aestheticizing" effect [48]. Research indicates that music is a factor influencing people's judgments on their environment, particularly in relation to their soundscape [49,50].

The present study uses the aforementioned modified SSQP, in addition to two appropriateness scales (appropriateness of soundscape for activity and appropriateness of overall sound level for the park), and identification and evaluation of heard sound sources.

2.2. Public Space Engagement

The next axis of QUPE explores the way users engage with public space.

Extensive research has been dedicated to exploring the "desirable qualities" of public spaces as well as how to encourage or achieve the well-documented social, health, environmental, and economic benefits that public spaces bring to the users they serve (see [51,52] for comprehensive reviews). However, central to many studies on public spaces are aspects of sociability, interaction, and use that straddle the lines between the physical dimensions of the space (focused on the materiality of space and how aspects of accessibility and usability are encoded in its morphology [53]) and the enactment of publicness in as part of what Yucesoy refers to as the "interactional and experiential space" [54] (p. 2). Research from a variety of human and social sciences have emphasized the deeply social nature of public spaces and much thought is put into their functionality and in the way they are appropriated by users in their everyday activities, with public spaces representing not only the physical but also the social and cultural context for the occurrence of interactions and developing a sense of community [55–63].

The ubiquity of digital technologies, personal mobile technologies, on the one hand [64–66] and interactive technologies (e.g., [67,68]), on the other, have been consistently transforming the ways in which people engage with their public spaces, how they interact with others and thus blurring the lines between the public and private realm, not only spatially but also acoustically [69,70]. This QUPE axis is operationalized in the present study through observed changes in behavior and interactivity with other users.

2.3. Psychological Outcomes

This axis focuses on three psychological outcomes affecting QUPE.

2.3.1. Mood

There is significant support from the literature for a relationship between mood and soundscape. There is a demonstrated negative relationship between sound pressure levels and some aspects of mood (e.g., [71,72]). A relationship between mood (measured in relation to overall annoyance) and evaluations of everyday sounds has been shown in relation to ratings of sound annoyance [73]. For work specifically linking urban soundscape evaluations, Steffens et al. [30,50] demonstrated a significant effect of mood on ratings of pleasantness, eventfulness, and familiarity; this effect was particularly pronounced when music was present during an evaluation.

2.3.2. Public Space Evaluation

The experience of public spaces is moderated at an individual, psychological level by the emotional engagement with the space [74], which in turn affects the future patterns of use, engagement with and evaluation of the space. The interaction with the physical, political, social, or cultural context in general, and with the other users of an urban space in particular can alter one's personal feelings of safety and security (see [75] for a review), of restoration [76], of leisure [77], of perceived control over the space [78,79], and of psychological comfort (see [57])—often related to one's perceived freedom of action in a space, of inclusiveness or being excluded from a space ([62], also see [80] for a study on women's experiences). Mood is measured in the present study with a single, self-reported scale rating.

2.3.3. Soundscape Restorativeness Evaluation

An important aspect of public space experience is the psychological restoration (measured on multiple *restorativeness* scales) that one may achieve from visiting the space [81,82]. Restorative environments enable users to recover from drained cognitive resources and to reflect upon daily- or life issues, and they decrease stress levels [83,84]. Restorative soundscapes, specifically, enable users to recover from the negative effect of noise exposure. The Perceived Restorativeness Soundscape Scale

(PRSS) was developed and validated [85,86] to measure the perceived qualities of soundscapes in terms of the four theoretical components considered necessary to create a restorative environment, namely Fascination, Being-Away, Compatibility, and Extent [83,87]. Fascination refers to involuntary, effortless attention. Being-Away involves a shift away from the present situation or problems, allowing tired cognitive structures to rest while activating others. Compatibility refers to the fit of the environment with the needs and inclinations of the user. It has been shown to relate to appropriateness for activity [86]. Extent refers to the richness and structure of the environment into a coherent whole. The first three of these components have been used in the present study due to their relevance in the context of a small urban park.

2.4. Spatial Context—Pocket Parks

Ample evidence shows that large urban parks dominated by greenery have measurable effects on aspects of the aforementioned restorativeness as well as stress relief for their users [88–90]. However, the question is whether the various health-related benefits apply at smaller scales. The smallest urban public parks, called "pocket parks" [91] by some in the literature, are often as busy as the surrounding city. While these pocket parks have received attention in the design literature, there is not much information available about their potential benefits; they have been left disproportionally understudied, despite intuitive or explicit knowledge on the functions that they serve for the local population [91], including acting as a setting for social interactions and encouraging physical activity in neighborhoods that otherwise lack access to public spaces [92]. A study by Peschardt and Stigsdotter [93] confirms the extensive use of pocket parks for socializing purposes, emphasizing also the effect on mental health and restoration, both for "average" and stressed users. For average users, aspects of socialization were essential, whereas for stressed users, nature was more important, corroborating, to a large extent, the findings for larger green urban parks. A follow up study by the same authors [94] investigated the features of the pocket park that could encourage their potential effect on the two aforementioned health benefits. They showed that different amenities are expected for encouraging socializing and restoration, with some amenities evaluated at times positively for one activity and negatively for the other (like tables or green groundcovers), demonstrating the difficult challenge of designing a small sized public space affording multiple simultaneous uses and purposes. A laboratory-based study [95] showed that, based on visual assessment of pocket parks, they have the potential to afford recovery and restoration-related activities. To our knowledge, the sonic dimension of pocket parks has not been studied; further the function and use of park amenities on the sound environment (and vice versa) is ripe for investigation, though one such study has taken place on a soundscape intervention in a larger public square [96].

2.5. Politico-Technological Context

This study also aims to bridge the gap toward understanding user-modified soundscapes. Enabling this study, technological developments of the last decade or two allow listeners to carry their musical choices "in their pocket" and to engage in mobile music listening behaviors in the ephemeral and personalized auditory private spaces delineated by headphones, usually in the context of physical public spaces. These new forms of engagement with urban public through mobile music listening subvert existing norms of social behavior by allowing public space users to control their own auditory experience on site and in real time [97,98]. Given the ample evidence on the effect of music over sociability and loitering behaviors in public spaces (e.g., [26,97–101]), control over music in a public context becomes "a source of social power" [102] (p. 20). Therefore, these behaviors are particularly interesting in light of increased controls set in place in highly monitored public spaces, where rules are continuously created to prohibit a growing list of such behaviors considered disruptive (including playing amplified music in public).

There is a well-documented relationship between music and identity (e.g., [103]), with music as a medium through which people from different cultures and backgrounds can communicate, share experiences and affirm their collective and individual identity. By deciding to bring their private musical behaviors in the public and play their music out loud in a public space setting, users appropriate their space and delineate auditory spaces of identity and belonging—or rejection [100]. In this context, users could engage in 'responsible listening' practices [104], complying with shared norms, regulations and behaviors or, on the contrary, defiant to these factors, based on a combination of internal needs (e.g., desire to impress friends or to listen to music) and external considerations (e.g., presence of others). Musikiosk, by encouraging space users to connect their mobile devices to a public output system that is free, accessible, unprogrammed and unsupervised, challenges the centrally set musical policies by promoting new forms of auditory democracy and appropriation. By allowing users to participate in the process of musical production and consumption in public spaces, we revisit the privateness of portable devices, which now become a tool for bringing the private into the public through public islands of music where others can join in.

3. Methods

Soundscape research favors qualitative and mixed approaches over quantitative-only approaches [7,105]. The mixed-methods research design developed here follows this trend and was designed to integrate seven different methods at four stages of data collection and a data analysis stage. This integrated approach to data collection and analysis was used to provide a multilayered and holistic understanding of the relationship between park users and their environment as well as the specific effects of Musikiosk on their engagement with the park. All methods were approved by McGill Research Ethics Board, #55-0615.

Figure 2 shows the different methods used at each of the five project phases. The sections below follow the same timeline.

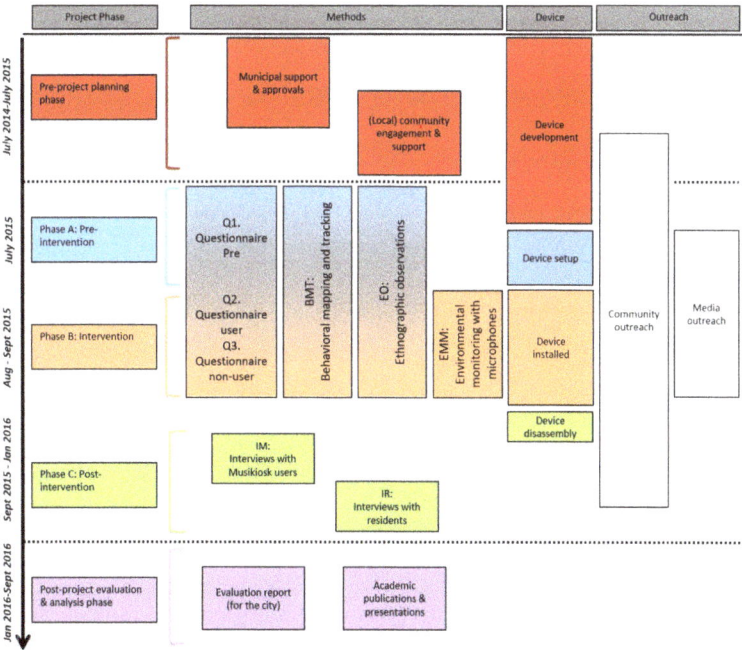

Figure 2. Musikiosk research timeline by phase. Legend indicates method type.

3.1. The Musikiosk Device and Parc Du Portugal

Users connected to Musikiosk with anything that had an audio jack (e.g., mp3 players, musical instruments) or a Bluetooth connection (e.g., phone). The device consisted of a Raspberry Pi (Raspberry PI, UK) equipped with a sound card, a Bluetooth module and a Wi-Fi USB antenna (see [106] for a detailed description of the device). It was coupled with an audio card and a calibrated electret microphone for acoustic monitoring. These measurements were used to automatically adjust playback levels to be appropriate based on the time-of-day, automatic system logs for the researchers to monitor usage frequencies, and automatic power down during predetermined nighttime hours (10 PM) as agreed with the city (see [106]).

The Parc du Portugal (see Figure 3) is situated in a lively, musical neighborhood with a history of Portuguese immigration and, more recently, has become one of the centers of Montreal nightlife. On one side of the park is the rue Saint-Laurent commercial artery, home to a large number of different kinds of businesses, active almost 24/7 with shops, cafes, bars, and companies. Yet, on its other side, it borders a quiet(er) residential area, therefore serving a mixed function to both residents and passers-by, like tourists and office workers. Due to the traffic artery and multipurpose activities, there is a rather high background noise level (i.e., 58.5–60.5 dBA during a typical afternoon. The World Health Organization, for example, strongly recommends an average road traffic noise level of below 53 decibels (dB) L_{den} (see: http://www.euro.who.int/__data/assets/pdf_file/0009/383922/noise-guidelines-exec-sum-eng.pdf). Because of its location, the park hosts a diverse combination of peacefully overlapping users: recurrent users—elderly members of a Portuguese community who chat with each other from late afternoon through evening, employees from businesses nearby—and also passers-by (see [107] for more details). On the quiet(er) side of this park, a gazebo structure is located, which was chosen for the Musikiosk, because of the history of gazebos as local focal points for music performance, and because of the observed relative lack of use of side of the park. Given this context, the Musikiosk team proposed that a lively musical intervention would not cause a disruption of the park's character.

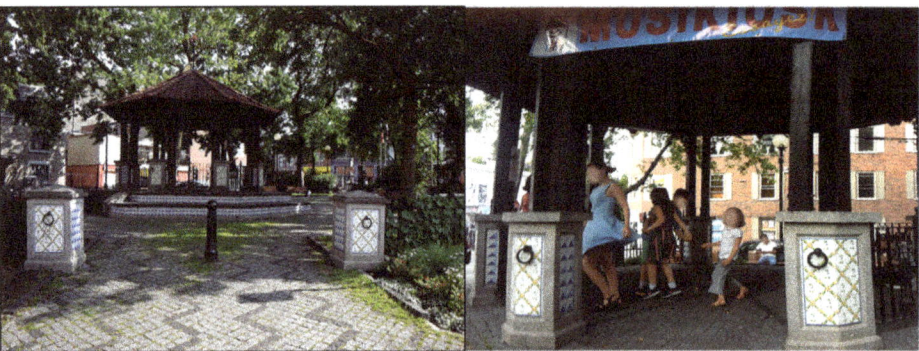

Figure 3. Left: gazebo in Parc du Portugal; right: users enjoying Musikiosk.

The Musikiosk device was unsupervised in that the researchers did not need to be present for it to be operational. Ample signage and instructions were placed around Musikiosk, in addition to a media outreach strategy, including a website and Facebook page, to allow users the opportunity to encounter and use the system. The device was free-of-charge and the democratic aspect of the installation ensured that all users were able to select their own audio content and use any device of their choosing.

3.2. Research Design and Timelines

The research project had five distinct phrases spanning more than 18 months: a pre-project, planning phase; Phase A: the pre-intervention; Phase B: intervention; phase C: post-intervention; and a post-project evaluation and analysis phase. The first four of these phases provided the core data reported in this paper. The central phases A, B, and C have been labeled using this separate nomenclature to facilitate comparisons between the experimental conditions arising from the installation of the Musikiosk.

3.2.1. Pre-Project Planning Phase

The project was conceived in the summer of 2014 and the technical aspects were in preparation throughout the following fall and winter. Generating technical and other practical specifications, building the device, selecting and garnering approvals for an installation site, and planning the research took approximately one year. Given Montreal's weather extremes (very warm summers and very cold winters) and the summer tourist season, the installation was elected to be in place for two months (August and September) in the late summer of 2015.

Given the unusual specifications of the Musikiosk, the permitting process included multiple meetings with municipal employee and elected official stakeholders, including multiple on-site visits, negotiations to liaison with local community and other stakeholders, and technical specifications such as functional hours to be written into the permit. We developed operations rules (e.g., hours of operation, maximal levels) with representatives of the city's Department of Culture, Sports, Leisure, and Social Development. The permit itself was, in fact, not a permit, but a temporary (2-month) exemption from the noise regulations. Stipulations were appended as conditions of the continued exemption.

During this phase, no formal data were collected; however, observations and accounts from the researchers and details of the permitting process are included to situate parts of the results section.

3.2.2. Phase A—Pre-Intervention

In this phase, formal data collection commenced. A timeframe of approximately one month was chosen for Phase A so that it could be of similar duration to the installation period (Phase B) but would still be in similar conditions for weather and frequency of neighborhood cultural events, enabling controlled comparisons.

In Phase A, three data collection methods were used simultaneously: pre-installation questionnaires (Q1), behavioral mapping and tracking (BMT), and ethnographic observations (EO). After piloting, we conducted 10 days of systematic observations (BMT and EO) in the park to document the patterns of daily park use, the groups of recurrent users and their profiles. Through questionnaires (Q1), we collected a baseline on users' on-site evaluations of their park and their on-site soundscapes during different times of day and weather conditions. This phase acted as a baseline (control) characterization of the park in terms of use and evaluation (both auditory and overall).

During this period, we also engaged in outreach activities and media engagement, to both advertise the Musikiosk system and the research project (and thus encourage visits and use and engagement of the system), as well as to ensure residents and the local community that their potential concerns on the effect of the system on the neighborhood had been heard and that their potential complaints would be addressed in a timely manner. Particular efforts were made to understand and ensure that existing park users, such as elderly Portuguese-Canadians, were not displaced.

3.2.3. Phase B—Intervention

In Phase B—or the intervention phase—we aimed to collect a detailed characterization of the relationship between park users and their space, with a focus on collecting evidence (if any) on the effect of the Musikiosk system on any potential changes in the aforementioned relationship.

We asked users of the system and non-users (present in the park while the system was in use) to complete questionnaires combining open and closed ended questions on their perception of the park, their evaluation of their soundscape as well as their opinion on the system and its appropriateness for the park (Q2 and Q3). We continued with systematic observations (BMT and EO) of the park to observe whether there were any noticeable changes in the dynamic of the park that could be related to the Musikiosk; these observations were conducted both when the system was in use and when it was not. While initially paper-based, during this phase the observations were conducted by trained data collectors using a handheld device equipped with specially designed software.

Throughout the intervention phase, we continued with our community outreach strategy, organizing special events to increase the visibility of Musikiosk in the neighborhood and demonstrating the usability of the system in an informal setting. The events took place on Tuesday evenings. During the events, through ethnographic observations, we focused on how users engaged with the system and others present, how they negotiated the use of Musikiosk, how other users of the park reacted to the system and what was the overall dynamic of the park during the events.

3.2.4. Phase C—The Post-Implementation Stage

Following the intervention phase, Phase C was an opportunity to speak more in-depth with Musikiosk users (IM) and nearby residents (IR) to reflect on their experience with Musikiosk. These observations were conducted via semi-structured interviews detailed below. In this time frame, Musikiosk was also removed from the park.

3.2.5. Post-Project Evaluation Phase

In this phase, direct feedback to the borough was provided via a written report. Also, feedback on the project outcomes was solicited via interactions with community and researchers. No data from this phase is reported in the present study.

3.3. Data Collection

The mixed-methods research protocol developed for this project was designed to be used in an integrated manner. The section that follows details the data collection methods by method and each subsection will describe the procedure, the data collection instrument, and the analysis techniques. Data collection methods have each been given a code (matched in Figure 2) and will be used throughout the document to reference findings specific to the method.

3.3.1. Questionnaires

The purpose of the questionnaires was to collect direct and momentary measurements of participants' evaluations in use of the park and/or Musikiosk. Questionnaires comprised a combination of open and closed-ended questions (see Appendix A). The questionnaire asked for insight on reported activity (Q1–3), demographic and psychological information (gender, age, noise sensitivity) and other contextual data about users' visits (e.g., whether they were alone), their evaluation of their soundscape as well as their opinion on the system and its appropriateness for the park.

All 3 questionnaires included 7 of the 8 SSQP scales (pleasant, unpleasant, eventful, vibrant, monotonous, calm, chaotic; Q4). Appropriateness (for activity) was included after the SSQP (Q5). All 3 questionnaires also asked for mood before and during, as self-reported (Q9–10). Mood was probed by directly asking for it ("What is your mood right now?"), and beside the momentary mood, they were asked to make a retrospective judgment ("What was your mood before coming to the park?"). As mood was not the main focus of this study, we feel that using a single mood scale was justified. All of the above scale were 7-point Likert scales.

We collected three types of questionnaires, based on the same template, to mirror the three available park-use conditions. The park baseline during Phase A represents the control condition and is called Q1. During Phase B, with the Musikiosk functioning, questionnaires were given both to those who used the Musikiosk (Q2) and to those who were in the park but did not use Musikiosk (Q3). The questionnaires all measured soundscape evaluation ratings, mood, and demographic data, but they differed only with relation to the details of the condition (degree of Musikiosk engagement). Eighty-eight Q1 questionnaires, 42 Q2 questionnaires, and 67 Q3 questionnaires were administered.

Consistent with the university's ethics policy, all participants were approached in the park by researchers and asked to take a voluntary, unpaid questionnaire of under 10 minutes. All materials were available in French and English and participants elected to take the questionnaire fully in one language or the other. Participants were approached only after they had already been in the park for a few minutes in order to ensure that they had been exposed the park and its soundscape before making judgments.

Q1: Pre-installation Questionnaire (Phase A)

This questionnaire, described above, was administered in the phase preceding the installation of Musikiosk and serves as a baseline condition for the other two conditions. See Appendix A, Table A1.

Q2: Musikiosk User Questionnaire (Phase B)

Musikiosk users were given a questionnaire about their experience using it, including who they had chosen to try it, whether it was appropriate for the park, what they liked about the system, and what they thought could be improved. Musikiosk users were not prompted to list the sound sources they heard around them, as were the participants of Q1 and Q3. Participants in this condition were recruited on the basis of having used the system themselves and interacted with their own device to control played content. See Appendix A, Table A2.

Q3: Non-MK User Questionnaire (Phase B)

This questionnaire was administered to park visitors who did not physically interact with Musikiosk. This included those who were friends of Musikiosk users as well as those seated on the other side of the park who were unaware of the installation, and all contexts in between. These questionnaires were also administered while the Musikiosk was not necessarily in use.

Participants in this condition were asked what they thought of an installation like this one in this park, how it changed their park experience and activities, whether they found it appropriate, whether it was in use, and whether they would like to use it themselves. See Appendix A, Table A3.

Analysis

ANOVA, MANOVA, t-tests, and chi-squared tests were performed on quantitative and/or categorized questionnaire data and were dependent on the data type. Relevant statistical methods, results, and significance levels are reported in line in the results text. Qualitative data are counted, categorized into emerging themes using the constant comparison method [108], quoted with descriptions of the analysis in-line and counted. Statistical tests are also reported in detail in Steele et al. [109].

3.3.2. EO: Ethnographic Observations

Ethnographic observations focused on documenting how the existence and use of Musikiosk affected people's use of their park, with a focus on the changes (if any) of patterns of use of the park by regular users and the patterns of new users. The ethnographic observations were completed both in Phase A (pre-intervention) and Phase B (intervention), concomitantly with the deployment of the other main data collection methods. To this end, we took field notes and photographs and engaged in informal discussions with regular park users.

3.3.3. BMT: Behavioral Mapping and Tracking

To observe the interactions between users of public spaces and their spaces in a non-intrusive yet systematic manner and document their patterns of use of the park, their engagement with amenities, their performed activities on an everyday basis, as well as the groups of recurrent users and their profiles, we used behavioral mapping as a data collection method. Behavioral mapping is the main type of structured observation used to systematically describe, on a map of the space, how its users use and move in it [31,110–112]. It allows researchers to integrate spatial and temporal dimensions of use of space and to visually represent changes in patterns of activities. Behavioral mapping was completed throughout the project duration, in each of its three lettered phases (A, B, and C).

For a detailed explanation of the behavioral mapping strategy, please consult [107]. The results of the behavioral mapping were used to offer a behavioral and spatial-temporal context in which we situate the other types of data that were collected, analyzed, and integrated, supplementing the results of the ethnographic observations.

3.3.4. Interviews

Interviews were conducted last, in Phase C (post-implementation), so that an interview guide could be developed in order to include, engage with, and understand emergent findings from the other methods. Residents are labeled R1 through R5 and Musikiosk users U1–U11.

IR: Interviews with Nearby Residents

A few weeks to months after the system was taken down, we completed interviews with residents living in the vicinity of the park in which Musikiosk was installed. This included five French-language interviews; two participants (R1 and R2) conducted their interview simultaneously. One of the interviewed residents used Musikiosk themselves and in their interview, we also addressed questions related to their experience of the system. Participants were selected on the basis of living within one block of the park. Their contact information had been collected primarily during outreach activities.

In the interview with residents, we addressed the perceived appropriateness of the Musikiosk system for the park and for the neighborhood as well as how the existence of such a system could change their use of the park. Emphasis was put on whether they observed or experienced any consequences in the use of the park (negative or positive). Questions were also posed as to the greater relationship of these residents with their soundscape for insight on how Musikiosk may have played a role in changing these perceptions.

For the complete interview guide instrument, consult the Appendix B, Table A4.

IM: Interviews to Expand on the Questionnaire with Musikiosk Users

Building on the data collected during the questionnaires and ethnographic observations we developed an interview guide aimed to go in depth on how the Musikiosk experience changed the Musikiosk users' perception and potential future use of the park (if at all) and whether Musikiosk was an appropriate addition for Parc du Portugal. The interview guide included questions in five thematic areas: use of Parc du Portugal, use of the Musikiosk system (including hypothetical scenarios), feedback about the Musikiosk system, a description of the park's soundscape, and demographic and other background information. Interviews were conducted with 11 users of the system (in English) who had engaged with it throughout the summer. These interviews were intended to be reflective of past uses of Musikiosk and were conducted outdoors in Parc du Portugal.

For the complete interview guide instrument, consult the Appendix C, Table A5.

Analysis

The interviews were transcribed and coded by bilingual researchers. They were analyzed using both a combination of deductive coding, based on the operationalization of QUPE, and inductive coding allowing for new themes to emerge. A preliminary list of the themes was originally detailed in [113] but has been updated to reflect the findings matched across methods.

3.4. Integrating Methods for Analysis

During the course of the study, some methods were used to inform the design of others. Questionnaires from the first part of Phase A (Q1) informed the variables collected in the behavioral mapping and tracking (BMT) and, to some extent, the recorded ethnographic observations (EO). Results from Q1, Q2, Q3, BMT, and EO informed the Musikiosk user interviews (IM), and each of these subsequently informed the resident interviews (IR).

We first processed and analyzed the data collected in our mixed-methods research design separately and then integrated the key findings along the main dimensions of QUPE (see Table 1), supplemented by additional themes emergent from the different data sources. Methods for each QUPE theme and sub-theme have been labeled as primary when results directly contribute to the theme at-hand and secondary when the results clarify or were informed by the primary methods.

Table 1. Research methods supporting QUPE analysis. Secondary methods support the results of the primary methods in this mixed-method study.

QUPE Theme	Sub-Theme	Supporting Methods
Soundscape evaluation	'Traditional' soundscape descriptors	Primary: Q1, Q2, Q3 Secondary: IM
	Soundscape appropriateness for activity	Primary: Q1, Q2, Q3 Secondary: IM, IR
Specific sounds		Primary: Q1, Q2, Q3 Secondary: IM
Behavior	Observed public space use	Primary: Q1, Q2, Q3 Secondary: IM
	Reported activity	Primary: BMT, EO Secondary: IR, EO, Q1, Q3
Interaction with others		Primary: IM, IR
Mood		Primary: Q1, Q2, Q3 Secondary: IM, IR
Public space evaluation		Primary: Q1, Q2, Q3 Secondary: IM
Restorativeness		Primary: Q1, Q2, Q3 Secondary: IM

In the presented analysis, themes are presented in sequence, organized roughly by the three QUPE dimensions (sound-related evaluation, public space engagement and psychological outcomes) and respective sub-dimensions. and corroborating findings from each method support the theme at-hand. These themes are detailed at the beginning of the results and form the structure of that section.

4. Results

Results Structure

We structure our results along the key psychological-behavioral themes of QUPE to illustrate the effects of Musikiosk on the experiences of both Musikiosk and other park users. The results and subsequent discussion are based on integrated analysis of the different methods. We group the aforementioned QUPE themes along three axes: sound-related evaluation; public space engagement; and psychological outcomes. We force, at times, a separation between certain themes for ease of presentation of results. Two additional results sub-sections follow concerning evaluations specifically of Musikiosk (rather than its effects on users) and the lasting effects of Musikiosk after it was uninstalled.

Note: Findings from individual methods indicate the method in parenthesis according to the codes described in Figure 2, e.g., *this finding comes from the pre-installation questionnaire (Q1)*. As some findings have already been published, they are summarized here in the results with references. Author-provided translations of French-language quotations are given in-line with the original in in Appendix D, Table A6, liked using the format *see Table A6–1* to direct the reader to quotation 1. Quotations are reported as, *"sample"* (participant ID, reported gender, age).

4.1. Park Profile

An initial integration of results (BMT, EO, Q1, Q2, and Q3) allowed for a characterization of the park in terms of its patterns of use and users, confirming initial observations that it was both a transition and a destination space, the latter particularly for neighborhood users.

BMT and EO pointed to the idea that there were strong differences in park use between the daytime and evening, as well as the weekday and the weekend (see [107] for a detailed analysis). The differences were visible in terms of profile of users, with younger users visiting the park more in the evening and a mix of regulars (elderly Portuguese-Canadians and returning users on their lunch break) during the day, but also for types of activities performed, with, perhaps unsurprisingly, fewer solitary users in the park in the evenings. In interviews (IM), participants claimed that it was quieter at night and they could hear more people.

Activities involving interacting with others dominate the park throughout times of day and the week, earning Parc du Portugal the label of a "social park" [109,114], however, the nature of the lingering, socially interactive activities changed from daytime to evening due to the profile and age of the users engaged in those activities.

The deeply social nature of the park has been emphasized by both residents and Musikiosk users in interviews; one resident (IR) stated of Parc du Portugal, "it's a park that seems to be used mostly for community meetings" (R5, M, 34, see Table A6–1), whereas a Musikiosk user (IM) emphasized that "it's a good place to socialize and meet up with friends, maybe stop for lunch, smoke" (U7, F, 18). Another user argued: "it just seems like a neighborhood park. People just come here, I don't know, maybe in-between places, but I don't feel like they come here just […] for the park itself" (U10, F, 27). This neighborhood-like quality, reinforced by the aforementioned presence of regular users, has been evaluated as unwelcoming for new users: "the fact that [the park is] very territorial and people seem to have their little clique and their eyes on the entrance, does make it feel less welcoming" (U2, F, 20s).

Some Musikiosk users debated the friendliness of the park, with one interviewee arguing that it was "a cold park […] It's a bit like a closed park, it's not super inviting" (U9, M, 26), while two others focused on its appeal or its potential for activities: "I never thought it was a friendly park because it doesn't have that much […] entertaining activities to do, I guess. It just it doesn't look very appealing." (U1, F, 27); "I just pass it on my way to some other places […] I don't have any particular reason to just stop here" (U8, M, 21).

Observations also determined that specifically the gazebo of the park was, previous to the installation of Musikiosk, used for very little (BMT). The findings set the stage for a soundscape intervention that, rather than disturbing the quiet, appears to take place in a space of negotiation.

4.2. Effects of Musikiosk on QUPE

The following sections step through the effects that Musikiosk had on each of the three QUPE dimensions and present emergent themes as they are supported from findings in various methods.

4.2.1. Sound-Related Evaluation

The first of these effects on QUPE pertains to evaluations the soundscape as well as individual sound sources.

Soundscape Evaluation

The section on soundscape evaluation has been divided into traditional soundscape descriptors and soundscape appropriateness for activity.

"Traditional" Descriptors

The first theme is centered specifically on evaluations of the soundscape using semantic scales. These essentially include 7 of the 8 SSQP descriptors (not including uneventful): pleasant, unpleasant, eventful, calm, monotonous, vibrant, and chaotic, evaluated using scales. Two additional descriptors, friendly and convivial, are also included.

In Phase B (including Q2 and Q3, users and non-users post intervention), compared to Phase A (Q1 pre-intervention), ratings of the soundscape as *pleasant*, *eventful*, and *vibrant* increased significantly, while *unpleasant* decreased significantly. Looking at Q3 alone, only *pleasantness* increased significantly compared to Q1; all other scales remained unchanged. Users of Musikiosk (Q2) found the park more *pleasant* (M = 6.20 vs. 5.72, $p < 0.01$) and *vibrant* (M = 5.29 vs. 4.48, $p < 0.01$) than non-users (Q3). These findings and associated statistical tests are detailed in [109].

To better evaluate the effect of Musikiosk on the evaluations, we divided non-users (Q3) into two categories, based on the self-reported characteristic of Musikiosk being in-use (ON) and not in-use (OFF). For, Musikiosk ON, the soundscape was evaluated significantly more *vibrant* and less *unpleasant*, than for Musikiosk OFF (vibrant: M(MSKon) = 4.92, M(MSKoff) 3.86, F = 6.46, $p = 0.014$) (unpleasant: M(MSKon) = 1.64, M(MSKoff) = 2.41, F = 4.85, $p = 0.032$). There was no significant difference between Musikiosk OFF and the pre-installation condition (Q1). Overall, the system had no significant effect on ratings of the soundscape as *monotonous*, *calm*, and *chaotic*.

Corroborating the scale ratings, in free-response sections of the questionnaires (Q2 and Q3), users claimed to like the *friendliness* and *conviviality* of the system in addition to its *pleasantness*. Five separate users (Q2) spontaneously described the park as being more eventful with the addition of Musikiosk, corroborating the scale ratings from the SSQP questions. In interviews, Musikiosk users (IM) describe a park baseline as either *pleasant*, *convivial*, or *nice* (e.g., "it's a really convivial park and it's really nice" (U3, M, 30)), as well as the experience of using Musikiosk: "having the music and the sounds of the city at the same time is really nice" (P3, M 30). This theme of "city sound as background" will be explored later in Section 4.2.1.

In summary, the effects of the Musikiosk on soundscape descriptors was very localized to the times when it was on; when it was not in use, the park returned to "normal".

Soundscape Appropriateness for Activity

Ratings of soundscape appropriateness for participants' activities did not change significantly as a result of Musikiosk (Q1, Q2, Q3). In other words, overall, the presence of Musikiosk likely did not change the perceived soundscape appropriateness (as directly rated) for activity across all park users. Appropriateness was consistently rated high (Mean = 5.71 of 7, across all conditions), and was the highest rated of all tested descriptors, including pleasantness. With Musikiosk in the park, the high appropriateness rating remained high.

Non-users (Q3) were asked if and why Musikiosk was appropriate for the park (also covered in Section 4.3). Out of 67 total non-users, the majority (55) found Musikiosk appropriate. Of the 12 non-users who did not find it appropriate for the park, only one had actually heard Musikiosk in use: an older man who indicated on his questionnaire that he was trying to read alone in the evening and found the music "a little too party" for his tastes. Interestingly, a resident (IR) who had used Musikiosk stated in their interview that:

> "If I was reading, music could indeed bother me at times. Although I didn't note that people who were reading around us were bothered. I don't know if it's loud enough to be disturbing". (R3, F, 49, see Table A6–2)

This suggests that users may not be good at judging whether people engaged in other activities find a soundscape appropriate. The same resident said, "it's a very diverse, lively neighborhood. I think it's placed so as not to disturb, it's not too close to the houses, so I think it's very well integrated"

(R3, F, 49, see Table A6–3). These findings suggest that Musikiosk was an appropriate installation for a park that was largely appropriate for its activities in terms of soundscape.

Musikiosk was also capable of enabling activity. One user (IM) described that "it's nice to have something conducive to conversation" (U11, M, 24).

One other facet of appropriateness what that of the sound level. Users almost uniformly rated the park's sound level as moderate (3 of 5) but considered that level appropriate (3 of 5), rather than too loud or too quiet (Q1, Q3). However, in both of the interview corpuses (IM, IR), participants spontaneously described the park as noisy, especially in relation to the commercial artery, but also from specific types of users (e.g., "it might be a bit noisy from St. Laurent but over here in general it's a nice place" [U1, F, 27]). This finding paints a picture of the park where people describe it as noisy, but not in a pejorative sense. Musikiosk thus was welcome in this context because it did not violate expectations, for example, of calm that may permeate in other park spaces. A dichotomy of *noisy* but *quiet* and *appropriate* is described by a Musikiosk user (IM):

> "I did not use [Musikiosk] the first time because, as I've mentioned, people come here together and enjoy the quiet—it seems like they were enjoying the silence and the quietness. Still, even if it's noisy all around, it's still an oasis of quietness in the big city". (U2, F, 20s)

Specific Sounds

The presence of Musikiosk had a two-part effect by (1) reducing the prominence of negative sound sources, and (2) being a positive sound source resulting in a soundscape made up of sources that promoted fascination, attention, and memories of the space.

Results from multiple methods show a positive effect of Musikiosk on reducing the identification and prominence of traffic sounds as negative sound sources. Non-users listed fewer negative mechanical sound sources (73 vs. 50) as well as fewer prominent unpleasant sounds (19 vs. 11) than did pre-installation participants (Q1, Q3), indicating a likely mix of energetic and informational sound masking. This evidence is corroborated in interviews (IR, IM):

> "Yes, in any case, the Saint Laurent [boulevard] is so noisy that music will certainly be more pleasant than the traffic noise"; (R5, M, 34, see Table A6–4)

> "You can definitely hear the cars, the street is there [...] you can hear bits of conversations here and there of people. What else do I hear? Birds, the wind a little bit, squirrels. Yeah, but mostly, what I hear the most are the cars if the music is not playing". (U10, F, 27)

Musikiosk not only reduced the impact of a negative sound source, namely traffic, but also improved the soundscape and the attention paid to it. Five separate users (Q2) described how the system engaged them to listen in the park when they otherwise may have not. Interviewees (IM) elaborated on their new perspective with Musikiosk as a sound source:

> "It's just really nice having the option to play music [...] It just adds a nice dimension to the sound environment". (U5, M, 28)

> "For me, it does really enhance the enjoyment of the park, because anywhere I go, I'm like "oh I should listen to music" and if it's on headphones, then I don't really mind but now I get cut off of the sounds around me so having the music and the sounds of the city at the same time is really nice." (U3, M, 30)

> "It really feels like—I kind of feel it's not a—it is a public place, but at the same time, it's intimate. It feels like an apartment or something, it feels like a party at someone's place" (U10, F, 27)

> "I feel like it turns your situation almost like a movie so whenever you hear music that's like not in a room but outside, it adds magic to the place I'd say, it feels really good". (U7, F, 18)

4.2.2. Public Space Engagement

The second QUPE dimension affected by the installation of Musikiosk was in terms of how users behaved in and engaged with the public space.

Behavior

Observed Public Space Use—Lingering Behavior

Multiple methods showed that the presence of Musikiosk increased lingering behavior in the park. In the free response portion of the questionnaire, 12 users spontaneously reported wanting to stay longer in the park because of the presence of the system (Q2). This was also confirmed by follow-up interviews (IM), where there was a direct relationship between lingering and whether Musikiosk was in use either by themselves or by others. All interviewees (IM) confirmed that Musikiosk and the opportunity to engage with the space sonically, encouraged them to linger in the park, irrespective of who was playing the music.

The lingering effect was robust across personality types, though the details of engagement were different. A self-defined introvert stated that: "I might find myself a little quiet spot nearby and enjoy […] in the periphery […] I'm allergic to interaction" (U2, F, 20s). In contrast, "[If people played something I liked] I'd probably just be inclined to dance or, [at least,] I would be inclined to certainly stay" (U5, M, 28). Looking back at the questionnaire participants, the average self-reported extraversion was no higher for users than for non-users or pre-installation participants, thus Musikiosk didn't attract extraversion, but extraversion did affect the details of the engagement.

Lingering behaviors are also directly related with the idea of sharing (discussed below), as Musikiosk is repeatedly evaluated as being best enjoyed with company: "it would definitely be a place to hang out with your friends […] I know some of the students who were there, who decided to leave the bar and come back here and hang out and just listen to some music until it closed" (U6, F, 36).

Observations also demonstrated that Musikiosk led to more dynamic and prolonged uses of the gazebo area of Parc du Portugal (EO), particularly during the evenings and when special events had been organized as part of the community outreach strategy.

Most surprisingly, one of the residents (IR) had used Musikiosk and hoped to have it back again the following year because: "It would be nice for it to come back. I think that, in the summer, it's all right, because we linger more during the summer, especially in this street. Yes, it can be fun to stop, take a break while shopping or between errands" (R3, F, 49, see Table A6–5).

Observed Public Space Use—Diversification

While lingering behaviors increased, changing the park demographic, it was necessary to observe whether existing park users were displaced by this new activity. This analysis begins with questionnaire data. To categorize self-reported activity data, a bottom-up approach elaborated six categories of activities: consuming, relaxing, interacting, moving, observing, and music (See Table 2). Prior to the installation of Musikiosk, there were no reported activities related to music. Once Musikiosk was installed, this number jumped to 14 (not including Musikiosk users). Among only the first five of these activities (without music), a chi-squared test revealed no significant difference, X^2 (4, $N = 251$) = 2.0014, $p = 0.736$, between the types of activities conducted before and after the installation of Musikiosk. This finding suggests that the installation of Musikiosk had little effect on the ongoing activities of the park, only superimposing musical activities on top of the existing uses.

Table 2. Activity categorization before and after Musikiosk installation. Note: if people reported multiple activities, it was coded more than once.

Activity	N (Q1)	N (Q3)
Consuming (eating, drinking, smoking)	42	43
Relaxing (resting, waiting, sitting, sunbathing)	39	28
Interacting (date, meeting friends)	31	35
Moving (walking around, biking)	12	13
Observing (people-watching)	4	4
Music (Musikiosk, dancing, listening)	0	14

These findings were corroborated and explained in more detail through other methods. For Musikiosk users (IM), diversification referred to two distinct aspects: diversification in terms of users as well as (potential) diversification in terms of activities to be performed in the park.

The diversification of users is related to the novel aspect of the system and the new opportunities it affords for park use: "it would attract more people […] if the project is there for long enough and the people know what's it about, cause surely you know, it takes time for people to learn about it, to know how to use it, to develop patterns" (U10, F, 27). Another added: "it brought people in, definitely […] When there's people in a park, people tend to want to be in that park too, which is nicer. And people stop by more, show more interest in it." (U9, M, 26). One other interviewee (IM) observed just this change in park users that Musikiosk brought about:

"normally, it's an ambiance of older people who are just kind of hanging out, and then there was a lot of 90s pop being played, which definitely changed it from an 'old-people-sitting-around' park to a 'youngish-but-not-too-young-people-dancing-around-to-cheesy-music-from-their-past' park". (U4, M, 25)

The diversification can also be understood in terms of how activities performed in the park could change, especially in the context of planned events:

"I see a lot of people that [go to organized events in parks in the city], and especially if all these young mothers are here all the time with their kids, I'm sure it would work really well amongst that group. It'd be nice for like a mix I guess, it's like a free-for-all and then sometimes organized". (U6, F, 36)

One interviewee combined these two ideas, saying, "I liked that there were events planned, so then I would know when to show up while other people would be there. I guessed it's not really something I would use on my own" (U4, M, 25).

While these insights collected from users (IM) may have suggest a shift in the park demographic, the questionnaire results presented above (Q1, Q3) corroborate observations (EO), showing that previously existing, frequent users were not displaced by Musikiosk; instead, Musikiosk added an extra layer of novel activities to the park. As observed, the regular users did not change their patterns of use of the park, performing the same activities during the same time frames and with more or less the same frequency. Furthermore, no one was observed to spontaneously approach Musikiosk, despite attempts to introduce and demonstrate the system during Community Outreach. When it was in use; there was no visible reaction either to the music played nor to the Musikiosk users, except for 'people-watching', which had already been observed as a key activity of these park users before the installation (EO).

These regular users' people-watching proved intimidating for some Musikiosk users (IM), one of which stated that:

"population-wise, you have regulars here who eye you every time you come in and you do feel like there's regular people who are sitting here and they like their park the way it is, as in you coming in out of curiosity, wanting to try out this toy […] it does feel intimidating to come into this park". (U2, F, 20s)

This sentiment was not shared by all Musikiosk users (IM): "I never noticed anyone giving me judge-y looks or any neighbors coming out with like dough-rolling pins being like "get out of here! You don't belong here!" (U6, F, 36).

However, for the elderly Portuguese users, who usually sat talking amongst each other, this lack of reaction could be related to the position of the Musikiosk system in relation to their "usual spot" (EO): while the system was installed in the gazebo on the quiet, residential side of the park, their usual spot was on the commercial, active side of the park, where the music played through the system was frequently not audible, allowing for the creation of separate soundscapes dominated by different sounds. This was confirmed by Musikiosk users (IM), who stated that: "the sound doesn't propagate to the surroundings, cause it's not a very loud sound, but it's just such an enjoyable part of being in a park" (U6, F, 36).

There were no measurable changes in the patterns of use of the park throughout Phase B (BMT), indicating that presence of Musikiosk did not lead to an observable transformation in the behavioural profile of the park (see [107] for a detailed analysis). However, observations (EO) did show that Musikiosk did increase the spontaneous use only of the gazebo on a daily basis, mostly by younger users, in small groups, engaging in lingering behaviours and using the system for hours at a time, sitting either in the gazebo or on its steps to maximize their listening experience (confirmed by IM). Also, the outreach events organized by the project team introduced new users to Musikiosk and increased the number of users performing socially interactive activities in the early and late evening in the park. Among the local users of Musikiosk, some of the participants who had come in the evenings returned, either as users of Musikiosk (alone or with a small or large group of people) or of the park itself (observed on different occasions e.g., reading on a bench or having lunch; EO).

One interviewee (IM) highlighted this dynamic between regular and new users, the way in which Musikiosk brings new people in without displacing the current users, while allowing for potential, but not mandatory interactions:

"I think they really didn't mind [us listening to music through Musikiosk]. Because they were just continuing to do what they were doing, sitting down, playing with kids, talking. It didn't really bother them. And I think that at the same time some of them were curious, like of what's happening inside, because of some nice people having fun". (U1, F, 27)

This diversification was largely perceived as a positive change, even by local community members, with one resident (IR) describing the process of how important it was to have new users for the viability of their community:

"and it also creates roots, the people who come, they know the neighborhood, maybe they'll shop, eat closer [...] It probably gathered more young people, who were pleasant, who were happy, and so people came to see what it was". (R1, F, 79, see Table A6–6)

Another resident explained that they didn't think this mix of people would have happened otherwise: "it's an opportunity to sit and take a break outside, to meet people that we wouldn't have met otherwise, indeed. No, it's nice and it adds to the neighborhood life" (R3, F, 49, see Table A6–7).

In summary, Musikiosk was observed to add a new layer of activity and users into the existing park without displacing existing users. An explanation, in part, is in the way Musikiosk gave existing users something to people-watch. Musikiosk also occupied, sonically and physically, a small, but unused section of the park.

Interaction with Others

Increased Interaction and Sharing

In addition to lingering and the diversification of users and activities, the presence of Musikiosk encouraged interaction between people and sharing of information, music, and space.

Nine Musikiosk users, when reporting something they liked about the system mentioned how they liked the improved interactions with others, while nine others reported enjoying the feeling of sharing a space and/or music (Q2). Even among non-users describing the system, 3 spontaneously mentioned how it was good for bringing people together, and 3 others mentioned how it was good for sharing (Q3), e.g., "when someone came, they could share what they were listening to" (R1, F, 79, see Table A6–8).

One of the residents had used the system and talked about dancing with her children (IR): "it was merry, we were dancing [...] And, the weather was nice, it was the end of summer, so it was festive" \ The same resident later explained, "I think it facilitated communication between us and the young people who were there before we arrived" (R3, F, 49, see Table A6–9 and 10).

A different resident (IR) explained in more detail:

"It's great to have interactive devices in the city like that that can create community spaces that are a bit broader compared to simply meeting up. I imagine we can carry a wider ambiance with such a system [...] It's more participatory obviously, because the majority of activities on the Saint Laurent [boulevard] are very passive". (R5, M, 34, see Table A6–11)

The aspects of increased interaction were visible when interviewees were asked about their Musikiosk experience or when they were asked about hypothetical situations in which others played music that they liked or not. They were generally open to actual or potential socialization with strangers brought upon by the sharing of music (IM): "If I play music out loud and someone else comes to me and talks to me, I guess I would talk to the person, that would be part of the whole experience, to meet people" (U3, M, 30). Two users described their encounters with other park users, curious about the system:

"A few people that were walking by came up and asked what the track was. One person wrote it down, and then two people that were sitting on a nearby bench, came up and were like 'what is this? How do we make it work?', and it was like 'you just plug it in and play your music and that's it apparently', and they were like 'cool, sweet.' And then that was—we were probably here for fifteen minutes maybe, so there wasn't tons of attraction but interactions with three–four people [...] and they were enthusiastic about it"; (U5, M, 28)

"I just ended up getting involved in a conversation with two people I'd met before at Musikiosk, and then one or two people I hadn't met and hung out for a while and then left". (U4, M, 25)

One interviewee, acknowledging their reticence of usually interacting with others in public settings, welcomed the possibility of using music as a topic of conversation to interact with strangers:

"(if people came in the gazebo) I would probably ask them what they thought of the music, or maybe not say that right away but, you know, I'm not really one to start talking to people in public, but I'm thinking if I were the one playing music in here, I would feel more open talking to people who came by and sat down, you know. It's obvious that they're interested in the same things as me [...] It changes the dynamic of approaching people in public a little bit in that case [...] hopefully, that would generate some kind of conversation". (U11, M, 24)

Interacting with others is described as an essential part of the music-listening process; as music is brought into the public sphere, the aspect of *sharing* the listening experience with others takes center stage:

"it's more the fact that it's a social experience of sharing the music that actually makes me enjoy being at the park. I'm not sure that if I just came here to read my book and I turn on the music, that I will actually enjoy the experience more. It's really a matter of this being a social experience of sharing music". (U2, F, 20s)

One interviewee explains this point in relation to her Musikiosk experience as shared with her coworkers:

> "It was a really fun moment between coworkers, because everyone just kinda came out with a song on an mp3 player, we'd just listen to it, and we'd kind of see the person who'd played it and they'd get a little embarrassed, and then everyone's laughing and listening to the song and discovering new music, which is super cool". (U6, F, 36)

The nature of the Musikiosk system was evaluated by park users and residents alike as intrinsically encouraging social interaction and sharing, both of the space itself and of music. Actual or potential interactions, mediated my music and listening in a social, public context, were appreciated or welcome across the board. Two particular points were emphasized: self-policing—of music played (in relation to the sharing aspect) and the idea of "passing the baton" and sharing the actual use of the system.

Increased Interaction and Sharing—Self-Policing

As part of the interaction and sharing theme, the idea of Musikiosk users' self-regulation of their musical behavior and choices emerged as a key finding. This was related to topics of "responsible listening" that have been addressed extensively elsewhere [113]. Musikiosk users (IM) intuited or "enforced" these rules on their own, relating them to being mindful of other park users and adjusting their content to an imagined "average other", as a member of a musical community that shares the same ideas on what music would be "universally appreciated" (U2, F, 20s) or "nice for people to hear" (U7, F, 18):

> "It turns off on its own so between those times, go for it, have fun, do whatever, as long as they understand there's rules there, don't be mean and loud and obnoxious cause there are people who live around it, but generally, live and let live, right?"; (U9, M, 26)

> "Well I wanted to play something that would show how awesome my music tastes were, but also be something that a lot of people would enjoy and dance to". (U4, M, 25)

Further demonstrating this idea of responsibility as part of sharing music and listening in public, interviewees were very sensitive to the possibility of someone *disliking* their music and quick in adjusting their content to the (perceived) preferences of the other listeners in the park, as well as to offer other the possibility to play their own music (IM):

> "(if they didn't like my music) I would ask if they have something else to play and they could play it after I'm playing my song or something"; (U3, M, 30)

> "I mean, if it's a music that is likely controversial, I would understand and I would turn it down. But if it's just regular classical music, that 90% of the population seems to like Bach, Beethoven, Brahms, this type of—stuff like that. I won't go with the hits because it really depends on the generation and I, myself, do not always agree with the charts but let's say something very soft, non-aggressive classical music". (U2, F, 20s)

Despite the open and democratic nature of the system that allowed its users to be free in their consumption of (musical) content, Musikiosk users self-policed and engaged in responsible listening practices as they emphasized the need to be mindful of other park users, their needs and tastes.

Increased Interaction and Sharing—Passing the Baton

In addition to self-policing, a sub-theme of interaction and sharing was the idea that Musikiosk users took on the responsibility of showing others how to use it. One of the residents (IR) who had used the system explained an interaction with a group that she was familiar with, but would have never interacted with:

"It had the potential of creating a nice ambiance, that could possibly gather the people who were a little in their individual world, it could unite maybe, because we started talking, actually with the young people who were drinking in their own corner, at any rate, it's not people we would have initially approached, but then we explained to them what to do because they were listening to their own music but didn't realize they could use [Musikiosk]". (R3, F, 49, see Table A6–12)

Passing the baton was emphasized by an interviewee (IM), who acknowledged that for some park users the idea of engaging with the system spontaneously would be unlikely without having someone introducing them to the experience:

"It's always fun to introduce people and it's an easier way to get people to come and actually experience it, if they can latch on to something that they're like 'okay, I can invite people, and there's gonna be a certain time, and there's gonna be people and we can chill and hang out and understand what's going on', because if it's just a thing, people might not touch it as much, if they don't understand there's something going on". (U9, M, 26)

However, as mentioned above in the theme on interaction, interaction with others and invitations to system use were welcomed by most users as being a natural consequence of the system: "generally people would talk to you (when you are using Musikiosk) and then after a little bit, they'd ask to put something on." (U9, M, 26). One interviewee described her experience:

"It wasn't just me and my friends. It was actually also some strangers, who I didn't know before and, not that I was planning to meet them, it's just that they were there too and you can share, it's not like it's someone's gazebo! Everybody can use it, so. I think one of the girls she played some Latin music so everybody just, all of a sudden, the mood just switched completely". (U1, F, 27)

The fact that anyone could use Musikiosk to play their preferred content made its users conscientious about ideas of sharing and "passing the baton"; they both reported and were observed to encourage and show others how to engage with the system in order to allow everyone to appropriate the park sonically with their own content.

4.2.3. Psychological Outcomes

The third and final dimension of QUPE on which Musikiosk had an effect was the category of psychological outcomes. The themes in this dimension pertained to individual effects on space users, which includes mood and restorativeness.

Mood

As was hinted in the previous section on passing the baton by a Musikiosk user, Musikiosk had a strong impact on moods. According to the questionnaires (Q1, Q2, Q3), users entering the park arrived with approximately the same mood across all contextual details (alone vs. others, age, etc.) and conditions (i.e., no significant effect was found on mood (before) for any variable.) Park visits increased reported moods significantly for all users (mood (after); see Steele et al. [109]), but the presence of Musikiosk boosted these moods even higher for both Musikiosk users and non-users (Q2, Q3). This effect was exaggerated for Musikiosk users (Q2), who saw yet significantly higher mood improvements.

Descriptions in the changes in mood from users (IM) varied from generic, "it put people in a good mood" (U8, M, 21), to the specific example above with the example of Latin music "switching the "mood". The mood improvement was noticed even by a resident (IR), who said "It increased the turnout of people who were happy, but I can't tell you the difference. People kept going there, families, children and all that" (R1, F, 79, see Table A6–13).

Public Space Evaluation—Post Musikiosk Lasting Effects

This part of the results section details findings from Phase C, when Musikiosk had been removed from the park. Memories and experience with the system and the park, as well as reflection on the engagement process lead us to some findings we term "lasting effects" of Musikiosk.

Interviewees (IM) cite their engagement with Musikiosk (both as system users and non-users) as a reason for a shift in their perception of Parc du Portugal:

> "now I know this is a place that is friendly to me at least and I know, I've been here, I've used it, I know how to behave here so now for me. It's a place where I can totally feel safe, I can come whenever I want, just sit down"; (U1, F, 27)

> "now [...] I have associations [...] that my friends would occasionally be (here), as opposed to, usually, when I would use this park before, I'd be by myself and I wouldn't really be talking to anybody". (U4, M, 25)

Thus, not only did Musikiosk increase the aforementioned lingering, but it also brought people to the park for the first time and created a lasting sense of belonging and safety.

Residents also described a positive change in their quality of life (IR):

> "The more we inhabit public spaces, the more the quality of life improves. I think neighborhoods need to be animated, otherwise it creates dead zones [...] It seems to me more pleasant to pass through a park with a few people playing music than nothing at all [...] I think that yes, it broadened the hours of park use, so in that way, yes. It's more pleasant and more convivial, a park with people compared to a dead park". (R5, M, 34, see Table A6–23)

Conversations that took place with researchers (EO) confirmed that the space served well as a unique and lasting memory of tourists' trips to Montreal, shaping their holistic impressions of the city.

Residents (IR) explained that Musikiosk brought a sense of safety:

> "It's a good use because it prevents other activities more [...] I would even say criminal, from happening"; (R1, F, 79, see Table A6–24)

> "There are a lot of areas like that, where it's a little scary to pass through at night. If there was a community playing music regularly, at any time of the day, it makes it more pleasant and safer for everyone". (R5, M, 34, see Table A6–25)

Resonating with the idea of safety, appropriateness for children came up often: "It's a place for children, it's safe" (R1, F, 79, see Table A6–26).

The lasting effects of Musikiosk thus revolved around a place and opportunity for making memories, and long-term impacts on feelings of belonging and safety.

Restorativeness

The final theme in the psychological outcomes dimension is soundscape restorativeness, described in the Review. Restoration contains five main elements, three of which applied to the study at-hand: fascination from sound sources, the soundscape offering a break from users' routines, and the perception that "it's easy to do what I want" in this soundscape. Note that Musikiosk questionnaire participants (Q2) were not directly asked to rate restorativeness.

Linked to the appropriateness of the soundscape for activity, Musikiosk had no effect on the perception of the park soundscape as being *easy to do what I want* (Q1, Q3), nor did Musikiosk have a significant effect across any other restorativeness scale; however, park restorativeness was already rated fairly highly, and it remained high with Musikiosk in place, demonstrating that the added sound sources did not compromise this aspect of the park's character.

Free response and verbal data tell a more detailed story. Musikiosk users (Q2) reported appreciating something new (5), dancing (4), improved relaxation (3), and being invited to think (2). In a separate section, 4 users remarked on the system's originality. Interviews (IM) elaborated many deeper, spontaneous mentions linking the system to increased restorativeness, particularly through a soundscape that makes it easy to do desired activities: "I can totally feel safe, I can come whenever I want, just sit down [...], have a coffee with a friend, chill, maybe read a book" (U1, F, 27). A resident commented, "It's out of the ordinary, it gives us an occasion to sit down and take a break outside, meet some people, some people we might not necessarily have met otherwise. No, it's nice and it adds to the life of the neighborhood" (R3, F, 49, see Table A6–14).

4.3. Evaluation of Musikiosk

We turn now from examining QUPE as affected by Musikiosk, and instead focus on the interactions and experiences with Musikiosk itself.

4.3.1. Engagement with Musikiosk

Musikiosk users (Q2) generally found Musikiosk easy to use and access, original, and found that it promoted activity. The simplicity and accessibility of the technology itself was appreciated by users:

"It's nice when you don't depend on anybody and you can just go there and enjoy it"; (U1, F, 27)

"So it's a little music system, a very, very humble music system, basically five zero, plugged on the roof of a gazebo in a little park somewhere in Montreal, where you can play your own music and enjoy your own music, in an amplifier". (U2, F, 20s)

User engagement has been discussed previously [113], employing O'Brien and Toms' [115] process model of engagement to understand users' approaches to music consumption through their engagement with Musikiosk as a free, democratic soundscape system. We showed how Musikiosk ultimately encouraged a feeling of temporary ownership of the space as well as a certain degree of complicity with the other users of the space, through the sharing of music as a social experience. Even outside of user engagement, one of the older residents (IR) described how the system made her want to engage more with technology:

"I want to come but I have a cellphone for emergencies [...] I don't know how, I'm not really equipped, I want to equip myself better, I would like to download all the music I like, and to be able to listen to it instead of on my little device, which is still cumbersome". (R1, F, 79, see Table A6–15)

4.3.2. Unrealized Fear of a Democratic Soundscape Intervention

One of the key challenges of Musikiosk was negotiating fears of the risks that residents, city authorities, and park users imagined would materialize as a result of the system. These fears were prominent particularly in the pre-project planning phase, as people imagined uses of Musikiosk that were contrary to their needs of the park. The borough authority was initially apprehensive of awarding the permit to install Musikiosk and required many rounds of negotiation and rule-setting, taking months (Municipal support and approvals). However, this process established a relationship of trust that was further solidified by the positive results of the system.

Elaborating on this unrealized fear from imagined system uses was a media outlet who had an interesting interpretation of what they believed the device would entail (Media Outreach): they photoshopped very large speakers facing outwards in every corner of the gazebo and claimed that "Montreal is getting a (massive sound system you can control with your phone" (https://www.mtlblog.com/news/montreal-park-is-getting-a-massive-sound-system-you-can-control-with-your-phone). After an exchange with the Musikiosk team, the news outlet removed the word "massive".

Despite and perhaps thanks to the planning and coordination between the municipality and other stakeholders, in addition to the community outreach, very few problems came to pass. No formal complaints were lodged with the municipal complaint hotline (311). Residents (IR) spoke of this unrealized fear:

> "It's a concern, that once people are done listening to music, they will settle in the gazebo together to talk, some might bring beers, and it can maybe end later. Which can be invasive, but also very welcoming. That's what we don't know. Our experience at this time is that we didn't have that, let's be honest, it didn't happen". (R1, F, 79, see Table A6–16)

Unrealized fears were also seen from non-users (Q3), but attitudes toward Musikiosk varied greatly with degree of exposure to the system. When Musikiosk was not in use, the idea of the system gave park users pause; of 67 non-users, there were 9 negative judgments and all of them came at a time when Musikiosk was not in-use (condition: Musikiosk OFF). One fear was "I'm afraid that there might be too many types of music at the same time" (see Table A6–17). Non-users who were exposed to the system (Musikiosk ON), however, reported satisfaction, generally found the system appropriate for the park, and appreciated the unique offering of music in the public space; for example, the mood benefits of the Musikiosk ON subgroup were almost as high as they were for users (Q2), and were higher than the control condition (Q1). Non-users (Q3) who responded during Musikiosk OFF showed mood benefits that were not significantly different from the pre-installation condition (Q1).

If Musikiosk was in use, non-users (Q3) had less abstract concerns, e.g., "great idea, but I think the use of 'public space' for my personal enjoyment gives me second thoughts about using it"; "I don't know if it's necessary" (see Table A6–18); "It's tricky because not everyone has the same musical taste"; and "good—as long as people are mindful of those nearby." The concerns tie in with ideas of self-policing and responsible listening referred to above:

> "If I was using the Musikiosk, it would be sort of with the understanding that it is a public place, and it's sort of like a public place that I'm using, so it sort of feel like I should include people who wanted to come hang out. As opposed to sort of privately appropriate it for my own ends.". (U4, M, 25)

In summary, we believe the "intuited" rules of Musikiosk involved the necessary negotiation of public space use such as to minimize the behaviors that were most feared.

4.3.3. Appropriateness of the System for the Park

In addition to the Musikiosk creating a soundscape that made new activities possible, there was also a research question on whether Musikiosk was appropriate for Parc du Portugal.

40 of 41 Musikiosk users (Q2) found it appropriate for the park. Reasons for its perceived appropriateness were that it is well located, not too loud or disturbing, that it was friendly, and most interestingly, that it added something to the park that was missing. The one user who did not say yes said "yes and no", and suggested that while it "bridges people together, some people like to meditate"—this reasoning did not appear to be associated with the park in question. One of the users who found it appropriate added that it was appropriate in the Parc du Portugal, but "not in my park".

Users also weighed in on appropriateness during their interviews (IM):

> "I guess that before it's a really convivial park and it's really nice, so I guess music is just a natural extension of the enjoyability of the park"; (U3, M, 30)

> "I think the area is very dynamic, you have a very wide range of people that come by and also there's a lot of noise coming from the city, you're on a commercial street, there's traffic, so it kind of gives a little serenity and it gives a little—it attributes almost like a, how would I say it, like to own part of the park or to feel part of it almost". (U6, F, 36)

There were two interviewees uncertain of the appropriateness of Musikiosk for the park precisely because of the risk of displacing or disrupting "regular users" referred to above:

> "[...] it's sort of an older neighborhood that I don't know if it's really the sort of thing that a lot of the people who regularly use the park would do. I feel like there are other small parks where there are fewer old Portuguese people talking to each other in Portuguese on benches"; (U4, M, 25)

One resident (IR) was not pleased with the presence of the Musikiosk, principally because the park had been the host of a number of other festivals in the preceding months: "I was annoyed because there wasn't only Musikiosk. All throughout the summer, we were bothered by the noise." (R4, F, 33, see Table A6–19). Yet, to contrast this, a different resident explained his reason for liking Musikiosk was actually that having it there protected them from these more disturbing events, alluded to by R4, that happened at other times during the season: "It would seem reasonable, this thing that the city did a few times, [...] to pretend to sing (The municipality had previously hosted a public karaoke event with a large speaker system.) ... Yes, well that was noisy." (R2, M, 95, see Table A6–20).

In line with the fair amount of agreement of the appropriateness of Musikiosk for this park, the above section on unrealized fears is also better contextualized. We again saw that those who had not interacted with Musikiosk were more likely to not find it appropriate. Also, the characterization of the park as previously "noisy" (as described in Section Soundscape Appropriateness for Activity) before the installation likely helped to prevent Musikiosk from disturbing a quiet environment.

4.3.4. Uniqueness of the System

The uniqueness of the system was a recurrent topic in interviewee's evaluation of Musikiosk, particularly in the context of its open, democratic, and political nature. "I think it's a great idea, it's the first time I've ever seen or heard of something like this, so I think it should become a permanent thing, for sure" (U7, F, 18); one resident summarized it: "It's something out of the ordinary" (R3, F, 49, see Table A6–21).

The open, egalitarian and participatory nature of the system was emphasized by a number of interviewees. A resident remarked on what aspect was so different: "It's the participatory aspect that's different" (R5, M, 34, see Table A6–22). A Musikiosk user argued that:

> "It's free, it's democratic, it's 'do whatever you want with that music.' You do have a time limit, 30 minutes, just so that everybody has equal access to the music. It seems like a lot of fun and the people that thought of it are geniuses". (U2, F, 20s)

A second Musikiosk user further focused on the political nature of the system in an urban context i.e., its democratic nature: "I feel like the whole nature, the whole point of Musikiosk is that it should be thought of as a public good [...] it's sort of a volunteering kind of public—everybody comes together to hang out. I feel that's part of civic-mindedness" (U4, M, 25).

A third user highlighted the aforementioned idea of responsible listening, but showing how the system flips the script and offers park users control and trust to appropriate their space acoustically:

> "I feel like it's such a strong message, giving power to those who use this park, because in a sense, you give a tool—there are limitations to that tool, but you tell people 'use it' and 'enjoy it' [...]—I think it makes it much more dynamic between the different types of people that use it. I'm really for that idea of good incentives, like being positive instead of negative and saying, 'you can't do this, you can't do that', just giving a tool to someone and being like 'do what you want with it, we trust you', it's nice". (U6, F, 36)

Musikiosk was also perceived as offering park users a unique way of interacting with the park, to do something that's normally not permitted, namely, play music out loud in a public space: "there are speakers available to anyone and a really nice park, and anyone can join and put their music on if they like and enjoy the park as they please, but with [...] added music of their liking. It's not like a program ... , you go to listen to your music in a park, officially, sanctioned by the city" (U3, M, 30).

5. Discussion

The goal of this paper was to investigate the effects of a democratic soundscape installation on various aspects of public space use and appropriation in an urban pocket park, utilizing the proposed concept of QUPE and its three axes. Considering that the nature of Musikiosk directly affected users' soundscapes in their public space, we started by focusing on the sound-related aspects of evaluation of one's experience, but then demonstrated that the effects of Musikiosk were more far reaching, as we studied broader changes in users' engagement with the park as well as potential outcomes at a psychological level.

We first discuss the effects of Musikiosk on each of the three-subthemes of QUPE, then reflect on methodological and theoretical contributions that this paper (and Musikiosk) brings.

5.1. Soundscape Evaluation

The appropriateness of the soundscape for the reported activity of users was in any case rated as high across conditions and remained unchanged (high) by Musikiosk; in fact, appropriateness of the soundscape was the highest rated of all descriptors (including pleasantness), further demonstrating the added value of a pocket park, even if with one side on a comparatively loud, busy street, for the urban public experience. Extending research that shows that the level of social interaction of one's activities influences their evaluation of soundscape [31,40], Musikiosk users stated that Musikiosk was best used with others, encouraging social interaction. Furthermore, in line with the questionnaire findings, interviews showed that the system was perceived to encourage interaction with strangers, as well as solitary enjoyment of the park, maintaining high appropriateness of the park for a range of activities.

The present study extends findings from Steffens et al. [50], which showed benefits in pleasantness and eventfulness when people were modifying their own sound environments with their own music. The difference is that these participants were usually modifying home or office environments with music, but Musikiosk brought these benefits to a public park

In terms of the effects of specific sounds, Musikiosk encouraged soundscape benefits in terms of, for example, masking of traffic [25,41,116]. Unlike other soundscape installations that achieved that with purposeful acoustic design [25,37,41–44], Musikiosk did not have pre-programmed content. However, users displayed care in the content they chose to play (generally, music), engaging in self-policing behaviors [113] in relation to the genres of music they played and what was considered appropriate for the setting of Parc du Portugal and its users.

5.2. Engagement with the Park

Our mixed-methods study confirmed the well-documented aspect of the sociability of public spaces, acting as contexts for different forms of social interaction [54,58,75]. Interviews with local residents, park users in general and Musikiosk users in particular, as well as behavioral mapping and ethnographic observations showed that Parc du Portugal was used (and evaluated as suitable) for socially interactive activities, but also for restoration-related activities, in line with the findings of Peschardt and Stigsdotter [93] on urban pocket parks. There were clear temporal patterns in how the park was used, that influenced the profile of users; there were elderly regulars that had been identified in the preparation stages of this study and recurrent users of various ages observed during lunchtime (usually middle aged) or in the evenings (usually younger). Considering that the soundscape in the park was evaluated as appropriate across users' diverse activities for all time periods, we employ Peschardt's findings [93,94] on the provision of park amenities. We show how the provision of an amenity that allowed for public music playing that encouraged socializing benefited park users, ensuring that restoration was also possible [95].

Musikiosk resulted in increased and diversified social interactions in the park without disrupting ongoing activities. It also brought new users while not displacing the regular ones. Musikiosk offered users control over the content played, which led to the creation of temporary public auditory communities based on shared listening practices, along the lines of the work of O'Hara and Brown [117]. These temporary communities were described to function under self-imposed rules of responsible listening, as described by Haake [104], as well as the need to share the access to Musikiosk and teach others how to use it by "passing the baton".

The engagement with the Musikiosk system itself, as mediated by mobile music listening technologies like smartphones [65,118] further encouraged aspects of interaction by e.g., offering the opportunity to exchange and share music, discuss musical tastes and opinions as well as listening together. The democratic and free nature of the system allowed them to bring their private (musical) identity to the foreground and into the public realm, along the lines of Thompson's [69] suggestion on the role of mobile music technologies in blurring the line between the private and the public realm.

5.3. Psychological Outcomes

The benefits of a park visit on psychological outcomes have been demonstrated in the literature [57,75–79]; the sounds of parks have also demonstrated a restorative effect [82,83]. In addition, the aforementioned Steffens et al. [50] study showed positive benefits of the presence of music on mood. In the present study, we saw a positively interacting effect on mood and restorativeness of both the park visit and the presence of one's own music, which may not have been predicted using a sound level-based approach [71,72].

The engagement with Musikiosk was reported to have affected park users' emotional engagement with Parc du Portugal [74], triggering (positive) long-term effects on their evaluation of the park, particularly in terms of psychological comfort [57] and perceptions of safety and appropriate behaviors for the space, shifting previous negative evaluations of the park. Some Musikiosk users specifically addressed issues of control over their public space, in relation to more general ideas of access to and expected behavior in public spaces in general (along the lines of the work of Atkinson [79]). Also, in relation to the (unique) opportunity to play and the (unique) opportunity to have control over their auditory spaces [102], Musikiosk users managed their soundscapes by playing their own amplified content in a public space context.

5.4. Contributions

On methodological grounds, we employed a mixed-method approach to better capture and understand the impact of Musikiosk as well as to situate the results and implications of different methods. Further, we needed a mixed-method design to be able to properly capture the three axes of QUPE. These methods came from a number of disciplines, as was necessary to adequately capture aspects of e.g., soundscape evaluation as well as the social, behavioral and psychological outcomes resulting from park users' interaction with Musikiosk. For example, while behavioral mapping did not show a substantial change in the patterns of use of the park, ethnographic observations showed a subtle yet clear diversification in terms of users and an increase in lingering times, particularly in the area around Musikiosk, driven by the engagement with the system. Interviews allowed us to go in depth in some of the topics that were touched upon in the questionnaires, to further investigate aspects of engagement with the park or evaluation of the system that could not be captured using quantitative data collection methods.

On theoretical grounds, we created the QUPE model to integrate the auditory and non-auditory aspects of a soundscape intervention and to make a connection to urban public experience and public health. Our findings converge to show that a democratic soundscape installation affected not just the soundscape in the park but broader aspects of use and engagement with the park as well as outcomes at a psychological level, increasing the perceived pleasantness and restorativeness of the park and intensifying as well as diversifying interaction in the park without displacing or disrupting existing users or patterns of use. From another angle, we also contribute to a growing body of work on the restorative, social, and cultural functions of small urban spaces, i.e., pocket parks, as distinct from the more studied large, green parks.

On practical grounds, the benefits to QUPE were achieved through a relatively modest, low-cost intervention. For future urban planning and design efforts, such interventions could extend the range of solutions available to address tensions between commercial, residential, and leisure uses in dense urban areas.

6. Conclusions

Our study provides insights into understanding how a democratic soundscape installation can affect the quality of the urban public experience of space users, and how goals of e.g., restoration and increased social interaction can be attained and accommodated in the context of a small, urban pocket park. The findings presented here highlight the integration between multiple data collection methods as they contribute, in a complex way, to the stated research question. Findings from individual methods have and will be presented in separate studies (see [22,108,110,114]). Future work will also include an analysis of acoustic measurements taken throughout the study. In preliminary analyses (e.g., descriptive statistics, mediation analysis), the acoustic measurements (referred to in Figure 2 as EMM: Environmental Monitoring with Microphones) did not prove predictive or descriptive of other themes, such as the soundscape evaluation scales and restorativeness. Future research will integrate the analyses of the EMM using, for example, manual annotation of recording data or computational auditory scene analysis. Future studies based on the Musikiosk model will attempt to address the constraint that the microphones were placed very close to the sound installation.

This paper illustrates a number of contributions put forward by Musikiosk as a democratic soundscape installation to both sound-related scientific knowledge as well as to city-making knowledge, particularly for designers and other city workers working on small-scale urban projects concerned with the quality of the urban public experience of city dwellers in their encounters with and use of public spaces. From a methodological perspective, Musikiosk was a proof of concept on the process of developing both a complex installation for use in an urban pocket park context and an integrated mixed-methods research strategy to document the effects (if any) of Musikiosk on park users' quality of their urban public experience. Considering that Musikiosk is an intervention that directly influenced the park soundscape, it was necessary to investigate the sound-related effects it had over users and their evaluations; however, its effects were farther reaching. QUPE, having been developed iteratively, could thus be a framework that stands for the missing link from quality of life to public experience and it could be extended to other aspects of the multisensory urban public experience; we focused on sound, but it could very well be applied to other aspects of it.

Partially going against mainstream policy-oriented quests for noise abatement where urban sound is conceptualized as "bad for public health", we confirmed the findings of previous initiatives centered on adding decibels through soundscape interventions in public spaces. However, unlike most known such initiatives, that are based on top-down processes of auditory output selection (in which usually sound artists, alone or with the support of local stakeholders, design the content to be played), Musikiosk was developed with ideas of democratizing the (auditory) appropriation of public spaces by allowing the public space—and system—users to choose their own content, musical or not. From a technological perspective, the aspect of interacting with the installation itself was not essential; the technology behind Musikiosk was developed to be simple and user-friendly, so as for it to be a means for city dwellers to engage with others and with the park itself through the aforementioned appropriation of the public space rather than an end in itself.

The democratic aspect of the installation represented the main source of both interest and apprehension for its users, and that brought with it complex negotiations with one's self in terms of "adequate" music to play for the other park users and the park itself while adhering to principles of mutual respect. We can thus argue that the availability of such a democratic sound system that allowed users to control (to an extent) their soundscape, contrary to expectations, tapped into an intuitive, perhaps empathetic understanding that sharing their music openly would make their private domain (and, to an extent, their identity as defined by musical taste) public; thus, potentially because they have had their auditory spaces invaded previously (by music blasting from cars, motorcycles revving, construction work), Musikiosk users were conscientious in their engagement with the system.

Despite repeated worries expressed by officials as well as acknowledged by multiple members of the public (particularly Musikiosk users), the minimally invasive nature of the system, combined with its conscientious use was confirmed in the results of questionnaires as well as the observed patterns of use of the park, which did not change significantly when the system was in use per se, nor overall, in the post-intervention phase. What Musikiosk did succeed in was diversifying the park i.e., bringing new users to the park by changing their previous impression of the park (as a consequence of their engagement with the installation), while not displacing the current users, particularly members of the local aging Portuguese community, who did not show signs of interest in engaging with it throughout the intervention stage.

Finally, the effects of Musikiosk on QUPE have been observed and recorded in a small spatial context i.e., Parc du Portugal, a pocket park in a residential area off a busy traffic artery in Montreal; while it is well known and accepted that access to and use of large urban parks have beneficial effects over the health and wellbeing of urbanites, this project demonstrated that similar benefits in terms of restorativeness, mood or diversification of users can be achieved from a small (pocket) park. Thus, key aspects in designing a restorative environment are that it has to match the activities envisaged, users should be granted more control over their environment, work closely with the community to make sure that they will be on board with plans. Furthermore, our findings indicate that the effects of the installation extend beyond only those who interact with the system. This insight is of particular interest for urban designers and other professionals intervening in city design because it demonstrates that increasing the quality of the urban public experience of city dwellers is an attainable goal at low costs by developing and providing sufficient access to small, yet plentiful and smartly distributed spaces of respite and enjoyment, exposed to the sounds of the city. In these contexts, given the spaces themselves and the types of activities either current or intended, installations like Musikiosk could be low cost yet democratic alternatives to more complex soundscape installations that can provide public space users with the responsibility of using and appropriating their spaces. The findings potentially suggest that this type of intervention may be appropriate for similar public spaces, i.e., those with a relatively noisy character and dense activity, where sound levels are elevated but not harmful, and there is no "quiet" to disturb. This approach is not intended as a replacement of noise mitigation measures, but rather could serve as a complement by addressing aspects of quality of public life and accounting more deeply for users' perceptions.

Author Contributions: Conceptualization, D.S., E.B., and C.G.; methodology, all authors.; formal analysis, D.S., E.B., and C.T.; writing—original draft preparation, D.S. and E.B.; writing—review and editing, all authors; project administration, D.S.; supervision, C.G.

Funding: This research received no external funding; the project team, however, did receive a small internal award (McGill Dean of Arts Development Fund) for materials. The writing of this manuscript was supported by a Grant from Canada's Social Sciences and Humanities Research Council (#430-2016-01198), awarded to C.G.

Acknowledgments: The authors would like to thank Romain Dumoulin, the technical lead for this project as well as Jaimie Cudmore, who began the outreach programs. We would also like to thank Jayne Engle for helping us establish a relationship with the project neighbors and Christine Gosselin for supporting our project internally at the municipality.

Conflicts of Interest: The authors declare no conflict of interest.

Appendix A

Table A1. Questionnaire Q1.

Section	Q#	Question	Type
Activity	1	■ What were you doing in the park today?	Free response
	2	■ In your opinion, what are the main activities that take place in this park?	Free response
	3	■ Park visit frequency	Multiple choice
Soundscape evaluation	4	■ SSQP—I find the soundscape to be:	
		a. Pleasant	Likert scale
		b. Unpleasant	Likert scale
		c. Eventful	Likert scale
		d. Vibrant	Likert scale
		e. Monotonous	Likert scale
		f. Calm	Likert scale
		g. Chaotic	Likert scale
	5	■ The soundscape I hear is appropriate for my activity	Likert scale
	6	■ Soundscape restorativeness scale:	
		a. I find these sounds fascinating	Likert scale
		b. Spending time in this soundscape gives me a break from my day-to-day routine	Likert scale
		c. It's easy to do what I want while I'm in this soundscape	Likert scale
	7	■ The sound level of the park is: (low to high)	Multiple choice
	8	■ I find that level to be: (appropriate)	Multiple choice
	9	■ What was your mood before coming to the park?	Likert scale
	10	■ What is your mood now?	Likert scale
	11	■ Can you list below some sounds that you hear here in the park?	
		a. Pleasant	Free response
		b. Unpleasant	Free response
		c. Neutral	Free response
		Noise sensitivity (short version)	
		Demographics	

Table A2. Questionnaire Q2, Musikiosk users, presented in addition to Q1 questions.

Section	Q#	Question	Type
Musikiosk	12	■ Did you know about Muskiosk before you came into the park today?	Y/N
		If so, how did you hear about it?	Multiple choice
	13	■ Why are you using Musikiosk today?	Free response
	14	■ While using Muskiosk, besides listening, I was/we were also:	Multiple choice
	15	■ What was the content of the audio you played (e.g., musical genre)?	Free response
	16	■ Did Musikiosk change what you did in the park? How?	Free response
	17	■ Did Musikiosk change your park experience? How?	Free response
	18	■ Is Musikiosk appropriate for this park?	Y/N—explain
	19	■ Did you find it easy to use Musikiosk?	Y/N—explain
	20	■ Would you like to use Musikiosk again?	Y/N—explain
	21	■ What did you like about using Musikiosk?	Free response
	22	■ Do you have any suggestions for improving Musikiosk?	Free response

Table A3. Questionnaire Q3, Musikiosk non-users, presented in addition to Q1 questions.

Section	Q#	Question	Type
Musikiosk	12	■ How do you feel about this type of installation in this park?	Free response
	13	■ Does the installation change your park experience? How?	Free response
	14	■ Does/Would it change what you do in the park? How?	Free response
	15	■ Is Musikiosk appropriate for this park?	Y/N
	16	■ Is Musikiosk currently in use?	Y/N/IDK
	17	■ Were you aware of Musikiosk before taking this questionnaire?	Y/N
If you answered **Yes** to the previous question		■ Have you ever used it yourself?	Y/N
		■ Have you ever seen or heard anyone else use it?	Y/N
		■ Did you like it?	Y/N
If you answered **No** to the previous question		■ Would you like to try it?	Y/N

Appendix B

Table A4. Resident interview guide.

Section	Topics	Question
Use of Parc du Portugal	frequency of use; familiarity with space; functionality of space; awareness	■ How often do you come to the Parc?
Overall experience with Musikiosk		■ This summer, there was an installation in the Parc du Portugal, called Musikiosk; were you aware of it? ■ What was your initial impression of the Musikiosk idea? What were your expectations/hopes/concerns? ■ Did you advertise/tell other people (friends, family, etc.) about Musikiosk? ■ Did you use it yourself? (If they did, they were also asked questions from Appendix C—see Table A5.)
	perceptions of project; experience; evaluation; user design; deliberation	■ How do you feel about Musikiosk now that it is over/finished? Has your initial impression changed in any way? ■ Do you think it's appropriate for this park? Would you want it to be a permanent system? Why? ■ Who do you think should be allowed to use the equipment? For what purposes? ■ Do you think that there should be programming of these spaces? Why? ■ Did you notice a change in the way in which the park is used and by whom? Please detail ■ Did you feel the Musikiosk had an effect on the ambiance of the park? the quality of life of the neighborhood? ■ Do you find the ambiance of Parc du Portugal convivial or friendly? Did Musikiosk have an effect on its conviviality or friendliness? ■ Did you feel like the researchers were available to you? ■ Did you feel like the city was available to you?
Soundscape description	perceived appropriateness of sounds for activity	■ How would you describe the soundscape of this park in this moment?
		Demographics, background and music habits

Appendix C

Table A5. Musikiosk user interview guide.

Section	Topic	Question
Use of Musikiosk system	perceived control; user engagement; motivation; interest; awareness; affect; attention; feedback; aesthetics and sensory appeal; activity response to sound; conviviality	*Use of Parc du Portugal* (see Appendix B—Table A4) ■ What music did you play? ■ Why did you choose that music? ■ Who did you play music/your sounds for? ■ How do you think other people in the park felt about what you played? ■ Did you notice people reacting to what you were playing? Could you give me some examples? ■ Does the fact that the system was free to use and publicly available contribute to your enjoyment of the park? Why? ■ How do you think the music you played influenced the ambiance of the park? ■ What would you do if a park user told you that they did not like the music you were playing? ■ If someone else was using Musikiosk, how do you think it would affect what you do in the park? ■ What would you do if a park user played a series of songs that you liked very much? ■ What would you do if you were using Musikiosk and other people came into the gazebo to join you?
		Overall experience with Musikiosk (see Appendix B—Table A4) Soundscape description (see Appendix B—Table A4) Demographics, background and music habits

Appendix D

Table A6. French quotations.

Note	Original in French	Participant
1	« c'est un parc qui semble surtout être utilisé pour de la rencontre communautaire »	R5, M, 34
2	« Si j'étais en train de lire, effectivement, la musique, parfois ça pourrait gêner. J'ai pas remarqué que ça avait gêné des personnes qui lisaient autour de nous par contre. Je sais pas si c'est suffisamment fort pour déranger »	R3, F, 49
3	« Oui, pour les mêmes raisons, parce que c'est un quartier qui est très diversifié, animé. Je pense que c'est placé de manière à ne pas déranger, c'est pas trop proche des habitations, donc je pense que c'est très bien intégré. »	R3, F, 49
4	« Oui, de toute façon le Saint Laurent, c'est tellement bruyant que la musique, ça peut être sûrement plus agréable que le bruit des voitures »	R5, M, 34
5	« Ce serait sympathique que ça revienne. Je pense que l'été c'est pas mal, parce qu'on flâne plus l'été, surtout dans cette rue-là. Oui ça peut être rigolo de s'arrêter, faire une pause en faisant du shopping ou entre les courses »	R3, F, 49
6	« puis ça crée des racines aussi, des gens qui viennent, ils connaissent le quartier, ils vont peut-être acheter, manger plus proche […] Ça a probablement rassemblé plus de jeunes gens, qui étaient bien agréables, qui étaient content, et puis les gens allaient voir qu'est-ce que c'était »	R1, F, 79
7	« c'est une occasion de s'asseoir et faire une pause dehors, de rencontrer du monde qu'on aurait pas rencontré forcément, effectivement. Non, c'est sympathique et ça ajoute à la vie de quartier »	R3, F, 49
8	« quand quelqu'un venait, ils pouvaient échanger un peu de ce qu'ils écoutaient »	R1, F, 79
9	« c'était gai, on dansait […] Et puis, il faisait beau, c'était la fin de l'été, donc c'était festif. »	R3, F, 49
10	« je pense que ça a facilité la communication entre nous et les jeunes qui étaient là avant qu'on arrive »	R3, F, 49
11	« C'est chouette d'avoir des bornes interactives dans la ville comme ça qui peuvent créer des espaces communautaires un peu élargis par rapport à simplement se rencontrer. On peut transporter une ambiance plus large, j'imagine, avec un système comme ça […] C'est plus participatif évidemment, parce que la majorité des activités sur le Saint Laurent sont très passives »	R5, M, 34
12	« Ça avait un potentiel de mettre une ambiance très sympathique, qui pouvait éventuellement réunir les personnes qui étaient un peu dans leur monde individuel, que ça pouvait fédérer peut-être, parce que nous on s'est mis à discuter, d'ailleurs, avec les jeunes qui buvaient dans leur coin, enfin, c'est pas des gens à priori on aurait approché, mais du coup on leur a expliqué comment faire, parce qu'il écoutait leur musique mais ils se rendaient pas compte qu'ils pouvaient s'en servir »	R3, F, 49
13	« Ça a augmenté une fréquentation de gens qui étaient contents, mais je peux pas vous dire la différence. Les gens continuaient d'y aller, les familles, les enfants et tout. »	R1, F, 79
14	« Ça sort de l'ordinaire, c'est une occasion de s'asseoir et faire une pause dehors, de rencontrer du monde qu'on aurait pas rencontré forcément, effectivement. Non, c'est sympathique et ça ajoute à la vie de quartier »	R3, F, 49
15	« Je veux y venir mais j'ai un téléphone cellulaire qui me sert pour les urgences […] Je sais pas comment, je suis pas vraiment équipée, je veux m'équiper mieux que ça, j'aimerais téléchargé toute la musique que j'aime, et pouvoir l'écouter au lieu d'écouter ça sur ma petite machine qui est quand même encombrante »	R1, F, 79
16	« C'est une crainte, que quand les gens ont fini d'écouter la musique, ils s'installent ensemble dans le kiosque pour parler, il y en a qui peuvent apporter des bières, et puis ça peut peut-être finir plus tard. Qui peut être envahissante et puis qui va être très chaleureuse aussi. C'est ce qu'on sait pas. L'expérience de maintenant c'est que on a pas ça, il faut être honnête, c'est pas arrivé »	R1, F, 79
17	« J'ai peur qu'il y ait trop de musiques différentes en même temps »	Q3
18	« Je ne sais pas si elle est nécessaire »	Q3
19	« J'étais agacée parce qu'il y avait pas que Musikiosk. Parce que tout l'été, on a été gênés par le bruit »	R4, F, 33
20	« Ça semblerait raisonnable, cette histoire que la ville a produit là quelques fois, comment ça s'appelle le […] de faire semblant. Les gens prétendent de chanter. [Le karaoké ?] Oui, alors c'était bruyant »	R2, M, 95
21	« Ça sort de l'ordinaire »	R3, F, 49
22	« c'est le côté participatif qui change »	R5, M, 34
23	« Plus on habite les espaces publics, plus la qualité de vie augmente, moi je pense faut animer les quartiers, sinon ça fait des zones mortes … Ça me parait plus agréable de passer dans un parc avec quelques personnes qui jouent de la musique que rien du tout […] Je pense que oui, ça a élargi les heures d'usage du parc, donc de ce point de vue là, oui. C'est plus agréable et c'est plus convivial, un parc où il y a des gens qu'un parc mort. »	R5, M, 34
24	« C'est une bonne utilisation parce que ça empêche d'autres activités plus […] je dirais même illicites, d'arriver. »	R1, F, 79
25	« Il y a plein de zones comme ça où ça fait un peu peur aux gens de passer le soir, s'il y avait une communauté qui jouait de la musique régulièrement, à toutes les heures de la journée, ça rend ça plus agréable et plus sécuritaire pour tout le monde. »	R5, M, 34
26	« C'est un endroit pour les enfants, c'est sécuritaire. »	R1, F, 79

References

1. Thompson, E. Noise, music and the Meaning of Modernity. *Arch. Sci.* **2005**, *58*, 65–72.
2. Dubois, D.; Guastavino, C.; Raimbault, M. A Cognitive Approach to Urban Soundscapes: Using Verbal Data to Access Everyday Life Auditory Categories. *Acta Acust. United Acust.* **2006**, *92*, 865–874.

3. Lercher, P.; Schulte-Fortkamp, B. The relevance of soundscape research to the assesment of annoyance at the community level. In Proceedings of the Proceedings of the 8th International Congress on Noise as a Public Health Problem, Rotterdam, The Netherlands, 29 June–3 July 2003.
4. Schulte-Fortkamp, B.; Brooks, B.M.; Bray, W.R. Soundscape: An approach to rely on human perception and expertise in the post-modern community noise era. *Acoust. Today* **2007**, *3*, 7–15. [CrossRef]
5. Hall, D.A.; Irwin, A.; Edmondson-Jones, M.; Phillips, S.; Poxon, J.E.W. An exploratory evaluation of perceptual, psychoacoustic and acoustical properties of urban soundscapes. *Appl. Acoust.* **2013**, *74*, 248–254. [CrossRef]
6. *ISO 12913-1:2014 - Acoustics—Soundscape—Part 1: Definition and Conceptual Framework*; International Organization for Standardization: Geneva, Switzerland, 2014.
7. Aletta, F.; Kang, J.; Axelsson, Ö. Soundscape descriptors and a conceptual framework for developing predictive soundscape models. *Landsc. Urban Plan.* **2016**, *149*, 65–74. [CrossRef]
8. Botteldooren, D.; Andringa, T.; Aspuru, I.; Brown, L.; Dubois, D.; Guastavino, C.; Lavandier, C.; Nilsson, M.; Preis, A. *Soundscape for European Cities and Landscape: Understanding and Exchanging*; Soundscape-COST: Oxford, UK, 2013; pp. 36–43.
9. Botteldooren, D.; Andringa, T.; Aspuru, I.; Brown, A.L.; Dubois, D.; Guastavino, C.; Kang, J.; Lavandier, C.; Nilsson, M.; Preis, A. From sonic environment to soundscape. *Soundscape Built Environ.* **2015**, *36*, 17–42.
10. Kang, J. *Urban Sound Environment*; CRC Press: Boca Raton, FL, USA, 2006; ISBN 0-203-00478-7.
11. Schulte-Fortkamp, B.; Voigt, K. Why soundscape? The new approach to "measure" quality of life. *J. Acoust. Soc. Am.* **2012**, *131*, 3437. [CrossRef]
12. Alvarsson, J.J.; Wiens, S.; Nilsson, M.E. Stress Recovery during Exposure to Nature Sound and Environmental Noise. *Int. J. Environ. Res. Public Health* **2010**, *7*, 1036–1046. [CrossRef]
13. Ratcliffe, E.; Gatersleben, B.; Sowden, P.T. Bird sounds and their contributions to perceived attention restoration and stress recovery. *J. Environ. Psychol.* **2013**, *36*, 221–228. [CrossRef]
14. Steele, D. Bridging the gap from soundscape research to urban planning and design practice: How do professionals conceptualize, work with, and seek information about sound? Ph.D. Thesis, McGill University, Montreal, QC, Canada, 2018.
15. Raimbault, M.; Dubois, D. Urban soundscapes: Experiences and knowledge. *Cities* **2005**, *22*, 339–350. [CrossRef]
16. Nilsson, M.E.; Botteldooren, D.; De Coensel, B. Acoustic indicators of soundscape quality and noise annoyance in outdoor urban areas. In Proceedings of the Proceedings of the 19th International Congress on Acoustics, Madrid, Spain, 2–7 September 2007.
17. Herranz-Pascual, K.; García, I.; Diez, I.; Santander, A.; Aspuru, I. Analysis of Field Data to Describe the Effect of Context (Acoustic and Non-Acoustic Factors) on Urban Soundscapes. *Appl. Sci.* **2017**, *7*, 173. [CrossRef]
18. Axelsson, Ö. How to Measure Soundscape Quality. In Proceedings of the Proceedings of Euronoise 2015, Maastricht, The Netherlands, 1–3 June 2015.
19. Axelsson, Ö.; Nilsson, M.E.; Berglund, B. A principal components model of soundscape perception. *J. Acoust. Soc. Am.* **2010**, *128*, 2836–2846. [CrossRef]
20. Axelsson, Ö.; Nilsson, M.E.; Berglund, B. The Swedish soundscape-quality protocol. *J. Acoust. Soc. Am.* **2012**, *131*, 3476. [CrossRef]
21. Tarlao, C.; Steele, D.; Fernandez, P.; Guastavino, C. Comparing soundscape evaluations in French and English across three studies in Montreal. In Proceedings of the Proceedings of INTER-NOISE 2016, Hamburg, Germany, 21–24 August 2016.
22. Brown, A.L. A review of progress in soundscapes and an approach to soundscape planning. *Int. J. Acoust. Vib.* **2012**, *17*, 73–81. [CrossRef]
23. Lavia, L.; Easteal, M.; Close, D.; Witchel, H.; Axelsson, Ö.; Ware, M.; Dixon, M. Sounding Brighton: Practical approaches towards better soundscapes. In Proceedings of the 41st International Congress and Exposition on Noise Control Engineering 2012 (INTER-NOISE 2012), New York, NY, USA, 19–22 August 2012.
24. Dubois, D. Categories as acts of meaning: The case of categories in olfaction and audition. *Cognit. Sci. Q.* **2000**, *1*, 35–68.
25. Brown, A.L.; Muhar, A. An approach to the acoustic design of outdoor space. *J. Environ. Plan. Manag.* **2004**, *47*, 827–842. [CrossRef]

26. Lavia, L.; Witchel, H.J.; Kang, J.; Aletta, F. *A Preliminary Soundscape Management Model for Added Sound in Public Spaces to Discourage Anti-Social and Support Pro-Social Effects on Public Behaviour*; DAGA: Aachen, Germany, 2016.
27. Steele, D.; Steffens, J.; Guastavino, C. The role of activity in urban soundscape evaluation. In Proceedings of the Proceedings of Euronoise 2015, Maastricht, The Netherlands, 1–3 June 2015; pp. 1507–1512.
28. Bild, E.; Coler, M.; Pfeffer, K.; Bertolini, L. Considering Sound in Planning and Designing Public Spaces A Review of Theory and Applications and a Proposed Framework for Integrating Research and Practice. *J. Plan. Lit.* **2016**, *31*, 419–434. [CrossRef]
29. Aletta, F.; Lepore, F.; Kostara-Konstantinou, E.; Kang, J.; Astolfi, A. An Experimental Study on the Influence of Soundscapes on People's Behaviour in an Open Public Space. *Appl. Sci.* **2016**, *6*, 276. [CrossRef]
30. Steffens, J.; Steele, D.; Guastavino, C. Situational and person-related factors influencing momentary and retrospective soundscape evaluations in day-to-day life. *J. Acoust. Soc. Am.* **2017**, *141*, 1414–1425. [CrossRef]
31. Bild, E.; Pfeffer, K.; Coler, M.; Rubin, O.; Bertolini, L. Public Space Users' Soundscape Evaluations in Relation to Their Activities. An Amsterdam-Based Study. *Front. Psychol.* **2018**, *9*. [CrossRef]
32. Guastavino, C. Categorization of environmental sounds. *Can. J. Exp. Psychol. /Revue Can. Psychol. Exp.* **2007**, *61*, 54–63. [CrossRef]
33. Davies, W.J.; Adams, M.D.; Bruce, N.S.; Cain, R.; Carlyle, A.; Cusack, P.; Hall, D.A.; Hume, K.I.; Irwin, A.; Jennings, P.; et al. Perception of soundscapes: An interdisciplinary approach. *Appl. Acoust.* **2013**, *74*, 224–231. [CrossRef]
34. Raimbault, M. Qualitative judgements of urban soundscapes: Questionning questionnaires and semantic scales. *Acta Acust. United Acust.* **2006**, *92*, 929–937.
35. Mzali, M.; Dubois, D.; Polack, J.-D.; Létourneaux, F.; Poisson, F. Mental representation of auditory comfort inside trains: Methodological and theoretical issues. In Proceedings of the Proceedings of INTER-NOISE 2001, The Hague, The Netherlands, 27–30 August 2001.
36. Delepaut, G. Contribution de la linguistique cognitive à l'identification du confort: Analyse des discours des passagers sur le confort en train. Ph.D. Thesis, Université de la Sorbonne nouvelle - Paris III, Paris, France, 2007.
37. Cerwén, G.; Pedersen, E.; Pálsdóttir, A.-M. The Role of Soundscape in Nature-Based Rehabilitation: A Patient Perspective. *Int. J. Environ. Res. Public Health* **2016**, *13*, 1229. [CrossRef]
38. Filipan, K.; Boes, M.; De Coensel, B.; Lavandier, C.; Delaitre, P.; Domitrović, H.; Botteldooren, D. The Personal Viewpoint on the Meaning of Tranquility Affects the Appraisal of the Urban Park Soundscape. *Appl. Sci.* **2017**, *7*, 91. [CrossRef]
39. Nielbo, F.L.; Steele, D.; Guastavino, C. Investigating soundscape affordances through activity appropriateness. *Proc. Meet. Acoust.* **2013**, *19*, 040059.
40. Bild, E.; Coler, M.; Dubois, D.; Pfeffer, K. A pilot experiment on effects of motor and cognitive activities on memories of soundscapes. In Proceedings of the Proceedings of Euronoise 2015, Maastricht, The Netherlands, 1–3 June 2015; p. 5.
41. Rådsten-Ekman, M.; Axelsson, Ö.; Nilsson, M.E. Effects of Sounds from Water on Perception of Acoustic Environments Dominated by Road-Traffic Noise. *Acta Acust. United Acust.* **2013**, *99*, 218–225. [CrossRef]
42. Arroyo, E.; Bonanni, L.; Valkanova, N. Embedded Interaction in a Water Fountain for Motivating Behavior Change in Public Space. In Proceedings of the Proceedings of the SIGCHI Conference on Human Factors in Computing Systems, New York, NY, USA, 5–10 May 2012; pp. 685–688.
43. Jambrošić, K.; Horvat, M.; Domitrović, H. Assessment of urban soundscapes with the focus on an architectural installation with musical features. *J. Acoust. Soc. Am.* **2013**, *134*, 869–879. [CrossRef] [PubMed]
44. Hellström, B. Acoustic design artifacts and methods for urban soundscapes: A case study on the qualitative dimensions of sounds. In Proceedings of the Proceedings of INTER-NOISE 2012, New York, NY, USA, 19–22 August 2012.
45. Di, G.; Li, Z.; Zhang, B.; Shi, Y. Adjustment on subjective annoyance of low frequency noise by adding additional sound. *J. Sound Vib.* **2011**, *330*, 5707–5715. [CrossRef]
46. Licitra, G.; Cobianchi, M.; Brusci, L. Artificial soundscape approach to noise pollution in urban areas. In Proceedings of the Proceedings of INTER-NOISE 2010, Lisbon, Portugal, 13–16 June 2010; p. 11.
47. Yang, W.; Kang, J. Acoustic comfort evaluation in urban open public spaces. *Appl. Acoust.* **2005**, *66*, 211–229. [CrossRef]

48. Lavia, L.; Witchel, H.J.; Aletta, F.; Steffens, J.; Fiebig, A.; Kang, J.; Howes, C.; Healey, P.G.T. Non-Participant Observation Methods for Soundscape Design and Urban Planning. In *Handbook of Research on Perception-Driven Approaches to Urban Assessment and Design*; Aletta, F., Xiao, J., Eds.; Advances in Civil and Industrial Engineering (ACIE); IGI Global: Hershey, PA, USA, 2018; pp. 73–99.
49. Yamasaki, T.; Yamada, K.; Laukka, P. Viewing the world through the prism of music: Effects of music on perceptions of the environment. *Psychol. Music* **2015**, *43*, 61–74. [CrossRef]
50. Steffens, J.; Steele, D.; Guastavino, C. Music influences the perception of our acoustic and visual environment. In Proceedings of the Proceedings of INTER-NOISE 2016; Institute of Noise Control Engineering, Hamburg, Germany, 21–24 August 2016.
51. Woolley, H. *Urban Open Spaces*; Taylor & Francis: Abingdon, UK, 2003; ISBN 978-1-135-80229-5.
52. Carmona, M.; de Magalhães, C.; Hammond, L. *Public Space: The Management Dimension*; Routledge: Abingdon-on-Thames, UK, 2008; ISBN 978-1-134-16664-0.
53. Nissen, S. Urban Transformation From Public and Private Space to Spaces of Hybrid Character. *Sociol. Čas. / Czech Sociol. Rev.* **2008**, *44*, 1129–1149.
54. Ünlü Yücesoy, E. Everyday urban public space: Turkish immigrant women's perspective. Ph.D. Thesis, Utrecht University, Utrecht, The Netherlands, 2006.
55. Whyte, W.H. *The Social Life of Small Urban Spaces*; Conservation Foundation: Washington, DC, USA, 1980; ISBN 978-0-89164-057-8.
56. Jacobs, J. *The Death and Life of Great American Cities*; Random House: New York, NY, USA, 1961; ISBN 978-0-679-74195-4.
57. Carr, S.; Francis, M.; Rivlin, L.G.; Stone, A.M. *Public Space*; Cambridge series in environment and behavior; Cambridge University Press: Cambridge, UK; New York, NY, USA, 1992; ISBN 978-0-521-35148-5.
58. Gehl, J.; Gemzøe, L. *New City Spaces*; Danish Architectural Press: Copenhagen, Denmark, 2001.
59. Given, L.M.; Leckie, G.J. "Sweeping" the library: Mapping the social activity space of the public library11A version of this article was presented at the Library Research Seminar II: Partners and Connections, Research and Practice, held at College Park, Maryland, November 2001. *Libr. Inf. Sci. Res.* **2003**, *25*, 365–385.
60. Kohn, M. *Brave New Neighborhoods: The Privatization of Public Space*; Routledge: Abingdon-on-Thames, UK, 2004; ISBN 978-1-135-94460-5.
61. Dines, N.T.; Cattell, V.; Gesler, W.M.; Curtis, S. *Public Spaces, Social Relations and Well-Being in East London*; Public spaces series; Published for the Joseph Rowntree Foundation by Policy Press: Bristol, UK, 2006; ISBN 978-1-86134-923-1.
62. Shaftoe, H. *Convivial Urban Spaces: Creating Effective Public Places*, 1st ed.; Routledge: London, UK, 2008; ISBN 978-1-84407-388-7.
63. Francis, J.; Giles-Corti, B.; Wood, L.; Knuiman, M. Creating sense of community: The role of public space. *J. Environ. Psychol.* **2012**, *32*, 401–409. [CrossRef]
64. Bull, M. No Dead Air! The iPod and the Culture of Mobile Listening. *Leis. Stud.* **2005**, *24*, 343–355. [CrossRef]
65. Humphreys, L. Cellphones in public: Social interactions in a wireless era. *New Media Soc.* **2005**, *7*, 810–833.
66. Beer, D. Mobile Music, Coded Objects and Everyday Spaces. *Mobilities* **2010**, *5*, 469–484. [CrossRef]
67. *Public and Situated Displays*; O'Hara, K.; Perry, M.; Churchill, E.; Russell, D. (Eds.) Springer: Dordrecht, The Netherlands, 2003; ISBN 978-90-481-6449-3.
68. Ylipulli, J.; Suopajärvi, T.; Ojala, T.; Kostakos, V.; Kukka, H. Municipal WiFi and interactive displays: Appropriation of new technologies in public urban spaces. *Technol. Forecast. Soc. Change* **2014**, *89*, 145–160. [CrossRef]
69. Thompson, J.B. Shifting Boundaries of Public and Private Life. *Theory Cult. Soc.* **2011**, *28*, 49–70.
70. Yu, H. The publicness of an urban space for cultural consumption: The case of Pingjiang Road in Suzhou. *Commun. Public* **2017**, *2*, 84–101. [CrossRef]
71. Aniansson, G.; Pettersson, K.; Peterson, Y. Traffic noise annoyance and noise sensitivity in persons with normal and impaired hearing. *J. Sound Vib.* **1983**, *88*, 85–97. [CrossRef]
72. Peterson, Y.; Aniansson, G. Noise sensitivity and annoyance caused by traffic noise in persons with impaired hearing. *J. Sound Vib.* **1988**, *127*, 543–548. [CrossRef]
73. Västfjäll, D. Influences of Current Mood and Noise Sensitivity on Judgments of Noise Annoyance. *J. Psychol.* **2002**, *136*, 357–370. [CrossRef]
74. Burns, A. Emotion and Urban Experience: Implications for Design. *Des. Issues* **2000**, *16*, 67–79. [CrossRef]

75. Carmona, M.; Heath, T.; Oc, T.; Tiesdell, S. *Public Places, Urban Spaces: The Dimensions of Urban Design*; Routledge: Abingdon-on-Thames, UK, 2003; ISBN 978-0-7506-3632-2.
76. Thwaites, K.; Helleur, E.; Simkins, I.M. Restorative urban open space: Exploring the spatial configuration of human emotional fulfilment in urban open space. *Landsc. Res.* **2005**, *30*, 525–547. [CrossRef]
77. Lloyd, K.; Auld, C. Leisure, public space and quality of life in the urban environment. *Urban Policy Res.* **2003**, *21*, 339–356. [CrossRef]
78. Francis, M. Control as a Dimension of Public-Space Quality. In *Public Places and Spaces*; Altman, I., Zube, E.H., Eds.; Human Behavior and Environment; Springer: Boston, MA, USA, 1989; pp. 147–172. ISBN 978-1-4684-5601-1.
79. Atkinson, R. Domestication by Cappuccino or a Revenge on Urban Space? Control and Empowerment in the Management of Public Spaces. *Urban Stud.* **2003**, *40*, 1829–1843. [CrossRef]
80. Franck, K.A.; Paxson, L. Women and Urban Public Space. In *Public Places and Spaces*; Altman, I., Zube, E.H., Eds.; Human Behavior and Environment; Springer: Boston, MA, USA, 1989; pp. 121–146. ISBN 978-1-4684-5601-1.
81. Gidlöf-Gunnarsson, A.; Öhrström, E. Noise and well-being in urban residential environments: The potential role of perceived availability to nearby green areas. *Landsc. Urban Plann.* **2007**, *83*, 115–126. [CrossRef]
82. Payne, S.R. Are perceived soundscapes within urban parks restorative. *J. Acoust. Soc. Am.* **2008**, *123*, 3809. [CrossRef]
83. Kaplan, R.; Kaplan, S. *The Experience of Nature: A Psychological Perspective*; Cambridge University Press: New York, NY, USA, 1989; ISBN 978-0-521-34139-4.
84. Herzog, T.R.; Black, A.M.; Fountaine, K.A.; Knotts, D.J. Reflection and attentional recovery as distinctive benefits of restorative environments. *J. Environ. Psychol.* **1997**, *17*, 165–170. [CrossRef]
85. Payne, S.R. The production of a Perceived Restorativeness Soundscape Scale. *Appl. Acoust.* **2013**, *74*, 255–263. [CrossRef]
86. Payne, S.R.; Guastavino, C. Exploring the Validity of the Perceived Restorativeness Soundscape Scale: A Psycholinguistic Approach. *Front. Psychol.* **2018**, *9*. [CrossRef]
87. Kaplan, S. The restorative benefits of nature: Toward an integrative framework. *J. Environ. Psychol.* **1995**, *15*, 169–182. [CrossRef]
88. Jansson, M. Attractive Playgrounds: Some Factors Affecting User Interest and Visiting Patterns. *Landsc. Res.* **2010**, *35*, 63–81. [CrossRef]
89. *Forests, Trees and Human Health*; Nilsson, K.; Sangster, M.; Gallis, C.; Hartig, T.; de Vries, S.; Seeland, K.; Schipperijn, J. (Eds.) Springer: Dordrecht, The Netherlands, 2011; ISBN 978-90-481-9805-4.
90. Refshauge, A.D.; Stigsdotter, U.K.; Cosco, N.G. Adults' motivation for bringing their children to park playgrounds. *Urban For. Urban Green.* **2012**, *11*, 396–405.
91. Blake, A. *Pocket Parks*; Open Space Seattle 2100: Seattle, WA, USA, 2005.
92. Cohen, D.A.; Lapham, S.; Evenson, K.R.; Williamson, S.; Golinelli, D.; Ward, P.; Hillier, A.; McKenzie, T.L. Use of neighbourhood parks: Does socio-economic status matter? A four-city study. *Public Health* **2013**, *127*, 325–332. [CrossRef]
93. Peschardt, K.K.; Stigsdotter, U.K. Associations between park characteristics and perceived restorativeness of small public urban green spaces. *Landsc. Urban Plan.* **2013**, *112*, 26–39. [CrossRef]
94. Peschardt, K.K.; Stigsdotter, U.K.; Schipperijn, J. Identifying Features of Pocket Parks that May Be Related to Health Promoting Use. *Landsc. Res.* **2016**, *41*, 79–94. [CrossRef]
95. Nordh, H.; Østby, K. Pocket parks for people—A study of park design and use. *Urban For. Urban Green.* **2013**, *12*, 12–17.
96. Kang, J.; Schulte-Fortkamp, B.; Fiebig, A.; Botteldooren, D. Mapping of Soundscape. In *Soundscape and the Built Environment*; CRC Press: Boca Raton, FL, USA, 2016; pp. 161–195.
97. Bull, M. Investigating the Culture of Mobile Listening: From Walkman to iPod. In *Consuming Music Together: Social and Collaborative Aspects of Music Consumption Technologies*; O'Hara, K., Brown, B., Eds.; Computer Supported Cooperative Work; Springer: Dordrecht, The Netherlands, 2006; pp. 131–149. ISBN 978-1-4020-4097-9.
98. Watson, A.; Drakeford-Allen, D. 'Tuning Out' or 'Tuning in'? Mobile Music Listening and Intensified Encounters with the City. *Int. J. Urban Reg. Res.* **2016**, *40*, 1036–1043.

99. Hargreaves, D.J.; North, A.C. The Functions of Music in Everyday Life: Redefining the Social in Music Psychology. *Psychol. Music* **1999**, *27*, 71–83. [CrossRef]
100. O'Hara, K.; Lipson, M.; Jansen, M.; Unger, A.; Jeffries, H.; Macer, P. Jukola: Democratic music choice in a public space. In Proceedings of the Proceedings of the 2004 Conference on Designing interactive systems processes, practices, methods, and techniques - DIS '04, Cambridge, MA, USA, 1–4 August 2004; pp. 145–154.
101. DeNora, T. Music and Emotion in Real Time. In *Consuming Music Together: Social and Collaborative Aspects of Music Consumption Technologies*; O'Hara, K., Brown, B., Eds.; Computer Supported Cooperative Work; Springer: Dordrecht, The Netherlands, 2006; pp. 19–33. ISBN 978-1-4020-4097-9.
102. DeNora, T. *Music in Everyday Life*; Cambridge-Obeikan: Cambridge, UK, 2000; ISBN 978-0-511-14915-3.
103. Connell, J.; Gibson, C.; Gibson, C. *Sound Tracks: Popular Music Identity and Place*; Routledge: Abingdon-on-Thames, UK, 2003; ISBN 978-1-134-69913-1.
104. Haake, A.B. Music listening in UK offices: Balancing internal needs and external considerations. Ph.D. Thesis, University of Sheffield, Sheffield, UK, 2010.
105. Aletta, F.; Kang, J. Towards an Urban Vibrancy Model: A Soundscape Approach. *Int. J. Environ. Res. Public Health* **2018**, *15*, 1712. [CrossRef]
106. Steele, D.; Dumoulin, R.; Voreux, L.; Gautier, N.; Glaus, M.; Guastavino, C.; Voix, J. Musikiosk: A Soundscape Intervention and Evaluation in an Urban Park. In Proceedings of the Audio Engineering Society Conference: 59th International Conference: Sound Reinforcement Engineering and Technology; Audio Engineering Society, Montreal, QC, Canada, 15–17 July 2015.
107. Bild, E.; Steele, D.; Pfeffer, K.; Bertolini, L.; Guastavino, C.; Bild, E. Activity as a Mediator Between Users and Their Auditory Environment in an Urban Pocket Park: A Case Study of Parc du Portugal (Montreal, Canada). In *Handbook of Research on Perception-Driven Approaches to Urban Assessment and Design*; Aletta, F., Xiao, J., Eds.; IGI Global: Hershey, PA, USA, 2018; pp. 100–125. ISBN 978-1-5225-3637-6.
108. Glaser, B.G.; Strauss, A.L. *The Discovery of Grounded Theory: Strategies for Qualitative Research*; AldineTransaction: New Brunswick, Canada, 1967; ISBN 978-0-202-30260-7.
109. Steele, D.; Tarlao, C.; Bild, E.; Guastavino, C. Evaluation of an urban soundscape intervention with music: Quantitative results from questionnaires. In Proceedings of the Proceedings of INTER-NOISE 2016; Institute of Noise Control Engineering, Hamburg, Germany, 21–24 August 2016.
110. Ostermann, F.O. Digital representation of park use and visual analysis of visitor activities. *Comput. Environ. Urban Syst.* **2010**, *34*, 452–464. [CrossRef]
111. Cosco, N.G.; Moore, R.C.; Islam, M.Z. Behavior Mapping: A Method for Linking Preschool Physical Activity and Outdoor Design. *Med. Sci. Sports Exerc.* **2010**, *42*, 513–519. [CrossRef]
112. Goličnik, B.; Ward Thompson, C. Emerging relationships between design and use of urban park spaces. *Landsc. Urban Plan.* **2010**, *94*, 38–53. [CrossRef]
113. Bild, E.; Steele, D.; Tarlao, C.; Guastavino, C.; Coler, M. Sharing music in public spaces: Social insights from the Musikiosk project (Montreal, CA). In Proceedings of the Proceedings of INTER NOISE 2016, Hamburg, Germany, 21–24 August 2016; Volume 16, pp. 21–24.
114. Peschardt, K.K.; Schipperijn, J.; Stigsdotter, U.K. Use of Small Public Urban Green Spaces (SPUGS). *Urban For. Urban Green.* **2012**, *11*, 235–244.
115. O'Brien, H.L.; Toms, E.G. What is user engagement? A conceptual framework for defining user engagement with technology. *J. Am. Soc. Inf. Sci.* **2008**, *59*, 938–955. [CrossRef]
116. Coensel, B.D.; Bockstael, A.; Dekoninck, L.; Botteldooren, D.; Schulte-Fortkamp, B.; Kang, J.; Nilsson, M.E. The soundscape approach for early stage urban planning: A case study. In Proceedings of the Noise Control Engineering, 39th International Congress, Proceedings, Lisbon, Portugal, 13–16 June 2010.
117. *Consuming Music Together: Social and Collaborative Aspects of Music Consumption Technologies*; O'Hara, K.; Brown, B. (Eds.) Computer Supported Cooperative Work; Springer: Dordrecht, The Netherlands, 2006; ISBN 978-1-4020-4031-3.
118. Bull, M. *Sound Moves: iPod Culture and Urban Experience*; Routledge: Abingdon, UK, 2007; ISBN 978-1-134-51699-5.

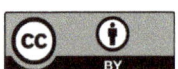

© 2019 by the authors. Licensee MDPI, Basel, Switzerland. This article is an open access article distributed under the terms and conditions of the Creative Commons Attribution (CC BY) license (http://creativecommons.org/licenses/by/4.0/).

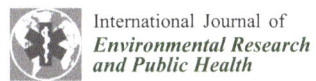

Brief Report

An Investigation of Soundscape Factors Influencing Perceptions of Square Dancing in Urban Streets: A Case Study in a County Level City in China

Jieling Xiao * and Andrew Hilton

Birmingham School of Architecture and Design, Birmingham City University, Birmingham, B47BD, UK; andrew.hilton@bcu.ac.uk
* Correspondence: jieling.xiao@bcu.ac.uk; Tel.: +44-0121-331-5984

Received: 1 January 2019; Accepted: 24 February 2019; Published: 7 March 2019

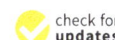

Abstract: Square dancing is a popular music-related group physical exercise for health benefits in China mainly participated by mid-aged women and elderly people. This paper investigates the soundscape and enjoyment of the square dancing in urban streets through a case study in Lichuan, a county level city in southwest China, in December 2017. It examines the impact of gender, age, participation and places on perceptions of square dancing soundscape. Two sites along two main urban streets in the city were selected to conduct onsite investigations where residents spontaneously perform square dancing on a daily basis. Ethnographical observations were conducted to identify the social-physical features and sounds of both sites during the dance and without dance. Sound pressure measurements (LAeq and LAmax) were also conducted under the two conditions. An off-site survey was distributed through the local social media groups to understand residents' everyday experiences and perceptions of square dancing in the city; 106 responses were received for the off-site survey. T-tests and Chi-squared tests were used for statistical analysis of the survey data. The results show gender does appear to be a factor influencing the regularity of participation in square dancing, with a bias towards more female participants. Participation frequency of square dance has an impact on the enjoyment of square dancing. There is no correlation between the dislike of watching square dancing, or dislike of the music and a desire to restrict locations for square dancing.

Keywords: square dancing; soundscape; public spaces; acoustic territory; enjoyment; appropriateness

1. Introduction

In the last decade, square dancing (known as grannies' dance) has gained vast popularity in Chinese cities [1,2]. Square dancing is a physical exercise combined with dancing movements in public spaces. There are three elements that make a square dancing scene: dance leader(s), music, a group of dancers in a paved urban space [3]. The dancing forms vary from gymnastic exercises to folk dance and disco. The music used for square dancing is edited with a plain soundtrack of drumbeats in similar rhythms. Often, the moves are made easy to follow the music. It is believed that the rise of square dancing originated from the historical folk dance, but more recently, Mao's promotion of sports to enhance people's health in China in the 1950s. The majority of people who practice square dance in China are middle-aged women and elderly people (both female and male). Square dancing serves as a social activity for people to enjoy themselves with low cost and maintain health. Estimated by the news centre of Chinese Central Television, over 100 million people in the country participate in square dancing everyday. It has become an undefeatable force in China to better understand the impacts and mechanism of square dancing to meet the demand of its large growing elderly population. Physical activities have been proven to bring health benefits, preventing chronic diseases and premature death [4]. The positive impacts of square dancing perceived by its participants are more than physical health benefits [5]. In a survey with square dancing participants in Shanghai, more than 60% of people believed square dancing enlarges their social networks and reduces the feeling of loneliness [6]. Group dancing serves as a tool to form a sense of community and generate collective experiences [7].

Criticism has been raised regarding square dancing for causing noise pollution [5,8]. The operating sound level during the dancing is often beyond the limits set by the national environmental noise control regulation (GB22337-2008) for urban streets - 70 dBA during daytime (10:00 pm–6:00 am) and 55 dBA at nighttime (6:00 am–10:00 pm) [9]. Responding such issues, the General Administration of Sport of China published legislations to force local authorities to manage the dancing groups, limit the time for dancing, create more activity spaces and control the noise and content of music used [10]. This has drawn attention to the sonic spatiality of public spaces that support music-related activities whilst not causing annoyance. Sounds generated by music-related activities such as street performance, taichi and skateboarding, are a common and important part of the sonic environment in the urban context [11]. A better understanding of the interrelationship between the music, perceptions of square dancing and place is needed to further promote this physical activity in open public spaces.

The soundscape concept provides a conceptual framework to understand the square dancing phenomenon. International Organization for Standardization defines soundscape as the acoustic environment perceived/understood or experienced by a person or people in context [12]. The sensation, interpretations and responses to the perceived acoustic environment play a central role in the concept. In recent studies of soundscapes in outdoor public spaces, activities have been considered as a key role in creating urban soundscapes whilst contextualizing the way people evaluated the perceived sound environment [8,13,14]. This dual effect has drawn attention to look at the activity-soundscape relations in spaces [15]. Positive soundscapes are considered to provide an acoustic environment to mediate site-specific activities and increase pleasantness of using the space [16]. The perception of sound is also considered as an aesthetic sensation that people constantly examine the pleasure in the listening process [17]. Expectations, familiarity and level of social interactions are considered key factors influencing soundscape evaluations of performed activities [18].

The spatial distribution and types of spaces are in the core debate of regulating square dancing. However, few studies have examined square dancing in urban streets. In many cases, for convenience and space shortage, people choose to dancing on busy street median strips and sidewalks [3]. A street has different layers forming a spatial sequence from buildings on the side to sidewalks for pedestrians and lanes for cyclists and vehicles. Sounds perceived from waling in urban streets are important to the kinaesthetic experiences of everyday cities [19]. Unlike parks or squares which are designed purposefully for active physical activities, sidewalks on urban streets seem to be less functional and appropriate for square dancing. Square dancing in inappropriate places will be perceived as noise and cause stress to its perceivers and decrease the quality of life. Regular exposure to uncontrollable noise in urban environments will cause after-exposure long-term health issues associated with depression and sleeping problems [20]. Thus, the impacts square dancing have on the acoustic environment in urban streets and whether types of places have an impact on people's perceptions of square dancing in everyday experience will be explored in this paper.

Gender and age play important roles in evaluating loudness and acoustic comfort in public spaces. Significant difference has been found in preferences of soundscape elements in urban spaces among different age groups [21]. Females are more sensitive to sounds than males [22]. The majority of square dancing participants are mid-aged females [10] which indicates favouritism of this activity in women and a certain age range. However, from the audience perspective in a recent study, female audiences rated lower on their evaluations of acoustic comfort in parks when square dancing took place [23]. Previous studies suggest the length of time people spent in a place and visiting frequencies influence their evaluations of acoustic comfort [24,25]. In the case of urban streets where the main function is conceived as transit and movement, the time people spent at a particular point is very limited. Thus, durations of stay are not essential in the context of square dancing in urban streets. Instead, participation of square dancing might have an impact on perceptions of square dancing and associated acoustic comfort in urban streets.

Square dancing brings dual perceptual evaluations of the space from both perspective of the audience and participants. Compared with non-music-associated activities, music-associated activities in urban spaces attract audiences through aural-visual interactions [16]. In particular, larger group activities (n > 6) have more significant influences on pedestrians' behaviours and the time they stop to watch [11]. The associations of sounds in streets are argued as the key to initiate the social interactions between the space and the moving body [19]. Music might have played an important role in the spontaneity of square dancing, breaking the boundaries between audience and dancers. Sound pressure levels have been used to as a key objective factor to examine acoustic comfort in public spaces. People in public spaces rated low acoustic comfort when the sound pressure level exceeds 73 dBA [24]. A recent study on square dancing in a park in Harbin China measured the sound pressure level difference in the park when square dancing occurred as well as surveyed the objective loudness perceived by visitors [23]. The results reveal the music of square dancing has no significant impact on users' subjective evaluations of soundscape comfort in the park. The sound pressure level difference in the case was only 3 dBA and the average sound pressure level was less than 70 dBA. However, in urban streets where the background noise level is relatively higher than in parks and squares, it is questionable whether the sound pressure level and perceptions of the square dancing music are similar.

Thus, this paper aims to answer the questions: (1) What influence does square dancing have on the acoustic environment in urban streets? (2) How do gender, age and participation influence the enjoyment of square dancing? (3) Are urban streets perceived appropriate for square dancing to occur? Mixed methods of onsite acoustic measurements, observations and off-site surveys were used to conduct the study in two sites in a selected case city.

2. Methods

2.1. Selection of Case Study

In metropolitan cities, like Beijing and Shanghai, square dancing has been banned in main streets and certain public spaces to deal with the noise compliance and public order. In order to investigate influences of square dancing in urban streets, a case study was conducted in a county-level city in southwest China (Lichuan) where square dancing is popular and relatively less controlled by the government compared to the metropolitan areas. The city has three main streets running through the urban area in parallel from west to east and a number of squares in front of key infrastructures such as government, hospitals and schools to facilitate the everyday public social activities. Square dancing spreads out in the city particularly along sidewalks in the three main streets. Two sites were selected in the case study city (Figure 1): site 1 along Qingjiang Road (high street) and site 2 along Binjiang Road (riverside). Qingjiang Road is mainly for commercial activities with buildings on both sides as shops, restaurants, hotels and a mixed-use residential complex. However, alongside Binjiang Road, there are mainly residential buildings and offices on one side and the Qingjiang river on the other side.

Site 1 is located outside a mixed-use residential building with shops on the ground floor. There is a paved space at the front of the building around 120 square metres (18 m × 6 m). A dance team starts dancing around 6:00 pm everyday there with a speaker positioned against the building façade projecting music towards the street. Site 2 is located along the paved riverside walk opposite the city's media and culture bureau. The site is stepped back from the pedestrian with a paved area around 300 square metres (30 m × 10 m). The speaker was positioned against the retaining wall projecting towards the open space facing the river.

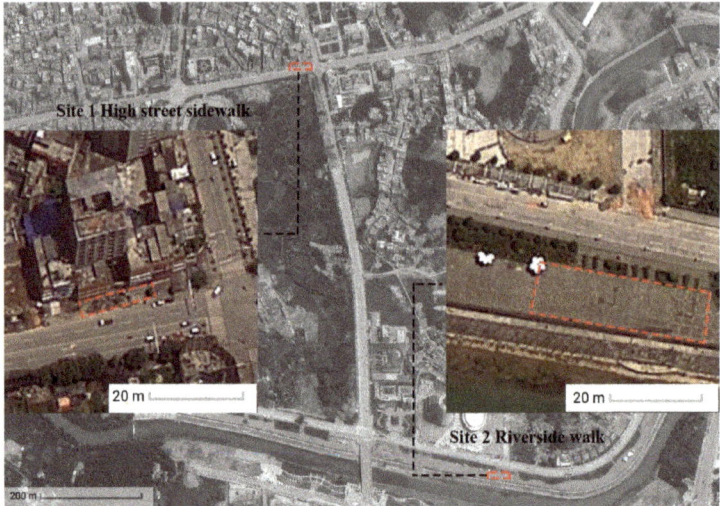

Figure 1. Map showing the two sites in the case study city and the urban morphology of the city.

2.2. Onsite Measurements

Data were collected in December 2017, using Castle-Group GA216L Sound Level Metre. During the measurements, the SLM was provided with a wind-screen and located on a tripod at a height of 1.50 m from the ground to reduce the effect of acoustic reflections (refer to [11]). Measurements were taken between 6:00 and 8:00 pm (the peak time for square dancing), conducted 30 min after the start when the size of group is more stable. A-weighted equivalent sound levels (L_{Aeq}) will be measured at slow-mode for 1-minute intervals three times in three different positions (as shown in Figure 2 where the red dot represents the location of the speaker and light grey dots represent participants in the square dancing):

a. 1 m from the loudspeaker (frontal position)
b. In the middle point of the area occupied by the square dancers (frontal position)
c. At the farthest point of the area occupied by the square dancers (side position).

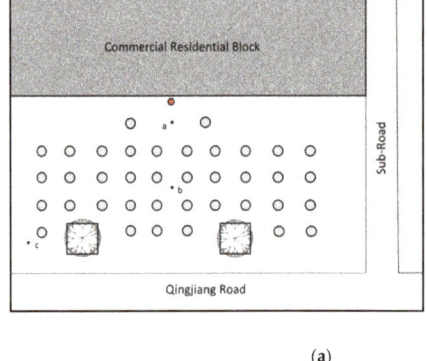

(a)

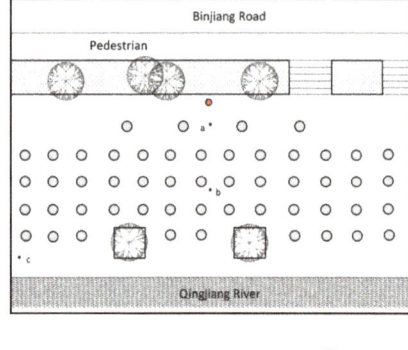

(b)

Figure 2. Illustrations of points for measurements onsite during the dance (where the red dot represents the location of the speaker and light grey dots represent participants in the square dancing): (**a**) layout of measuring settings in relation to the speaker at site 1; (**b**) layout of measuring settings in relation to the speaker at site 2.

Rather than noise monitoring, repeated recordings in short intervals are useful to capture the characteristics of the acoustic environment in an urban context [26]. In order to compare with no dancing conditions, a set of three 1-minute recordings were performed in position a and c as taken in in-session measurements to obtain an A-weighted equivalent sound level. The measurements outside the session were conducted between 1:00 and 2:00 p.m. to get a representative acoustic environment in streets for normal everyday city life. Considering the fluctuating sound features of square dancing music, the peak levels (L_{Amax}) will also be recorded to reflect on attractions of attentions during the dance.

2.3. Ethnographical Observations

Observations were conducted by the principle investigator onsite along with the measurements in order to map out the settings of square dancing on two sites (Table 1). The purpose was to note the size of the dancing group, built forms of the space and the engagement with the audience.

2.4. Off-Site Survey

Unlike previous studies, an off-site survey was conducted to understand how people perceive square dancing in a general sense in their everyday life rather than constrained to the site and temporary conditions. The survey was distributed online through local social media networks between 23 December 2017 and 23 January 2018 in the case study city. In total, 106 responses were received within the month when the measurements were conducted with an age range from twenty years old to seventy. Of those participants 69% were female, 78% were local residents with a further 17% originating from other county level cities and 4.7% from larger provincial cities. The age ranges from 20 through to 70, with 23% aged 20–30, 14% aged 30–40, 30% aged 40–50, 30% aged 50–60 and 3% aged 60+. Five questions were designed to gather data for statistic analysis on interrelationships between gender, age, participation, place and enjoyment of square dancing:

(1) Do you enjoy watching square dancing?
(2) How often do you participate in square dancing?
(3) How would you describe square dancing?
(4) Do you find the square dancing music unpleasant?
(5) What places are appropriate for square dancing?

Participants were given options to choose from for each question. Those options were developed based on the existing perceptual indicators, which focused more on the comfort and unique soundscape features of square dancing. Thus, three bipolar psycho-acoustic descriptors were chosen from previous studies [27–29] as multiple options to select in the survey for subjective perceptions of square dance: annoying-pleasing, noisy-rhythmic, boring-interesting.

2.5. Ethics

The study was conducted in accordance with the Declaration of Helsinki, and the protocol was approved by the Research Ethics Committee in Faculty of Arts, Media and Design at Birmingham City University on 20th December 2017. The survey is anonymised and has gained consent from the participants to use the data for academic research and publications.

Table 1. Observation notes and photos of sites during square dancing at 6–8:00 pm and without square dancing at 1–2:00 pm.

Site 1 Qingjiang Road (High Street)			
Time	Observations		Photo of the site
1–2:00 pm without square dancing	Dominant sounds onsite:	traffic	
	Other sounds:	people talking, advertisement music from shops on the side	
	Activities onsite:	People walking pass and walking in/out of the shops	
6–8:00 pm during square dancing	Dominant sounds onsite:	square dancing music	
	Other sounds:	people talking, traffic	
	Activities onsite:	square dancing, people walking pass and walking in/out of shops, people watching square dance	
	Size of the dancing group:	started with 12 and increased to 25 after 30 min	
Site 2 Binjiang Road (Riverside walk)			
Time	Observations		Photo of the site
1–2:00 pm without square dancing	Dominant sounds onsite:	traffic, people talking	
	Other sounds:	music from the other side of the river, people talking	
	Activities onsite:	People walking pass, children play	
6–8:00 pm during square dancing	Dominant sounds onsite:	square dance music	
	Other sounds:	Children playing	
	Activities onsite:	people walking pass, people watching square dancing	
	Size of the dancing group:	started with 18 and increased to 45 after 30 min	

3. Results

3.1. The Objective Loudness and Acoustic Environments

Mean values of sound pressure level measurements at the identified points were used to assess the change of objective loudness in urban streets during square dance compared to midday normal everyday conditions (see Table 2). The background noise level between 1 and 2:00 pm on site 2 is 2–5 dBA lower than at site 1. Significantly increased sound pressure levels were found at point a during the dance on both sites compared to midday without square dance. The most dominant sounds observed on both sites during the square dance were the square dance music from the audience side whilst the sound of traffic was dominant during midday. There is a significant drop from the speaker (point a) to the edge (point c) of the dancing group on both sites: 10 dBA difference at site1 whilst 30 dBA difference at site 2 during the dance. However, no significant difference was found at point c compared to normal conditions with only 2 dBA increase in site 1 and 5 dBA in site 2.

Table 2. Measurements of sound pressure levels (LAeq and LAmax) at two sites during and without square dance.

Site	Condition	Point	LAeq (mean)	LAmax (mean)
Site 1 Qingjiang Road sidewalk (High street)	Without square dance 1:00–2:00 pm	a	64.03	74.50
		b	n/a	n/a
		c	71.43	85.63
	During square dance 6:00–8:00 pm	a	87.50	94.20
		b	76.07	83.43
		c	75.10	80.43
Site 2 Bingjiang Road side walk (Riverside)	Without square dance 1:00–2:00 pm	a	59.57	65.40
		b	n/a	n/a
		c	69.03	79.40
	During square dance 6:00–8:00 pm	a	104.43	109.27
		b	93.03	99.73
		c	74.30	79.50

Although the background noise level at site 1 was higher than that at site 2, the sound pressure level of the broadcasting music during the dance at site 2 was much higher (17 dBA more) than at site 1. The scale of space and intensity of commercial activities onsite seem to have an impact on the background noise and loudness of the music broadcasted to reach to the edge of the group. The space of site 2 was twice the size of site 1 and without any solid construction within 30 m from the edges. Peak levels during the dance on both sites were found to be only 5–6 dBA different from the continuous equivalent levels. It seems unlikely that people will be attracted by the incident sound from the speaker.

3.2. Perceptions of Square Dance and Square Dance Music

Based on the survey data collected, a standard 95% confidence interval calculation was conducted to determine the true proportions of participants' responses to different factors. The true proportion of participants in the survey who regularly (more than once a week) participate in square dancing is between 24% and 41.9%. Over half of participants in the survey never practiced square dance. There is a variation in preference of watching square dance and listening to the square dance music among different age groups (see Figure 3).

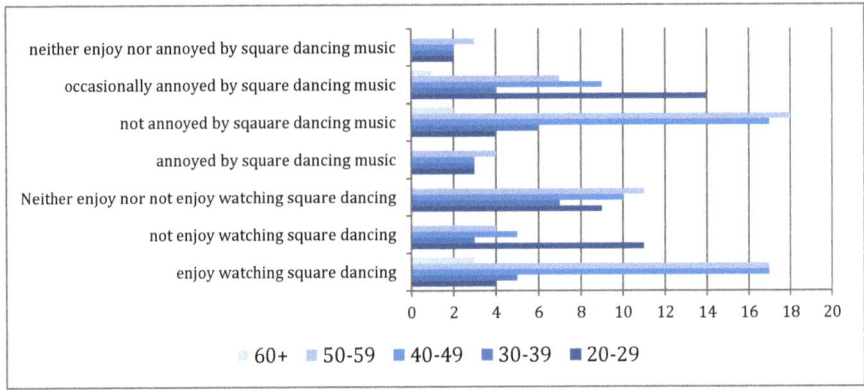

Figure 3. Responses from different age groups on the enjoyment of watching square dancing and the annoyance of square dancing music.

A series of T-tests were carried out to determine factors influencing the enjoyment of square dancing. A correlation was found between those who described square dancing in negative terms and those who find the music unpleasant (see Table 3). This correlation also held true between those not enjoying watching square dancing and those finding the music unpleasant

Table 3. Two-Sample t test with unequal variances comparing the description of square dancing with pleasantness of music.

Heading	n	Mean	Description of Square Dancing			
			Std. Deviation	Std. Error Mean	95% Confidence Interval	
					Lower	Upper
Describe Square Dancing as Pleasant	78	5.71	1.19	0.053	5.446	5.974
Describe Square Dancing as unpleasant	65	4.83	1.85	0.018	4.38	5.28
Pr ($|T| > |t|$) = 0.001, t = 3.2885.						

It can be concluded that with at least a 95% degree of certainty that perceived comfort of the music has an influence of whether people enjoy watching square dancing (see Table 4). Furthermore, there was a significant difference between the mean ages of those who enjoy watching square dancing and those who do not enjoy watching square dancing (see Table 5). This correlation with mean age also held true for the unpleasantness of the music (see Table 6) and the regularity of participation (see Table 7).

However we found *no significant difference* in gender associated with these preferences. Using a Chi-squared test (χ^2) we can conclude that with a 95% degree of certainty, gender has no significant impact on the enjoyment of watching square dance (χ^2 = 3.80 which is not > 5.991 for 95% with 2 degrees of freedom Table 8), of finding the music pleasant (χ^2 = 6.20 which is not > 7.815 for 95% with 3 degrees of freedom, Table 9).

Table 4. Two-Sample T test with unequal variances comparing enjoyment of watching square dance with pleasantness of music.

	Enjoyment of Watching Square Dance					
	n	Mean	Std. Deviation	Std. Error Mean	95% Confidence Interval	
					Lower	Upper
Describe Square Dancing Music as Pleasant	57	2.42	0.68	0.09	2.2436	2.5964
Describe Square Dancing Music as unpleasant	49	1.98	0.83	0.12	1.7448	2.2152

Pr(|T| > |t|) = 0.004, t = 2.9673.

Table 5. Two-Sample t test with unequal variances comparing Mean Age with enjoyment of watching square dance.

	Mean Age					
	n	Mean	Std. Deviation	Std. Error Mean	95% Confidence Interval	
					Lower	Upper
Enjoy Watching Square Dancing Yes	46	47.17	10.32	1.522	44.19	50.15
Enjoy Watching Square Dancing NO	23	35.87	12.03	2.51	30.95	40.79

Pr(|T| > |t|) = 0.0004, t = 3.8547.

Table 6. Two-Sample t test with unequal variances comparing Mean Age with unpleasantness of square dance music.

	Mean Age					
	n	Mean	Std. Deviation	Std. Error Mean	95% Confidence Interval	
					Lower	Upper
Unpleasantness of Square Dancing Music Yes	71	44.01	11.36	1.348	41.3676	46.652
Unpleasantness of Square Dancing Music No	15	35.67	12.23	3.158	29.481	41.859

Pr(|T| > |t|) = 0.025, t = 2.4315.

Table 7. Two-Sample t test with unequal variances comparing Mean Age with regularity of square dancing participation.

	Mean Age					
	n	Mean	Std. Deviation	Std. Error Mean	95% Confidence Interval	
					Lower	Upper
Regularly Participate in Square Dancing Yes	29	50.86	8.25	1.532	47.86	53.86
Regularly Participate in Square Dancing No	77	39.55	11.65	1.328	36.95	42.15

Pr(|T| > |t|) = 0.0000 t = 5.5849.

Table 8. Chi Squared Test comparing gender to enjoyment of watching square dance.

Enjoyment of Watching Square Dancing	Gender (n = 106)		χ^2	ϕ
	Male	Female		
Yes	10	36	3.80	0.036
Do not Know	13	24		
No	10	13		

$p = 0.1495$, df = 2.

Table 9. Chi Squared Test comparing gender to unpleasantness of square dance music.

Unpleasantness of Square Dancing Music	Gender (n = 106)		χ^2	ϕ
	Male	Female		
Yes	8	6	6.20	0.058
Do not Know	4	6		
Occasionally	10	25		
No	11	36		

$p = 0.1023$, df = 3.

However, our research did find some correlation between gender and the regularity of participation in square dance activities (χ^2 = 4.77 which is > 3.841 for 95% with 1 degree of freedom, Table 10), suggesting that females are more likely to participate more regularly.

Table 10. Chi Squared Test comparing gender to regularity of participation in Square Dance Activities.

Regularity of Participation in Square Dancing	Gender (N = 106)		χ^2	ϕ
	Male	Female		
Regularly *	6	29	4.77	0.045
Rarely **	27	44		

$p = 0.029$, df = 1, * Participation at least once per month. ** participation less than twice per year.

From the t-test data it can also be concluded to at least the same degree of certainty that age does in fact have a significant impact on the enjoyment of and participation in square dance. However, the distribution of online surveys might have an impact on the age groups who have access to the survey. This needs further investigation through a larger sampling survey through other methods.

A strong correlation was found between those who participate regularly with both the perceived unpleasantness of the music (see Table 11) and the enjoyment of watching square dance (see Table 12)

Table 11. Chi Squared Test comparing regularity of participation in Square Dance Activities to the perceived unpleasantness of the square dance music.

Unpleasantness of Square Dance Music	Regularity of Participation (n = 106)		χ^2	ϕ
	Regularly *	Rarely **		
Yes	3	11	10.26	0.097
Do not Know	1	9		
Occasionally	8	27		
No	23	24		

$p = 0.0165$, df = 3, * Participation least once per month. ** participation less than twice per year.

Table 12. Chi Squared Test comparing regularity of participation in Square Dance Activities to the enjoyment of watching square dance.

Enjoyment of Watching Square Dance	Regularity of Participation (n = 106)		χ^2	ϕ
	Regularly *	Rarely **		
Yes	30	16	39.27	0.37
Do not Know	5	32		
No	0	23		

p = 0.000, df = 2, * Participation at least once per month, ** participation less than twice per year.

However, there are 30% who occasionally are annoyed by the square dance music. The reasons for the occasional annoyance might come from personal conditions which are difficult to predict or control. Unlike previous literature, the overall perceptions of square dance in the survey are not negative particularly from the audience's perspectives (32.4% of those who rarely or never participate in square dance identified as not enjoying watching square dance). The music of square dance plays important roles in their perceptions where rhythm was the most frequently selected psycho-acoustic descriptor (see Figure 4). The percentage (based on 95% confidence intervals) of people who find square dancing music pleasant is between 63.6% and 78.4%.

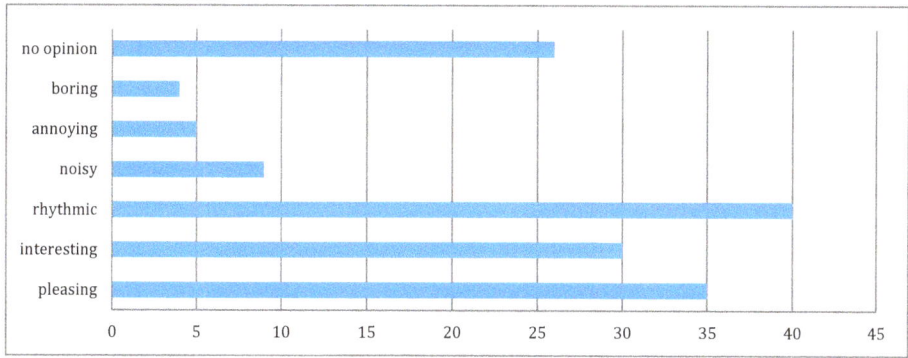

Figure 4. Frequencies of psycho-acoustic descriptors selected by participants in the survey to describe their perceptions of square dancing soundscape.

3.3. Perceptions of Appropriate Places for Square Dance

The majority of respondents (82%) suggested that external spaces are most appropriate for square dance, with only 18% suggesting that the interior spaces of gymnasium are most appropriate (see Figure 5). The percentage of participants (based on 95% confidence intervals) in the survey who think interior spaces are most appropriate for square dancing is between 11.8% and 24%. The percentage of participants who identified themselves enjoy the square dancing music and prefer square dance to occur in public urban spaces (i.e., urban squares and streets), rather than parks or community open spaces which are usually in gated enclaves, is between 27.6% and 46.2%. However, only a few considered sidewalks in urban streets like the case studies are appropriate for square dance. Park and squares are most frequently selected places which are appropriate for square dance to occur.

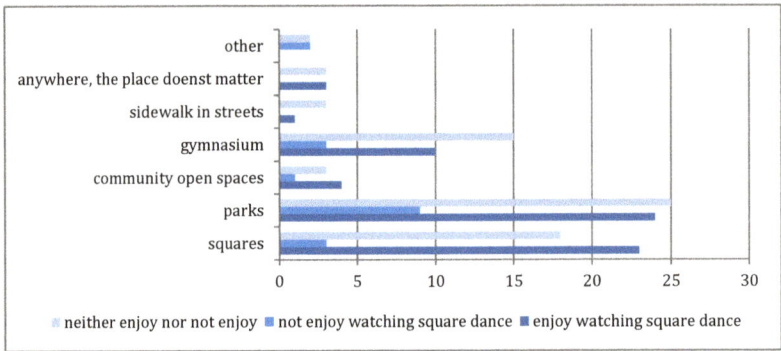

Figure 5. Participants' responses for appropriate places for practicing square dancing and their preferences of watching square dancing.

A range of T-tests and Chi Squared Tests were conducted to ascertain any correlation between spatial preferences for the performance of square dance. The majority of respondents (82%) suggested that external spaces are most appropriate for square dance, with only 18% suggesting that the interior spaces of gymnasium are most appropriate. Using a Chi Squared Test, there was no correlation between those who do not identify as enjoying square dance and a preference for interior spaces (see Table 13, χ^2 = 3.28 which is not > 5.991 for 95% with 2 degrees of freedom).

Table 13. Chi Squared Test comparing the description of square dance to the preferred location of Square Dance.

Preferred Location of Square Dance	Description of Square Dance (n = 144)		χ^2	ϕ
	Positive	Negative		
Public Space	38	9	3.28	0.023
Interior	17	10		
Non Urban	48	22		

$p = 0.194$, df = 2.

Using a T-test we found no correlation between those who described the music as being unpleasant and the preference for square dancing to be outside public urban areas (t = 0.8518 which is not >1.96 for the 95%, Table 14).

Table 14. Two-Sample T-test with unequal variances comparing unpleasantness of Square Dance Music with preferences for urban or non-urban spaces.

	Unpleasantness of Square Dancing Music					
	n	Mean	Std. Deviation	Std. Error Mean	95% Confidence Interval	
					Lower	Upper
Preference for Urban Space	47	3.00	1.08	0.157	2.691	3.309
Preference for Non Urban Space	96	2.83	1.13	0.115	2.604	3.056

$Pr(|T| > |t|) = 0.3964$, t = 0.8518.

However there was a tentative correlation (90–95% significance) between those who describe square dancing in negative terms (boring, noisy or annoying) and a preference for dancing to occur outside public urban spaces (t = 01.9082 which is not >1.96 for the 95% but is >1.645 for the 90% see Table 15).

Table 15. Two-Sample T-test with unequal variances comparing a negative description of Square Dance Music with preferences for urban or non urban spaces.

					Description of Square Dancing	
			Std.	Std. Error	95% Confidence Interval	
	n	Mean	Deviation	Mean	Lower	Upper
Preference for Urban Space	76	5.70	1.30	0.149	5.666	5.733
Preference for Non Urban Space	148	5.32	1.54	0.1266	5.300	5.34
		Pr($|T| > |t|$) = 0.05799, t = 1.9082.				

Using a Chi Squared Test, there was no significant difference between respondents description of square dance and the preference for public urban spaces (see Table 16), suggesting that people do not mind square dancing in urban spaces even if they do not enjoy participating, watching or listening to the music. No significant difference was found between those who participate regularly or rarely and a preference for square dances to occur in public urban spaces (see Table 17).

Table 16. Chi Squared Test comparing description of square dance to the preferred location of Square Dance.

Description of Square Dancing	Preferred Space for Square Dancing (n = 232)		χ^2	ϕ
	Urban	Other		
Pleasing	28	37	4.75	0.02
Rhythmic	26	43		
Interesting	19	32		
No opinion	6	19		
Boring	1	5		
Noisy	4	8		
Annoying	0	4		
	$p = 0.576$, df = 6.			

Table 17. Chi Squared Test comparing preferred location of Square Dance with regularity of participation.

Preferred Space for Square Dancing	Regularity of Participation in Square Dancing (n = 143)		χ^2	ϕ
	Rare	Regular		
Parks & Other	43	18	2.17	0.0152
Gymnasium	19	8		
Community open Space	6	2		
Urban Squares	28	16		
Urban Streets	3	0		
	$p = 0.704$, df = 4.			

Thus, participation of square dancing has no influence on perceptions of the physical settings of the soundscape and visual interactions of square dances. There is also no significant difference in preference of spaces for square dance to occur between those who described square dancing in a positive way and those who described it in more negative terms.

4. Discussion

4.1. Acoustic Boundaries between Square Dancers and Audience in Streets

The square dancing music also redefines acoustic territories in urban streets. Perception of sounds in public spaces is a dynamic process of disintegration and reconfiguration shifting between personal and shared experiences [17]. Sounds in streets create temporary territories for specific activities and attract attention from the outside. However, what defines the boundaries of acoustic territories is arguable.

The objective loudness is not decisive in defining the acoustic boundaries of square dancing in urban streets. In the case explored, there is only a 2-5 dBA difference at the audience side (edge of the dance group) during the dance which causes no significant contrast of loudness in the streets. The background sound level influences soundscape evaluations in urban open public spaces and a lower background level makes people feel quieter [24].

Although a 17 dBA difference was found near the speaker during the dance, similar sound levels were found at the edge of the dance group around 73 dBA. With a similar background noise level, 73 dBA might be the threshold sound level for participants to engage in the dance with the music. This territory is different from the audience's. It is suggested that people within 10 meters from edge of the music related activity group often will be attracted to stay and watch [11]. However, this might not be true for square dancing in urban streets. The significant correlation between the enjoyment of square dance music and watching square dance indicates the acoustic boundaries of the audience are set by the audible level of the square dance music. This might also relate to the scale of the space and visual distance between dancers and the dance leaders at the front.

4.2. Impacts of Age and Gender on Perceptions of Square Dancing

A previous study found differences in different age groups when evaluating acoustic comforts [21]. Personal preferences of different sounds play an important role in this evaluation. The older age groups in the survey enjoy watching square dancing or listening to the music which reveals a generational gap in preferences of musical sounds and activities in public urban spaces. Most participants in the age range between 20 and 30 rarely practice square dancing. The involvement and appreciation of square dancing seem to have an impact on their perceptions. The social context of the city (being a county level city, there are fewer options of leisure activities whilst closer social relationships) explored might also have impacts on people's perceptions and participation of square dancing.

Although square dance in China is commonly perceived as an exercise or leisure for mid-aged women [10], there is no difference in gender of perceiving square dances and the music in the case study. However, the types of square dance music in the city explored are quite singular and mostly based on popular folk music commonly heard on television without gender bias. This might be different if the types of music and dance are more gender targeted.

4.3. Impacts of Place Context on Perceptions of Square Dance

The preconceptions of soundscapes in different types of places might have impacts on perceptions of square dance and the music. The perceptions of a park being suitable for physical exercises with low background noise and squares for music-related activities with a loud background sound level have a significant impact on people's choices of square and parks as the most appropriate places for square dance. However, sidewalks in urban streets as explored in the case are not in preference for square dance. The expectations of space for square dancing to be a large flat area [3] might have influenced their evaluations of street sidewalks for square dancing. However, this is also related to the type and size of square dancing groups occurring frequently in participants' everyday experiences.

However, people do not seem to be influenced by the appearance of the physical space when evaluating their perceptions of square dance. No correlations were found between enjoyment of square dance and the choices of places. In the city explored, the time when square dance happens (between 6:00 pm and 8:00 pm) is often after sunset. The visual appearance of the physical space does not have much influence. This might be different in other places where there is a late sunset in some seasons.

4.4. Limitation of this Study

This study explored square dancing soundscape in a singular case which cannot represent the diversity of square dancing in other cities in a different context. The study was conducted in winter where the participation, clothing factor and background noise levels might be different from other seasons. The off-site survey based on people's everyday experiences retrieved from memories might be different from in-situational experiences. Onsite survey will be needed to explore the in-situ experiences from both perceivers' and dancers' views to further investigate the acoustic territories.

A previous study suggests that one potentially effective solution to control noise from square dancing is to use Bluetooth earphones [10]. The level of social interactions will be reduced in this sense. It might also cause safety issues since no sound signals will be received by other users in the street. Further investigations might be useful to examine this assumption through an initiated Bluetooth earphone aided square dancing.

5. Conclusions

It can be concluded from this study the main factor influencing the enjoyment of square dancing was age rather than gender. However, gender does appear to be a factor influencing the regularity of participation in square dancing, with a bias towards more female participants. Participation in square dancing has an impact on the enjoyment of square dancing. Those who participate in square dancing regularly and those who enjoy watching square dancing are more likely to find the music pleasant.

Similarly, those who found square dancing music unpleasant were less likely to participate in or watch square dancing; however, this dislike did not influence their preferences for square dancing to occur outside public urban spaces.

There is no correlation between the dislike of watching square dancing, or dislike of the music and a desire to restrict locations for square dancing. Likewise, no correlation was found between enjoyment of any aspect of square dancing and the desire for specifically urban spaces.

It can be seen from the results that the enjoyment of the music of square dancing has no significant influence on the preferred spatial location for square dancing.

Author Contributions: Conceptualization, J.X. and A.H.; Methodology, J.X; Statistic Analysis, A.H.; Investigation, J.X.; Writing-Original Draft Preparation J.X.; Writing-Review & Editing, A.H.

Funding: This research received no external funding.

Acknowledgments: Support was given by the local media and culture bureau in the case city for permission for the onsite measurements and distribution of surveys in the local residents' social media groups.

Conflicts of Interest: The authors declare no conflict of interest.

References

1. NBC News. China's Grooving Grannies: All They Want to Do Isd. 2014. Available online: https://www.nbcnews.com/news/asian-america/chinas-grooving-grannies-all-they-want-do-dance-n147246 (accessed on 20 January 2019).
2. BBC News. China Blog: Dancing Grannies Raise a Ruckus. 2013. Available online: https://www.bbc.com/news/blogs-china-blog-25330651 (accessed on 20 January 2019).
3. Chen, C. Dancing in the Streets of Beijing. In *Insurgent Public Space: Guerrilla Urbanism and the Remaking of Contemporary Cities*; Hou, J., Ed.; Routledge: London, UK, 2010.
4. Warburton, D.E.; Nicol, C.W.; Bredin, S.S. Health benefits of physical activity: The evidence. *CMAJ* **2006**, *174*, 801–809. [CrossRef] [PubMed]
5. Kirkpatric, N. China's War on Square Dancing Grannies. 2015. Available online: https://www.washingtonpost.com/news/morning-mix/wp/2015/03/25/chinas-war-on-square-dancing-grannies/?noredirect=on&utm_term=.d12e7f8260c1 (accessed on 22 January 2019).
6. Wong, H. Shanghai Citizens 'Support' Square Dancers. 2014. Available online: http://www.chinadaily.com.cn/china/2014-07/18/content_17830503.htm (accessed on 23 January 2019).
7. Dueck, B. 'Suddenly a sense of being a community': Aboriginal square dancing and the experience of collecPvity. *Musiké* **2006**, *1*, 41–58.
8. Hu, Q. Dancing with Danger. 2013. Available online: http://en.people.cn/90782/8455170.html (accessed on 22 January 2019).

9. National Standards of People's Republic of China. *GB22337-2008: Emission Standard for Community Noise*; The State Council, PRC: Beijing, China, 2008.
10. Zhou, L. Music is not our enemy, but noise should be regulated: Thoughts on shooting/conflicts related to dama square dance in China. *Res. Q. Exerc. Sport* **2014**, *85*, 279–281. [CrossRef] [PubMed]
11. Meng, Q.; Kang, J. Effect of sound-related activities on human behaviours and acoustic comfort in urban open spaces. *Sci. Total Environ.* **2016**, *573*, 481–493. [CrossRef] [PubMed]
12. ISO. *FDIS 12913-1:2014 Acoustics—Soundscape—Part 1: Definition and Conceptual Framework*; International Organization for Standardization: Geneva, Switzerland, 2014.
13. Aletta, F.; Lepore, F.; Kostara-Konstantinou, E.; Kang, J.; Astolfi, A. An experimental study on the influence of soundscapes on people's behaviour in an open public space. *Appl. Sci.* **2016**, *6*, 276. [CrossRef]
14. Estévez-Mauriz, L.; Forssén, J.; Dohmen, M.E. Is the sound environment relevant for how people use common spaces? *Build. Acoust.* **2018**, *25*, 307–337. [CrossRef]
15. Bild, E.; Steele, D.; Pfeffer, K.; Bertolini, L.; Guastavino, C. Activity as a mediator between users and their auditory environment in an urban pocket park: A case study of Parc du Portugal (Montreal, Canada). In *Handbook of Research on Perception-Driven Approaches to Urban Assessment and Design*; Aletta, F., Xiao, J., Eds.; IGI Global: Hershey, PA, USA, 2018; pp. 100–125.
16. Prato, P. Music in the streets: The example of Washington Square Park in New York City. *Pop. Music* **1984**, *4*, 151–163. [CrossRef]
17. Aucouturier, J.J.; Defreville, B.; Pachet, F. The bag-of-frames approach to audio pattern recognition: A sufficient model for urban soundscapes but not for polyphonic music. *J. Acoust. Soc. Am.* **2007**, *122*, 881–891. [CrossRef] [PubMed]
18. Bild, E.; Pfeffer, K.; Coler, M.; Rubin, O.; Bertoloni, L. Public Space Users' Soundscape Evaluations in Relation to Their Activities. An Amsterdam-Based Study. *Front. Psychol.* **2018**. [CrossRef] [PubMed]
19. Labelle, B. *Acoustic Territories: Sound Culture and Everyday Life*; Bloomsbury Publishing: New York, NY, USA, 2010.
20. Stansfeld, S.; Haines, M.; Brown, B. Noise and health in the urban environment. *Rev. Environ. Health* **2000**, *15*, 43–82. [CrossRef] [PubMed]
21. Yang, W.; Kang, J. Soundscape and sound preferences in urban squares: A case study in Sheffield. *J. Urban Des.* **2007**, *10*, 61–80. [CrossRef]
22. Mehrabian, A.; Russell, J.A. *An Approach to Environmental Psychology*; The MIT Press: Cambridge, MA, USA, 1974.
23. Ba, H.; Zhang, X.; Kang, J. On the influence of square dance in the park on the evaluation of soundscape. *Urban. Archit.* **2017**, *20*, 9–12.
24. Yang, W.; Kang, J. Acoustic comfort evaluation in urban open public spaces. *Appl. Acoust.* **2005**, *66*, 211–229. [CrossRef]
25. Schulte-Fortkamp, B.; Nitsch, W. On soundscapes and their meaning regarding noise annoyance measurements. In *INTERNOISE*; New Zealand Acoustical Society: Auckland, New Zealand, 1999; Volume 3, pp. 1387–1394.
26. Kang, J.; Aletta, F.; Margaritis, E.; Yang, M. A model for implementing soundscape maps in smart cities. *Noise Mapp.* **2018**, *5*, 46–59. [CrossRef]
27. Axelsson, Ö.; Nilsson, M.E.; Berglund, B. A principal components model of soundscape perception. *J. Acoust. Soc. Am.* **2010**, *128*, 2836–2846. [CrossRef] [PubMed]
28. Maculewicz, J.; Erkut, C.; Serafin, S. How can soundscapes affect the preferred walking pace? *Appl. Acoust.* **2016**, *114*, 230–239. [CrossRef]
29. Davies, W.J.; Adams, M.D.; Bruce, N.S.; Cain, R.; Carlyle, A.; Cusack, P.; Hall, D.A.; Hume, K.I.; Irwin, A.; Jennings, P.; et al. Perception of soundscapes: An interdisciplinary approach. *Appl. Acoust.* **2013**, *74*, 224–231. [CrossRef]

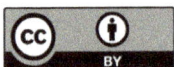

© 2019 by the authors. Licensee MDPI, Basel, Switzerland. This article is an open access article distributed under the terms and conditions of the Creative Commons Attribution (CC BY) license (http://creativecommons.org/licenses/by/4.0/).

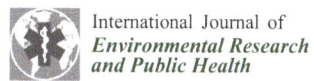

Article

On the Person-Place Interaction and Its Relationship with the Responses/Outcomes of Listeners of Urban Soundscape (Compared Cases of Lisbon and Bogotá): Contextual and Semiotic Aspects

Luis Hermida [1,2,*], Ignacio Pavón [1], Antonio Carlos Lobo Soares [3,4] and J. Luis Bento-Coelho [3]

1. Department of Mechanical Engineering, Escuela Técnica Superior de Ingenieros Industriales, Universidad Politécnica de Madrid, 28006 Madrid, Spain; ignacio.pavon@upm.es
2. Faculty of Engineering, Universidad de San Buenaventura-Bogotá, 110141 Bogotá, Colombia
3. Instituto Superior Técnico, University of Lisbon, 1049-001 Lisboa, Portugal; lobosoares@hotmail.com (A.C.L.S.); bcoelho@ist.utl.pt (J.L.B.-C.)
4. Ministério da Ciência, Tecnologia, Inovações e Comunicações, Museu Paraense Emílio Goeldi, 66.040-170 Belém, Pará, Brazil
* Correspondence: lhermida@usbbog.edu.co; Tel.: +57-320-818-5317

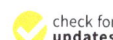

Received: 26 December 2018; Accepted: 12 February 2019; Published: 14 February 2019

Abstract: Design, planning, and management of the urban soundscape require various interacting fields of knowledge given the fact that it is the human person that experiences and provides meaning to the urban places and their acoustic environments. The process of environmental perception involves contextual information that conditions people's responses and outcomes through the relationship between the variables Person, Activity, and Place. This research focuses on the interaction between Person and Place and its impact on responses and outcomes from listeners with different geographical origin and background. Laboratory studies were conducted in the cities of Lisbon (Portugal) and Bogotá (Colombia), where local listeners were introduced to known and unknown acoustic environments. Sound data recorded in the two cities allowed comparison of responses and outcomes of the listeners according to the Person-Place Interaction, leading to different meanings depending on the contextual variables. The results clearly show a relationship between site, acoustic environment, soundscape, Person-Place Interaction, and meaning of the place. This information can be useful for urban technicians and designers dealing with planning and management of urban soundscapes.

Keywords: urban environments; soundscape; semiosis model

1. Introduction

The traditional approach to environmental acoustics management has mainly revolved around the control of sound energy levels, according to criteria established by governmental environmental agencies in each country. Nonetheless, considering the impact of the acoustics environments on people's health and life quality [1–5], and the need to promote and preserve quiet areas [6,7], the conventional approach has had to broaden its scope and to redirect the focus where the human being is considered the center [8–15], which has led to the strengthening of the soundscape concept.

Soundscape only exist through human perception, therefore its study, evaluation, and design require an interdisciplinary work, where in addition to dealing with aspects of characterization of the acoustic environment, it is also necessary to analyze the way human beings perceive and understand their acoustic environment [1,16,17]. Therefore, in order to approach the soundscape concept, research has been conducted in different lines, such as the description and classification of different taxonomic aspects of acoustic environments [1,18,19] and to determine acoustic descriptors and perceptual models that may prove useful in the assessment of soundscapes [20–25].

Regarding the perceptual processes, they are mediated by sociocultural and psychological aspects which in turn are conditioned by context [26,27]. In the conceptual framework proposed in the standard ISO 12913-1, the context influences the sound sources, the auditory sensation, and the cognitive process, thereby conditioning the person's responses and outcomes [28,29]. Given the preceding, it can be determined that the design, management, and planning of soundscape not only comprises aspects of design and engineering, but also encompasses a different kind of view based on ecological perception, environmental experience, and communication.

Under an ecological approach, human beings have a direct relation with their environment [30,31], where they find a varied affordance of stimuli that trigger a high number of physiological and psychological aspects, allowing them to collect and obtain information about their surrounding environment. This information enables experiencing sensations or emotions and consequently determines a response [32]. Likewise, a relation can be established between the social psychology approach and the perceptual model of soundscape in the standard ISO 12913-1, due to the fact that responses and outcomes represent, respectively, attitudes (referring to the degree to which people tend to judge aspects of reality) and behaviors (considered the set of responses or decisions resulting from the relation between the people and the environment) of the human being [33,34]. In other words, during one's immersion in an acoustic environment, human attitudes are generated (e.g., how quiet, pleasant or annoying is the place) and from there actions follow (e.g., perform a specific activity or decide to leave the place).

Regarding the process of environmental experience, Herranz-Pascual et al. have been developing work in the soundscape field following this approach, proposing a model of environmental experience for studying soundscape, based in the psychological process of environmental experience [32,34–36]. This model comprises three fundamental aspects: *Person*, *Activity*, and *Place*. These three elements generate four entities that can influence the experience of the acoustic environment: *Person*, *Activity*, *Place* and *Person-Place Interaction*. Nevertheless, taking the model of environmental experience of soundscapes to an effective practice of evaluation and design involve many variables (e.g., security, climate, previous experiences, place function, urban aspects, visual and olfactory stimuli, etc.), so it is necessary to determine which variables are the most influential in the environmental sound experience, as well as establishing processes and procedures for this type of analysis. Currently, most studies in this field focus on the influence of alternative stimuli to sound [35,37–43], detecting that one of the most influential stimulus in the perception of the acoustic environment is the vision. With regard to the study of contextual elements related to the *Person-Place Interaction*, reference is made in the cross-national comparison in assessment of urban park soundscapes, in the analysis and assessment of soundscapes in commonly used sightseeing sites (comparison between tourists and non-tourists), as well as comparison between responses of experts and non-experts [27,44–46].

Conversely, according to Blauert "the behavior of human beings is not guided directly by the acoustical signals that we provide them with, e.g., like a reflex, but rather by the "meaning" which is transferred via these signals" [47], which implies that acoustic environments also carry an important informational load when they are considered as "carrier" of meaning. In semiotics, the science of signs and languages, a sign can be defined as the mental representation processed as a reference of something else [48–50]. The study of urban environments under this approach has allowed analyzing the impact of different kind of information (mainly visual) in the identity of the place and the acquired meaning depending on the context of the person [51–54]. Now consider the question: What is the meaning that designers, administrators, and urban planners want to convey to people from acoustic environments? Note that the meaning depends on the repertoire and context of the listener, thus the study of contextual variables in the formation of meaning of acoustic environments becomes necessary.

Considering that: (1) A direct interaction between the person and the acoustic environment generates an *environmental experience*, when responses and outputs are mediated by the context, and (2) that acoustic environments can be analyzed as carrier of meaning that also depends on the context, this research seeks to deepen in the study of the relationship between the responses (attitudes) and outcomes (behaviors) of the listeners and the contextual element *Person-Place Interaction*, as well as to analyze the importance of semiotic aspects in the design, management, and assessment process of soundscapes. For this purpose, laboratory tests were developed in the cities of Lisbon (Portugal) and Bogotá (Colombia), where data on acoustic environments were presented to two groups of listeners from their own city and from a city that they haven't previously experienced. Differences were found in the *outcomes* according to the origin places of the listeners, allowing to establish a relationship between the use of places, their meaning (or lack of it) and the soundscapes.

2. Method

2.1. Sites of Study

Considering that the objective of this work was not to compare the acoustic environments of two different cities, but to analyze the responses and outcomes of people according to the variable Place-Person and its impact on the formation of meaning, eight places were chosen from the cities of Bogotá and Lisbon. The site selection was aimed at capturing the city's diverse acoustic environments, including high-speed road, city center, square with a water source, urban parks, and quiet areas.

The sites in Lisbon consisted of urban public places of great recognition among the inhabitants:

- Jardim da Estrela (LJES),
- Jardim da Fundação Calouste Gulbenkian (LJFG),
- Jardim do Príncipe Real (LJPR).

The selected sites in Bogotá were:

- Autopista norte estación Alcalá (BOAPA),
- Calle 19 con Cra. 7 (BOC197),
- Fuente de agua edificio Tequendama (BOFAET),
- Plaza de Lourdes (BOPL),
- Simón Bolívar park (BOPSB).

The Lisbon sites have different uses, characteristics, and locations, with urban areas of 7.5 ha (LJFG), 4.6 ha (LJES) and 1.15 ha (LJPR). They feature water fountains, diverse vegetation, children playgrounds, good infrastructure, cleanliness, security, and are located in privileged areas of the city, surrounded by buildings of aligned storefronts with a maximum of six floor-to-ceiling-height, where noise (traffic, road, and aerial) can be perceived by the inhabitants. Like the Lisbon sites, the Bogotá sites offer a great diversity of acoustic environments, presented the most important roadway of the city (BOAPA); the downtown area (with vehicular traffic and street vendors) (BOC197); a square with a water fountain (BOFAET); one of the most representative squares of the city of Bogotá (BOPL) and one of the largest urban parks in South America with 113 ha (BOPSB). Figure 1a–h depict the urban spaces in Lisbon and Bogotá.

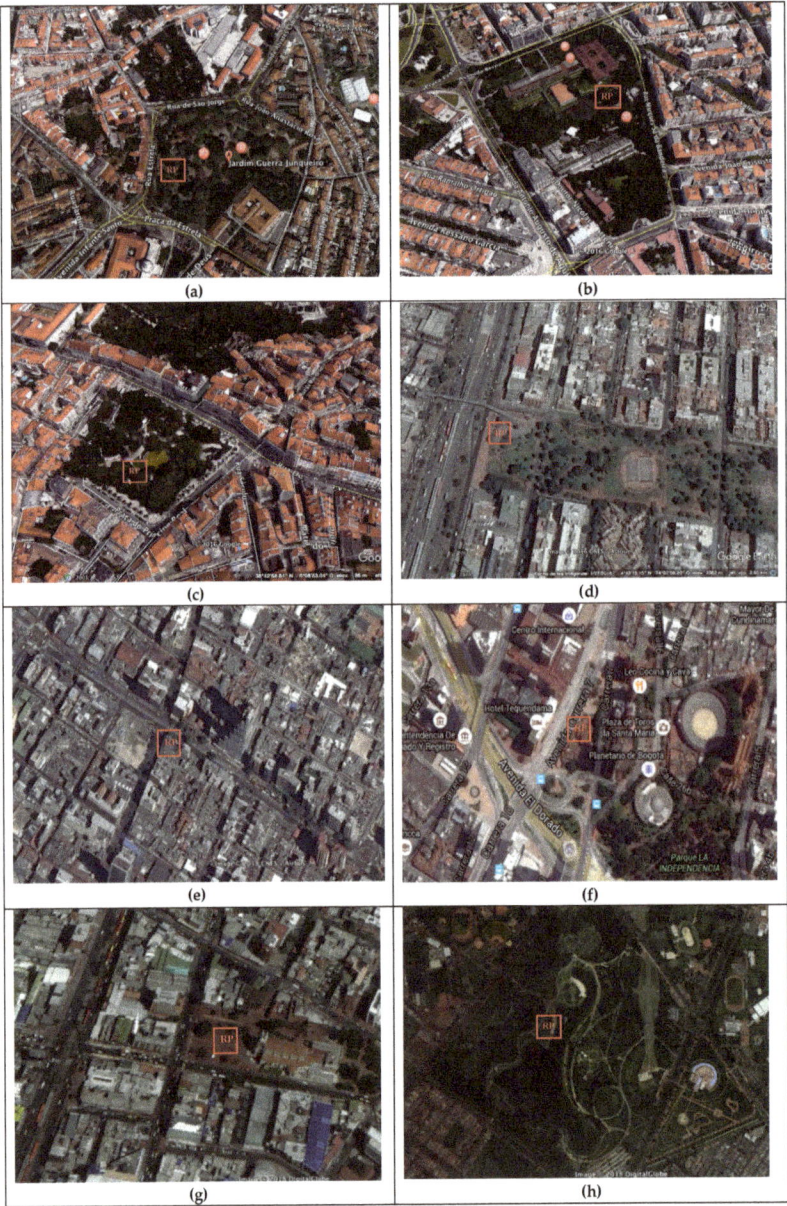

Figure 1. Urban Spaces in Lisbon and Bogotá cities. (**a**) Jardim da Estrela (LJES); (**b**) Jardim da Fundação Calouste Gulbenkian (LJFG); (**c**) Jardim do Príncipe Real (LJPR); (**d**) Autopista norte estación Alcalá (BOAPA); (**e**) Calle 19 con Cra. 7 (BOC197); (**f**) Fuente de agua edificio Tequendama (BOFAET); (**g**) Plaza de Lourdes (BOPL); (**h**) Simón Bolívar park (BOPSB).

As the analysis of the human perception of acoustic environments is required for soundscape studies, binaural recordings were made. This type of recordings allow an image of the spatial distribution of the sound sources, and generate sound immersion in the listeners [55–58]. While each recording is unique and unrepeatable due to the renewable temporal characteristics of the acoustic environments, it was sought that each recording would present to the listeners sounds of the most common and representative activities in each place. For this purpose, prior to the recording process, the places under study were visited, to gather *in-situ* information on the usual on-going activities. These data were used in the process of selection and edition of the audio fragments presented to the listeners in the laboratory test.

A portable binaural recording system was used with the purpose of not interfering with the free development of everyday activities or to draw the passers-by's attention to foreign elements oblivious to their daily lives (e.g., binaural heads). The recordings were made in each place at fixed points parallel to the main sound sources, each with a duration of 15 min.

2.2. Descriptive Aspects of the Acoustic Environments

Keynote sounds were used to analyze some descriptive aspects of the acoustic environments. This concept refers to sounds that are continually heard or that have a constant presence strong in the acoustic environment [59]. To identify the keynote sounds of the eight places, the subjective test included a list of sounds, and participants were asked to indicate how dominant they perceived each one. The response options were "non-dominant", "little dominant", "moderately dominant", "very dominant" and "totally dominant" and each option corresponds to values of −1, −0.5, 0, 0.5 and 1 respectively.

Although the objective of this work focuses on deepening the study of contextual and semiotic aspects in management and planning processes of urban soundscapes, it was considered relevant to include an acoustic indicator to complement descriptive aspects of the acoustic environments. In this study, the equivalent continuous A-weighted sound pressure level L_{Aeq} was used, since it is a widely sound descriptor and shows good correlations with perceptual attributes as pleasant and comfort [21,24,57,60,61].

2.3. Subjective Evaluation

The work focuses on the analysis of the influence of the *Person-Place Interaction* with input variables such as responses and outcomes. For this purpose, a test was applied where listeners evaluated unknown sites and places with which they had interacted. Figure 2 describes the general design of the subjective tests.

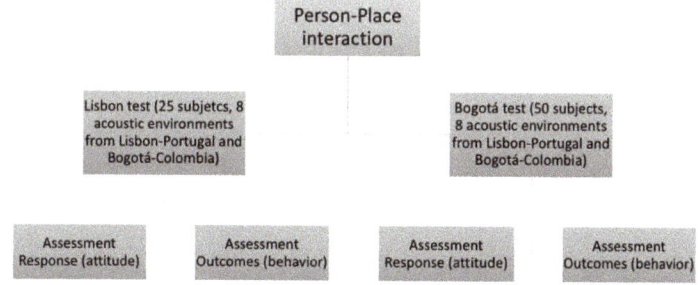

Figure 2. General design of the subjective evaluation test.

The laboratory tests were attended by 75 listeners (25 in Lisbon and 50 in Bogotá), in line with other similar previous works [62,63], all aged between 18 and 60 years old. The participants knew the places of their respective cities and had advanced knowledge in the acoustics field (sound engineering students and professors from Universidad de San Buenaventura-Bogotá and students and professors of the architecture and acoustics from Instituto Superior Técnico, University of Lisbon). No distinction is made between experts and non-experts because the interaction of listeners with acoustic environments can generate a natural process of training of the listeners mediated by context [46]. All participants contributed voluntarily to the test and were informed in writing and orally about the research's objectives and methodology. They also authorized the use of the collected information for strictly academic purposes.

From the fifteen minutes of the binaural recording obtained in each location, thirty seconds of audio for each urban acoustic environment in study were selected. For the audio edition, the information obtained in the previous visits and sound walks to each place was considered, trying that the audio samples represented some of the observed activities. Eight audio fragments of 30 seconds duration corresponding to the sites were then presented to each listener, with a maximum total duration of 15 min. The time length of each audio fragment was chosen taking into account previously works (which presented audios between 6 seconds and 1 min [20,21,38,46,64–68]) and sound quality recommendations (tests were designed of 30 min maximum concerning the importance of not tiring the listener [62,63,69]). The playback order was randomized for each tested subject to avoid bias by playing order [63]. The listeners played each sample at a time and responded to the different questions of the test according to the self-paced methodology. The separation between each audio fragment varied between one minute and one minute and a half depending on the speed of response of the participants. Headphones were used by the listeners. Both the recording and the playback systems were duly calibrated, using an artificial head to ensure that the sound pressure levels presented to the listeners were as close as possible to those they would perceive at the recording location (see Figure 3). The tests were carried out in the recording studios of the Universidad San Buenaventura, Bogotá and in the anechoic chamber of the Instituto Superior Técnico (IST), Lisbon, University of Lisbon.

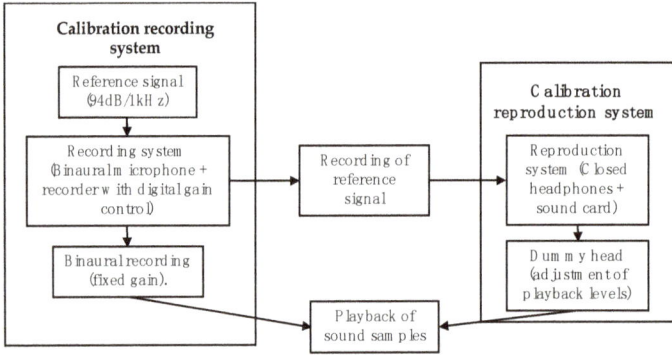

Figure 3. Calibration process diagram for the recording and reproduction of acoustic environments in laboratory test.

The subjective test was divided into two parts, the first related to the responses (attitudes) and the second related to the outcomes (behaviors) according to the model depicted in the depicted in the ISO 12913-1 standard. For the assessment of responses Axelsson's model was used, considering the eight perceptual attributes: *pleasant, chaotic, exciting, uneventful, calm, annoying, eventful,* and *monotonous* [21,70,71]. These attributes allow the estimation of the main components of the ortho-normalized bidimensional model: *Pleasantness* and *Eventfulness* [71]. For the assessment of each attribute the technique of the semantic response scale (response scale) was followed asking the subjects "to what extent do you consider that the following eight factors describe the sound environment heard?". Each attribute had five levels of response: fully agree, partially agree, disagree, partially disagree, and strongly disagree. For the data processing, each of these levels took values between +1 to a step of 0.5, being +1 completely agree and −1 totally disagree. Considering that the participants' native language was Spanish and Portuguese, the Axelsson attributes were translated from English into Spanish and Portuguese. In the translation process, the eight attributes were considered as related (orthogonal model), so the words used in the test were the product of the combination of the two main components (Pleasantness and Eventfulness).

Concerning the outcomes (behaviors), this study deepened in the decisions that the listeners would take in a site with an acoustic environment like was presented in the audio sample. For this, questions related to the *Permanency Time* and the *Possible Use* were established. The permanency times were presented by ranges (less than 10 min, between 10 and 30 min, between 30 and 60 min, between 1 and 2 h, and more than two hours), while the possible uses were presented from a list of activities (physical activity, place of transit, contemplation, reading and meditation, general rest, and other activities).

For the data obtained from responses (attitudes), Shapiro-Wilk's normality tests were applied, finding that the data do not present a normal distribution. In the comparative study between Lisbon and Bogotá listeners, the data were analyzed on the basis of the U Mann-Whitney tests for numerical data (responses resulting from the evaluation of perceptual attributes) and contingency tables for nominal data (in the case of questions related to outcomes), where the Pearson's statistical significance Chi-square and the likelihood-ratio chi-square tests were carried out.

Finally, from the results obtained from the responses and outputs of the evaluators, a discussion is proposed in the light of the anthropological concept of "non-places" [72], as well as semiotic aspects (Use-Meaning relationship) and models of semiosis based on the Peirce model [50].

3. Results

3.1. Keynote Sounds and Sound Pressure Levels

Table 1 presents information on the keynote sounds and the L_{Aeq} of the different places under study. Regarding the keynote sounds of the eight places, both Lisbon and Bogota evaluators determined that the keynote sounds are road traffic for the BOAPA and BOC197 places, sounds of nature for LJFG and BOPSB, the human voice for LJES and LJPR, and the water source for the BOFAET. Only BOPL presented differences for the keynote sounds between the evaluators of Bogota and Lisbon, where the panel of Bogotá considered that the keynote sound of this space is speech, while the panel of Lisbon considered that the keynote sound of this space it's road traffic.

Table 1. Keynote sound and L_{Aeq} of the acoustic environments in study.

Place	City	Keynote Sound	L_{Aeq} (dBA)
LJES	Bogotá Lisbon	Speech (mean value 0.57 and 88% of detection) Speech (mean value 0.54 and 84% of detection)	65.6
LJFG	Bogotá Lisbon	Nature (mean value 0.43 and 80% of detection) Nature (mean value 0.46 and 76% of detection)	58.4
LJPR	Bogotá Lisbon	Speech (mean value 0.49 and 78% of detection) Speech (mean value 0.38 and 60% of detection)	56.6
BOAPA	Bogotá Lisbon	Road Traffic (mean value 0.66 and 96% of detection) Road Traffic (mean value 0.70 and 96% of detection)	63.9
BOC197	Bogotá Lisbon	Road Traffic (mean value 0.94 and 100% of detection) Road Traffic (mean value 0.94 and 100% of detection)	74.6
BOFAET	Bogotá Lisbon	Water (mean value 0.80 and 93% of detection) Water (mean value 0.90 and 100% of detection)	75.4
BOPL	Bogotá Lisbon	Speech (mean value 0.56 and 88% of detection) Road Traffic (mean value 0.50 and 92% of detection)	68.7
BOPSB	Bogotá Lisbon	Nature (mean value 0.50 and 80% of detection) Nature (mean value 0.42 and 68% of detection)	51.4

Regarding the sound pressure levels, the table shows that those with higher levels are BOFAET (75.4 dBA and keynote sound water) and BOC197 (74.6 dBA and keynote sound road traffic), while the lowest levels are from the BOPSB (51.4 dBA and keynote sound of nature) and LJPR (56.6 dBA and keynote sound of speech). It can be seen that the higher levels do not correspond only to places with keynote sound of road traffic, as well as the places with the lowest L_{Aeq} does not correspond only to the keynote sound of nature.

3.2. Listeners' Responses

Differences between Lisbon and Bogotá Responses

Figure 4a,b present the results obtained for the eight attributes of the Axelsson model, as well as for the general assessment according to the place of origin of the evaluators. It is possible to appreciate differences according to the listener's Test Site for attributes such as Exciting, Monotonous, Eventful, Annoying, among others, although to determine if these differences are statistically significant it is necessary to apply the U Mann-Whitney nonparametric test. Table 2 presents these results.

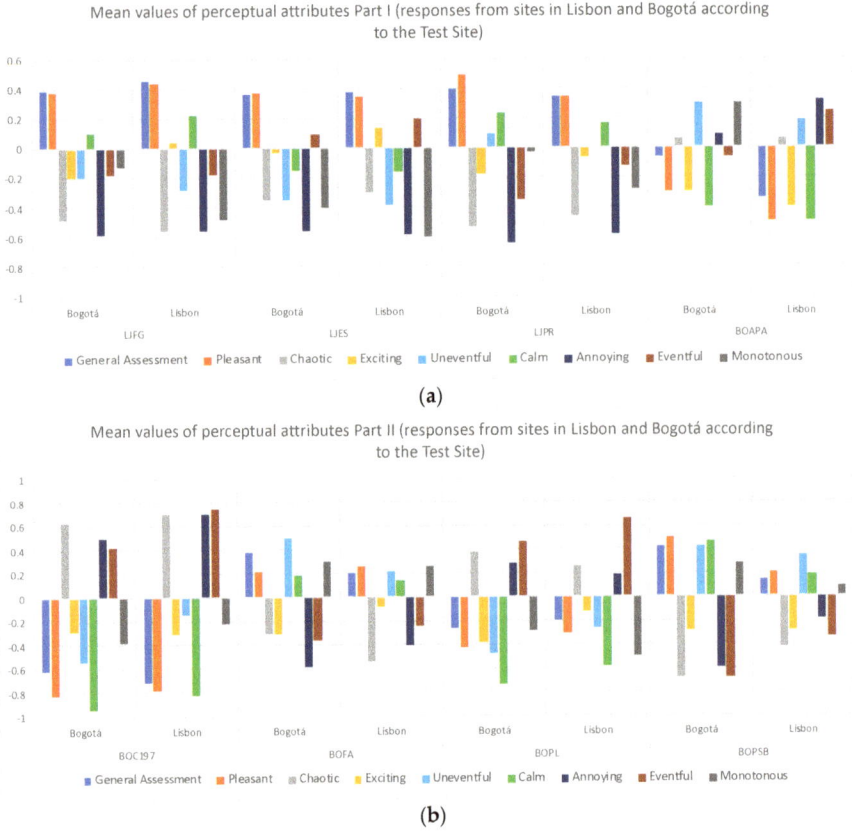

Figure 4. (a) Mean values of perceptual attributes Part I (responses from sites in Lisbon and Bogotá according to the listener's Test Site); (b) Mean values of perceptual attributes Part II (responses from sites in Lisbon and Bogotá according to the listener's Test Site).

Table 2. Results of the U Mann-Whitney test with α = 0.05 for evaluators from Bogotá and from Lisbon. Green values represent statistically significant differences in the responses according to listener origin. Shaded values represent the highest average rank value between listeners in Bogotá and Lisbon.

Place	Statistics	General Assessment	Pleasant	Chaotic	Exciting	Uneventful	Calm	Annoying	Eventful	Monotonous
LJFG	U	540.0	537.0	577.5	437.5	577.5	535.5	620.0	625.0	338.0
	p value	0.282	0.286	0.571	0.024	0.575	0.281	0.952	1.000	0.001
	Mean Rank Bogotá	36.30	36.24	38.95	34.25	38.95	36.21	37.90	38.00	43.74
	Mean Rank Lisbon	41.40	41.52	36.10	45.50	36.10	41.58	38.20	38.00	26.52
LJES	U	597.0	624.5	594.5	497.0	612.5	615.0	622.5	570.0	499.5
	p value	0.731	0.995	0.722	0.126	0.882	0.906	0.976	0.504	0.128
	Mean Rank Bogotá	37.44	38.01	37.39	35.44	38.25	38.20	38.05	36.90	40.51
	Mean Rank Lisbon	39.12	37.98	39.22	43.12	37.50	37.60	37.90	40.20	32.98
LJPR	U	569.0	500.5	530.0	542.0	569.5	550.0	543.0	469.0	433.5
	p value	0.474	0.137	0.258	0.324	0.517	0.375	0.319	0.068	0.025
	Mean Rank Bogotá	39.12	40.49	36.10	36.34	39.11	39.50	36.36	34.88	41.83
	Mean Rank Lisbon	35.76	33.02	41.80	41.32	35.78	35.00	41.28	44.24	30.34
BOAPA	U	207.5	258.0	309.5	278.5	271.5	293.0	237.0	212.0	218.0
	p value	0.030	0.265	0.951	0.489	0.395	0.690	0.127	0.040	0.058
	Mean Rank Bogotá	29.70	27.68	25.62	26.86	27.14	26.28	22.48	21.48	29.28
	Mean Rank Lisbon	21.30	23.32	25.38	24.14	23.86	24.72	28.52	29.52	21.72
BOC197	U	278.5	280.5	302.5	306.5	193.5	229.5	222.5	204.5	256.5
	p value	0.466	0.463	0.830	0.904	0.017	0.025	0.055	0.022	0.261
	Mean Rank Bogotá	26.86	24.22	25.10	25.74	20.74	22.18	21.90	21.18	23.26
	Mean Rank Lisbon	24.14	26.78	25.90	25.26	30.26	28.82	29.10	29.82	27.74
BOFA	U	264.0	288.5	244.5	243.0	243.5	285.0	247.0	264.5	303.5
	p value	0.317	0.613	0.168	0.156	0.160	0.580	0.165	0.332	0.856
	Mean Rank Bogotá	27.44	24.54	28.22	22.72	28.26	26.60	22.88	23.58	25.86
	Mean Rank Lisbon	23.56	26.46	22.78	28.28	22.74	24.40	28.12	27.42	25.14
BOPL	U	286.5	269.5	268.5	229.5	242.5	236.5	276.5	230.5	242.5
	p value	0.595	0.375	0.371	0.095	0.151	0.100	0.467	0.075	0.154
	Mean Rank Bogotá	24.46	23.78	27.26	22.18	22.70	22.46	26.94	22.22	28.3
	Mean Rank Lisbon	26.54	27.22	23.74	28.82	28.30	28.54	24.06	28.78	22.70
BOPSB	U	208.5	213.5	203.5	305.5	263.5	218.5	196.0	183.0	233.0
	p value	0.034	0.045	0.025	0.887	0.314	0.057	0.019	0.008	0.108
	Mean Rank Bogotá	29.66	29.46	21.14	25.22	27.46	29.26	20.84	20.32	28.68
	Mean Rank Lisbon	21.34	21.54	29.86	25.78	23.54	21.74	30.16	30.68	22.32

For the LJFG site, statistically significant differences were found only for the *Exciting* and *Monotonous* attributes and according to the mean rank values: the Lisbon listeners considered this place more Exciting, while evaluators from Colombia rated it as Monotonous. The LJES site did not show statistically significant differences in any perceptual attribute, while the LJPR site showed statistically significant difference only in the *Monotonous* attribute (judged as more *Monotonous* in Bogotá than in Lisbon).

Regarding the Colombian sites, the BOAPA presents statistically significant differences in the *General Assessment* and in the *Eventful* attribute (a better General Assessment was found in Bogotá though it was judged more Agitated by the Lisbon listeners). The BOC197 site presented statistically significant differences in the *Uneventful, Calm, Annoying,* and *Eventful* attributes (higher mean rank values were found in the evaluations in Lisbon for the four attributes), while the sites BOFA and BOPL did not present statistically significant differences in none of their attributes. Finally, the BOPSB site was the one with the highest number of attributes with statistically significant differences in *The General Assessment, Pleasant, Chaotic, Annoying,* and *Eventful* (mean rank values in *General assessment* and *Pleasant* were found by Bogotá listeners, while higher mean ranks values were found in *Chaotic, Annoying,* and *Eventful* by Lisbon listeners).

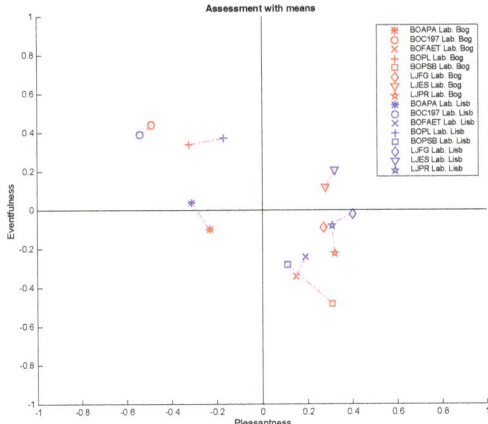

Figure 5. Application of Axelsson's two-dimensional model. In red, places evaluated in Bogotá-Colombia. In blue, places evaluated in Lisbon-Portugal.

Figure 5 presents the Cartesian representation of the Axelsson's model according to the evaluations carried out in Lisbon and Bogotá. One can see that, although small shifts are found in the x and y axes for the different places under study according to their Test Site, the shifts are not considerable. In fact, only one of the eight places under study (BOAPA) showed a slight change of quadrant, represented in the change of the main component Eventfulness.

3.3. Outcomes: Permanency Time and Possible Uses

Figure 6a,b and Figure 7a,b show the outcomes of the evaluators, represented in the hypothetic *Permanency Time* and the *Possible Uses* of Bogotá and Lisbon listeners in sites with acoustic environments such as those that are presented in the recordings. There are some notable differences according to the place of origin of the listener in the outcome *Permanency Time*, as in BOC197 where for the seventy-six percent of the listeners in Lisbon it would only be less than 10 min, compared to the forty-nine percent of listeners from Bogotá that would be that same amount of time. However, in BOAPA or LJPR these differences are not so simple to appreciate. Regarding the *Possible Uses*, the LJFG results reveal differences between the listeners in Lisbon and in Bogotá, but similarly to the variable Permanency Time, in places such as BOAPA or BOFAET differences are not easily appreciated regarding the listener's place of origin. To determine whether these differences are statistically significant, the Pearson's statistical significance Chi-square and the likelihood-ratio Chi-square tests were applied. The results are depicted in Table 3.

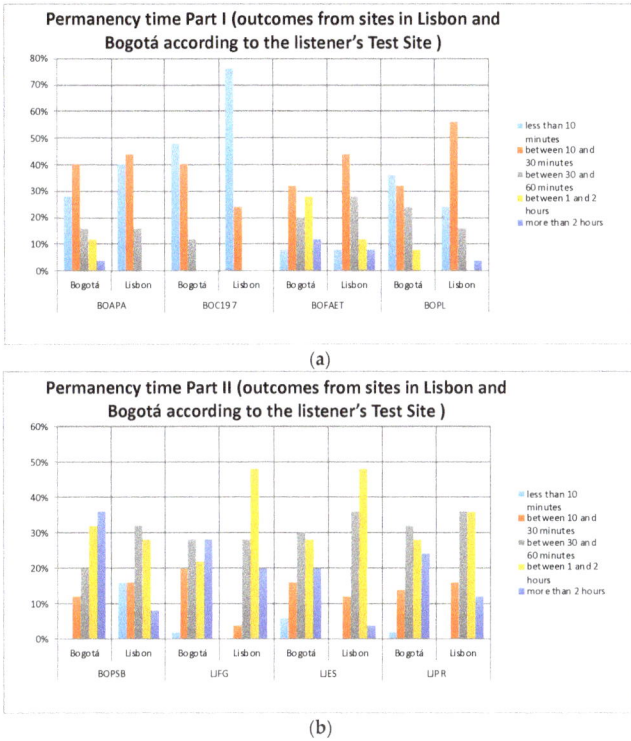

Figure 6. (**a**) Outcomes: permanency time of the listener according to test sites in Lisbon and Bogotá places (Part I); (**b**) Outcomes: permanency time of the listener according to test sites in Lisbon and Bogotá places (Part II).

Table 3. X^2 and the likelihood-ratio tests with a $\alpha = 0.05$ for the eight soundscapes for both the evaluators from Bogotá and from Lisbon. Green values represent statistically significant association between the outcomes and the listener origin.

Test Site		Permanency Time			Possible Use		
	Statistics	Value	df	p Value (2-Sided)	Value	df	p Value (2-Sided)
BOAPA	X^2	4.577	4	0.376	3.026(a)	4	0.77
	Likelihood Ratio	6.125	4	0.301	3.818	4	0.77
BOC197	X^2	5.581	2	0.056	6.364(a)	2	0.05
	Likelihood Ratio	6.764	2	0.044	8.682	2	0.05
BOFA	X^2	2.607	4	0.643	11.493(a)	6	0.05
	Likelihood Ratio	2.658	4	0.658	13.66	6	0.051
BOPL	X^2	5.636	4	0.198	11.026(a)	4	0.008
	Likelihood Ratio	6.823	4	0.181	15.275	4	0.006
BOPSB	X^2	9.356	4	0.049	10.273(a)	6	0.094
	Likelihood Ratio	11.272	4	0.038	11.785	6	0.093
LJFG	X^2	7.504	4	0.096	22.646(a)	6	0
	Likelihood Ratio	8.3	4	0.086	24.59	6	0.001
LJES	X^2	6.701	4	0.155	25.736(a)	6	0
	Likelihood Ratio	8.239	4	0.11	28.267	6	0
LJPR	X^2	2.173	4	0.773	17.942(a)	6	0.004
	Likelihood Ratio	2.584	4	0.74	18.474	6	0.009

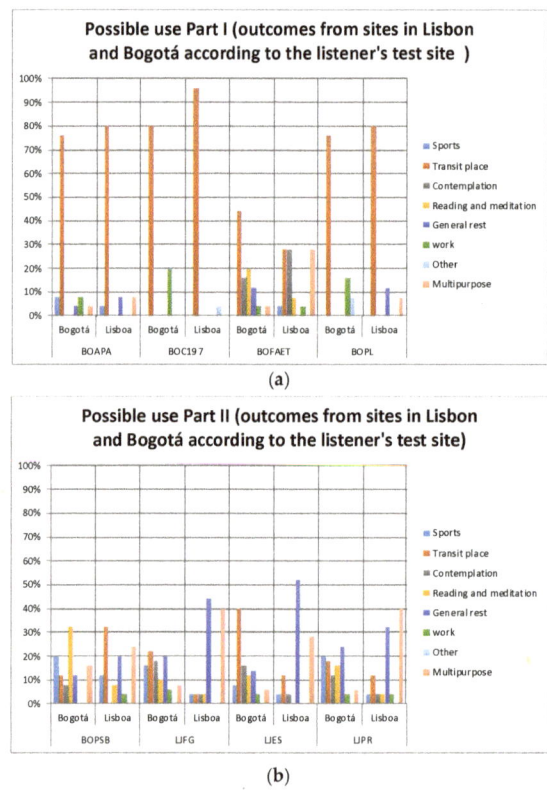

Figure 7. (**a**) Possible use that might be given by the evaluators in places with acoustic environments such as the ones presented in the recordings (Part I); (**b**) Possible use that might be given by the evaluators in places with acoustic environments such as the ones presented in the recordings (Part II).

Regarding the *Permanency Time*, of the eight test sites under study, only two revealed a statistically significant association between the listener's Test Site and this variable in particular. Evaluators from Bogotá would stay longer in the BOC197 and BOPSB sites than Lisbon evaluators.

As for the *Possible Use*, five of the eight sites under study showed a statistically significant association between this variable and the listener's Test Site. It is interesting to note that of the three sites that did not show a statistically significant association between the variables listener's Test Site and Possible Uses, two can be considered common places in any city (a water fountain in BOFAET and a BOAPA highway), while the third one, the BOPSB park, does not present an association between these variables, though as mentioned before, this site shows an association between the variables of *Permanency Time* and listener's Test Site.

Carrying on with the analysis of the variables *Possible Use* and Listener's *Test Site* variables, the results allow the appreciation of a second group of sites (the Lisbon LJFG, LJES, and LJPR places, and the BOC197 and BOPL Bogotá places), which do present statistically significant association between the variables Test Site and Possible Use. Although the BOPL site has the highest percentages for Transit Site within the variable Possible Use for the two evaluation sites (76% in Bogotá and 80% in Lisbon), evaluators from Bogotá would also use this site for Work, while evaluators from Lisbon would use it for General Rest. The same phenomenon was also found for the BOC197 site. In the LJFG site, strong differences were found, given that responses of the Lisbon listeners showing that this site would be used mainly as a place of General Rest and a Multipurpose place, while in Bogotá the main percentages were scattered between Place of Transit, General Rest, and Contemplation. Similar results were found for the LJES site, where the evaluations of Lisbon show the use to be mainly related to General Rest, while once again in Bogotá it would be used mainly as a Site of Transit. Finally, the LJPR site for the evaluators of Lisbon would be used mostly as a Multipurpose place and General Resting place, while in Bogotá it would be used as a place of Transit and a General Resting site as well.

4. Discussion

The discussion herein is based on descriptive aspects of the acoustic environments, Person-Place interaction and contextual as well as semiotic aspects. The results show that the listeners of the two countries identified the same keynote sounds for seven out of the eight places under study. This may mean that, for the cases under study, the possibility of identifying the keynote sound is not affected by the Person-Place relationship. However, it is interesting that although no differences were found in this descriptive aspect, some differences in responses and outcomes were found according to the place of origin of the listener. This may indicate that one thing is the ability to detect and identify the keynote sound of the acoustic environments and another is the meaning that is given to them by the listeners (meaning that is mediated by the context).

Likewise, while it is clear that high levels of L_{Aeq} affect people's health (which implies that a first step for urban acoustic management is the control and reduction of these sound levels), not necessarily low energy levels may ensure a longer permanency time in places, or a specific use (outcomes). For example, BOFAET presented the highest values of L_{Aeq}, but it was a place where most people would be between 10 and 30 min. However, the places with higher L_{Aeq} if they were considered more annoying by the listeners what agrees with previous findings, where parameters associated with energy levels influence the degree of comfort and/or discomfort [21,25,57,61,73].

Moreover, three out of the eight sites under test presented statistically significant differences for the variable *Responses* (perceptual attributes) according to the listener's *Test Site* in the *Eventful* perceptual attribute, while the *Monotonous*, *Calm*, and *Unpleasant* attributes presented significant differences in only two sites. The general assessment also presented differences in two places, while attributes such as *Pleasant*, *Chaotic*, *Exciting* and *Uneventful* only showed statistically significant differences in one of the sites under study. As previously discussed, these eight components directly impact the estimation of the main components Eventfulness and Pleasantness of Axelsson's model. Therefore, if there are few associations between the listeners' Test Site and the perceptual attributes, there will be little impact on the cartesian representation by quadrants on this model.

Since the variable *Test Site* implies a previous knowledge of the places by the people involved in the experiments, there is, consequently, an interaction between Person and Test Site (activities and characteristics), hence it can be said that, under the conditions of these tests, there is a relation between the *responses* (attitudinal aspects) and the *Person-Place Interaction*. Therefore, from previous knowledge and experiences in places, it is possible to generate differences in listeners' responses (e.g., for the LJFG place, Lisbon listeners considered it as more Exciting, while evaluators from Colombia rated it as Monotonous).

Regarding the *Outcomes* (Permanency Time and Possible use) and place of testing, it was found that five out of the eight sites under study had an association between the variables *Test Site* and the *Possible Uses*, although only two were dependent on the variables *listener's Test Site* and *Permanency Time*. These results show that, under the conditions proposed during the development of this experiment, the outcomes (or behaviors) have a dependency according to the Person-Place interaction. To better understand these results, the semiotics approach seems useful, where sites, usage, sound, and meaning have a direct relationship.

The meaning of the places depends on the use given to the places (meaning = use) [74], which is why users are able to read a place and assign it a meaning. Therefore, a place can be considered a "center of meaning" that feeds on the experiences and attachments of the people [75]. For this reason, it is not possible that representative places of each city (such as Lisbon and Bogotá parks) can have the same use and consequently the same meaning for evaluators of different countries, when the evaluators do not have previous knowledge, or have not used these places or do not have the same practices and activities. In view of the above, although it is true that the recordings of the acoustic environment provide an idea of the activities and practices developed on the place, the recordings do not yield information related to the use of the place according to the context, conveying information from the practices or activities that are common. The *Person-Place Interaction* is the product of the direct experience of the person, which generates memories and previous background that raise the expectations about the activities to be carried out in such place. Under laboratory conditions and without such previous experiences, the listeners will associate the acoustic environments with experiences of their own, with places of different characteristics, which might generate a difference of "meanings" according to the place of origin of the listener.

Likewise, it is interesting to see the emergence of sites that can be considered common or mainstream to any city (a highway or a water fountain, for example), since there is no association between the variables *Possible Use* and the *Listener's Test Sites*, which means that its "meaning" is the same regardless of the Listener's Test Site. It is here that the concept of *"the non-place"* arises and becomes relevant. A place can be defined as "an identity, relational and historical site" so that a space that "can not be defined either as an identity, relational or historical site is considered a non-place" [72]. Bringing this concept to the soundscape field, acoustic environments that do not represent or generate identity, evoke a memory or awake some sense of belonging in the listener can be considered as *sonorous non-places*. To delve into this concept, two out of the eight cases presented in this study will be shown: the BOAPA site (north highway of Bogotá) and LJES site (urban park of the city of Lisbon).

The BOAPA site is the main highway of Bogotá and it communicates the Colombian capital with the north of the country. It crosses part of the city in south-north and north-south directions with around 14,000 vehicles transiting through it every hour (both directions are considered for this estimation). It should be noted, as a main feature of this specific highway, that part of its layout has exclusive lanes where biarticulated buses belonging to the Bogotá mass transportation system circulate. Summarizing, it is a common highway that, although located in Bogotá, Colombia, could also be anywhere else in the world. Its use is just like that of any other highway: a main road where vehicles circulate. It could be the perfect example of a *sonorous non-place*, given that the sound sources that compose it and the uses that are given to this space do not vary significantly depending on the city. When the association tests for the variables *Possible Use* and *Listener's Test Site* were applied, it was found that the use that would be given to an acoustic environment like the one presented in the recording, would be the Place of Transit both for the evaluators of Lisbon and for those of Bogotá. This implies that for the two groups of evaluators the place has the same use and therefore the same meaning, which exemplifies a sonorous non-place.

Conversely, the LJES park is located in the Lapa neighborhood of the city of Lisbon, built at the end of the 19th century. Its 4.6 hectares feature two lakes, children playgrounds, kiosks and equipment for physical exercise. In the lakes one can see ducks, swans and geese, and prowling around the garden a majestic peacock can sometimes be spotted. There is a kiosk that is usually used for philharmonic concert and overall enjoyment. One of its streets adjoins the Basilica da Estrela in Lisbon, a must see for tourists who can also get to the place on the legendary E28 wooden tram. In the summertime, concerts and picnics are common for tourists and residents. The binaural recordings presented to the evaluators registered the sound of the bells of the Estrela Basilica, the sounds of birds and nature, as well as the sound of public transportation. When the results for the variables *Possible Use* and *Listener's Test Site* were analyzed, it was found that they have a statistically significant association: while the people from Bogotá would identify it mostly as a Place of Transit, people from Lisbon would identify it as a General Resting place. Therefore, the results suggest in this case that the history and the direct contact with the place impact the perceived "meaning" and, due to the decontextualization of the evaluators of Bogotá, and the multiple "meanings" that can be assigned by the people of Lisbon, such "meanings" are very different depending on the listener's Test Site.

Contextual and Semiotic Aspects Applied to Urban Soundscapes Management, Design and Planning Processes

The cities are a reflex of their inhabitants and their culture, and thus different forms of expression can be found, represented by different languages. Therefore, every action potentially becomes a sign that will be deciphered by the people according to their repertoire and context. In this sense, the city speaks, transmits information [76], and the sonorous language is a powerful carrier of meaning. Since the acoustic environments are the product of practices and activities developed by people, the soundscape concept constitutes another approach for relating and understanding the city. The aim thus, in processes of design, planning, and management of urban spaces, consists of designing and implementing urban acoustic environments that carry coherent information to the people in order that they assign a meaning to the signs according to space.

Likewise, if a place acquires "meaning" according to its use, the "meaning" of the acoustic environment will be influenced by the *Person-Place Interaction* (contextual aspects). When performing an inverse exercise in design, planning and management processes, it is worth asking: what is the "Use-Meaning" of the place? This exercise involves the understanding of the semiotic process where three aspects, *Place*, *Acoustic Environment* and *Soundscape*, are related to the context to generate a "meaning", that is, it implies a semiosis model applied to urban soundscape.

Considering the concept of semiosis as a process of selection, organization, coordination, and structuring of the items of perception and objects of experience [48], Figure 8 depicts the core of a semiosis model adjusted for soundscapes. The model's purpose is fed by previous findings in the fields of sound quality, semiotics, and soundscape design [15,48–50,77], where the *Place*, the *Acoustic Environment* and the *Soundscape* are related, with *the Person* as the central axis. The semiosis model is based on the general triadic model proposed by Peirce, which was adapted by Jekosch for sound quality processes. In this adaptation, the acoustic environment is a sign carrier that represents a specific place (object), the soundscape is the result of the cognitive process developed by a person, which acquires meaning from the context (which in turn influences the city, the persons and the acoustic environments).

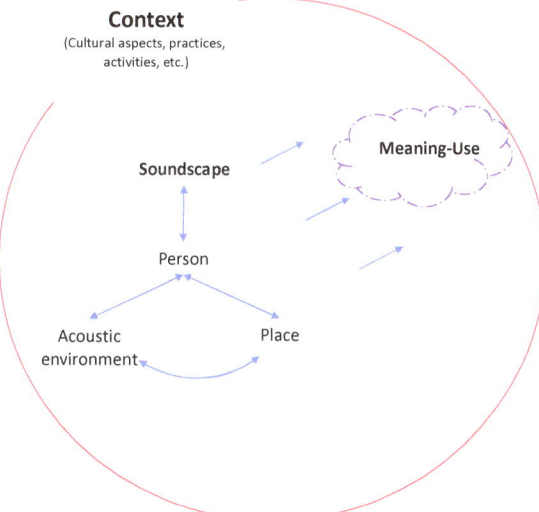

Figure 8. Semiosis model for urban soundscapes.

The process presented in Figure 8, establishes a connection between the Place, the Acoustic environment and the resulting Soundscape, and go in the same line of previous works, that indicate the need to relate the use of the spaces to the soundscapes [43,77]. Persons interact with places, so the acoustic environment is configured from the *affordance* place, the activities and practices developed. The soundscape is, therefore, a product of the interaction of Person with their Place and their Acoustic environment, which in turn feeds on the context and contributes to the meaning of places.

Based on the fact that the soundscape management approach broadens traditional acoustic management, due to the fact that its main objective is the well-being of people, this work deepens the need to manage soundscapes that improve the environmental experience of people (according to the place's use, and the desired responses and outcomes) and contribute to the strengthening of the meaning of places.

The soundscape design process can thus be deepened by putting forward questions related to the contextual and semiotic aspects. Their answers may provide input for the criteria of evaluation, design, management, and planning of acoustic environments, according to Bento-Coelho's soundscape design roadmap (Table 4) [77]:

Table 4. Contextual and semiotic aspects in the Bento Coelho's soundscape design roadmap.

Define purpose and activities
• What is the desired objective and/or meaning of the place?
Define acoustic objectives according to purpose and activities
• How does the acoustic environment contribute to the environmental experience and/or the meaning of the place?
• What is the Person-Place relationship? (including expectations, use, and appropriation of people)?
Identify listening places and listening itineraries
• What activities take place in the places? (according to the time of year, hour, etc.)
Identify sound sources and sound components
• Which sounds identify or represent the most characteristic activities of the place?
• Which sounds enhance the environmental experience and are coherent with the context, the meaning and use of the place?
Identify sound propagation paths
• How do sounds and sound sources interact with their environment?
Identify preferred and unwanted preferred and unwanted sounds
• Which sounds do not favor the environmental experience, are incoherent with the context, the meaning and use of the place?
Manage sound components (Diminish unwanted sounds, enhance preferred sounds, and identify wanted sounds in context)
• How to enhance and/or create sounds that favor the environmental experience, the use and meaning of the place?
• How to reduce sounds that do not favor environmental experience, to the detriment of the use and meaning of the place?

5. Conclusions

The recent developments on the concept of soundscape as a needed alternative in the analysis, assessment, and design of urban acoustic environments has led to new challenges, since an interdisciplinary approach is required that broadens the perspective of the environmental acoustic management. Specifically, in this work aspects related to *Person-Place Interaction* and its impact on people's responses and outcomes were studied, building a discussion based on concepts from the fields of psychology, anthropology, and semiotics.

In this study, the laboratory tests showed that the *responses* (perceptual attributes indicating attitudes) did not generate considerable associations with respect to the Listener's Test Site (*Person-Place Interaction*). However, the *outcomes* (associated with the behavior = possible use) revealed associations with the Listener's Test Site, generating two effects: (1) the association of the "place meaning" to the Possible Use and (2) the emergence of a *sonorous non-place*.

The association of the Place Meaning to the Possible Use, as well as the relation of these aspects with the soundscapes, prove the need to carry out studies with multidisciplinary approaches in this field. In this work, in addition to considering aspects of ecological perception, acoustic environments were analyzed as carriers of meaning, which acquire meaning from contextual aspects. Under the conditions of this study, it was established that for the formation of meaning of an acoustic environment the previous experiences of the people, the activities for which that space was created, and the cultural and spatial aspects that influence the practices developed in the places must be taken into consideration. That is, the *Person-Place Interaction* impacts the meaning of acoustic environments from its use.

Likewise, the homogenization of places also impacts soundscapes, and if there are similar sound sources and similar site uses, the soundscapes will also be similar. This leads to the consideration of *sonorous non-places*, places that have no difference in their "meaning" independently of the *Person-Place Interaction*. Of course, it is not possible or necessary to think that all places must have a unique identity, although it is important to preserve the spaces that require so.

Therefore, in processes of design, planning, and management of environmental acoustics, not only taxonomic, energetic, temporal, and spatial analysis of the acoustic environments are necessary, but a contextual and semiotic study of urban space is also required. In this sense, the analysis of the use of the place, of the people who will use the space, of the coherence between the space and the acoustic environment and the desired meaning, are key to the success of the project. When considering the soundscape as part of a semiosis process, it is important to emphasize in the interaction of the triad *Place*, *Acoustic environment* and *Soundscape*, the *Person* as the central axis.

This work's results seem to suggest the need to continue expanding the processes of management, design, and planning of urban soundscapes, by considering contextual and semiotic aspects that allow a better understanding of the environmental experience and strengthen the meaning of the places, so as to further ensure the people's well-being. In this way, the questions opened up in this work can complement the traditional approaches and enrich the acoustic design and management processes. These questions together with the proposed semiosis model can contribute concretely to create inputs required for such processes.

Finally, urban acoustic designers have the responsibility to present coherent information between the acoustic environment and the use of the place. This, in turn, implies defining multidisciplinary strategies that establish how and when information is generated, to help in the process of formation of meaning of the places by the listeners.

Author Contributions: Conceptualization, L.H.; methodology, L.H., I.P., A.C.L.S. and J.L.B.-C.; writing—original draft preparation, L.H.; writing—review and editing, I.P., A.C.L.S. and J.L.B.-C.; investigation, I.P. and Bento Coelho, J.L.; supervision, I.P. and J.L.B.-C.

Funding: This research received no external funding.

Acknowledgments: Part of this work was financially supported by the Instrumentation and Applied Acoustic Research Group (I2A2) of the Universidad Politécnica de Madrid, by the Brazilian National Council for Scientific and Technological Development–CNPq, by the University of San Buenaventura, and by the Portuguese Foundation for Science and Technology (FCT) which are greatly acknowledged.

Conflicts of Interest: The authors declare no conflict of interest.

References

1. Brown, A.L.; Kang, J.; Gjestland, T. Towards standardization in soundscape preference assessment. *Appl. Acoust.* **2011**, *72*, 387–392. [CrossRef]
2. Van Kamp, I.; Klaeboe, R.; Brown, A.L.; Lercher, P. Soundscapes, Human Restoration and Quality of life. In *Soundscape and the Built Environment*; Kang, J., Schulte-Fortkamp, B., Eds.; CRC Press: Boca Raton, FL, USA, 2016; pp. 43–68.
3. Lercher, P.; Van Kamp, I.; Von Lindern, E.; Botteldooren, D. Perceived Soundscapes and Health-Related Quality of Life, Context, Restoration, and Personal Characteristics. In *Soundscape and the Built Environment*; Kang, J., Schulte-Fortkamp, B., Eds.; CRC Press: Boca Raton, FL, USA, 2016; pp. 133–160.
4. Clark, C.; Paunovic, K. Who Environmental Noise Guidelines for the European Region: A Systematic Review on Environmental Noise and Quality of Life, Wellbeing and Mental Health. *Int. J. Environ. Res. Public Health* **2018**, *15*, 2400. [CrossRef] [PubMed]

5. Medvedev, O.; Shepherd, D.; Hautus, M.J. The restorative potential of soundscapes: A physiological investigation. *Appl. Acoust.* **2015**, *96*. [CrossRef]
6. *World Health Organization (WHO) Environmental Noise Guidelines for the European Region*; World Health Organization Regional Office for Europe: Copenhagen, Denmark, 2018; ISBN 9789289053563.
7. European Environmental Agency. *Good Practice Guide on Quiet Areas*; European Environmental Agency: Luxembourg, 2014; ISBN 9789292134242.
8. Bento Coelho, J.L. A paisagem sonora como instrumento de design e engenharia em meio urbano. In Proceedings of the XXIII Encontro da Sociedade Brasileira de Acústica (SOBRAC), Salvador, Brazil, 19–21 May 2010.
9. Adams, M.; Cox, T.; Moore, G.; Croxford, B.; Refaee, M.; Sharples, S. Sustainable soundscapes: Noise policy and the urban experience. *Urban Stud.* **2006**, *43*, 2385–2398. [CrossRef]
10. Jennings, P.; Cain, R. A framework for improving urban soundscapes. *Appl. Acoust.* **2013**, *74*, 293–299. [CrossRef]
11. Kang, J. From understanding to designing soundscapes. *Front. Archit. Civ. Eng. China* **2010**, *4*, 403–417. [CrossRef]
12. Brown, A.L. Soundscape planning as a complement to environmental noise management. In Proceedings of the Internoise 2014—43rd International Congress on Noise Control Engineering: Improving the World Through Noise Control, Melbourne, Australia, 16–19 July 2014; pp. 1–10.
13. Bento Coelho, J.L.; Remy, N.; Vogiatzis, K. Urban Sound Planning in the City Centre of Thessaloniki. In Proceedings of the ICSV 2015—22 International Congress on Sound and Vibration, Florence, Italy, 12–16 July 2015; pp. 12–16.
14. Remy, N.; Vogiatzis, K. Soundscape & Land Uses Management As Comprehensive Environmental Protection Action Policy Tool Within the Strategic Environmental Noise Mapping in Greece. In Proceedings of the ICSV 2016—23rd International Congress on Sound and Vibration: From Ancient to Modern Acoustics, Athens, Greece, 10–14 July 2016; pp. 1–8.
15. Kang, J.; Aletta, F.; Gjestland, T.T.; Brown, L.A.; Botteldooren, D.; Schulte-fortkamp, B.; Lercher, P.; Van Kamp, I.; Genuit, K.; Luis, J.; et al. Ten questions on the soundscapes of the built environment. *Build. Environ.* **2016**, *108*, 284–294. [CrossRef]
16. Davies, W.J.; Adams, M.D.; Bruce, N.S.; Marselle, M.; Cain, R.; Jennings, P.A.; Poxon, J.; Carlyle, A.; Cusack, P.; Hall, D.A.; et al. The Positive Soundscape Project: A synthesis of results from many disciplines. In Proceedings of the 38th International Congress and Exposition on Noise Control Engineering 2009, INTER-NOISE 2009, Ottawa, ON, Canada, 23–26 August 2009; Volume 1, pp. 663–672.
17. Davies, W.J.; Adams, M.D.; Bruce, N.S.; Cain, R.; Carlyle, A.; Cusack, P.; Hall, D.A.; Hume, K.I.; Irwin, A.; Jennings, P.; et al. Perception of soundscapes: An interdisciplinary approach. *Appl. Acoust.* **2013**, *74*, 224–231. [CrossRef]
18. Kogan, P.; Turra, B.; Arenas, J.P.; Hinalaf, M. A comprehensive methodology for the multidimensional and synchronic data collecting in soundscape. *Sci. Total Environ.* **2017**, *580*, 1068–1077. [CrossRef]
19. Rychtáriková, M.; Vermeir, G. Soundscape categorization on the basis of objective acoustical parameters. *Appl. Acoust.* **2013**, *74*, 240–247. [CrossRef]
20. Cain, R.; Jennings, P.; Poxon, J. The development and application of the emotional dimensions of a soundscape. *Appl. Acoust.* **2013**, *74*, 232–239. [CrossRef]
21. Axelsson, Ö.; Nilsson, M.E.; Berglund, B. A principal components model of soundscape perception. *J. Acoust. Soc. Am.* **2010**, *128*, 2836–2846. [CrossRef]
22. López, I.; Guillén, J. Calidad acústica urbana: Influencia de las interacciones audiovisuales en la valoración del ambiente sonoro. *Medio Ambient. Comport. Hum.* **2005**, *6*, 101–117.
23. Kawai, K.; Kojima, T.; Hirate, K.; Yasuoka, M. Personal evaluation structure of environmental sounds: Experiments of subjective evaluation using subjects' own terms. *J. Sound Vib.* **2004**, *277*, 523–533. [CrossRef]
24. Hermida, L.; Pavón, I. Spatial aspects in urban soundscapes: Binaural parameters application in the study of soundscapes from Bogotá-Colombia and Brasília-Brazil. *Appl. Acoust.* **2019**, *145*, 420–430. [CrossRef]
25. Maristany, A.; Recuero López, M.; Asencio Rivera, C. Soundscape quality analysis by fuzzy logic: A field study in Cordoba, Argentina. *Appl. Acoust.* **2016**, *111*, 106–115. [CrossRef]
26. Schulte-Fortkamp, B.; Fiebig, A. Impact of Soundscape in Terms of Perception. In *Soundscape and the Built Environment*; Kang, J., Schulte-Fortkamp, B., Eds.; CRC Press: Boca Raton, FL, USA, 2016; pp. 69–88.

27. Jeon, J.Y.; Hong, J.Y.; Lavandier, C.; Lafon, J.; Axelsson, Ö.; Hurtig, M. A cross-national comparison in assessment of urban park soundscapes in France, Korea, and Sweden through laboratory experiments. *Appl. Acoust.* **2018**, *133*. [CrossRef]
28. International Standard Organization (ISO) 12913-1 Acoustics-Soundscape—Part 1: Definition and Conceptual Framework. International Standard Organization: Geneva, Switzerland, 2013. Available online: https://www.iso.org/standard/52161.html (accessed on 26 December 2018).
29. Brown, A.L.; Gjestlan, T.; Dubois, D. Acoustic Environments and soundscapes. In *Soundscape and the Built Environment*; Kang, J., Schulte-Fortkamp, B., Eds.; CRC Press: Boca Raton, FL, USA, 2016; pp. 1–16.
30. Gibson, J.J. *The Ecological Approach to Visual Perception*; Taylor & Francis: New York, NY, USA, 1986.
31. Gibson, J.J. The Ecological Approach to the Visual Perception of Pictures. *Leonardo* **1978**, *11*, 227–235. [CrossRef]
32. Herranz-Pascual, K.; Aspuru, I.; García, I. Proposed conceptual model of environmental experience as framework to study the soundscape. In Proceedings of the Internoise 2010. Noise and Sustainability, Lisbon, Portugal, 13–16 June 2010.
33. Javaloy, F.; Vidal, T. Bases ambientales del comportamiento. In *Psicología Social*; Morales, J.F., Moya, M., Gaviria, E., Cuadrado, I., Eds.; McGraw-Hill: Madrid, Spain, 2007; ISBN 978-84-481-5608-4.
34. Pol, E.; Valera, S.; Vidal, T. Psicología ambiental y procesos psicosociales. In *Psicología Social*; Morales, F., Huici, C., Eds.; McGraw-Hill: Madrid, Spain, 1999; pp. 235–252. ISBN 8448124359.
35. Herranz-Pascual, K.; García, I.; Aspuru, I.; Díez, I.; Santander, Á. Progress in the understanding of soundscape: objective variables and objectifiable criteria that predict acoustic comfort in urban places. *Noise Mapp.* **2016**, *3*, 247–263. [CrossRef]
36. Garcia, I.; Herranz-Pascual, K.; Aspuru, I.; Gutierrez, L.; Acero, J.A.; Santander, A. Indicators of Environmental Comfort Sensitive to Human Perception. In *Handbook of Research on Perception-Driven Approaches to Urban Assessment and Design*; Aletta, F., Xiao, J., Eds.; IGI Global: Hershey, PA, USA, 2018; pp. 508–533. ISBN 9781522536376.
37. Jeon, J.Y.; Lee, P.J.; Hong, J.Y.; Cabrera, D. Non-auditory factors affecting urban soundscape evaluation. *J. Acoust. Soc. Am.* **2011**, *130*, 3761–3770. [CrossRef]
38. Pheasant, R.; Horoshenkov, K.; Watts, G.; Barrett, B. The acoustic and visual factors influencing the construction of tranquil space in urban and rural environments tranquil spaces-quiet places? *J. Acoust. Soc. Am.* **2008**, *123*, 1446–1457. [CrossRef]
39. Liu, J.; Kang, J.; Behm, H.; Luo, T. Effects of landscape on soundscape perception: Soundwalks in city parks. *Landsc. Urban Plan.* **2014**, *123*, 30–40. [CrossRef]
40. Truax, B.; Barrett, G.W. Soundscape in a context of acoustic and landscape ecology. *Landsc. Ecol.* **2011**, *26*, 1201–1207. [CrossRef]
41. Liu, J.; Kang, J.; Luo, T.; Behm, H. Landscape effects on soundscape experience in city parks. *Sci. Total Environ.* **2013**, *454–455*, 474–481. [CrossRef]
42. Herranz-Pascual, K.; García, I.; Diez, I.; Santander, A.; Aspuru, I. Analysis of Field Data to Describe the Effect of Context (Acoustic and Non-Acoustic Factors) on Urban Soundscape. *Appl. Sci.* **2017**, *7*, 173. [CrossRef]
43. Hong, J.Y.; Jeon, J.Y. Landscape and Urban Planning Influence of urban contexts on soundscape perceptions: A structural equation modeling approach. *Landsc. Urban Plan.* **2015**, *141*, 78–87. [CrossRef]
44. Romero, V.P.; Brambilla, G.; Gabriele, M.D.; Gallo, V.; Maffei, L. The influence of the soundscape on the tourists' environmental quality perception. In Proceedings of the Euronoise 2015, Maastrícht, Belgium, 31 May–3 June 2015; pp. 1535–1540.
45. Liu, A.; Liu, F.; Deng, Z.; Chen, W. Relationship between soundscape and historical-cultural elements of Historical Areas in Beijing: A case study of Qianmen Avenue. In Proceedings of the Internoise 2014—43rd International Congress on Noise Control Engineering: Improving the World Through Noise Control, Melbourne, Australia, 16–19 November 2014; pp. 1–7.
46. Hermida, L.; Lobo Soares, A.C.; Pavón, I.; Bento Coelho, J.L. Assessing soundscape: Comparison between in situ and laboratory methodologies. *Noise Mapp.* **2017**, *4*, 57–66. [CrossRef]
47. Blauert, J. Analysis and Synthesis of Auditory Scenes. In *Communication Acoustics*; Blauert, J., Ed.; Springer: Berlin, Germany, 2005; pp. 1–20. ISBN 3-540-22162-X.
48. Jekosch, U. Assigning Meaning to Sounds—Semiotics in the Context of Product-Sound Design. In *Acoustics Comunication*; Blauert, J., Ed.; Springer: Berlin, Germany, 2005; pp. 193–219. ISBN 3-540-22162-X.

49. Santaella, L. *Matrizes da Linguagem e o Pensamento*; Iluminarias: São Paulo, Brazil, 2013.
50. Peirce, C.S. *Semiótica*, 4th ed.; Perspectiva: São Paulo, Brazil, 2015; ISBN 9788527301947.
51. Santos, F.A. dos Design: A conexão do corpo com o ambiente e a sintaxe do pensamento humano. *Triades* **2010**, *1*, 1–18.
52. Santos, F.A. dos Comunicação visual e design como índice da complexidade semiótica do espaço urbano. In *Urbanidades: mediações*; Santos, F.A., Camara, R., Eds.; Estereográfica Editorial: Brasilia, Brazil, 2017; pp. 45–68.
53. Saleh, M.A.E. Place identity: The visual image of Saudi Arabian cities. *Habitat Int.* **1998**, *22*, 149–164. [CrossRef]
54. Wagner, A. French Urban Space Management: A Visual Semiotic Approach Behind Power and Control. *Int. J. Semiot. Law* **2011**, *24*, 227–241. [CrossRef]
55. Genuit, K.; Fiebig, A. The measurement of soundscapes—Is it standardizable? In Proceedings of the Internoise 2014—43rd International Congress on Noise Control Engineering: Improving the World through Noise Control, Melbourne, Australia, 16–19 July 2014; p. 9.
56. Genuit, K.; Fiebig, A. Human Hearing-Related Measurement and Analysis of Acoustics Environments: Requisite for Soundscape Investigations. In *Soundscape and the Built Environment*; Kang, J., Schulte-Fortkamp, B., Eds.; CRC Press: Boca Raton, FL, USA, 2016; pp. 133–160.
57. Rey Gozalo, G.; Trujillo Carmona, J.; Barrigón Morillas, J.M.; Vílchez-Gómez, R.; Gómez Escobar, V. Relationship between objective acoustic indices and subjective assessments for the quality of soundscapes. *Appl. Acoust.* **2015**, *97*, 1–10. [CrossRef]
58. Jeon, J.Y.; Hong, J.Y. Classification of urban park soundscapes through perceptions of the acoustical environments. *Landsc. Urban Plan.* **2015**, *141*, 100–111. [CrossRef]
59. Schafer, R.M. *The Tuning of the World*; Random House, Knopf: New York, NY, USA, 1977; ISBN 0394409663.
60. Marry, S.; Defrance, J. Analysis of the perception and representation of sonic public spaces through on site survey, acoustic indicators and in-depth interviews. *Appl. Acoust.* **2013**, *74*, 282–292. [CrossRef]
61. Ricciardi, P.; Delaitre, P.; Lavandier, C.; Torchia, F.; Aumond, P. Sound quality indicators for urban places in Paris cross-validated by Milan data. *J. Acoust. Soc. Am.* **2015**, *138*, 2337–2348. [CrossRef] [PubMed]
62. Otto, N.C. Listening test methods for automotive sound quality. In *Audio Engineering Society*; Audio Engineering Society: New York, NY, USA, 1997.
63. Otto, N.; Amman, S.; Eaton, C.; Lake, S. *Guidelines for Jury Evaluations of Automotive Sounds*; Society of Automotive Engineers SAE: Traverse City, MI, USA, 1999; Volume 4.
64. Guillén, J.; López, I. Importance of personal, attitudinal and contextual variables in the assessment of pleasantness of the urban sound environment. In Proceedings of the 19th International Congress on Acoustics ICA, Madrid, Spain, 2–7 September 2007; pp. 1–6.
65. Hall, D.A.; Irwin, A.; Edmondson-Jones, M.; Phillips, S.; Poxon, J.E.W. An exploratory evaluation of perceptual, psychoacoustic and acoustical properties of urban soundscapes. *Appl. Acoust.* **2013**, *74*, 248–254. [CrossRef]
66. Hong, J.Y.; Jeon, J.Y. Designing sound and visual components for enhancement of urban soundscapes. *J. Acoust. Soc. Am.* **2013**, *134*, 2026–2036. [CrossRef] [PubMed]
67. Viollon, S.; Lavandier, C.; Drake, C. Influence of visual setting on sound ratings in an urban environment. *Appl. Acoust.* **2002**, *63*, 493–511. [CrossRef]
68. Hume, K.; Ahtamad, M. Physiological responses to and subjective estimates of soundscape elements. *Appl. Acoust.* **2013**, *74*, 275–281. [CrossRef]
69. Lyon, R.H. Product sound quality: From perception to design. *Sound Vib.* **2003**, *108*, 2471. [CrossRef]
70. Axelsson, Ö. How to measure soundscape quality. In Proceedings of the Euronoise 2015, Maastrícht, Belgium, 31 May–3 June 2015; pp. 1477–1481.
71. Axelsson, Ö.; Nilsson, M.E.; Berglund, B. The Swedish soundscape-quality protocol. *J. Acoust. Soc. Am.* **2012**, *131*, 3476. [CrossRef]
72. Auge, M. *Los no Lugares. Espacios del Anonimato*; Gedisa: Barcelona, Spain, 2009; ISBN 9788474324594.
73. Jeon, J.Y.; Lee, P.J.; You, J.; Kang, J. Perceptual assessment of quality of urban soundscapes with combined noise sources and water sounds. *J. Acoust. Soc. Am.* **2010**, *127*, 1357–1366. [CrossRef] [PubMed]
74. Ferrara, L.D. *A Estratégia dos Signos: Linguagem, Espaço, Ambiente Urbano*; Perspectiva: São Paulo, Brazil, 2009; ISBN 8527308398.

75. Tuan, Y.-F. *Space and Place: The Perspective of Experience*, 25th ed.; University of Minnesota Press: Minneapolis, MN, USA, 1977; ISBN 0816638772.
76. Santos, F.A. dos Urbanidades mediações-Apresentação. In *Urbanidades: Mediações*; Santos, F.A., Camara, R., Eds.; Estereográfica Editorial: Brasilia, Brazil, 2017; pp. 7–10.
77. Bento Coelho, J.L. Approaches to Urban Soundscape management, planning and design. In *Soundscape and the Built Environment*; Kang, J., Schulte-Fortkamp, B., Eds.; CRC Press: Boca Raton, FL, USA, 2016; pp. 197–214.

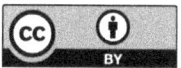

© 2019 by the authors. Licensee MDPI, Basel, Switzerland. This article is an open access article distributed under the terms and conditions of the Creative Commons Attribution (CC BY) license (http://creativecommons.org/licenses/by/4.0/).

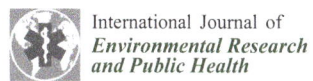
International Journal of
Environmental Research and Public Health

Review

Associations between Positive Health-Related Effects and Soundscapes Perceptual Constructs: A Systematic Review

Francesco Aletta, Tin Oberman and Jian Kang *

UCL Institute for Environmental Design and Engineering, The Bartlett, University College London (UCL), Central House, 14 Upper Woburn Place, London WC1H 0NN, UK; f.aletta@ucl.ac.uk (F.A.); t.oberman@ucl.ac.uk (T.O.)
* Correspondence: j.kang@ucl.ac.uk; Tel.: +44-(0)20-3108-7338

Received: 10 September 2018; Accepted: 22 October 2018; Published: 29 October 2018

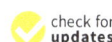

Abstract: In policy-making and research alike, environmental sounds are often considered only as psychophysical stressors, leading to adverse health effects. The soundscape approach, on the other hand, aims to extend the scope of sound-related research to consider sounds as resources, promoting healthy and supportive environments. The ISO 12913-1 standard defined soundscapes as acoustic environments "as perceived by people, in context." The aim of this study was assessing associations between positive soundscapes (e.g., pleasant, calm, less annoying) and positive health-related effects (e.g., increased restoration, reduced stress-inducing mechanisms, etc.). Studies collecting data about individual responses to urban acoustic environments, and individual responses on psychophysical well-being were selected, looking at cases where positive effects were observed. The Web of Science, Scopus and PubMed databases were searched for peer-reviewed journal papers published in English between 1 January 1991 and 31 May 2018, with combinations of the keywords "soundscape" and at least one among "health", "well-being" or "quality of life." An additional manual search was performed on the reference lists of the retrieved items. Inclusion criteria were: (1) including at least one measure of soundscape dimensions as per the ISO 12913-1 definition; (2) including at least one health-related measure (either physiological or psychological); (3) observing/discussing a "positive" effect of the soundscape on the health-related outcome. The search returned 130 results; after removing duplicates, two authors screened titles and abstracts and selected 19 papers for further analysis. Seven studies were eventually included, with 2783 participants in total. Each study included at least a valence-related soundscape measure. Regarding the health-related measures, four studies included physiological monitoring and the remaining three included self-reported psychological measures. Positive soundscapes were associated with faster stress-recovery processes in laboratory experiments, and better self-reported health conditions in large-scale surveys. Due to the limited number of items and differences in measures across studies, no statistical analysis was performed, and a qualitative approach to data synthesis was sought. Results support the claim that, in contrast with looking at noise only as an environmental stressor, sound perception can act as an enhancer of the human experience in the urban realm, from a health-related point of view.

Keywords: soundscape; environmental noise; public health; well-being; quality of life; restoration

1. Introduction

The adverse health effects of environmental noise on people and communities have been thoroughly investigated by world-wide research institutions and international health organizations over the past decades [1–3]. Particularly in cities, excessive exposure to noise has been proved to account for a wide range of psychophysical detrimental health effects, such as: Increased risk of ischaemic heart disease, sleep disturbance, cognitive impairment among children, annoyance, stress-related mental health risks, and tinnitus [4,5]. As this is a substantial public health issue, regulatory bodies, public authorities, and policy makers have put a lot of effort into reducing environmental noise exposures, and noise levels more generally. In the European Union, such efforts are reflected in the "Environmental Noise Directive" (END) [6] and a number of other technical reports and documents issued by EU agencies [7,8], which constitute the references for Member States for the "assessment and management of environmental noise" [6]. The END deals with the management of specific sources; in particular: Road and rail vehicles and infrastructure, aircraft, outdoor and industrial equipment and mobile machinery. As it can be observed, the focus is on typically "unwanted" sound sources and possible nuisance they generate: Little is said in the document about "wanted" sounds, the sounds of "preference", or the possibility that being exposed to certain acoustic environments can actually induce positive rather than negative moods.

While reducing environmental noise in cities can certainly generate economic and social benefits, in principle it did not always lead straightforwardly to improved well-being and quality of life for people [9–11], as sounds might also be important because they transfer information, and loudness can even be desirable in some contexts [12].

Being underpinned by a more holistic approach, soundscape research aims indeed to compensate for this issue, by shifting the research focus from the negative to the positive effects of environmental sounds [13–16]. The ISO 12913-1 standard defines the term soundscape as "an acoustic environment as perceived or experienced and/or understood by a person or people, in context" [17]. Sometimes "soundscape" is used in community noise literature as an equivalent for "acoustic environment" [16], but the ISO 12913-1 definition highlights that they can be treated as separate concepts: The former relates to the perceptual outcome of the individuals, the latter relates to the whole set of sources generating sounds in a specific space and its physical implications. As such, acoustic environments are neither good nor bad: When the sound sources composing them become "wanted" or "unwanted" for a listener, they are likely to elicit positive or negative soundscapes, accordingly.

The corpus of soundscape studies is growing steadily, and their outreach is increasing accordingly [18], which is promising evidence that the course of this research field is changing. Several studies have tried to provide scientific evidence of the benefits of the "soundscape approach" for public engagement, health, and well-being [19–22]; however, the lack of empirical and analytical evidence to support that claim is still perceived as a crucial issue by the scientific community [23].

To the best of the authors' knowledge, no review has been performed so far on the association between the individuals' positive perception of acoustic environments (i.e., positive soundscapes) and positive health-related effects. Thus, the aim of this paper is to explore such relationships and to identify potential paths to extend the scope of the soundscape approach towards environmental and public health research [23]. For this purpose, we carried out a systematic review of the literature in main scientific databases. The underpinning research question was whether statistically significant associations exist between positive soundscape dimensions and positive health-related effects. It is worth pointing out that, as a perceptual outcome, any soundscape can either be positive or negative. The main theoretical reference of this review to define a positive soundscape is the circumplex model for soundscape characterisation proposed by Axelsson and colleagues [24]. This model has two orthogonal components: The horizontal component is a valence-related dimension (annoying-pleasant), while the vertical component is an activation-related dimension (uneventful-eventful). A soundscape that is both: Pleasant and eventful will be vibrant; pleasant and uneventful will be calm; annoying and uneventful will be monotonous; annoying and eventful will be chaotic. Having this two-dimensional space as reference, any perceptual outcome that can be located in the pleasant region of the model (e.g., pleasant, calm, vibrant, or similar) can be considered as a positive soundscape, while any perceptual outcome that can be located in the annoying region of the model can be considered as a negative soundscape (e.g., annoying, monotonous, chaotic, or similar). Regarding the health-related effects, the definition of "positive" is somewhat more intuitive: It can be assumed that positive health effects occur when, either in a measured or self-reported configuration, enhanced restoration and recovery mechanisms or reduced stress-inducing mechanisms are observed.

2. Methods

Given the exploratory nature of this study, there was no pre-defined protocol registration for this review. The basic process and data extraction forms were agreed upon at the beginning of the review work. The study was performed and reported in accordance with the PRISMA (Preferred Reporting Items for Systematic Reviews and Meta-Analyses) guidelines for systematic reviews [25].

2.1. Search Strategy and Eligibility Criteria

Studies were selected if they collected data about individual responses to (urban) acoustic environments, and individual responses on psychophysical well-being, looking at positive effects of the former on the latter. The specific inclusion criteria were: (1) Including at least one measure of soundscape dimensions as per the ISO 12913-1 definition [17]; (2) including at least one health-related measure (either physiological or psychological); (3) observing/discussing a "positive" effect of the soundscape on the health-related outcome. Only peer-reviewed journal articles published in English were considered.

The ISO 12913-1 standard highlights that soundscape is a perceptual outcome, deriving from the experience of a physical phenomenon (the acoustic environment) [17]. Thus, any perceptual construct (e.g., calmness, excitement, pleasantness, annoyance, etc.) related to the experience of an acoustic environment could be seen as a potential item on which it is possible to gather individual responses [24,26,27]. These perceptual constructs (soundscape dimensions), when clearly identified and/or formalised, have indeed previously been defined in literature as "soundscape descriptors", which are "measures of how people perceive the acoustic environment" [10]. Soundscape researchers typically make use of soundscape descriptors associated to scales (e.g., numerical scales, Likert scales, etc.) and ask people to assess their experience of the acoustic environment on those [28–30]: Within the framework of this review, soundscape descriptors associated with scales (or other metrics/observations) will therefore be considered as "soundscape measures."

Regarding the well-being and health-related measures, these were in turn considered to relate to two main groups, namely: (1) Physiological measures: e.g., heart rate, respiratory rate, electrodermal activity or skin conductance level, etc.; (2) psychological measures: e.g., self-reported health condition, satisfaction, quality of life, etc. The rationale for selecting the former group is that most of them are related to the autonomic function (parasympathetic and sympathetic activation) and consequently stress recovery and relaxation or excitement and arousal, which influence health and well-being, and have been reported to be influenced by the acoustic environment [31,32]. The sympathetic system is responsible for stimulating the body's "fight-or-flight" response, whilst the parasympathetic system is responsible for the stimulation of "rest-and-digest" or "feed and breed" activities, which occur when the body is at rest, or preparing for relaxation. Studies of this kind are typically performed in laboratory settings and include small samples of participants. On the other hand, psychological measures of the latter group are instead more often included within broader (large-scale) socio-acoustic surveys.

Studies were identified by searching Web of Science, Scopus and PubMed electronic databases, by manually scanning the reference lists of retrieved items and through consultation with experts in the field. A combination of the following keywords was used: Soundscape; and at least one among: Health, well-being, or "quality of life". The search was applied between 1 January 1991 and present. The last search was performed on 31 May 2018. Using two or three databases is a common approach in systematic reviews [25]; the three mentioned above have been shown to be effective in covering most of the relevant soundscape literature [16,18,33].

The assessment about the eligibility of the study was performed independently in a non-blinded standardized manner by two reviewers; a few disagreements between reviewers about inclusion/exclusion of some items were resolved by consensus.

2.2. Data Extraction

Information was extracted from each included study on: (1) Soundscape measure(s); (2) health-related measure(s); (3) number of participants of the study; (4) study design; (5) sound levels (or range thereof) and corresponding metrics considered to define exposure conditions; and (6) main observed positive effect(s) of soundscapes on health and well-being.

Considering the unresolvable differences in the metrics across the selected studies, a quality assessment and quantitative meta-analysis under the quality-effects model were not possible [34]. Therefore, a qualitative approach to data synthesis was adopted to answer the review question.

2.3. Rationale for the Review

The main aim of this review was supporting the claim that the positive perception of acoustic environments might be beneficial for human health and promote more positive living experiences: Both the health effects and the soundscapes can be seen as outcomes of the exposure to a specific acoustic environment. In order to support this hypothesis, it was then necessary to include studies that drew clear associations between these two domains, in the most objective possible way. Figure 1 summarises the general theoretical framework for this review. A considerable amount of literature has looked at this topic only from one side: Either by checking for differences in perceptual outcomes between groups experiencing different acoustic environments, but without considering the health implications on the sample [29,35,36]; or by investigating the health impacts (either supportive or detrimental) of exposure to different acoustic environments on different populations, but dismissing the perceptual constructs being elicited [37,38]. The novelty of this review lays in the fact of looking at associations between health effects and perceptual responses directly (regardless of the acoustic environments inducing them) and focusing on the positive outcomes (instead of detrimental effects) deriving from the interactions between these two. Therefore, among the inclusion criteria of this review, two of them were the most crucial ones: Having considered a health-related measure, and having considered a soundscape measure on the same sample of participants. Those two types of measures were conceived by the reviewers in the broadest possible fashion.

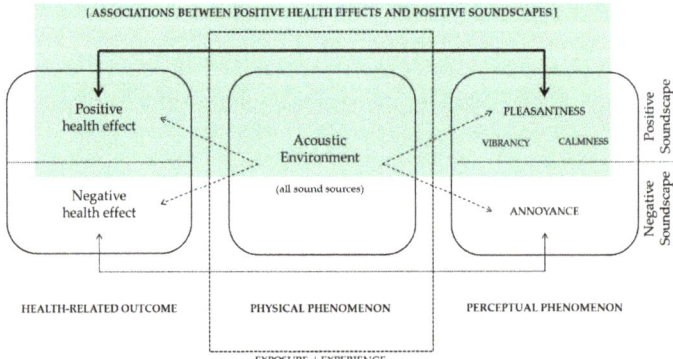

Figure 1. Schematic representation of the theoretical framework underpinning the systematic review: The inclusion criteria were defined to detect studies that established clear associations positive soundscapes and positive health-related effects (area highlighted in green), instead of negative soundscapes and negative health effects (bottom part of the figure), and to dismiss those focusing only on either the perceptual outcome or the health-related outcome (dashed arrows).

3. Results

The search through the three databases and the additional manual search returned 130 results. After removing duplicates, the abstract of 113 records were read by two authors and 94 items were excluded because the topic of the papers was not relevant (e.g., different research field) and/or did not address the review research question. The full-texts of the remaining 19 papers were accessed and 13 of them were excluded because they failed to meet the eligibility criteria (e.g., lack of either the soundscape or the health-related measure, the paper did not actually include data collection, etc.). The remaining six papers were included in the review; one of those reported on two separate studies, thus seven studies were eventually considered. Figure 2 summarises the selection process of the review records.

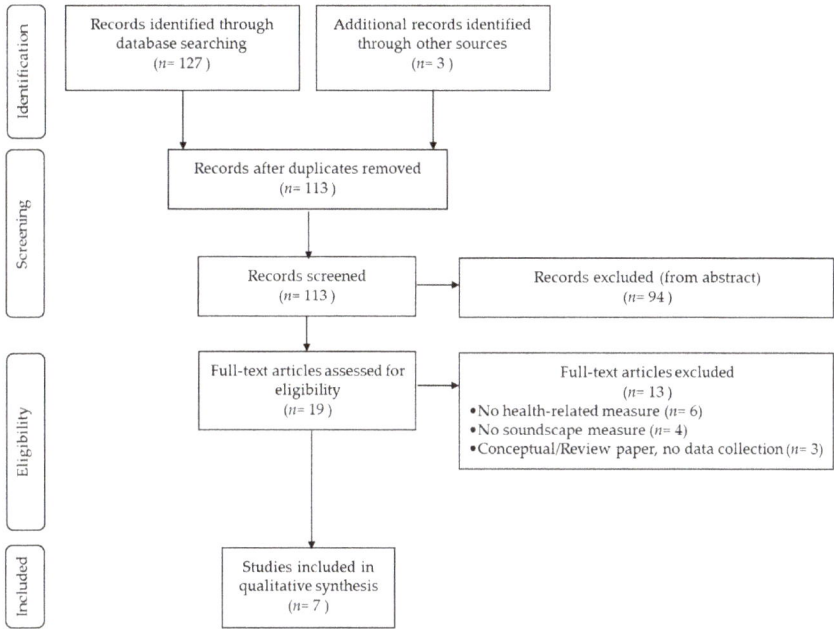

Figure 2. Flow of information through the different phases of the systematic review [25]. The number of studies included in the qualitative synthesis does not equal the difference between the articles assessed and those excluded ($n = 6$), because one of the selected articles included two separate studies, both meeting the eligibility criteria.

Table 1 shows the data extracted from the seven studies considered in the review, reported according to the chronological order of publication. It is important to notice that, due to the differences in study designs, the selected studies used substantially different metrics for the characterisation of the acoustic environments and/or auditory stimuli. Laboratory studies typically referred to equivalent levels (L_{eq}) while socio-acoustic surveys made use of daily-averaged levels (e.g., L_{day}, L_{den}). This makes it difficult to compare sound levels or exposure across studies, but they are reported in any case for descriptive purposes.

Four studies [39–41] included soundscape measures that are either standardized or well-established in soundscape literature [24,27,30]; all these studies referred to physiological health-related measures and made use of laboratory experiments, thus using relatively small samples of participants. The other three studies included in the review [42–44], on the other hand, referred to annoyance-related soundscape measures [10,45,46]. In this review "annoyance" is also considered a soundscape measure, consistently with the model proposed by Axelsson and colleagues [24]; reduced annoyance can be interpreted as a positive soundscape outcome. These three studies included psychological health-related measures instead and were performed within large-scale environmental surveys (the acoustic aspects of which were not necessarily the main ones); thus, they typically included larger samples of participants than the laboratory studies.

For the sake of reporting and discussion, the studies were grouped according to the abovementioned sample size criterion (large- and small-scale) and their main characteristics; methods and results are described in the two following sub-sections, accordingly.

3.1. The Large-Scale Studies

Öhrström, et al. [42] investigated the benefit of access to quietness in reducing the annoyance from road traffic noise through a set of large-scale socio-acoustic surveys about environmental perception at home in Gothenburg and Stockholm. Their study included 956 participants who were asked several groups of questions about (among others): Noise annoyance, general physical health, and mental well-being. The soundscape-related question (i.e., noise annoyance) was evaluated through two standardized annoyance scales [46]: A five-point categorical scale and numeric 0–10 scale (ranging from "not at all annoyed" to "extremely annoyed"). The verbal standardized annoyance question was: "Thinking about the last (12 months or so), when you are at home, how much does noise from road traffic bother, disturb, or annoy you?". The health-related part of the questionnaire consisted of a number of items, asking how often ("seldom/never"; "a few times a month"; "a few times a week"; or "everyday") participants experienced/felt: "Very tired", "headache", "stressed", "unsociable and preferred to be alone", "irritated and angry", "stomach discomfort", "worried and nervous", and "sad and depressed." The sample was stratified by "access to a quiet side at home" (i.e., low or high exposure to road traffic noise). For the purpose of the review, this variable is not relevant, as it only relates to the authors' experimental design and transcends its main aim, which is seeking the association between the health items and soundscape annoyance. Indeed, the authors reported that, in any case (regardless of low or high exposure), lower noise annoyance was associated with improved (i.e., less occurring) experience of health-related issues. Statistically significant relationships ($p < 0.01$, Spearman correlation coefficient, r_s) were observed between noise annoyance (soundscape dimension) and heath items: "Very tired", $r_s = 0.246$; "stressed", $r_s = 0.224$; "irritated/angry", $r_s = 0.216$, "headache", $r_s = 0.197$; and "unsociable", $r_s = 0.191$.

Booi and van den Berg [43] conducted another socio-acoustic survey that included 809 participants, within a broader study about quiet areas in Amsterdam. For the soundscape measure the authors developed a "Need for Quietness" construct, which was based on two scales: "How important is quietness to you: (1) In/around home; (2) in the neighbourhood. Answers were provided for each item on a five-point scale ranging from 1 ("not at all important") to 5 ("very important"). The internal consistency of the two scales for the Need for Quietness perceptual construct was tested through a Cronbach's α test (0.711). According to the ISO 12913-1 definition, the Need for Quietness can be considered as a soundscape measure, as it is a perceptual outcome emerging from the experience of an acoustic environment. In this context, lower scores of Need for Quietness can be interpreted as a positive soundscape, as it implies lower psychological burden on the subjects. The health-related measure was based on a single question: "How is your health in general?". The categorical answers were: "Excellent"; "very good"; "good"; "reasonable"; "poor". The scores for this question were then recoded into a simpler two-level "health" variable (i.e., good; poor/bad). An independent-sample t-test revealed statistically significant differences ($p < 0.05$) in terms of Need for Quietness between the good (M = 3.7) and poor/bad (M = 4.0) groups of the health variable. Thus, the authors concluded that, for their sample, a better health condition was associated with greater satisfaction with everyday soundscape experience (i.e., lower need for quietness).

Shepherd et al. [44] carried out a study in New Zealand including 823 participants in total, residing across a different gradient of urbanization (i.e., rural areas of New Zealand's North Island, areas around Auckland International Airport, and Auckland city). For the health-related dimensions, the surveys referred to the standardized protocol for Health-Related Quality of Life (HRQOL), as a proxy for the influence of the individuals' health status on their global well-being. The HRQOL was assessed using the reduced version of the World Health Organization quality of life protocol, the WHOQOL-BREF (World Health Organization Quality of Life) [47,48]. This instrument includes two general items on self-reported health and quality of life, and 24 items representing four HRQOL domains; namely: Physical health (seven items), psychological wellbeing (six items), social relationships (three items), and environmental factors (eight items). In this protocol items are rated using a five-point scale, ranging from negative (1) to positive (5) evaluations of HRQOL domains. As a soundscape measure, the dimension of "annoyance" was assessed also in this case. Questions referred to noise from road traffic, neighbours, or other sources and participants could assess them on a five-point scale ranging from "Not annoyed at all" (1) to "Extremely annoyed" (5). The annoyance scores were pooled and dichotomised into a new variable (i.e., "not annoyed" and "most annoyed") to identify two groups within the sample. The most annoyed group had lower mean scores than the not annoyed group for the HRQOL domains. A set of ANCOVA tests [49] revealed statistically significant differences between the most annoyed and not annoyed groups for all the HRQOL domains: Physical ($F = 41.799$, $p < 0.001$); psychological ($F = 36.02$, $p < 0.001$); social ($F = 14.984$, $p < 0.001$), and environmental ($F = 64.83$, $p < 0.001$). The authors concluded that, while unpleasant soundscapes can induce annoyance, positively evaluated soundscapes can support restoration and quality of life.

3.2. The Small-Scale Studies

Alvarsson et al. [39] carried out a laboratory experiment where 40 participants were exposed to four different environmental sounds after a stressful mental arithmetic task to see what sounds would provide a faster recovery from the stressor event. The four sounds were: Nature sound (i.e., tweeting birds mixed with sounds from a fountain—50 dB); high traffic noise (i.e., road traffic noise recorded close to a densely used road—80 dB); low traffic noise (same stimulus as the previous one, set at a lower sound level—50 dB); and ambient noise (i.e., sound from a quiet backyard, mixed with constant and low ventilation noise—40 dB). During the recovery phase of the experimental design, while the auditory stimulus was being provided, the health-related measures were taken. They consisted of the skin conductance level (SCL), which was used as a proxy for sympathetic activation, and high frequency heart rate (HR) variability, which was used as a proxy for parasympathetic activation. In terms of soundscape measures, the participants were asked to assess the four environmental sounds used during the experiment in terms of pleasantness, eventfulness, and familiarity. The authors reported that these descriptors were assessed through bipolar categorical scales, but no further details were provided; thus, it is assumed the question was posed on a scale related to each item, ranging from "not at all" to "completely", or similar. While HR variability showed no effect, SCL decrease (interpreted as stress recovery) tended to be faster during exposure to natural sound compared to noisy environments. In an ANCOVA test, with baseline (i.e., silence) as covariate, the interaction between sound type and stress recovery time was found to be statistically significant ($F = 1.34$, $p = 0.034$). Likewise, nature sounds were assessed as being the most pleasant and familiar (positive dimensions of soundscape appraisal). These results suggest that positive soundscapes can facilitate recovery from sympathetic activation after a psychological stressor.

A similar laboratory setting was prepared by Hume and Ahtamad [40]. Their experiment included 80 participants. The participants were exposed to eight different auditory stimuli (e.g., kids playing, fire siren, birdsong, etc.) in a randomized sequence. The health-related measures consisted of heart rate (HR), respiration rate (RR) and electromyography (EMG); these were taken immediately before (baseline) and during the participants' exposure to each stimulus. The soundscape measures were instead taken subsequently to the exposure: Immediately after listening to the audio excerpt, participants had to score the pleasantness and arousal of the stimuli on two nine-point scales ranging from "extremely unpleasant" and "no arousal" (1) to "extremely pleasant" and "extremely aroused" (9), accordingly. The associations between the three health-related measures and soundscape measures were tested separately through linear mixed model ANOVAs. For the health variables, the change (i.e., increase or decrease) of the physiological measures during the sound exposure was considered, rather than absolute values. The pleasantness scores were recoded into a new three-level ordinal variable: Most unpleasant (scores 1–3), neutral (scores 4–6), and most pleasant (scores 7–9). The authors report it was not possible to draw conclusions on the arousal dimension, since the sample of participants failed to achieve a full range of arousal estimates (possibly due to an incomplete understanding of the concept, compared to pleasantness). In terms of heart rate, the more unpleasantly scored sounds resulted in the largest HR decrease, whilst the most pleasant sounds were associated with the smallest HR decrease. These differences were found to be statistically significant ($F = 2.153$, $p = 0.029$). For the respiration rate, a positive relationship was observed: An increased RR was associated with an increase in pleasantness. These differences were statistically significant too ($F = 107.8$, $p < 0.001$). For the electromyography, there was no general separation measured between the baseline and the exposure, as observed instead for the HR and RR results; thus, the authors did not report any statistical test on this last variable. Although no detailed interpretation is provided about the health implications of the observed physiological profiles, the authors generally concluded that soundscapes have the potential to (positively) affect health by observing that for soundscapes assessed as unpleasant, there was a trend for HR to decrease and RR to slightly increase, while for soundscapes assessed as pleasant, there was a minimal HR decrease and a clear RR increase. To some extent, this issue is left unsolved by the authors who did establish the association but did not offer further insights into its causal connections, and more research would be desirable to explain that particular physiological response.

The paper by Medvedev et al. [41] reported on two separate studies, which addressed similar research questions from slightly different perspectives, to support the authors' research hypothesis. The listening experiments shared the same methodology (i.e., exposure of participants to sound, physiological monitoring, and self-reported soundscape appraisal), but were independent of one another (different samples of participants, different stimuli and procedure, etc.); therefore, for the sake of this review, they were considered as separate items, since Study 1 and Study 2 alike met the inclusion criteria alone. The health-related measures consisted of continuous monitoring of heart rate (HR) and skin conductance level (SCL). The soundscape measures consisted of self-reported appraisals based on seven-point Likert scales ranging from "not at all" to "completely" for the following soundscape dimensions: Pleasantness, arousal, familiarity, eventfulness, and dominance. In Study 1, participants were asked to perform a stressful arithmetic task, and for the recovery phase they were exposed to four different environmental sounds (i.e., birdsong, ocean, road noise, and construction). On the other hand, in Study 2, there were six slightly different stimuli (i.e., aviation, motorcycle, construction, ocean, birdsong, classical music) and the scenarios started "at rest" (no cognitive task): Participants were asked to listen passively to the stimuli and to assess the soundscape after each scenario. The same health and soundscape measures were taken as in Study 1. The authors performed a set of paired comparison tests to explore the effects of soundscapes on stress recovery (i.e., decrease of SCL). A statistically significantly faster decrease of SCL ($p < 0.01$) was observed for soundscapes rated as the most pleasant and the least eventful, compared to the least pleasant and most eventful. Furthermore, a statistically significant difference ($p < 0.05$) was observed between sounds assessed as most and least familiar. Study 2 looked at the same issue, from a "symmetric" perspective. Paired comparison tests showed that soundscapes assessed as the least pleasant and familiar, and the most dominant, were associated with significantly larger ($p < 0.05$) increases of the SCL, compared to the soundscapes ranked as the most pleasant and familiar, and the least dominant, accordingly. By integrating the results from the two studies, the authors concluded that the experience of pleasant soundscapes would facilitate faster recovery from stress, compared to unpleasant soundscapes.

Table 1. List of studies included in the systematic review in chronological order of publication. The main soundscape and health-related measures, the study design, the sound levels, the number of participants and main conclusions of the studies are reported. Since the studies often included several experimental conditions and sound levels, these are reported as levels range (e.g., 40–80 dB, might include several experimental conditions of 40, 50 and 80 dB: For more specific information it is possible to refer to the original studies).

Reference	Soundscape Measure	Health-Related Measure	Study Design	Sound Levels (Metric)	Participants	Main Conclusion(s)—Observed Positive Effect(s)
Alvarsson et al. [39]	Pleasantness, Eventfulness, Familiarity	Autonomic function (HR, SCL)	Laboratory experiment	40–80 dB ($L_{Aeq4min}$)	40	Nature sounds facilitate recovery after a psychological stressor.
Booi and van den Berg [43]	Need for Quietness	Self-reported health condition	Socio-acoustic survey	30–75 dBA (L_{day})	809	People with good health have a lower need for quietness.
Medvedev et al. [1] [40]	Pleasantness, Eventfulness, Familiarity, Arousal, Dominance	Autonomic function (HR, SCL)	Laboratory experiment	64 dB (SPL)	45	Pleasant soundscapes facilitate faster recovery from stress compared to unpleasant soundscapes.
Medvedev et al. [1] [40]	Pleasantness, Eventfulness, Familiarity, Arousal, Dominance	Autonomic function (HR, SCL)	Laboratory experiment	64 dB (SPL)	30	Experience of unpleasant soundscapes at rest produces greater stress than pleasant soundscapes.
Öhrström et al. [42]	Noise Annoyance	Self-reported health and well-being condition	Socio-acoustic survey	35–65 dB (L_{Aeq24h})	956	Experience of quietness supports health and results in a lower degree of annoyance, disturbed relaxation and sleep, and contributes to physiological and psychological well-being.
Shepherd et al. [44]	Noise Annoyance	Self-reported health and well-being condition	Socio-acoustic survey	55–76 dBA (L_{den})	823	Quiet soundscapes facilitate restoration, and/or impede insult to health.
Hume and Ahtamad [40]	Pleasantness, Arousal	Autonomic function (HR, RR, EMG)	Laboratory experiment	60–74 dBA (SPL)	80	The more pleasant the soundscape, the greater the increase in respiratory rate and the smaller the decrease in heart rate.

[1] Reference [41] included two separate studies and they are treated as separate items within the current review.

4. Discussion

4.1. Differences in the Methodological Backgrounds of the Reviewed Studies

The review identified studies that could approximately be sorted into two categories: The large-scale studies (see Section 3.1) and the small-scale studies (see Section 3.2); the two categories were underpinned by substantially different methodological approaches. Studies from the former group tend to be led by annoyance-related analyses. It should be noted that, being a valence measure and a perceptual construct itself, noise annoyance can be considered a soundscape dimension in its own right (thus, meeting the inclusion criteria). However, such studies are possibly inspired by different principles. In general, they aim at estimating long-term effects (e.g., "thinking about the last 12 months ... " and similar questions), focus on specific contexts (e.g., experience of sound/noise at home or at work), and consequently need large samples of participants to achieve reasonable robustness. On the other hand, studies from the latter group were found to be more soundscape-oriented. They are the outcomes of projects that typically had the perceptual domain as a driving research component. They are more aligned to the soundscape approach of contextual experience (i.e., "right here, right now") and are more focused on the immediate response of participants to auditory stimulation, thus mainly disregarding long-term effects.

Globally, the number of soundscapes studies is increasing with time [18]. Although, interestingly enough, the type of studies one usually retrieves in "classical" soundscape literature did not emerge within the context of this systematic review [16]. Indeed, the vast majority of soundscape studies nowadays tend to refer to data collection on individual responses about the acoustic environments experienced by people on site, with a relatively limited set of methods, such as: Soundwalks, questionnaires/interviews, non-participant behavioural observations, etc. [10,13,50,51]. These approaches encounter growing consensus in the soundscape research community, because of the ecological validity provided by their results, which is often compromised in laboratory settings [52], or unattended large-scale socio-acoustic surveys. Notwithstanding, none of such studies was detected by the review criteria, as they failed to include any health-related measure. A future direction for research that is possibly worth exploring, therefore, could be the inclusion of additional items related to health, well-being and quality of life, in the protocols of soundscape studies. Currently, standardized questionnaires do not consider this aspect [26,27], even if a number of reduced health-related protocols have already been validated in public health research and proved to properly relate also to psychometric properties in sound-related research [48,53,54]. This would offer further materials and analysis to establish stronger associations between soundscapes experience and positive effects on human health.

4.2. Key Results

The results from the items of the first group (large-scale studies) all show a consistent trend; that is: Better self-reported health-related conditions were always associated with reduced noise annoyance. In the specific case of Booi and van den Berg [43], the less urging need for quietness was interpreted as being expression of a reduced noise annoyance (i.e., no need for remediation means). In all studies, the associations were statistically significant with at least a $p < 0.05$ significance level.

Results from the items of the second group (small-scale studies) also show positive effects of experiencing good soundscapes on well-being. The health measures in these studies referred to the autonomic function; i.e., sympathetic or parasympathetic activation. In general, the studies looked at the parasympathetic activation, from a restoration perspective, observing that pleasant soundscapes are associated with more effective stress-recovery, and all those relationships were found to be statistically significant with at least a $p < 0.05$ significance level. The study by Hume and Ahtamad [40] did not provide a detailed interpretation about the relationship between the physiological measures and the soundscape measures, but it specified that the influence of context should be further investigated by considering "contextually supportive" sounds for health.

Taken together, the outcomes of this review support the claim that, both for short-term and long-term (as well as small-scale and large-scale) perspectives, positive perceptions of acoustic environments (soundscapes) can be associated to positive health effects.

4.3. Limitations

Due to the substantial differences in measures across studies, it was not possible to perform any statistical or quantitative meta-analysis, and a qualitative approach to data synthesis had to be sought instead. However, this is a common approach in noise-related public health research [34].

Furthermore, the relatively small number of items retrieved might raise some concerns. Notwithstanding, the choice to exclude studies that only collected soundscape data (but did not consider health-related measures) and studies that only assessed health effects of exposure/experience for different sound environments (but did not investigate the actual "perception" of those) was justified in Section 2.3. For both sub-groups, small-scale and large-scale studies, it was not always possible to "quantify" and compare the positive effects in the association between soundscapes and health measures. This was either because of a reporting bias (no means reported, only statistical significance) or because of substantial differences in the experimental designs of the studies (e.g., within-group or between-group designs, etc.).

Apart from that, the two sub-groups identified by the review had then their own characteristics related to the methodological approach. For the large-scale studies, it is almost never reported how the questionnaires were submitted to the participants; for instance: Whether the interview was attended/unattended by the researchers, the forms sent/returned by post, etc. This has the potential to introduce a bias in such a way that it is not possible to gather how participants were instructed and/or what was their understanding of the study. Furthermore, in this case, it is hard to control for objective exposure (noise levels), as metrics vary greatly across studies. However, all studies deal with sound levels that ranged between 30 and 80 dB; that is: Excluding cases of extremely low or high exposures.

The small-scale studies have the limitation of having a very specific scope, as they looked at the soundscape efficiency in supporting stress-recovery mechanisms (e.g., relaxing or calming down). There is indeed ongoing research aimed at reviewing the positive effects of specific sounds (e.g., natural sounds) on health and restoration [55]. However, some other sound sources (e.g., human sounds) could also be considered, as well as the soundscape's potential to elicit the positive perceptual constructs of excitement, liveliness and, more generally, engaging behaviours [12].

Overall, it is important to acknowledge that, especially for self-reported measures, the association between perception and health related to sound is a complex issue in terms of potential confounding factors, such as the sound level itself (which was not possible to control for in this review, due to the substantial differences of metrics between studies) or other personal elements (e.g., expectation, preconception, familiarity, etc.). Studies dealing with physiological measures are of course less vulnerable to this type of bias. However, more approaches are becoming relevant in soundscape studies to try to overcome the "experimenter bias" and self-reported data, by relying on behavioural observations and covert methods for data collection [50,51].

5. Conclusions

This paper reported on the positive health-related effects of experiencing positive soundscapes. For this purpose, a systematic review in accordance with the PRISMA guidelines was performed on three major scientific databases. After the screening process, the dataset resulted in seven items that were sorted into two groups, depending on the scale (i.e., large or small) of the investigation. Having substantially different methodological approaches, the studies were qualitatively analysed. The review pointed out that, regardless of the scale, statistically significant associations exist between positive soundscape perceptual constructs and health benefits. The main conclusions are:

- For the large-scale studies, positively assessed soundscapes (e.g., reduced noise annoyance) are statistically significantly associated with better self-reported health conditions.
- For the small-scale studies, positively assessed soundscapes (e.g., pleasant, calm) are statistically significantly associated with faster recovery from environmental stressors.

The review qualitatively showed that a trend is clearly observable, and more research efforts should be deployed in that direction to support the application of the soundscape approach at a planning and design level [56,57]. The ongoing standardization in soundscape studies [58] will hopefully help better position the discipline in the broader context of environmental research and public health.

Author Contributions: F.A., T.O. and J.K. designed and developed the study. F.A. and J.K. screened the items for the review. F.A. wrote the first draft of the manuscript. All authors revised the paper.

Funding: This research was funded through the European Research Council (ERC) Advanced Grant (no. 740696) on "Soundscape Indices" (SSID).

Acknowledgments: The authors are grateful to Andrew Mitchell for the comments on the first draft of this manuscript.

Conflicts of Interest: The authors declare no conflict of interest. The funder had no role in the design of the study; in the collection, analyses, or interpretation of data; in the writing of the manuscript, and in the decision to publish the results.

References

1. Wothge, J.; Belke, C.; Möhler, U.; Guski, R.; Schreckenberg, D. The Combined Effects of Aircraft and Road Traffic Noise and Aircraft and Railway Noise on Noise Annoyance—An Analysis in the Context of the Joint Research Initiative NORAH. *Int. J. Environ. Res. Public Health* **2017**, *14*, 871. [CrossRef] [PubMed]
2. World Health Organization. *Guidelines for Community Noise*; World Health Organization: Geneve, Switzerland, 1999.
3. European Commission—WG2 Dose/Effect. *Position Paper on Dose Response Relationships between Transportation Noise and Annoyance*; Office for Official Publications of the European Communities: Luxembourg, 2002.
4. Śliwińska-Kowalska, M.; Zaborowski, K. WHO Environmental Noise Guidelines for the European Region: A Systematic Review on Environmental Noise and Permanent Hearing Loss and Tinnitus. *Int. J. Environ. Res. Public Health* **2017**, *14*, 1139. [CrossRef] [PubMed]
5. De Paiva Vianna, K.M.; Alves Cardoso, M.R.; Calejo Rodrigues, R.M. Noise pollution and annoyance: An urban soundscapes study. *Noise Health* **2015**, *17*, 125–133. [CrossRef] [PubMed]
6. European Parliament and Council. *Directive 2002/49/EC Relating to the Assessment and Management of Environmental Noise*; Publications Office of the European Union: Brussels, Belgium, 2002.
7. European Environment Agency. *Good Practice Guide on Quiet Areas*; Publications Office of the European Union: Luxembourg, 2014.
8. European Environment Agency. *Noise in Europe 2014*; Publications Office of the European Union: Luxembourg, 2014.
9. Andringa, T.C.; Weber, M.; Payne, S.R.; Krijnders, J.D.; Dixon, M.N.; Linden, R.V.D.; de Kock, E.G.; Lanser, J.J. Positioning soundscape research and management. *J. Acoust. Soc. Am.* **2013**, *134*, 2739–2747. [CrossRef] [PubMed]
10. Aletta, F.; Kang, J.; Axelsson, Ö. Soundscape descriptors and a conceptual framework for developing predictive soundscape models. *Landsc. Urban Plan.* **2016**, *149*, 65–74. [CrossRef]
11. Kang, J. From dBA to soundscape indices: Managing our sound environment. *Front. Eng. Manag.* **2017**, *4*, 184–192. [CrossRef]
12. Aletta, F.; Kang, J. Towards an Urban Vibrancy Model: A Soundscape Approach. *Int. J. Environ. Res. Public Health* **2018**, *15*, 1712. [CrossRef] [PubMed]

13. Schulte-Fortkamp, B.; Fiebig, A. Soundscape analysis in a residential area: An evaluation of noise and people's mind. *Acta Acust United Acust.* **2006**, *92*, 875–880.
14. Schulte-Fortkamp, B.; Kang, J. Introduction to the special issue on soundscapes. *J. Acoust. Soc. Am.* **2013**, *134*, 765–766. [CrossRef] [PubMed]
15. Botteldooren, D.; Andringa, T.; Aspuru, I.; Brown, A.L.; Dubois, D.; Guastavino, C.; Kang, J.; Lavandier, C.; Nilsson, M.E.; Preis, A.; et al. From Sonic Environment to Soundscape. In *Soundscape and the Built Environment*; Kang, J., Schulte-Fortkamp, B., Eds.; CRC Press: Boca Raton, FL, USA, 2015.
16. Kang, J.; Aletta, F.; Gjestland, T.T.; Brown, L.A.; Botteldooren, D.; Schulte-Fortkamp, B.; Lercher, P.; van Kamp, I.; Genuit, K.; Fiebig, A.; et al. Ten questions on the soundscapes of the built environment. *Build. Environ.* **2016**, *108*, 284–294. [CrossRef]
17. International Organization for Standardization. *ISO 12913-1:2014 Acoustics—Soundscape—Part 1: Definition and Conceptual Framework*; ISO: Geneva, Switzerland, 2014.
18. Kang, J.; Aletta, F. The Impact and Outreach of Soundscape Research. *Environments* **2018**, *5*, 58. [CrossRef]
19. Lercher, P.; van Kamp, I.; von Lindern, E.; Botteldooren, D. Perceived Soundscapes and Health-Related Quality of Life, Context, Restoration, and Personal Characteristics. In *Soundscape and the Built Environment*; Kang, J., Schulte-Fortkamp, B., Eds.; CRC Press: Boca Raton, FL, USA, 2015.
20. Cerwén, G. Urban soundscapes: A quasi-experiment in landscape architecture. *Landsc. Res.* **2016**, *41*, 481–494. [CrossRef]
21. Xiao, J.; Lavia, L.; Kang, J. Towards an agile participatory urban soundscape planning framework. *J. Environ. Plan. Manag.* **2018**, *61*, 677–698. [CrossRef]
22. Bild, E.; Pfeffer, K.; Coler, M.; Rubin, O.; Bertolini, L. Public Space Users' Soundscape Evaluations in Relation to Their Activities. An Amsterdam-Based Study. *Front. Psychol.* **2018**, *9*, 1593. [CrossRef] [PubMed]
23. Aletta, F.; Oberman, T.; Kang, J. Positive Health-Related Effects of Perceiving Urban Soundscapes: A Systematic Review. In *Public Health Science—A National Conference Dedicated to New Research in UK Public Health*; The Lancet: Belfast, Ireland, 2018.
24. Axelsson, Ö.; Nilsson, M.; Berglund, B. A principal components model of soundscape perception. *J. Acoust. Soc. Am.* **2010**, *128*, 2836–2846. [CrossRef] [PubMed]
25. Liberati, A.; Altman, D.G.; Tetzlaff, J.; Mulrow, C.; Gøtzsche, P.C.; Ioannidis, J.P.A.; Clarke, M.; Devereaux, P.J.; Kleijnen, J.; Moher, D. The PRISMA Statement for Reporting Systematic Reviews and Meta-Analyses of Studies That Evaluate Health Care Interventions: Explanation and Elaboration. *PLoS Med.* **2009**, *6*, e1000100. [CrossRef] [PubMed]
26. Axelsson, Ö.; Nilsson, M.E.; Berglund, B. A Swedish Instrument for Measuring Soundscape Quality. In Proceedings of the Euronoise 2009, Edinburgh, UK, 26–28 October 2009.
27. International Organization for Standardization. *ISO/TS 12913-2:2018 Acoustics—Soundscape—Part 2: Data Collection and Reporting Requirements*; ISO: Geneva, Switzerland, 2018.
28. Berglund, B.; Nilsson, M.E. On a tool for measuring soundscape quality in urban residential areas. *Acta Acust. United Acust.* **2006**, *92*, 938–944.
29. Aletta, F.; Kang, J. Soundscape approach integrating noise mapping techniques: A case study in Brighton, UK. *Noise Map.* **2015**, *2*, 1–12. [CrossRef]
30. Axelsson, Ö. How to measure soundscape quality. In Proceedings of the Euronoise 2015, Maastricht, The Netherlands, 1–3 June 2015; pp. 1477–1481.
31. Park, B.J.; Tsunetsugu, Y.; Kasetani, T.; Hirano, H.; Kagawa, T.; Sato, M.; Miyazaki, Y. Physiological Effects of Shinrin-yoku (Taking in the Atmosphere of the Forest)—Using Salivary Cortisol and Cerebral Activity as Indicators. *J. Physiol. Anthropol.* **2007**, *26*, 123–128. [CrossRef] [PubMed]
32. Irwin, A.; Hall, D.A.; Peters, A.; Plack, C.J. Listening to urban soundscapes: Physiological validity of perceptual dimensions. *Psychophysiology* **2011**, *48*, 258–268. [CrossRef] [PubMed]
33. Aletta, F.; Xiao, J. What are the Current Priorities and Challenges for (Urban) Soundscape Research? *Challenges* **2018**, *9*, 16. [CrossRef]
34. Dzhambov, A.M.; Dimitrova, D.D. Occupational Noise and Ischemic Heart Disease: A Systematic Review. *Noise Health* **2016**, *18*, 167–177. [CrossRef] [PubMed]
35. Cassina, L.; Fredianelli, L.; Menichini, I.; Chiari, C.; Licitra, G. Audio-Visual Preferences and Tranquillity Ratings in Urban Areas. *Environments* **2018**, *5*, 1. [CrossRef]

36. Minichilli, F.; Gorini, F.; Ascari, E.; Bianchi, F.; Coi, A.; Fredianelli, L.; Licitra, G.; Manzoli, F.; Mezzasalma, L.; Cori, L. Annoyance Judgment and Measurements of Environmental Noise: A Focus on Italian Secondary Schools. *Int. J. Environ. Res. Public Health* **2018**, *15*, 208. [CrossRef] [PubMed]
37. Zhang, Y.; Kang, J.; Kang, J. Effects of Soundscape on the Environmental Restoration in Urban Natural Environments. *Noise Health* **2017**, *19*, 65–72. [PubMed]
38. Benfield, J.A.; Taff, B.D.; Newman, P.; Smyth, J. Natural Sound Facilitates Mood Recovery. *Ecopsychology* **2014**, *6*, 183–188.
39. Alvarsson, J.J.; Wiens, S.; Nilsson, M.E. Stress recovery during exposure to nature sound and environmental noise. *Int. J. Environ. Res. Public Health* **2010**, *7*, 1036–1046. [CrossRef] [PubMed]
40. Hume, K.; Ahtamad, M. Physiological responses to and subjective estimates of soundscape elements. *Appl. Acoust.* **2013**, *74*, 275–281. [CrossRef]
41. Medvedev, O.; Shepherd, D.; Hautus, M.J. The restorative potential of soundscapes: A physiological investigation. *Appl. Acoust.* **2015**, *96*, 20–26. [CrossRef]
42. Öhrström, E.; Skånberg, A.; Svensson, H.; Gidlöf-Gunnarsson, A. Effects of road traffic noise and the benefit of access to quietness. *J. Sound Vib.* **2006**, *295*, 40–59. [CrossRef]
43. Booi, H.; van den Berg, F. Quiet Areas and the Need for Quietness in Amsterdam. *Int. J. Environ. Res. Public Health* **2012**, *9*, 1030–1050. [CrossRef] [PubMed]
44. Shepherd, D.; Welch, D.; Dirks, K.N.; McBride, D. Do Quiet Areas Afford Greater Health-Related Quality of Life than Noisy Areas? *Int. J. Environ. Res. Public Health* **2013**, *10*, 1284–1303. [CrossRef] [PubMed]
45. Guski, R.; Felscher-Suhr, R.; Schuemer, R. The concept of noise annoyance: How international experts see it. *J. Sound Vib.* **1999**, *223*, 513–527. [CrossRef]
46. International Organization for Standardization. *ISO/TS 15666: 2003 Acoustics—Assessment of Noise Annoyance by Means of Social and Socio-Acoustic Surveys*; International Organization for Standardization: Geneva, Switzerland, 2003.
47. Skevington, S.M.; Lotfy, M.; O'Connell, K.A. The World Health Organization's WHOQOL-BREF quality of life assessment: Psychometric properties and results of the international field trial—A report from the WHOQOL group. *Qual. Life Res.* **2004**, *13*, 299–310. [CrossRef] [PubMed]
48. Krägeloh, C.U.; Kersten, P.; Billington, R.; Hsu, P.; Shepherd, D.; Landon, J.; Feng, X. Validation of the WHOQOL-BREF quality of life questionnaire for general use in New Zealand: Confirmatory factor analysis and Rasch analysis. *Qual. Life Res.* **2013**, *22*, 1451–1457. [CrossRef] [PubMed]
49. Rutherford, A. *ANOVA and ANCOVA: A GLM Approach*, 2nd ed.; John Wiley & Sons, Inc.: Hoboken, NJ, USA, 2011.
50. Aletta, F.; Lepore, F.; Kostara-Konstantinou, E.; Kang, J.; Astolfi, A. An experimental study on the influence of soundscapes on people's behaviour in an open public space. *Appl. Sci.* **2016**, *6*, 276. [CrossRef]
51. Lavia, L.; Witchel, H.J.; Aletta, F.; Steffens, J.; Fiebig, A.; Kang, J.; Howes, C.; Healey, P.G. Non-Participant Observation Methods for Soundscape Design and Urban Panning. In *Handbook of Research on Perception-Driven Approaches to Urban Assessment and Design*; Aletta, F., Xiao, J., Eds; IGI Global: Hershey, PA, USA, 2018; pp. 73–99.
52. Guastavino, C.; Katz, B.F.; Polack, J.; Levitin, D.J.; Dubois, D. Ecological validity of soundscape reproduction. *Acta Acust. United Acust.* **2005**, *91*, 333–341.
53. Lercher, P. Environmental noise and health: An integrated research perspective. *Environ. Int.* **1996**, *22*, 117–129. [CrossRef]
54. Welch, D.; Shepherd, D.; Dirks, K.N.; McBride, D. Road traffic noise and health-related quality of life: A cross-sectional study. *Noise Health* **2013**, *15*, 224230. [CrossRef] [PubMed]
55. Allou, C.; Pearson, A.; Rzotkiewicz, A.; Buxton, R. Positive Effects of Natural Sounds on Human Health and Well-Being: A Systematic Review. Available online: http://www.crd.york.ac.uk/PROSPERO/display_record.php?ID=CRD42018095537 (accessed on 22 October 2018).
56. Alves, S.; Estévez-Mauriz, L.; Aletta, F.; Echevarria-Sanchez, G.M.; Puyana Romero, V. Towards the integration of urban sound planning in urban development processes: The study of four test sites within the SONORUS project. *Noise Map.* **2015**, *2*, 57–85.

57. Echevarria Sanchez, G.M.; Alves, S.; Botteldooren, D. Urban Sound Planning: An Essential Component in Urbanism and Landscape Architecture. In *Handbook of Research on Perception-Driven Approaches to Urban Assessment and Design*; Aletta, F., Xiao, J., Eds.; IGI Global: Hershey, PA, USA, 2018; pp. 1–22.
58. Brown, A.L.; Kang, J.; Gjestland, T. Towards standardization in soundscape preference assessment. *Appl. Acoust.* **2011**, *72*, 387–392. [CrossRef]

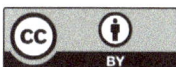

© 2018 by the authors. Licensee MDPI, Basel, Switzerland. This article is an open access article distributed under the terms and conditions of the Creative Commons Attribution (CC BY) license (http://creativecommons.org/licenses/by/4.0/).

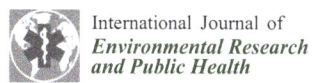

Review

The Psychophysiological Implications of Soundscape: A Systematic Review of Empirical Literature and a Research Agenda

Mercede Erfanian *, Andrew J. Mitchell, Jian Kang * and Francesco Aletta

UCL Institute for Environmental Design and Engineering, The Bartlett, University College London (UCL), Central House, 14 Upper Woburn Place, London WC1H 0NN, UK; andrew.mitchell.18@ucl.ac.uk (A.J.M.); f.aletta@ucl.ac.uk (F.A.)

* Correspondence: mercede.erfanianghasab.18@ucl.ac.uk (M.E.); j.kang@ucl.ac.uk (J.K.); Tel.: +44-(0)20-3108-7338 (J.K.)

Received: 16 September 2019; Accepted: 19 September 2019; Published: 21 September 2019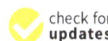

Abstract: The soundscape is defined by the International Standard Organization (ISO) 12913-1 as the human's perception of the acoustic environment, in context, accompanying physiological and psychological responses. Previous research is synthesized with studies designed to investigate soundscape at the 'unconscious' level in an effort to more specifically conceptualize biomarkers of the soundscape. This review aims firstly, to investigate the consistency of methodologies applied for the investigation of physiological aspects of soundscape; secondly, to underline the feasibility of physiological markers as biomarkers of soundscape; and finally, to explore the association between the physiological responses and the well-founded psychological components of the soundscape which are continually advancing. For this review, Web of Science, PubMed, Scopus, and PsycINFO were searched for peer-reviewed articles published in English with combinations of the keywords 'soundscape', 'environmental noise/sound', 'physiology/physiological', 'psychology/psychological', and 'perceptual attributes/affective/subjective assessment/appraisals'. Previous research suggests that Electrocardiography (ECG) and Vectorcardiography (VCG) biometrics quantifying Heart Rate (HR), stimulus-locked experimental design, and passive listening with homogeneous populations are predominantly applied to characterize the psychophysiology underlying the soundscape. Pleasantness and arousal are the most frequent psychological descriptors for soundscape subjective appraisals. Likewise, acoustic environments are reported to inconsistently evoke physiological responses with great variability among studies. The link between the perceptual attributes and physiological responses of soundscape vary within and among existing literature. While a few studies detected a link between physiological manifestations of soundscape and the perceptual attributes, the others failed to validate this link. Additionally, the majority of the study findings were limited to one or two physiological responses.

Keywords: soundscape; physiology; acoustic environment; perceptual attributes; auditory; noise

---

1. Introduction

Sound is capable of generating powerful reactions in human beings which inform how they interact with and interpret their everyday environments. There is accumulating research indicating how sound affects the activity and functionality of the Central Nervous System (CNS) and the Peripheral Nervous System (PNS) in response to various forms of sounds, such as music [1,2], natural sounds [3,4], and urban sounds (or anthropogenic) [4,5] throughout a person's lifetime [6,7].

From a physiological point of view, a sound signal is a detectable change in our external environment that can elicit a series of unconscious responses, unbalancing our homeostasis (the dynamic state of equilibrium). These responses are similar among populations in a similar situation, are automatic, and regulated by the Sympathetic Nervous System (SNS). The Parasympathetic Nervous System (PSNS), on the contrary, is constantly active to maintain homeostasis. It has been long established that both SNS and PSNS are part of the Autonomic Nervous System (ANS), which is per se a division of the Peripheral Nervous System (PNS) [8]. At the neural level, there appear to be segregated pathways, carrying the auditory signals and brain regions that orchestrate the way the brain responds to the auditory stimuli. The ascending auditory system, from the cochlea to the auditory cortex, is proven to respond to physical or acoustic properties of sound regardless of the emotional content or context of the sound (arousal) (the descending auditory pathway follows a similar path but in reverse) [9]. However, regions in the limbic system (emotional brain), such as amygdala and insula (known as a core hub of the "salience network"), are involved in processing the emotional magnitude of the auditory stimuli (valence), as a part of the CNS response [10,11]. The integration of the acquired auditory information from both ascending pathways results in the perception of the sound signals.

The soundscape, conceived as the acoustic equivalent of the landscape, is defined as the human's perception of the acoustic environment, in context [12–15]. The soundscape can be the result of a single sound or a combination of sounds that arises from an engaging environment. The Canadian composer and naturalist R. Murray Schafer led much of the original work to advance research in the area [15], borrowing the term originally from work carried out by city planner Michael Southworth [16]. Since Schafer, there have been several multi-dimensional classifications for soundscapes. However, according to Schafer, the main components of the soundscape consist of keynote sounds, sound signals, and soundmarks [15]. The soundscape ecologist Bernie Krause characterized soundscapes into three main domains based on the source of the sound. According to his classification, the soundscape refers to a wide spectrum of sounds, encompassing natural sounds relating to non-organic elements of nature such as waterfalls (geophony), organic but non-human sources such as animals' copulatory vocalizations (known as biophony), and all environmental sounds generated by human sources (anthrophony) such as human voices or human activity-related sounds [17–19].

Humans and soundscapes have a dynamic bidirectional relationship—while humans and their behaviour directly influence their soundscape, humans and their behaviour are in turn influenced by their soundscape. Several scientific communities in the area of neuroscience and psychology, therefore, have begun to pay close attention to our day-to-day exposure to particular sounds and their impact on the mental and physical health of individuals. Researchers in the areas of acoustics, environmental psychology, and auditory neuroscience outline the adverse impact of noise or negative sounds on well-being in an attempt to improve modern living standards [20–24]. In this regard, evidence indicates that positively perceived sounds (e.g., natural sounds) are tied with a high quality of life and enhanced psychological and physical health [5,25–27]. Subsequently, Attention Restoration Theory (ART) argues the impact of nature (e.g., being exposed to natural sounds such as waterfalls) on humans improved cognitive performance and stress recovery [28–31]. Not only has spending time in nature been demonstrated to have positive effects on humans' nervous system but it has also been shown that humans innately tend to seek connections with nature, a hypothesis known as Biophilia [32].

Within many acoustics-related fields, noise is defined specifically as *unwanted sound* [33,34]. However, the term has been used inconsistently and interchangeably across the studies reviewed here. Additionally, we refer to 'soundscape' as the perception of the acoustic environment in context. In order to maintain consistency within the field and for ease of understanding within this review noise and soundscape will be used only to refer to the definitions above.

Despite the accumulating evidence of the effects of sound on the human nervous system, the candidate peripheral and central mechanisms underlying its elicitation are far from understood. Although there is a line of robust literature in the areas of urban planning, architecture, noise control and health (linking noise to adverse mental and physical health which necessitates noise mitigation) pertaining to the assessment and design of soundscapes, the soundscape concept has only recently been introduced to the areas of psychophysiology and neuroscience.

As the development of the newly emerging body of psychophysiology and neuroscience research is a necessity, it does not trivialize the psychological approach that has considerably served to enhance our knowledge in the soundscape research domain.

The physiological and psychological approaches are two sides of the same coin in the realm of soundscape research, strongly interconnected and equally important. The psychological approach, in soundscape research, strives to depict the acoustic environment through the human behavioural pattern by borrowing a more deductive approach. It translates the underlying mechanisms into explicit behavioural manifestations, resulting from the perception of the acoustic environment.

The physiological approach investigates the impact of the acoustic environment through the investigation of fundamental mechanisms of CNS and PNS by adopting a more inductive inferential approach. The physiological approach delineates the causation of the particular behaviour evoked by the environmental sounds.

The soundscape is composed of three main components—human interaction, acoustic environment, and perception—so it potentially draws attention across several life-science disciplines such as environmental psychology and public health, psychophysiology and auditory neuroscience. To the best of authors' knowledge, no previous work has highlighted the explicit psychophysiological underpinnings of the soundscape. The current review of literature is the first work that reflects the fundamental mechanisms of the soundscape rather than its behavioural expressions.

Hence, the main research questions are (a) whether consistent methodologies were applied for the investigation of physiological aspects of soundscape; (b) secondly, what were the physiological markers as biomarkers of soundscape; and (c) finally, whether there was an association between the physiological responses and the perceptual attributes evoked by the acoustic environment.

2. Materials and Methods

The present literature review followed and was reported in accordance with PRISMA, Preferred Reporting Items for Systematic Review and Meta-Analysis (PRISMA) [35].

The inclusion criteria were: (a) including at least one measure of psychological dimensions or perceptual attributes of the soundscape as defined in ISO 12913-2; (b) including at least one physiological measure; and (c) published in English, excluding conference proceedings and books. The rationale of including these journal articles was that they all investigate the SNS and PSNS responses evoked by the acoustic environment.

The databases Thomson Reuters Web of Science, MEDLINE/PubMed, Scopus, and PsycINFO were searched for electronic records and studies related to the physiology of soundscape or the perception of environmental sounds, using the following Boolean search terms: 'soundscape' OR 'environmental noise/sound' AND 'physiology/physiological' AND 'psychology/psychological' OR 'perceptual attributes' OR 'affective/subjective assessment/appraisals' mentioned in either the title or the abstract. The time limitation was considered from 1 January 1990 to 1 February 2019, since the existing research is scarce. Journal articles were identified if they collected physiological responses to acoustic environments, regardless of whether they were investigating positive or negative soundscapes. One of the main theoretical frameworks on perceptual attributes has been proposed by Axelsson and his colleagues. Their circumplex model entails two horizontal and vertical axes, representing two different components of the soundscape. The vertical axis demonstrates the eventfulness component, which implies the intensity of soundscapes (i.e., eventful vs. uneventful). The horizontal axis refers to the emotional magnitude of soundscapes, representing the annoyance or pleasantness components (i.e., annoying vs. pleasant) [36]. The perceptual attributes proposed in this model have recently been adopted as a recommended standard in ISO 12913-2. In this review of the literature, the authors elucidate the perceptual attributes of soundscapes according to the circumplex model, where arousal is line with eventfulness on the vertical axis and valence is in line with pleasantness on the horizontal axis.

The search results were exported to Mendeley, which identified 122 published research articles. Then, the duplicates were removed (n = 29). Next, if the title or abstract did not provide sufficient information or did not meet the selection criteria, they were removed (n = 71). Then, the remaining 22 full-text articles were assessed for eligibility—of which, 17 were excluded from further inclusion as they were deemed irrelevant (e.g., physiology of noise). Finally, the exclusion resulted in five relevant journal papers which were read and analysed manually for method and content—of which, the oldest article was published in 2004 [5,10,37–39]. Figure 1 shows the process of inclusion of reviewed papers.

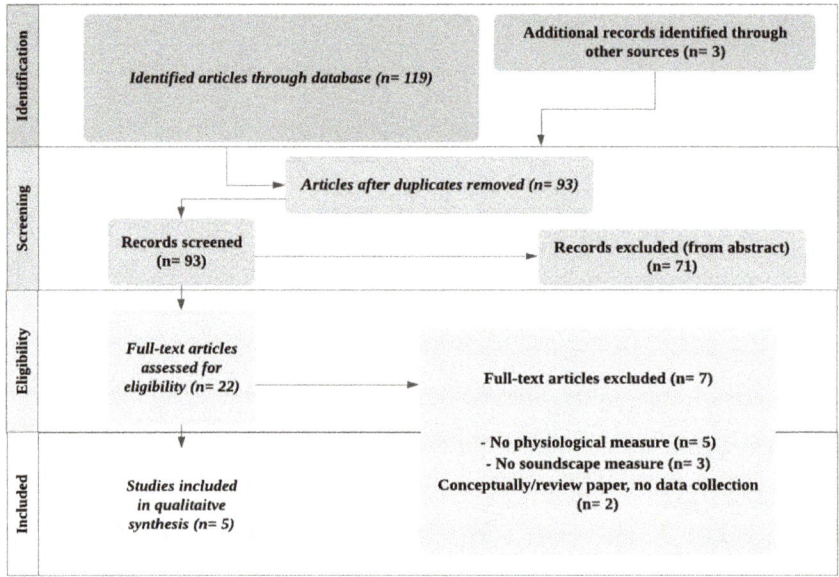

Figure 1. The flow of information through the different phases of the systematic review. The number of studies included in the qualitative synthesis (n = 5).

In the first step of the screening process, the first author (ME) reviewed the titles and abstracts of the journal articles and manually excluded the articles that did not meet the above-mentioned criteria. The second step was selecting the studies in which (ME) assessed the full-text articles for eligibility in accordance with the method outlined in PRISMA. Disagreements between the authors regarding the study selection were resolved by consensus.

3. Methodology in the Reviewed Studies

Although there is a long line of multidisciplinary research on soundscape, the majority of the available literature on soundscape and well-being has focused on the perceptual attributes and psychological components, lacking the conceptualization of its underlying physiological and neural mechanisms' validity [5,40,41]. In other words, the current understanding of the entanglement of psychology and soundscape is mostly limited to the relationship between acoustic characteristics and the subjective appraisal of soundscapes, without the clarification of corresponding responses in the CNS or PNS. Studies focusing on identification of the physiological and neural mechanisms underlying soundscape are scarce and this mode of study warrants deeper and more elaborate investigation. In this section, we review the aims and methodologies of the included studies. The methodology includes the type of individuals included as the study sample, the experimental design, the auditory stimuli, and the subjective and objective measurements. Table 1 demonstrates the summary of the articles included in the review with detailed information on methods and the materials.

Table 1. Summary of the review studies ($n = 5$).

Reviewed Articles	Stimuli Length	Number of Stimuli	Metrics	Sound Source Category				Physiological Metrics	Perceptual Attributes		
				Human	Natural	Mechanical	Music		Valence	Arousal	Other
Gomez and Danuser, 2004	30 s	32	52.2–77.5 dB (A) **	e.g., people playing tennis	-	e.g., siren	Ranging from low to high, e.g., Black arrows by Manowar	HR, SCL, RR	Valence	Arousal	-
Alvarsson et al., 2010 †	4 min	N/A	40–80 dB (A)	-	from fountain and tweeting birds	road traffic (high, low and ambient)	-	HF HRV, SCL	Pleasantness	Eventfulness	Familiarity
Irwin et al., 2011	8 s	150	71 dB (A) *,**	e.g., giggling	e.g., wind	e.g., construction	-	HR, fMRI, PET	Pleasantness	Vibrancy	-
Hume and Ahtamad, 2013 ***	8 s	18	60–74 dB (A) **	e.g., vomiting	e.g., horse hooves on road	e.g., traffic noise	-	HR, RR, EMG	Pleasantness	Arousal	-
Medvedev et al., 2015	4 min	4	64 dB (A) *,**	-	e.g., ocean	e.g., road noise	-	HR, SCL	Pleasantness	Arousal, eventfulness	Dominance, familiarity
Medvedev et al., 2015	2 min	6	64 dB (A) *,**	-	e.g., ocean	e.g., road noise	-	HR, SCL	Pleasantness	Arousal, eventfulness	Dominance, familiarity

* Normalized Auditory Stimuli. ** L_{eq} Sound Pressure Level (SPL). *** Used sound-clips with mix sources. † Binaural Recording. HR, Heart Rate; HF HRV, High Frequency Heart Rate Variability; fMRI, Functional Magnetic Resonance Imaging; PET, Positron Emission Tomography; SCL, Skin Conductance Level; RR, Respiration Rate; EMG, Electromyography.

3.1. Study 1

Alvarsson et al. [5] were the first to report that the SNS gains a faster recovery while exposed to nature sounds compared to other sounds. This study aimed at comparing the effects of different sounds on the physiological recovery of individuals with induced psychological stress.

In this study, Alvarsson et al. tested university students in a three-part study. The first part began with one 5 min silence baseline, then five 2 min sections of testing or stressor, each followed by a 4 min period of relaxation or recovery. The authors made a 4 × 4 mixed design with relaxation sound as the within-subject variable and the order of the four different sounds as the between-subject variable. A Latin square matrix was applied in which the participants were assigned at random. The participants were given a mental arithmetic task as a stressor. In the task, the participants should decide whether the equation which appeared on the screen was true or false and received feedback as to whether their answer was 'false', 'correct', or 'too late'.

The participants were exposed to 4 min samples of nature sounds (mixture of fountain and bird sounds, 50 dB $L_{Aeq,\ 4\ min}$), high noise (traffic noise, 80 dB $L_{Aeq,\ 4\ min}$), low noise (the same traffic noise adjusted to 50 dB $L_{Aeq,\ 4\ min}$), and ambient sound (referred to in the text as 'ambient noise') such as backyard sound including ventilation noise, 40 dB $L_{Aeq,\ 4\ min}$) during the recovery periods.

The indication of SNS activation was measured by Skin Conductance Level (SCL) and the recovery period or PSNS activity was measured by High-Frequency Heart Rate Variability (HF HRV). The perceptual attributes assessment was measured by a scale on three dimensions of pleasantness, eventfulness, and familiarity.

We should note that the exponential function coefficients in this work as part of the regression analysis produce a curve which is a factor of 10 off from the data. It is assumed this is a typographical error in the figure (where, e.g., $b_3 = -0.1111$ should be $b_3 = -0.01111$) that does not substantially impact the conclusions of the analysis.

3.2. Study 2

Gomez and Danuser [37] investigated the link between physiological parameters with subjective reports evoked by the acoustic environment. The main aim of this study was to evaluate the link between the judgment of affective arousal and valence and physiological responses.

The participants were selected mostly among university students. The authors exposed subjects to 30 s of mixed auditory stimuli that varied in emotional valence and arousal, representing environmental acoustic stimuli (referred to in the text as 'environmental noises') such as people playing tennis, sirens, as well as Western instrumental music (ranging from quiet Classical music, 'Adagio assai', M. Ravel, to loud Metal, 'Black Arrows', Manowar) with little acoustic variation over their 30 s, in order to maintain high intra-stimulus homogeneity.

All the environmental sounds and music excerpts were ranked from low to high based on a combination of the mean valence and mean arousal level, into groups (1–4, 5–8, 9–12, 13–16). Importantly, to ensure ecological validity of the auditory stimuli (ecological validity refers to methods and materials and the setting of the study that is close to the 'real world'), the authors did not change or modulate the intensity of the soundscapes presented in the experiments.

The physiological responses were extrapolated from SCL, Respiration Rate (RR), and ECG. The affective rating was probed by a 9-point self-assessment Manikin on two dimensions of arousal and valence.

3.3. Study 3

Irwin et al. [10] explored the physiological validity of perceptual aspects of the acoustic environment. The purpose of the study was to assess the visceral and neural basis of cognitive and emotional responses to positive or 'naturalistic urban soundscapes' and their association with the perceptual dimensions (here, 'naturalistic urban soundscapes' refers to realistically recorded sound environments, not to urban soundscapes with a high proportion of natural sounds).

In this study, only native English speakers were selected. Here, we will only report the results of the physiological investigation as the outcome of neural responses is not in the scope of this review. For the physiological experiments, the authors selected a set of 8 s stimuli that would broadly range over the pleasantness and vibrancy scales.

A set of 219 recordings were selected from different archives and a selected set of 150 sounds was presented to the subjects in a randomized fashion and -in four sequential blocks lasting about 10 min each. Each block comprised a set of sounds with a duration of 8 s followed by 8 s or 16 s of silence. This study did not include any active task and subjects were instructed merely to remain still and listen to the samples. The visceral changes were registered by measuring HR. The perceptual attributes were tested by a self-report assessment on two dimensions of vibrancy and pleasantness.

3.4. Study 4

A more recent study by Hume and Ahtamad [38] employed a similar stimulus selection and presentation technique towards developing a better understanding of the physiological manifestation of soundscape and its possible relationship with subjective reporting of pleasantness and arousal. This study entailed three main objectives: to investigate (a) whether there is a change in registered physiological responses to different soundscapes; (b) whether there is a link between the pattern of physiological changes and the subjective rating of the pleasantness and arousal of the sound excerpt; and (c) whether there is a gender difference in any physiological responses.

They selected their participants among unpaid volunteers. The authors state that a key experimental design consideration was to limit the total time needed for each subject's experiment to 20 min in order to mitigate potential issues with the experiment and listening fatigue. They also state that the presentation of 8 s sound stimuli was carefully considered in order to limit the prompting of the startle reflex in response to sudden loud sounds. The stimuli consisted of a range of sound-clips with a wide variety or source types such as 'horses hooves on the road' and 'jackhammer plus traffic noise'. The physiological alteration was measured by recording HR, RR, and Electromyography (EMG). The pleasantness and arousal were evaluated by a 9-scale self-report.

3.5. Study 5

Another study by Medvedev et al. [39] investigated the restorative potential of acoustic environment perception. The first objective was to examine the variations of physiological responses to a number of auditory stimuli after a stressful task.

In their first study, they included unpaid postgraduate students or members of staff. Initially, Medvedev et al. exposed participants to a thirty-minute sequence with 4 min stimuli. Each sequence entailed five stress periods of 2 min, followed by a stress recovery period of four minutes. During each stress recovery period, the participants were randomly exposed to one of the four different environmental sounds or a silence condition. The stimuli consisted of the sounds of a forest, sea wave, busy motorway, and construction site.

In their second study, the objective was to measure the same physiological responses of soundscape during the rest state. Only university students were involved in the second phase of the study. The authors, therefore, exposed their subjects to different 2 min sounds to determine the effects on the ANS by exposing the subjects to unpleasant sounds during the rest period.

The sound samples selected for the second part of the study were three unnatural, two natural, and one orchestra piece.

The participants' SCL and HR, representing the 'fight, flight, or freeze' response, were measured in both phases of the study, followed by participants' subjective ratings of their perception of the four presented sound samples. The perceptual attributes in this study were arousal, dominance, eventfulness, familiarity, and pleasantness which were measured by a self-rating questionnaire.

3.6. Overall Methodological Approaches

The research on the physiological underpinnings of the soundscape is limited and so is the methodology. With respect to the available literature, the majority of the reviewed studies focused on the impact of the acoustic environment on ANS arousal by looking at specific physiological indicators within homogeneous populations, e.g., university students. The most commonly administered study design was passive listening with event-related responses (also known as stimulus-locked design) in which the participants' physiological and perceptual responses, evoked by environmental sounds, were monitored. In the event-related design, the physiological arousal in response to environmental sounds is measured and evaluated in comparison with their baseline (silence condition). This response is generally more accurately related to the event in higher-frequency measures such as Electroencephalography (EEG), and less so in slower measures such as HR and Electrodermal Activity (EDA). Human, natural, and mechanical sounds reported being commonly used in most of the studies. HR is predominately applied for the quantification of ANS reactivity to environmental sounds. Analysis of heart rate (variability) is acknowledged as a cost-effective method with high validity and reliability, independent of risk factors of any cardiovascular diseases [42]. It has been commonly used in several studies to investigate the ANS reactivity to sounds [10,11,37]. The perceptual attributes of pleasantness (valence) vs. eventfulness (arousal) were mostly used among the existing literature.

4. Physiological Manifestations of Soundscapes

Beyond studies with a primary aim of investigating the psychological markers of the soundscape, a small body of research offers important insights toward a better understanding of the biomarkers of soundscapes by quantifying the physiological manifestations induced by ANS reactivity such as HR/HF HRV, EDA, RR, and musculoskeletal responses.

4.1. Heart Rate (HR) and Heart Rate Variability (HRV)

HR is a primary indication of ANS activation which is regulated by SNS and PNS. HR (V) are widely used in medical examinations and can be evoked in response to a variety of factors such as exercise, emotional arousal, and stimulant exposure. Although the outcome of HR and HRV are closely interconnected, they differ from each other in terms of pre-processing and analysis. While HR is measured in beats per minutes, or the average of the beats in a specific the time period (e.g., 1 min), HRV measures the specific change/variability in the time between the beats [43,44]. Only Alvarsson et al. applied HRV in the study. Notably, Bradley and Lang, in their 2000 study, pointed out a consistent 'triphasic' heart rate waveform across valence categories, in which an initial deceleration was followed by acceleration and then a secondary deceleration. When limited only to high-arousal sounds, the characteristics of the triphasic response varied across the valence categories [43].

In the 2004 study by Gomez and Danuser [37], the outcome of a mixed regression analysis of ECG indicated that high-arousal sounds (e.g., siren) evoked higher HR than low-arousal sounds (e.g., people playing tennis) ($\beta = 1.18$, $SE = 0.48$, $p = 0.05$), although the association was not found between music and HR [37]. On the other hand, Medvedev et al., 2015 [39] in the second phase of their study found no relationship between HR and environmental sounds regardless of the sound source type (music, mechanical sounds, or natural sounds) and the findings of Irwin et al. [10] were shown to be limited to the immediate rise of HR right after the onset of the stimulus. However, the HR was then shown to have declined by a sustained reduction after a few seconds. Surprisingly, the outcome from Hume and Ahtamad's study [38] is contrary to the previous works, showing a lowered HR in response to the sound stimuli, with a more prominent response to unpleasant sounds.

Although there are inconsistent findings with respect to HR response to soundscapes given a passive listening condition, there is a consensus between the two available studies which employed a stress task condition. Neither Medvedev et al.'s first study nor Alvarsson et al. could validate a significant link between HR and sound exposure during the recovery period after presenting a stress task [5,39].

4.2. Respiration Rate (RR)

Respiration rate (RR) is a vital sign and a widely used metric in medical research as a measurement of SNS reactivity and physiological stability of individuals with high accuracy. Abnormal RR is a serious indication of an imminent health crisis [45].

The study by Hume and Ahtamad [38] demonstrated an increased RR, to differing degrees, in response to all soundscapes except 'man hiccupping'. Further investigation pointed to a gender difference in RR response in which men exhibited a greater increase of RR to all soundscapes compared to women [38]. These findings were in line with the previous study by Gomez and Danuser in which they discovered increased RR in both music and environmental sounds conditions [37]. A conclusion can be drawn when considering the small number of reviewed studies using the RR measure. These two studies mainly showed a consistent RR outcome, and they do highlight the respiratory candidate process for further research in peripheral nervous system activity associated with exposure to environmental sounds.

4.3. Electrodermal Activity (EDA)

EDA is a reliable and valid psychophysiological expression of SNS arousal. Physiologically, the activation of the endocrinology system is driven by the interconnection between CNS and PNS, especially by the sympathetic branch of ANS. The increased reactivity of SNS in the epidermis changes its electrical conductance, forming the basis of the EDA that is measured by Skin Conductance Response (SCR) (also known as Galvanic Skin Response (GSR)) and/or Skin Conductance Level (SCL) [46]. However, SCR reflects the rapid phasic component of EDA and SCL is derived from the slow and background tonic component.

The second study by Medvedev et al. showed no significant effect of sounds on SCL [39] which is almost in agreement with the study by Gomez and Danuser. In the latter study, the results of SCL showed that only 'high' music pieces (e.g., heavy metal) cued higher SCL compared to 'low' music (e.g., classical music), while SCL showed no significant relationship with environmental sounds [37].

The results of SCL in stress task studies are in less agreement than those with no stress task. Medvedev et al. failed to show significance in measured SCL changes in response to sounds after stress tasks, similar to their findings with no stress task. On the other hand, Alvarsson et al. demonstrated that subjects exposed to natural sounds recovered significantly faster (9–36% faster) from psychological stress in comparison to when they were exposed to 'high noise' (traffic noise, 80 dB $L_{Aeq, 4\ min}$). The authors reported that during exposure to high noise, a minor upturn in SCL was observed during the last 50 s of the 4 min recovery period, implying long exposure to the unpleasant sounds increased arousal [5]. All in all, studies into EDA response have been more consistent than other indications of ANS arousal in response to sound. However, the implications of EDA in the context of public health and well-being is still not clear.

4.4. Musculoskeletal Activity

The SNS modulates the functions in the musculoskeletal system (e.g., metabolism and locomotion). EMG measures musculoskeletal activity, from which SNS activity can be derived. The research on musculoskeletal response to soundscape has been confined to Hume and Ahtamad's work. They showed that there was a significant relationship between attenuated muscle tone and pleasant sounds (e.g., evening bird songs with some traffic sounds). However, the significant difference was not consistent among all soundscape excerpts, and no difference between male and female participants could be detected [38].

5. The Association between Perceptual Attributes and Physiological Responses

The ANS is sensitive and responsive to external stimuli such as olfactory, textile, gustatory, vision, and auditory. The reactivity of ANS, triggered by environmental sensory stimulation, manifests in the variation of several systems in vivo, for instance, cardiovascular systems [47]. However, the representation of ANS reactivity does not always identify the type of emotion or perception, arising from this reactivation. It is therefore fundamental to make sense of the alteration of ANS through the subjective assessments which can be inconsistent. Table 2 shows the main objectives of the reviewed studies and their key findings.

5.1. Study 1

The outcome of the perceptual evaluation of the sounds in the study by Alvarsson et al. indicated that natural sounds were perceived as more pleasant than human and mechanical sounds. Among the latter, low traffic noise and the ambient sound were reported to be perceived as equally pleasant whereas the high traffic noise was reported to be the least pleasant sound. Further analysis showed that the high traffic noise was reported to be the most eventful while the ambient sound was rated as the least eventful and least familiar among all. The rationale of the authors for this finding was that the ambient noise contained no distinctive sound sources and may not be sufficiently salient to be differentiated [5]. This suggests that sympathetic arousal is influenced by the type of sound present in the environment with the largest observed differences between natural sounds and high traffic noise [5].

5.2. Study 2

The results of emotional magnitude ratings of both environmental sounds and music in the study by Gomez and Danuser showed wide variability in subjective ratings of valence and arousal. For the environmental stimuli, the subjective appraisals tended toward negative valence and high arousal. On the contrary, for the music condition, the subjective appraisals tended toward positive valence ratings and high arousal. In both conditions, faster breathing and high minute ventilation (MV) were related to increased arousal. While this association was reported to be present within the whole emotional magnitude (valence) for music, it was limited to only positive stimuli for the environmental sounds. However, their findings showed that slower breathing, as well as declined MV, were attributed to low-arousal sounds.

The thoracic breathing responses to environmental sounds and musical excerpts were demonstrated to be regulated moderately in line with valence ratings and arousal. The authors did not find any link between other physiological responses and perceptual attributes [37].

5.3. Study 3

Irwin et al. could not find a significant HR change associated with pleasantness and vibrancy. The results stayed the same for the association between pleasantness and the length of the sounds [10].

5.4. Study 4

In Hume and Ahtamad's study, the HR and RR outcomes were reported to be greater in response to increased pleasantness and showed a clear gender difference with larger RR and HR responses observed for males [38]. Furthermore, the results indicated that decreased muscle activity derived from EMG was associated with more pleasant sounds with no gender effect.

Table 2. Studies from 1990 to 2019 of the outcome of the psychophysiology of soundscape.

Reviewed Articles	Objective (s)	Research Design	No of Participants	Key Findings
Gomez and Danuser, 2004	(A) Evaluation of the link between the judgment of affective arousal and valence and physiological response	Stimulus locked	31	(A) Only RR in response to environmental sounds and music is in line with valence and arousal to a certain extent
Alvarsson et al., 2010 *	(A) Comparison of the effects of different sounds on the physiological recovery of individuals with induced psychological stress	Latin square matrix	40	(A) Nature sound accelerates the physiological recovery of SNS after psychological stress
Irwin et al., 2011	(A) Assessment of the visceral basis of cognitive and emotional responses to positive or 'naturalistic urban soundscapes' (B) Their association with the perceptual dimensions	Stimulus locked	16	(A) Increment of HR in response to the onset of auditory stimuli (B) No association was found
Hume and Ahtamad, 2013	(A) Investigation of variation in registered physiological responses to different soundscapes (B) Investigation of the link between the pattern of physiological changes and the subjective rating the pleasantness and arousal of the sound excerpt (C) Investigation of a gender difference in any physiological responses	Stimulus locked	80	(A) Decrement of HR, increment of RR, decrement of EMG limited to pleasant sounds (B) Increment of HR, and RR but decrement of EMG to rise of pleasantness, no association between physiological responses and valence reported (C) A significant rise in HR and RR responses in men but not in EMG
Medvedev et al., 2015 *	(A) Examining the variations of physiological responses to a number of auditory stimuli after a stressful task	Latin square matrix	45	(A) Faster recovery of SCL in response to the most pleasant and the least eventful sounds and a significant difference in mean HR only during the eventful sound
Medvedev et al., 2015	(A) Measuring the same physiological responses of soundscape during rest state	Stimulus locked	30	(A) SCL linked to the least pleasant, familiar, and dominating sounds specially in the first 10 s; the increase of SCL associated with the least pleasant, familiar and the most dominant; no SCL change in response to the most and the least arousing and eventful sounds; a fall in HR associated with the least pleasant and the most familiar sounds

* Stress Task.

5.5. Study 5

The outcome of the self-reported subjective ratings of the sound stimuli in the study by Medvedev et al. showed substantial variability of the mean response in the perceptual dimension assessing the appropriateness of the selected sounds. Among the presented sounds, ocean and birdsong were reported to be the most pleasant and arousing while construction and traffic were rated as the most dominating and eventful. The results of SCL in the first phase of the study, showed a faster decline in electrodermal activity in response to the more pleasant and less eventful sounds, although the perception of eventfulness and pleasantness differed among the participants. Likewise, sounds associated with the most familiarity and least eventfulness were linked to a decline of SCL. In addition, there was a significant difference in mean HR for the recovery period limited to only the eventfulness domain [39]. In the second phase of their study, the augmentation of SCL was reported to be attributed to the least pleasant and familiar as well as the most dominant sounds. Eventfulness and arousal showed no significant relationship with SCL change. Lower HR was significantly related to the least pleasant and the most familiar sounds.

5.6. Overall Association between Perceptual Attributes and Physiological Responses

Altogether, physiological expressions of the soundscape are not always aligned with the perceptual attributes and may remain inconclusive. Notably, it appears auditory stimuli length makes a major contribution to physiological expression and their link with perceptual attributes.

6. Discussion

The perception of the acoustic environment is the result of ongoing, meticulous, and unconscious interactions between subcortical and cortical brain structures. Consequently, the perception of the acoustic environment is closely correlated with the physiological properties elicited by the acoustic environment. There is a pressing deficiency in the existing soundscape research in which the implication of physiological changes in the context of human health and well-being is missing.

6.1. Soundscape and Noise Studies

Physiological studies have constituted a vital underpinning of conventional approaches to environmental noise control. As the direction of noise control has become progressively more holistic and begun incorporating the soundscape approach, an equivalent understanding of the physiological manifestations of the soundscape is needed. Since research on the physiology of noise pollution is generally more advanced than within the realm of the soundscape, in order to elucidate the physiological underpinnings of environmental sounds the authors briefly look into the physiology of noise exposure and its implications in soundscape research.

6.1.1. Heart Rate

The majority of the existing body of literature in the physiology of soundscape is limited to HR, which currently indicates that noise or negatively perceived sound exposure significantly contributes to causing tachycardia [10,37]. However, the results are not consistent throughout the studies [5,38,39]. Looking back at the long-established literature in the area of noise pollution and health, we find similar findings. A study by Hsu et al. on forty patients recovering from anaesthesia underlines a positive significant association between an increase in noise intensity and HR [48]. It is important to note that in this study, the sound level was the only considered physical factor irrespective of other acoustic characteristics of the considered sounds.

Another study by Elbaz et al. investigating the effect of aircraft noise on HR during sleep shows that increased HR is linked to an increase in Sound Pressure Level (SPL) [49]. These findings are also in agreement with more prolonged conditions such as individuals exposed to occupational noise such as those investigated in a study by Burns and her colleagues. In this study, the test results of

57 electronic waste recycling workers indicated a significant rise in HR associated with work-related noise [50]. Abdelraziq et al. conducted another study investigating the effects of noise pollution on HR of school children. A strong positive correlation was found between augmented HR and noise pollution level [51]. In all, it seems that the amplitude level plays a crucial role in the magnitude of an evoked increase in HR as long as the sound is considered/labeled as noise.

6.1.2. Respiration Rate

RR is a physiological metric with mainly consistent results in response to positively and negatively perceived extrinsic auditory stimuli. Regardless of the intensity of the sound, soundscape studies point to an increase of RR evoked by the acoustic environment [37,38]. Seemingly, RR alteration is a fundamental physiological parameter, indicating the impact of noise on homeostasis. Hassanein et al. studied the impact of interrupted loud noise in the Neonatal Intensive Care Unit (NICU). In this study, they registered the neonatal physiological responses at a different time of day and during different sound events. The findings revealed a significant increment of RR in pre-term neonates in comparison with full-term neonates when exposed to sound events during the day [52].

The existing literature also looked into the long-term effects of noise (e.g., road traffic) on physical health in which an association between traffic noise exposure and respiratory morbidities [53] was demonstrated. According to the literature, the adverse effects of exposure to noise are a high risk of developing diseases such as bronchitis and asthma and pneumonia in children that was attributed to an increase of 1 dB (A) of daily noise levels, as a short-term association [54].

6.1.3. Skin Conductance Response/Level

The essence of SCL response in soundscape research is to infer psychological descriptors from measured induced EDA. Whereas EDA has been proved to be an accurate manifestation of SNS activation, it does not always show a consistent outcome throughout the soundscape physiology research [5,35,37]. On the other hand, the majority of the findings on EDA when restricted to the response to noise is in agreement. A study by Park and Lee tested the effects of 'floor impact noise' on the physiological responses. Although the floor noise seems to be a trivial sound and not salient enough to be perceived as annoying, it leads to a significant increase in EDA of the subjects [55]. Similarly, Glass and Singer found a rise in the SCR evoked by noise in more than 90% of their participants which was irrespective of the amplitude and unpredictability of the sound. However, some further and deeper investigation revealed a drop in SCR which was an indication of the habituation in almost 90% of their participants, while only 4% seemed to be unable to adapt physiologically [56].

6.1.4. Musculoskeletal Responses

The potential for the examination of soundscape via musculoskeletal system activity is far from limited and understanding it should be deemed highly necessary. EMG, an electrodiagnostic technique which can help to better understand the possible effect of sounds in the musculoskeletal system is limited to one study in the context of soundscape but has been shown to increase in response to pleasant soundscapes [38]. The large body of literature on skeletal muscle activity provoked by noise is in line with the responses found by Hume and Ahtamad. A study by Trapanotto and colleagues in the Paediatric Intensive Care Unit (PICU) revealed an increase in skeletal muscle tone detected by EMG, in particular during exposure to highly intense noise [57].

In short, the literature on soundscape and noise appear to have consensus regarding the increase in HR, with less consistency in results among soundscape studies. The RR and EMG outcomes showed more steady patterns in both areas of research indicating the increment of RR in response to sound stimuli, with consideration of the limitation of RR application among soundscape research. On the other hand, there is less agreement on the results of EDA between soundscape and noise research domains since the findings are uncertain among soundscape literature.

6.2. Suggestions for the Research Agenda

6.2.1. Soundscape Characterization

The limited studies on physiological indices predominantly focus either on the adverse or the favourable aspects of soundscapes. Consequently, an interdisciplinary and holistic probe is deemed necessary to shed light on the entire spectrum spanning positive and negative soundscapes in order to better understand the impact of soundscapes in a general context. Since there is no sufficient evidence to make conclusions about either physiological manifestation related to soundscapes, we suggest that future investigations classify/categorize the types of sound sources. These categories (e.g., human, nature, and mechanical) would function as a steady baseline to which we can attribute the negative and positive responses [58,59]. Investigating soundscapes based on the source of the sound and not how positive or negative they are perceived will facilitate the researchers to characterize the physiological and neural responses regardless of the variability in the listeners [60].

Considering distinctions in the physiological responses to single or complex sound sources would also enable future research to better grasp the differences in potential evoked biological responses when considering the different source type characterizations suggested above.

Another essential aspect of soundscapes that may lead to invaluable findings and which could strongly reflect on human physiology is the duration of exposure and temporal variation of the acoustic environment, in an experimental context, reflecting in physiological responses [61,62]. The outcome could be potentially translated to how ANS habituates or sensitizes to sounds in the real world. Future research should take these factors into consideration because the current body of research strongly implies that sound duration and variation, in general, are well-established contributors to nervous system adaptation and the resulting habituation or sensitization. Although the habituation or sensitization of the nervous system to sounds relies upon acoustic features of the presented sound [63], to date they have not been addressed in the context of soundscapes.

6.2.2. Recording and Reproduction of Soundscapes

Given that many of the most promising physiological metrics must be performed in a laboratory setting (e.g., RR), the ecological validity of reproduced soundscapes is a vital consideration. Toward this, much work has been carried out within the field of soundscape studies toward reducing artificiality of the controlled acoustic environment and achieving immersion. Two main methods are used: binaural recordings and ambisonic recordings which use multiple microphones to record a sound field at a single point in full-sphere surround. Binaural audio has long been used in soundscape studies, but its use has generally been limited in physiological studies of soundscape and ambisonic audio has not yet been applied to physiological studies. Both binaural and ambisonic audio, which allows the full spherical sound field to be reproduced very close to what would be experienced in situ, can improve immersion and add ecological validity to laboratory studies [64].

In addition to the ecological validity of the acoustic environment, in order to fully research soundscape, it is highly recommended [65] to take the effects of other sensory modalities into account such as vision, olfactory, and environmental components such as temperature. The inclusion of other modalities represents another step toward understanding the cross-modalities interaction of perception of acoustic environment and how the interpretation of acoustic information is an integral part of this process by introducing new methods such as Virtual Reality (VR), Augmented Reality (AR) [66,67]. Toward this aim, virtual reality reproductions are increasingly being used to create an immersive and soundscape reproduction which can incorporate multiple sensory modalities [68].

6.2.3. Physiological and Neural Models

The conceptual framework of the physiological and neural network may be fruitful in order to develop specific candidate physiological and neural mechanisms of soundscape. This approach emphasizes an understanding of basic brain processes at the network level. Applying a network level approach would allow testing hypotheses about different brain regions working in an integrated and coordinated fashion. While the majority of our knowledge of how the brain implements soundscape processing is based on the assumption of assigning a certain role to each region of the brain, there is an emerging realization that shows this approach is not pragmatic in understanding brain function. Instead, it is suggested that functions of the brain in response to soundscape should be understood at the network level. In order to precisely pinpoint the physiological and neural mechanisms behind soundscape, it will not be enough to determine which brain substrates are activated by different sounds. We must also understand how those brain areas work together at a network level.

6.2.4. Physiological and Psychological Models/Body–Mind Integration Model

The integration of physiological and psychological approaches known as the 'body–mind' model can substantially strengthen our understanding of how and why we experience the soundscape the way that we do. In this model, the mind and body are not seen as separately functioning entities, but as one holistic bidirectional unit, driven by top–down and bottom–up factors. It is for this reason that they consolidate each other's results as a more complete scientific method. While the psychological component of the soundscape model relies on a wide range of environmental variables such as socio-cultural factors [69–71], the physiological aspect holds more consistency among different populations [37–39]. Also, the methods of data collection for each approach are considerably different. The psychological studies of soundscape revolve around narrative interviews, soundwalks, and uncontrolled behavioural observations [69,72,73]. The physiological is limited to controlled lab experiments [5,10,37–39]. Put together, these two approaches are as complementary as they are mutually reflective and the necessity to develop both in parallel is self-evident.

6.2.5. Relation to Health and Well-Being

Soundscape research could also benefit from ameliorating clarity and consistency in the description of the physiological and neurophysiological processes attributed to the soundscape in the context of human well-being. Notwithstanding a few existing studies which strove to unveil the physiological and neurophysiological indications of soundscapes [5,9,37–39], there is still very little known about what these research outcomes mean in terms of health and well-being. In other words, more research is needed to interpret the fundamental physiological alterations evoked by the acoustic environment in terms of acoustic comfort, health, and well-being to enable policy makers and professionals to extrapolate solid results. In addition, further research is needed toward 'reverse translation', in which characteristics of the acoustic environment can be extrapolated from the 'unconscious mechanisms' identified in physiological responses [74]. The success of this reverse translation approach could enable researchers to better predict physiological responses to measured sound environments and, finally, to predict overall health and well-being outcomes independent of subjective ratings.

7. Conclusions

The present literature review reported on the established psychophysiological outcomes of the soundscape within the existing research, such as HR, HRV, SCL, RR, and musculoskeletal activity underlying soundscape. Hence, a systematic review in accordance with the PRISMA guidelines was performed on four principle databases in the areas of psychophysiology and neuroscience. In this review, we raised three questions: what metrics were used to detect the physiological manifestations of soundscape; whether significant physiological changes occur in response to the acoustic environment; and ultimately, whether the detected changes correspond with perceptual attributes.

The outcome of the review indicates that HR measurement and an event-related or stimulus-locked design with passive listening are commonly applied among the existing soundscape physiology research, mostly with homogeneous subject populations. The most frequent subjective assessments used among the studies were based on two perceptual attributes of valence and arousal.

The reviewed literature showed the physiological manifestations of the soundscape with wide variability, ranging from rising to fall, which were inconsistently associated with the perceptual attributes. Based on the scope of the discussion provided in the papers themselves and the inconsistency of the results, conclusions cannot currently be drawn about a broader discussion regarding the implementation of the soundscape approach to the design of environments based on physiological manifestations or responses.

To advance the research on the psychophysiology of soundscape, we propose a potential classification for the environmental sounds with single and complex sources. It is worthwhile to look into the link of environmental sounds' temporal variation and length and how they may affect the adaptation, habituation or sensitization of ANS. It is recommended to investigate the psychophysiology aspect of the soundscape in a network level, taking into account all the contributing CNS and PNS factors and how they interact with each other, particularly in the context of health and wellbeing.

While the study of physiology and neurophysiology of soundscape is still in its infancy and inconclusive, cross-disciplinary team collaboration is highly recommended to propose an optimum biomarker multi-model for the soundscape investigation. As acoustic design moves further toward the soundscape approach, so should the psychophysiology of soundscape advance, to provide the same underpinning as the physiology of noise provided for conventional noise control.

Author Contributions: All authors contributed to the intellectual development and writing of this manuscript. M.E. conceptualized, wrote, revised, and synthesized revisions of this manuscript. A.J.M. wrote sections and helped with revisions of the manuscript. J.K. reviewed and supervised the structure and framework of the manuscript. F.A. reviewed and commented on the manuscript.

Funding: The authors disclosed receipt of the following financial support for this review. The current review was funded by the European Research Council (ERC) Advanced Grant (no. 740696) on Soundscape Indices (SSID).

Conflicts of Interest: The authors declare no conflict of interest. The funder had no role in the design of the study; in the collection, analyses, or interpretation of data; in the writing of the manuscript, and in the decision to publish the results.

Abbreviations

The following abbreviations are used in this manuscript:

AR	Augmented Reality
CNS	Central Nervous System
PNS	Peripheral Nervous System
SNS	Sympathetic Nervous System
PSNS	Parasympathetic Nervous System
HR	Heart Rate
HRV	Heart Rate Variability
HF HRV	High-Frequency Heart Rate Variability
RR	Respiration Rate
EDA	Electrodermal Activation
EMG	Electromyography
PRISMA	Preferred Reporting Items for Systematic Review and Meta-Analysis
MV	Minute Ventilation
SCL	Skin Conductance Level
SCR	Skin Conductance Response
VR	Virtual Reality

References

1. Kuan, G.; Morris, T.; Kueh, Y.C.; Terry, P.C. Effects of relaxing and arousing music during imagery training on dart-throwing performance, physiological arousal indices, and competitive state anxiety. *Front. Psychol.* **2018**, *9*, 14. [CrossRef] [PubMed]

2. Lim, H.A.; Park, H. The effect of music on arousal, enjoyment, and cognitive performance. *Psychol. Music* **2018**. [CrossRef]
3. Benfield, J.; Taff, B.D.; Weinzimmer, D.; Newman, P. Motorized recreation sounds influence nature scene evaluations: The role of attitude moderators. *Front. Psychol.* **2018**, *9*, 495. [CrossRef] [PubMed]
4. Zhao, Y.; Sun, Q.; Chen, G.; Yang, J. Hearing emotional sounds: Category representation in the human amygdala. *Soc. Neurosci.* **2018**, *13*, 117–128. [CrossRef] [PubMed]
5. Alvarsson, J.J.; Wiens, S.; Nilsson, M.E. Stress recovery during exposure to nature sound and environmental noise. *Int. J. Environ. Res. Public Health* **2010**, *7*, 1036–1046. [CrossRef]
6. Frenzilli, G.; Ryskalin, L.; Ferrucci, M.; Cantafora, E.; Chelazzi, S.; Giorgi, F.S.; Lenzi, P.; Scarcelli, V.; Frati, A.; Biagioni, F.; et al. Loud noise exposure produces DNA, neurotransmitter and morphological damage within specific brain areas. *Front. Neuroanat.* **2017**, *11*, 49. [CrossRef]
7. Brattico, E.; Kujala, T.; Tervaniemi, M.; Alku, P.; Ambrosi, L.; Monitillo, V. Long-term exposure to occupational noise alters the cortical organization of sound processing. *Clin. Neurophysiol.* **2005**, *116*, 190–203. [CrossRef]
8. Lewis, J.W.; Wightman, F.L.; Brefczynski, J.A.; Phinney, R.E.; Binder, J.R.; De Yoe, E.A. Human brain regions involved in recognizing environmental sounds. *Cereb. Cortex* **2004**, *14*, 1008–1021. [CrossRef]
9. McCorry, L.K. Teachers' topics: Physiology of the Autonomic Nervous System. *Am. J. Pharm. Educ.* **2007**, *71*, 1–11. [CrossRef]
10. Irwin, A.; Hall, D.A.; Peters, A.; Plack, C.J. Listening to urban soundscapes: Physiological validity of perceptual dimensions. *Psychophysiology* **2011**, *48*, 258–268. [CrossRef]
11. Kumar, S.; Tansley-Hancock, O.; Sedley, W.; Winston, J.S.; Callaghan, M.F.; Allen, M.; Griffiths, T.D. The Brain Basis for Misophonia. *Curr. Biol.* **2017**, *27*, 527–533. [CrossRef]
12. ISO. ISO 12913-1:2014: *Acoustics—Soundscape Part 1: Definition and Conceptual Framework*; ISO: Geneva, Switzerland, 2014.
13. Kang, J. From understanding to designing soundscapes. *Front. Archit. Civ. Eng. China* **2010**, *4*, 403–417. [CrossRef]
14. Meng, Q.; Kang, J. Effect of sound-related activities on human behaviours and acoustic comfort in urban open spaces. *Sci. Total Environ.* **2016**, *573*, 481–493. [CrossRef]
15. Schafer, R.M. *The Soundscape: Our Sonic Environment and the Tuning of the World*; Simon and Schuster: New York, NY, USA, 1977.
16. Southworth, M.; Ichae, M. The sonic environment of cities. *Environ. Behav.* **1969**, *1*, 49–70. [CrossRef]
17. Kang, J.; Schulte-Fortkamp, B.; Fiebig, A.; Botteldooren, D. *Mapping of Soundscape. Soundscape and the Built Environment*; CRC Press: Boca Raton, FL, USA, 2016; pp. 161–195. [CrossRef]
18. Liu, J.; Kang, J.; Behm, H.; Luo, T. Effects of landscape on soundscape perception: Soundwalks in city parks. *Landsc. Urban Plan.* **2013**, *123*, 30–40. [CrossRef]
19. Pijanowski, B.C.; Villanueva-Rivera, L.J.; Dumyahn, S.L.; Farina, A.; Krause, B.L.; Napoletano, B.M.; Pieretti, N. Soundscape Ecology: The Science of Sound in the Landscape. *BioScience* **2011**, *61*, 203–216. [CrossRef]
20. Ising, H.; Kruppa, B. Health effects caused by noise: Evidence in the literature from the past 25 years. *Noise Health* **2004**, *6*, 5.
21. Lawton, R.N.; Fujiwara, D. Living with aircraft noise: Airport proximity, aviation noise and subjective wellbeing in England. *Transp. Res. Part D Transp. Environ.* **2016**, *42*, 104–118. [CrossRef]
22. Pedersen, E.; Waye, K.P. Wind turbine noise, annoyance and self-reported health and well-being in different living environments. *Occup. Environ. Med.* **2007**, *64*, 480–486. [CrossRef]
23. Solet, J.M.; Dang-Vu, T.T.; McKinney, S.M.; Ellenbogen, J.M.; Buxton, O.M. Spontaneous brain rhythms predict sleep stability in the face of noise. *Curr. Biol.* **2010**, *20*, R626–R627. [CrossRef]
24. Hao, Y.; Kang, J.; Wörtche, H. Assessment of the masking effects of birdsong on the road traffic noise environment. *J. Acoust. Soc. Am.* **2016**, *140*, 978–987. [CrossRef]
25. Aletta, F.; Oberman, T.; Kang, J. Associations between positive health-related effects and soundscapes perceptual constructs: A systematic review. *Int. J. Environ. Res. Public Health* **2018**, *15*, 2392. [CrossRef]
26. Jeon, J.Y.; Lee, P.J.; You, J.; Kang, J. Perceptual assessment of quality of urban soundscapes with combined noise sources and water sounds. *J. Acoust. Soc. Am.* **2010**, *127*, 1357–1366. [CrossRef]
27. Shepherd, D.; Welch, D.; Dirks, K.; McBride, D. Do quiet areas afford greater health-related quality of life than noisy areas? *Int. J. Environ. Res. Public Health* **2013**, *10*, 1284–1303. [CrossRef]

28. Kaplan, S. The restorative benefits of nature: Toward an integrative framework. *J. Environ. Psychol.* **1995**, *15*, 169–182. [CrossRef]
29. Gill, C.; Packer, J.; Ballantyne, R. Applying Attention Restoration Theory to Understand and Address Clergy's Need to Restore Cognitive Capacity. *J. Relig. Health* **2018**, *57*, 1779–1792. [CrossRef]
30. Krzywicka, P.; Byrka, K. Restorative qualities of and preference for natural and urban soundscapes. *Front. Psychol.* **2017**, *8*, 1705. [CrossRef]
31. Zhang, Y.; Kang, J.; Kang, J. Effects of Soundscape on the Environmental Restoration in Urban Natural Environments. *Noise Health* **2017**, *19*, 65–72. [CrossRef]
32. Benfield, J.; Taff, B.; Newman, P.; Smyth, J. Natural sound facilitates mood recovery. *Ecopsychology* **2014**, *6*, 183–188. [CrossRef]
33. Harris, C.M. (Ed.) Introduction. In *Handbook of Acoustical Measurements and Noise Control*, 3rd ed.; Acoustical Society of America: Woodbury, NY, USA, 1998; p. 23.
34. Kliuchko, M.; Heinonen-Guzejev, M.; Vuust, P.; Tervaniemi, M.; Brattico, E. A window into the brain mechanisms associated with noise sensitivity. *Sci. Rep.* **2016**, *6*, 39236. [CrossRef]
35. Moher, D.; Liberati, A.; Tetzlaff, J.; Altman, D.G.; PRISMA Group. Preferred Reporting Items for Systematic Reviews and Meta-Analyses: The PRISMA Statement. *Ann. Intern. Med.* **2009**, *151*, 264–269. [CrossRef]
36. Axelsson, Ö.; Nilsson, M.E.; Berglund, B. A principal components model of soundscape perception. *J. Acoust. Soc. Am.* **2010**, *128*, 2836–2846. [CrossRef]
37. Gomez, P.; Danuser, B. Affective and physiological responses to environmental noises and music. *Int. J. Psychophysiol.* **2004**, *53*, 91–103. [CrossRef]
38. Hume, K.; Ahtamad, M. Physiological responses to and subjective estimates of soundscape elements. *Appl. Acoust.* **2013**, *74*, 275–281. [CrossRef]
39. Medvedev, O.; Shepherd, D.; Hautus, M.J. The restorative potential of soundscapes: A physiological investigation. *Appl. Acoust.* **2015**, *96*, 20–26. [CrossRef]
40. Berglund, B.; Eriksen, C.; Nilsson, M. *Exploring Perceptual Content in Soundscapes*; Fechner Day; Pabst Science Publishers: Lengerich, Germany, 2001; Volume 100, pp. 279–284. Available online: http://citeseerx.ist.psu.edu/viewdoc/download?doi=10.1.1.11.3335&rep=rep1&type=pdf (accessed on 16 September 2019).
41. Hall, D.A.; Irwin, A.; Edmondson-Jones, M.; Phillips, S.; Poxon, J.E. An exploratory evaluation of perceptual, psychoacoustic and acoustical properties of urban soundscapes. *Appl. Acoust.* **2013**, *74*, 248–254. [CrossRef]
42. Zygmunt, A.; Stanczyk, J. Methods of evaluation of autonomic nervous system function. *Arch. Med Sci. AMS* **2010**, *6*, 11. [CrossRef]
43. Bradley, M.M.; Lang, P.J. Emotion and motivation. In *Handbook of Psychophysiology*; Cambridge University Press: Cambridge, UK, 2000; Volume 2, pp. 602–642.
44. Schmidt-Nielsen, K. *Animal Physiology: Adaptation and Environment*, 5th ed.; Cambridge University Press: Cambridge, UK, 1997; Available online: https://www.amazon.com/Animal-Physiology-Environment-Knut-Schmidt-Nielsen-ebook/dp/B00D2WQ7XC (accessed on 10 April 1997).
45. Droitcour, A.D.; Seto, T.B.; Park, B.; Yamada, S.; Vergara, A.; el Hourani, C.; Shing, T.; Yuen, A.; Lubecke, V.M.; Boric-Lubecke, O. Non-Contact Respiratory Rate Measurement Validation for Hospitalized Patients. In Proceedings of the 2009 Annual International Conference of the IEEE Engineering in Medicine and Biology Society, Minneapolis, MN, USA, 3–6 September 2009; pp. 4812–4815. [CrossRef]
46. Allen, M. *The Sage Encyclopedia of Communication Research Methods*; SAGE Publications, Inc.: Thousand Oaks, CA, USA, 2017; Volumes 1–4. [CrossRef]
47. Buijs, R.M.; Swaab, D.F. (Eds.) *Autonomic Nervous System*; Newnes, Elsevier: Amsterdam, The Netherlands, 2013; Volume 117.
48. Hsu, S.-M.; Ko, W.-J.; Liao, W.-C.; Huang, S.-J.; Chen, R.J.; Li, C.-Y.; Hwang, S.-L. Associations of exposure to noise with physiological and psychological outcomes among post-cardiac surgery patients in ICUs. *Clinics* **2010**, *65*, 985–989. [CrossRef]
49. Elbaz, M.; Mietlicki, F.; Nguyen, P.; Lefèvre, M.; Sineau, M.; Laumon, B.; Léger, D. Effects of Aircraft Noise Exposure on Heart Rate during Sleep in the Population Living Near Airports. *Int. J. Environ. Res. Public Health* **2019**, *16*, 269. [CrossRef]
50. Burns, K.N.; Sun, K.; Fobil, J.N.; Neitzel, R.L. Heart rate, stress, and occupational noise exposure among electronic waste recycling workers. *Int. J. Environ. Res. Public Health* **2016**, *13*, 140. [CrossRef]

51. Abdel-Raziq, I.R.; Qamhieh, Z.N.; Abdel-Ali, M.M. Noise Pollution in Factories in Nablus City. *Acta Acust.* **2003**, *89*, 913–916.
52. Hassanein, S.M.; El Raggal, N.M.; Shalaby, A.A. Neonatal nursery noise: Practice-based learning and improvement. *J. Matern. Fetal Neonatal Med.* **2013**, *26*, 392–395. [CrossRef]
53. Recio, A.; Linares, C.; Banegas, J.R.; Díaz, J. Road traffic noise effects on cardiovascular, respiratory, and metabolic health: An integrative model of biological mechanisms. *Environ. Res.* **2016**, *146*, 359–370. [CrossRef]
54. Linares, C.; Díaz, J.; Tobías, A.; de Miguel, J.M.; Otero, A. Impact of urban air pollutants and noise levels over daily hospital admissions in children in Madrid: A time series analysis. *Int. Arch. Occup. Environ. Health* **2006**, *79*, 143–152. [CrossRef]
55. Park, S.H.; Lee, P.J. Effects of floor impact noise on psychophysiological responses. *Build. Environ.* **2017**, *116*, 173–181. [CrossRef]
56. Glass, D.C.; Singer, J.E. *Urban Stress: Experiments on Noise and Social Stressors*; Academic Press: New York, NY, USA, 1972.
57. Trapanotto, M.; Benini, F.; Farina, M.; Gobber, D.; Magnavita, V.; Zacchello, F. Behavioural and physiological reactivity to noise in the newborn. *J. Paediatr. Child Health* **2004**, *40*, 275–281. [CrossRef]
58. Bones, O.; Cox, T.J.; Davies, W.J. Sound categories: Category formation and evidence- based taxonomies. *Front. Psychol.* **2018**, *9*, 1277. [CrossRef]
59. Liu, J.; Kang, J.; Luo, T.; Behm, H.; Coppack, T. Spatiotemporal variability of soundscapes in a multiple functional urban area. *Landsc. Urban Plan.* **2013**, *115*, 1–9. [CrossRef]
60. Kang, J.; Meng, Q.; Jin, H. Effects of individual sound sources on the subjective loudness and acoustic comfort in underground shopping streets. *Sci. Total Environ.* **2012**, *435*, 80–89. [CrossRef]
61. Pantev, C.; Okamoto, H.; Ross, B.; Stoll, W.; Ciurlia-Guy, E.; Kakigi, R.; Kubo, T. Lateral inhibition and habituation of the human auditory cortex. *Eur. J. Neurosci.* **2004**, *19*, 2337–2344. [CrossRef]
62. Lehoczki, F.; Szamosvölgyi, Z.; Miklósi, Á.; Faragó, T. Dogs' sensitivity to strange pup separation calls: Pitch instability increases attention regardless of sex and experience. *Anim. Behav.* **2019**, *153*, 115–129. [CrossRef]
63. Prosser, R.T. Formal solutions of inverse scattering problems. IV. Error estimates. *J. Math. Phys.* **2003**, *23*, 2127–2130. [CrossRef]
64. Aletta, F.; Kang, J.; Axelsson, Ö. Soundscape descriptors and a conceptual framework for developing predictive soundscape models. *Landsc. Urban Plan.* **2016**, *149*, 65–74. [CrossRef]
65. Aletta, F.; Xiao, J. What are the Current Priorities and Challenges for (Urban) Soundscape Research? *Challenges* **2018**, *9*, 16. [CrossRef]
66. Hong, J.Y.; Lam, B.; Ong, Z.T.; Ooi, K.; Gan, W.S.; Kang, J.; Tan, S.T. Quality assessment of acoustic environment reproduction methods for cinematic virtual reality in soundscape applications. *Build. Environ.* **2019**, *149*, 1–14. [CrossRef]
67. Jurica, D.; Matija, P.; Mladen, R.; Marjan, S. Comparison of Two Methods of Soundscape Evaluation. In Proceedings of the 2019 2nd International Colloquium on Smart Grid Metrology (SMAGRIMET), Split, Croatia, 9–12 April 2019; pp. 1–5.
68. Echevarria Sanchez, G.M.; Van Renterghem, T.; Sun, K.; De Coensel, B.; Botteldooren, D. Using Virtual Reality for assessing the role of noise in the audio-visual design of an urban public space. *Landsc. Urban Plan.* **2017**, *167*, 98–107. [CrossRef]
69. Kang, J.; Aletta, F.; Gjestland, T.T.; Brown, L.A.; Botteldooren, D.; Schulte-Fortkamp, B.; Lavia, L. Ten questions on the soundscapes of the built environment. *Build. Environ.* **2016**, *108*, 284–294. [CrossRef]
70. Moscoso, P.; Peck, M.; Eldridge, A. Systematic literature review on the association between soundscape and ecological/human wellbeing. *PeerJ Prepr.* **2018**, *6*, e6570v2.
71. Engel, M.S.; Fiebig, A.; Pfaffenbach, C.; Fels, J. A review of socio-acoustic surveys for soundscape studies. *Curr. Pollut. Rep.* **2018**, *4*, 220–239. [CrossRef]
72. Radicchi, A.; Henckel, D.; Memmel, M. Citizens as smart, active sensors for the quiet and just city. The case of the "open source soundscapes" approach to identify, assess and plan "everyday quiet areas" in cities. *Noise Mapp.* **2018**, *5*, 1–20. [CrossRef]

73. Cassina, L.; Fredianelli, L.; Menichini, I.; Chiari, C.; Licitra, G. Audio-visual preferences and tranquillity ratings in urban areas. *Environments* **2018**, *5*, 1. [CrossRef]
74. Seals, D.R. Translational physiology: From molecules to public health. *J. Physiol.* **2013**, *591*, 3457–3469. [CrossRef]

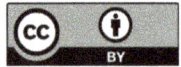

© 2019 by the authors. Licensee MDPI, Basel, Switzerland. This article is an open access article distributed under the terms and conditions of the Creative Commons Attribution (CC BY) license (http://creativecommons.org/licenses/by/4.0/).

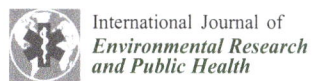

Article

Acoustic Comfort in Virtual Inner Yards with Various Building Facades

Armin Taghipour *, Tessa Sievers and Kurt Eggenschwiler

Empa, Swiss Federal Laboratories for Materials Science and Technology, Laboratory for Acoustics/Noise Control, Überlandstrasse 129, 8600 Dübendorf, Switzerland; tessa-sievers@gmx.de (T.S.); kurt.eggenschwiler@empa.ch (K.E.)
* Correspondence: armin.taghipour@empa.ch

Received: 28 November 2018; Accepted: 14 January 2019; Published: 16 January 2019

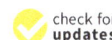

Abstract: Housing complex residents in urban areas are not only confronted with typical noise sources, but also everyday life sounds, e.g., in the yards. Therefore, they might benefit from the increasing interest in soundscape design and acoustic comfort improvement. Three laboratory experiments (with repeated-measures complete block designs) are reported here, in which effects of several variables on short-term acoustic comfort were investigated. A virtual reference inner yard in the ODEON software environment was systematically modified by absorbers on building facades, whereby single-channel recordings were spatialized for a 2D playback in laboratory. Facade absorption was found, generally, to increase acoustic comfort. Too much absorption, however, was not found to be helpful. In the absence of any absorbers on the facade, absorbing balcony ceilings tended to improve acoustic comfort, however, non-significantly. Pleasant and unpleasant sounds were associated with comfort and discomfort, accordingly. This should encourage architects and acousticians to create comfortable inner yard sound environments, where pleasant and unpleasant sound occurrence probabilities are designed to be high and low, respectively. Furthermore, significant differences were observed between acoustic comfort at distinct observer positions, which could be exploited when designing inner yards.

Keywords: acoustic comfort; inner yard acoustics; soundscape pleasantness; sound perception; virtual room acoustics; virtual audio; quality of experience

---

1. Introduction

Urban living in areas with a high population density is affected by classic noise sources, such as road traffic, railways, and aircraft noise, as well as by surrounding everyday life sounds. Conventional environmental and construction acoustics deal with noise assessment and noise control with the goal to reduce the noise immission at the living space of the residents [1–3]. Beyond the topic of noise immission, however, there has been an increasing interest in soundscape design with the aim to improve the soundscape and acoustic comfort [4–8]. Despite some overlap between both topics, the main goal of soundscape design and acoustic comfort improvement is not only to reduce relatively unpleasant sounds (such as noise), but also to design and enable a relatively pleasant sound environment. Residents of housing complexes might benefit from the latter, e.g., by controlled absorptions and reflections of the facade. Whereas sound absorbing materials have been frequently used to improve acoustic comfort in closed rooms [9–11], little is known about the influences of sound absorbers on the (outside) facade to improve acoustic comfort for residents of housing complexes with shared inner yards.

One of the challenges in soundscape and acoustic design for housing complexes is that it involves collaboration of people from various backgrounds, such as acousticians, engineers, planners, architects, urbanists and sound quality experts, who—based on their different backgrounds—not only have different understandings of acoustic phenomena related to such a housing project, but also, sometimes, different goals [12–14]. Even the definition of the term "acoustic comfort" is vague and colorful in the literature. While, in many studies, an "improvement in acoustic comfort" meant a general improvement of acoustics and was measured by different sets of objective acoustical or room acoustical parameters (such as lower sound pressure level, SPL) [10,11], other studies used a subjective evaluation of acoustic comfort [9,15,16]. Furthermore, a series of studies measured an improvement in acoustic comfort directly with a decrease in noise annoyance (associated with corresponding decrease in SPL) [17]. While acoustic comfort has been found to be related to the SPL—i.e., L_{eq} (equivalent continuous sound level) or L_{dn} (day-night sound level)—[15], reducing SPL alone might not be a sufficient measure for improving acoustic comfort in urban areas [15,18,19]. Acoustic comfort seems to be rather determined by more factors than just the sound level [15,16]. For a review of the variety of definitions, descriptions, and indicators of acoustic comfort, see [20–22]. The study reported in this paper uses a subjective evaluation of acoustic comfort and discomfort.

Similar to other urban areas around the world, also in Switzerland, soundscape evaluation and improvement of acoustic comfort have gained interest [14,23–25] and the problem of finding a unique language, understanding, and goals between people from different backgrounds is evident. One of the areas under investigation is sounds in inner yards, whereby examples of inner yards of housing complexes have been investigated in order to find capacities for improvement of the sound environment and acoustic comfort [14].

In housing complexes, the presence of buildings induces complicating acoustic effects such as multiple reflections, diffraction, and diffusion, which depend, among others, on the material properties of building facades [26]. By using acoustic absorbers, for example, SPL in outside areas of housing complexes might be reduced [27], which can increase acoustic comfort. Compared to the semi-free field situation, Yang et al. [26] reported up to 8 dB increase in SPL due to multiple reflections outside of an apartment complex. This indicates potential acoustic performance improvements.

Yu and Kang [28] investigated sustainability of different facade materials on several building types with the aim to reduce the (negative) environmental impact while reserving similar acoustic performance. It was found that suitable selection of acoustic material can increase sustainability. Given that the aim of the study was to investigate sustainability at comparable levels of acoustic performance—and not to improve acoustic performance–, only negligible acoustical differences were reported between usage of different materials.

Generally, building facade absorption was found to affect acoustics of the outer space, for example, at public squares [27] or alongside streets [29,30]. Combined with a proper balcony design, building facades seem to be effective in mitigating noise immission [29]. Tang [31] reviewed complex behavior of facade balconies with different designs, whereby absorbers were found to be significant or insignificant based on their position and angle [31,32]. With a noise source on the ground or from the roadway, generally, balconies on a building facade provide significant acoustical protection to the areas beyond them [31,33]. This protective effect is, however, partially canceled by reflecting balcony ceilings [34,35]. In addition, multiple rectangular balconies were found to be problematic reflectors [32].

The above literature review shows a potential to improve acoustic performance (also) for housing complexes with inner yards. There seems to be a need to link the design (and the physical or acoustical parameters) directly to the acoustic comfort, rather than to the SPL. Possible contributions of absorbing materials on facades and balcony ceilings in enhancing acoustic comfort should be investigated.

This paper deals with short-term (momentary) acoustic comfort in the presence of sound from an inner yard in a housing complex. The study was carried out by means of three experiments, whereby only acoustic stimuli and no visual representation was used. Laboratory experiments with audio [36–41] or audio-visual [17,42–44] stimuli have been increasingly used to investigate questions related to noise annoyance, soundscape, and/or acoustic comfort, partially because models of reality are extremely helpful in the planning and design stage [44]. Furthermore, for comparison studies, laboratory experiments offer a controlled setup, which is not easily practicable in the field. It should be mentioned that portions of this study were Presented at the DAGA 2018 (44. Jahrestagung für Akustik) [45], Munich, Germany, 19–22 March 2018.

Sections 2 and 3 of this paper give an introduction to the experimental concept, design and setup. Three experiments and their results are presented in Sections 4–6. Sections 7 and 8 offer a discussion of the results and conclude the paper.

2. Experimental Concept

In this study, short-term or acute comfort and discomfort reactions to sounds in virtual acoustic rooms were investigated under laboratory conditions. The term "short-term" refers to the time period during and after an acoustic stimulus' playback and before the next stimulus is presented. The observed "short-term" comfort or discomfort ratings were, hence, related to acute comfort in response to each stimulus, rather than long-term comfort or well-being.

To investigate possible differences in short-term comfort in inner yards with distinct building facades, sound propagation was simulated in virtual rooms, whereby single-channel recordings were auralized for a multi-channel playback system (see Section 3). To that aim, several design variables, such as categorical variables sound source type and observer position as well as continuous variables such as absorption coefficient were systematically varied to study their individual and combined associations with short-term acoustic comfort ratings. Observer positions were either outside in the yard, outside on the balcony or at open windows. That is, inner room acoustics (such as in [28]) were not investigated here.

The authors would also like to note that throughout this paper the terminology "acoustic comfort" will be used. That is, the German terminology in the questionnaire *sich wohl fühlen* was translated to "to feel comfortable" or "to be comfortable."

3. Experimental Design and Setup

This section reports a subset of the information related to the experimental setup and method, which was similar for all three experiments. Further method-related information specific to each experiment (such as stimuli or subjects) will be reported later in the respective sections.

3.1. Listening Test Facility

The experiments presented in this paper were conducted in the listening test facility of the Empa (Swiss Federal Laboratories for Materials Science and Technology), named AuraLab, which has a separate listening and control room allowing for audio-visual supervision to comply with ethical requirements.

AuraLab satisfies room acoustical requirements for high-quality audio reproduction in terms of its background noise and reverberation time. For the present experiments, the carpeted floor was covered with additional absorbers on the floor. The experimental setup in AuraLab is shown in Figure 1. Subjects were seated in the central listening spot. A 3D immersive sound system with 16 separate audio channels is installed in AuraLab. Fifteen loudspeakers "KH 120 A" (Georg Neumann GmbH, Berlin, Germany) are located in a hemispherical arrangement on three levels (0, 30, and 60° vertically) at a distance of 2 m from the central listening spot. Bass management by means of two subwoofers "KH 805" (Georg Neumann GmbH, Berlin, Germany) and a digital signal processor complete the playback system. Stimuli of the experiment presented here were played back by a 2D setup over the five loudspeakers at 0° elevation (subject's ear level) and both subwoofers.

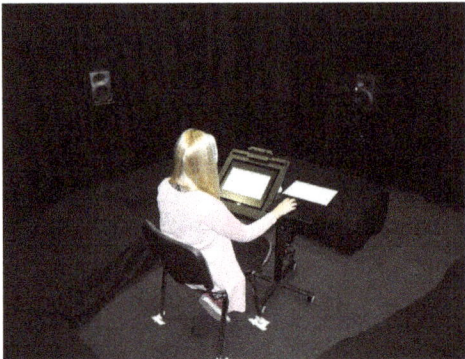

Figure 1. Experimental setup in AuraLab with five loudspeakers and additional porous floor absorbers.

3.2. Signal Processing and Room Acoustic Simulation

A block diagram of signal processing—from recording to playback—is given in Figure 2. Single-channel recordings were carried out in a semi-anechoic chamber. A B&K 2006 microphone (Brüel & Kjaer, Nærum, Denmark) was positioned on the reflecting floor. Recorded individuals (or, in case of children, their parents) were informed about the purpose of the recordings and signed a consent form, which was prepared under supervision and with approval of Empa's Ethics Committee Office.

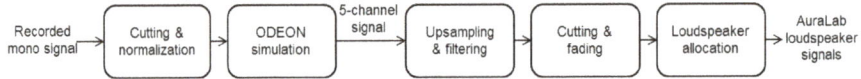

Figure 2. Block diagram of the signal processing steps from recording to playback.

Suitable 8-s extracts were made for the purpose of this study. The extracts were normalized to the A-weighted level (i.e., A-weighted equivalent continuous sound level, L_{Aeq}) of the signal with the largest maximum absolute amplitude.

Room acoustic simulations were done with ODEON software version 14.03 (Odeon A/S, Kgs. Lyngby, Denmark), which uses the image-source method and a ray tracing algorithm. A 2D auralization (2D surround sound) was chosen for five loudspeakers such as the AuraLab setup. Although the ODEON input signals (of different sources) had the same L_{Aeq} (see above), the ODEON outputs exhibited diverging L_{Aeq}, as they possessed unequal spectral and temporal characteristics, which reacted differently to the virtual rooms. The stimuli reported in this paper were simulated considering a single source, one source position, and several observer positions.

The multi-channel ODEON output signal was upsampled from 44.1 to 48 kHz, as this is a requirement of the playback system. It was then low pass ($f_c = 10$ kHz) and high pass ($f_c = 20$ Hz) filtered. After being gated with squared-cosine ramps, the multi-channel signal was allocated to the corresponding loudspeakers: front, front-left, front-right, back-left, and back-right.

All the processing steps (with exception of ODEON simulations) were carried out with MATLAB R2016b (MathWorks, Natick, MA, USA).

3.3. Reference Inner Yard

The reference inner yard used in the course of this study was a simplified 3D model of an existing housing complex in Dübendorf, Switzerland (see Figure 3). The geometric model was built in the SketchUp software environment (Trimble Inc., Sunnyvale, CA, USA) and was imported into the ODEON software environment using the plug-in SU2Odeon. The walls were of brick with large glass windows. Since ODEON works with bounded/closed room models, the inner yard was modelled as a ceiling-less room (100 m × 20 m × 20 m), which was inserted in a larger box (10 m away from each side) with a perfect absorbing inner surface, representing free field.

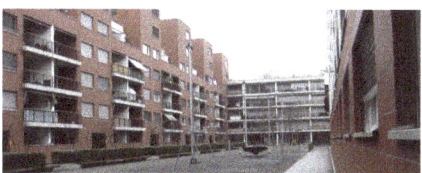

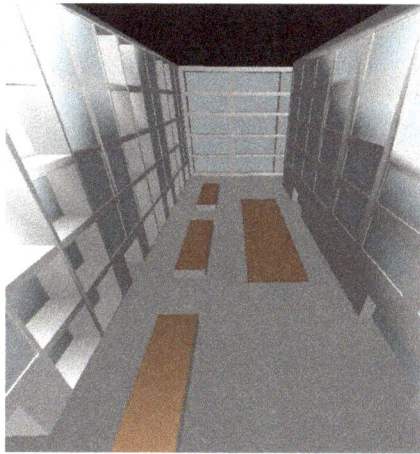

Figure 3. Reference inner yard in original (**above**) and as a simplified geometric model for the ODEON room acoustic simulation (**below**). Absorption coefficient of the materials is coded by their colors, whereby, black stands for the fully absorbing encasing box. Blue and gray represent the reflecting glass or brickwork facade, respectively. The floor is either reflecting smooth unpainted concrete (gray) or absorbing grass (brown).

3.4. Validation

In order to validate the system (i.e., the simulation-playback chain), a series of evaluation tests was carried out in AuraLab. Sound pressure levels (L_{Aeq}, L_{AFmax}), level reductions for several simulated distances (from a point source), and localization tests were carried out for single and/or multiple source(s) and several virtual source positions. This was done either by level measurement in AuraLab or, in the case of the source localization tests, by five expert listeners, who were acousticians.

3.5. Experimental Sessions

All three experiments were conducted as focused listening tests with repeated measures and a complete block design; i.e., each subject listened to all the stimuli of the experiment they participated in and rated the acoustic comfort they associated with each stimulus during or directly after its playback.

Subjects did the tests individually (i.e., one by one). After reading study information, they signed a consent form to participate, after which they answered the first part of the questionnaire about hearing and well-being. The subjects were then introduced to the listening test and the test software which guided them through the test. After the listening test, the subjects filled out the rest of the questionnaire (demographic data).

Whereas Experiment 1 was conducted as a single listening test, Experiments 2 and 3 were conducted as two listening tests in one experimental session (after each other). That is, there were two groups of subjects: those who participated in Experiment 1 and those who participated in

Experiments 2 and 3. For the latter experimental session, the order of the Experiments 2 and 3 was (randomly) counterbalanced between the subjects.

3.6. Listening Test Software, Procedure, and the Comfort Scale

The listening tests were done by means of a software (and its graphical user interface) which guided the subjects through the test. To familiarize the subjects with the sounds (incl. virtual rooms) and the test software, the subjects listened to several orienting and training stimuli. The main listening test began thereafter. For each stimulus, subjects completed the following statement: "In this virtual inner yard and in the presence of this sound, I feel …". Their short-term acoustic comfort was recorded during or after stimulus playback on a verbal bipolar 7-point scale: very uncomfortable (-3), uncomfortable (-2), to some extent uncomfortable (-1), neither comfortable nor uncomfortable (0), to some extent comfortable (+1), comfortable (+2), and very comfortable (+3). For the statistical analysis, the ratings were coded from -3 to 3, respectively.

To support the neutral category "neither uncomfortable nor comfortable" in its actual function as the scale center and to avoid its misuse as an avoiding or diverting answer [46], an additional "don't know" push button was made available to the subjects. This option was, however, never used by the subjects.

The stimuli were played in a random order after one another, with a 1.2-s break between stimuli after complete playback. By means of a push button, an option was given to the subjects to listen to each stimulus (only) one more time, if they wished to. The subjects rarely made use of this option.

3.7. Pilot Experiments

Prior to the experiments presented here, a number of pilot tests were carried out, based on which the number of stimuli, the selection of stimuli, and minor changes in the design were carried out. To avoid an unnecessarily long text, the design and the results of the pilot tests will not be reported in this paper. Effort was made to ensure that subjects from the pilot test, as well as other people aware of the study, did not participate in the main experiments. Fewer than 10% of interested pilot subjects were allowed to participate in the main experiments.

3.8. Statistical Analysis

The statistical analysis was carried out with IBM SPSS Statistics, version 25 (IBM Corporation, Armonk, NY, USA). Tested effects were considered significant if the probability, p, of the observed results under the null hypothesis (H0) was ≤ 0.05.

The individual and combined associations of the independent variables (i.e., experimental design variables) on short-term acoustic comfort was investigated as follows:

- Repeated-measures multi-factorial analysis of variance (ANOVA), corrected by the Greenhouse–Geisser method.
- Post hoc pairwise comparisons by Fisher's protected least significant difference (LSD) test, corrected by the Bonferroni method.
- Linear mixed-effects models for further combined analysis of variables of different types; i.e., categorical variables, covariates, and random intercept (comparison of the models by means of Akaike information criterion (AIC) [47] and Bayesian information criterion (BIC) [48]; i.e., choosing the model with the lowest AIC/BIC).

4. Experiment 1

Before testing different absorbing materials on the building facade, Experiment 1 dealt with the question, whether usage of (any) absorbers on the facade would change the inner yard soundscape such that the subjective acoustic comfort would be affected. There is evidence for such an effect in the case of outer spaces in urban areas (a small urban square) [27]. Furthermore, it was to assume that, at a given sound level, subjects would have a different perception of relatively pleasant and unpleasant sounds [15]. Therefore, since—in contrast to the unipolar (negative) 11-point ICBEN (International Commission on Biological Effects of Noise) noise annoyance scale [49]—the bipolar 7-point comfort/discomfort scale was to be associated with comfort (i.e., positive) or discomfort (i.e., negative), relatively pleasant as well as relatively unpleasant stimuli were presented to the subjects. Relative pleasantness and unpleasantness of sounds was evaluated after a statistical analysis of data of a pilot experiment (not reported here) and by environmental acousticians. The chosen sounds throughout this study were aimed to be representative for human-made (i.e., neighborhood) sounds occurring in typical inner yards.

4.1. Method

4.1.1. Hypotheses

The following three experimental hypotheses were to be tested in Experiment 1 [45]:

- Facade changes affect short-term acoustic comfort.
- Short-term acoustic comfort depends on sound source.
- Short-term acoustic comfort depends on observer position.

4.1.2. Experimental Design

Three design variables (i.e., independent variables) were considered in the design of Experiment 1: inner yard (four levels), source type (five levels), and observer position (three levels) [45].

Four inner yards were modelled in ODEON: the **reference** inner yard, an inner yard with one complete (long) side of the housing complex covered with a reflecting **glass facade**, an inner yard with **absorbing facade**, and an inner yard with **exaggerated absorption** of the housing complex whereby a number of glass windows and doors on the ground floor were covered by absorbing materials. Five different sources were used: a bouncing ball (**basketball 1**), a **doll's pram** (played/pushed by a child), a German conversation (**conversation 1**), and two sounds of (happily) playing and laughing children (**children 1** and **children 2**). An omni-directional sound source was placed in the yard 1.2 m above the ground. Three observer points were chosen: two observer points in the yard (1.2 m above the ground, representing the position of someone sitting on a bench), **5** and **20** m away from the source, and one observer point on a balcony (**balcony 2**) about 25 m away from the source (second floor, 9 m above the ground). Note that, on average, $L_{Aeq,Balcony2} < L_{Aeq,20m} < L_{Aeq,5m}$ and that the observer position at the balcony was considerably more affected by echos and flutter echos.

4.1.3. Stimuli

Based on the combination of four inner yards, five sources, and three observer positions, a total number of 60 stimuli were prepared for this experiment: $4 \times 5 \times 3 = 60$. It was mentioned that the input signals for the auralization in ODEON were 8 s long. Because of the reverberation time in the simulated inner yards, ODEON output audio files were of a length of up to 11 seconds. To have a unique length for all the stimuli used in the experiment, all ODEON outputs were cut down to 9 s. Fade-in and -out was realized with squared-cosine ramps of 200 and 600 ms, respectively. A-weighted equivalent continuous sound levels, L_{Aeq}, were between 42 to 59 dB(A) (mean $L_{Aeq} = 52$ dB(A)).

4.1.4. Subjects

Twenty-seven subjects (7 females and 20 males) participated in Experiment 1. All subjects declared to have normal hearing (self judgment) and to feel well. They were aged between 19 and 57 years (median 38 years). The majority of the participants worked at the Empa.

4.2. Results

Figure 4 shows the results of Experiment 1. A repeated-measures three-way ANOVA (corrected by the Greenhouse–Geisser method) revealed significant main effects of all three design variables inner yard ($F(2.2, 57.2) = 49.6$), sound source ($F(1.2, 31.9) = 25.8$), and observer position ($F(3.1, 79.3) = 33.1$) on short-term acoustic comfort (all $p < 0.001$) [45].

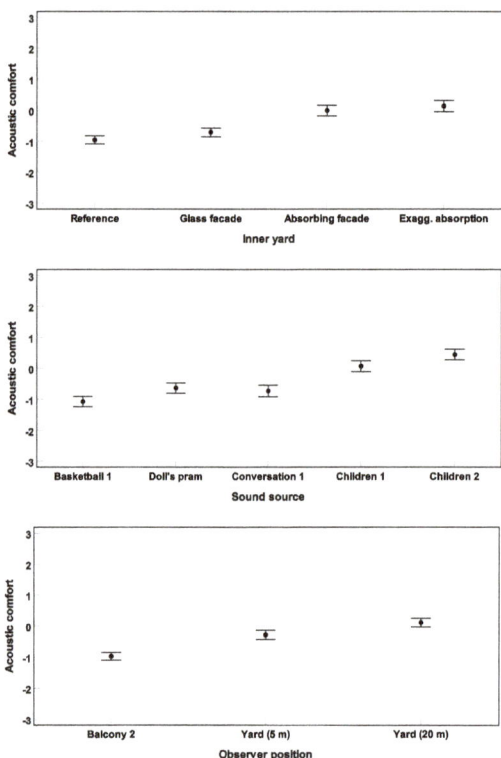

Figure 4. Results of Experiment 1: Mean acoustic comfort ratings across subjects and their 95% confidence intervals are shown for different inner yards (**above**), sound sources (**middle**), and observer positions (**below**).

Post hoc pairwise comparisons by an LSD test (corrected by the Bonferroni method) revealed no significant difference between the reference and glass facade yards ($p > 0.05$). No significant difference was found between the two absorbing yards ($p > 0.05$). However, in comparison to the non-absorbing yards, short-term acoustic comfort was rated significantly higher for the absorbing yards (all $p < 0.001$). With respect to sound sources, pairwise comparisons revealed that short-term acoustic comfort was rated higher for the two **children** sounds than for the three other sound sources (all $p < 0.001$). No further significant differences were found (all $p > 0.05$). Furthermore, comfort ratings for the three observer positions found to be significantly different from each other (all $p < 0.01$). The observer positions at 20 m distance in the yard and at the second floor balcony were found to be "more" and "less" comfortable than the position at 5 m distance in the yard, respectively (see Figure 4).

The repeated-measures ANOVA revealed two significant interactions between yard and position ($F(3.8, 97.5) = 52.8$) and between source and position ($F(6.0, 155.4) = 11.5$) (all $p < 0.001$). These interactions are shown in Figure 5. Whereas absorption improved the acoustics—with respect to acoustic comfort—for the observer positions in the yard, the observer point on the balcony did not benefit from the absorbing materials. The balcony stimuli revealed much more flutter echo than for the other positions (The authors would like to report an error in the case of stimuli with one inner yard, namely the glass front, and one observer position, i.e., on the balcony. All five of these stimuli were, by mistake, set on the first balcony. That explains less flutter echo and higher acoustic comfort ratings in this case. Had this been correct, would the already significant differences—and the explanation given in the text—have been even stronger. Therefore, the authors can assure that this mistake did not affect the conclusions of this study.). The interaction between sound source and observer position indicates several points. First, whereas for the human sounds (conversation 1 and the two playing **children** stimuli), acoustic comfort ratings were similar at 5 m and 20 m away in the yard, they were significantly lower on the balcony, where more echo and more flutter echo was present. Second, for basketball 1 and doll's pram—as examples of relatively unpleasant sounds—the 20 m position in the yard was significantly more comfortable than the two other observer positions. Note that, while $L_{Aeq,Balcony2} < L_{Aeq,5m}$, at the balcony echo and flutter echo were more dominant. That is, only at the yard position 20 m away from the source both $L_{Aeq,20m}$ and echos or flatter echos were less dominant.

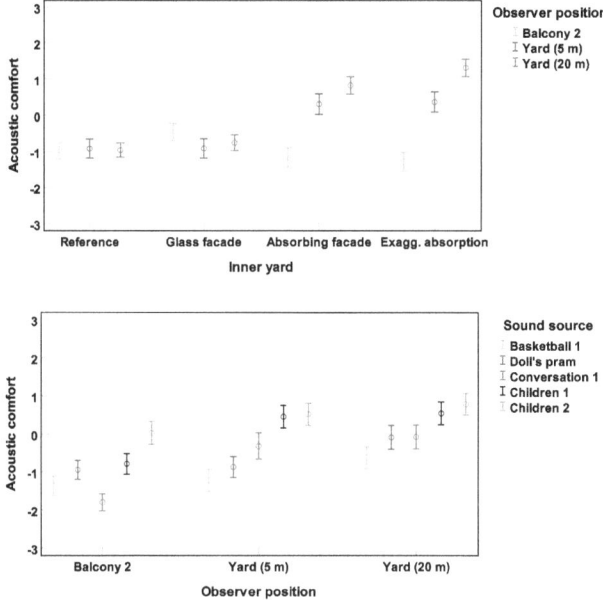

Figure 5. Significant interactions (Experiment 1) between inner yard and observer position (**above**) and between source and observer position (**below**). Mean acoustic comfort ratings across subjects and their 95% confidence intervals are depicted.

5. Experiment 2

The results from Experiment 1 showed that using absorbing materials on building facades increased short-term acoustic comfort. Experiment 2 aimed to focus on the effect of the absorption coefficient. 63% of the total facade of the reference building was non-glass material. This portion of the surface was varied from being a concrete reflecting facade to an absorbing facade. The main question under test was to what degree absorbing facade would improve acoustic comfort. Would there be saturation effects? Could too much absorption even lead to a decreased acoustic comfort?

5.1. Method

5.1.1. Hypotheses

The following three experimental hypotheses were established for Experiment 2:

- Short-term acoustic comfort depends on the absorption coefficient.
- Short-term acoustic comfort depends on the sound source.
- Short-term acoustic comfort is different at different balconies (i.e., floors).

5.1.2. Experimental Design

Three design variables (i.e., independent variables) were considered in the design of Experiment 2: the weighted absorption coefficient α_w [50] (five levels), source type (four levels), and observer location (two levels).

The two modelled inner yards **reference** and **absorbing facade** in Section 4.1.2 exhibited α_w values of nearly 0 and 1. Having these two cases in mind as extreme (realistic) cases of reflection and absorption, α_w was varied for Experiment 2 from 0.05 to 0.95 with an approximately exponential progression (i.e., approximately equidistant on a logarithmic axis). In order to avoid major frequency-dependent differences in absorption properties of the materials—because that would have led to a tremendously more complicated interpretation of the results—a simple material model was chosen, for which the frequency dependency of α remained approximately constant, as α_w was increased. Figure 6 shows the absorption coefficient as a function of frequency as α_w increases. Doing so, the facade was covered with absorbing materials exhibiting α_w values of **0.05, 0.15, 0.30, 0.55,** and **0.95**.

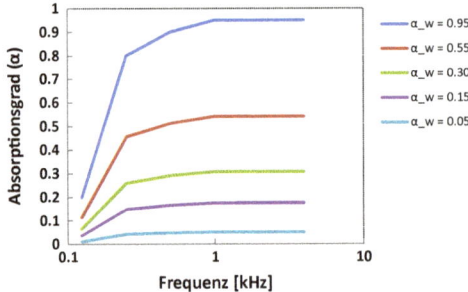

Figure 6. Absorption coefficient as a function of frequency (logarithmic horizontal axis).

Four different sources were used: a bouncing ball (**basketball 1**), a crying **baby**, a Swiss German conversation (**conversation 2**), and a sound of playing children (**children 2**). As in Experiment 1, an omni-directional sound source was placed in the yard 1.2 m above the ground. Two observer points were chosen on the **balcony 0** (patio) and **balcony 2** (second floor balcony). Compared to the level at **balcony 0**, **balcony 2** exhibited lower L_{Aeq} (i.e., mean $L_{Aeq,balcony2}$ < mean $L_{Aeq,balcony0}$).

5.1.3. Stimuli

Based on the combination of five absorption degrees (α_w), four sources, and two observer positions, a total number of 40 stimuli were prepared for Experiment 2: 4 × 5 × 2 = 40. ODEON outputs were cut down to 10 s. Fade-in and -out was realized with squared-cosine ramps of 400 and 1000 ms, respectively. A-weighted equivalent continuous sound levels, L_{Aeq}, were between 49 to 64 dB(A) (mean L_{Aeq} = 60 dB(A)).

5.1.4. Subjects

Forty-two subjects (13 females and 29 males) participated in Experiment 2. All subjects declared having normal hearing (self judgment) and to feel well. They were aged between 18 and 64 years (median 41 years). The majority of the participants worked at the Empa.

5.2. Results

Figure 7 shows the results of Experiment 2. A repeated-measures three-way ANOVA (corrected by the Greenhouse–Geisser method) revealed significant main effects of all three design variables α_w (F(3.0, 121.8) = 21.0), sound source (F(2.7, 112.1) = 71.6), and observer position (F(1.0, 41.0) = 29.3) on short-term acoustic comfort (all $p < 0.001$).

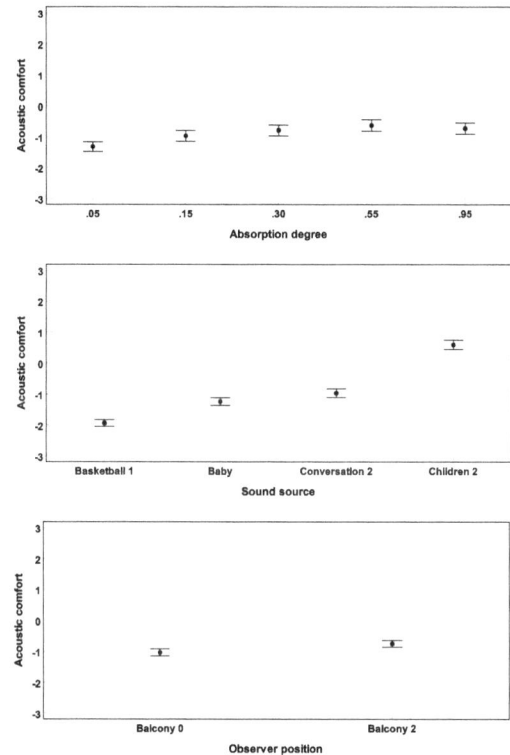

Figure 7. Results of Experiment 2: Mean acoustic comfort ratings across subjects and their 95% confidence intervals are shown for different absorption degrees α_w (**above**), sound sources (**middle**), and observer positions (**below**).

A linear mixed-effect model was established considering the covariates absorption coefficient (α_w) and playback number, categorical variables sound source and observer position, as well as random intercept. Since the effect of α_w seemed to have a parabolic shape here (and in a pilot experiment), also α_w^2 was considered in the model. The estimate of the model for the effect of α_w is depicted in Figure 8.

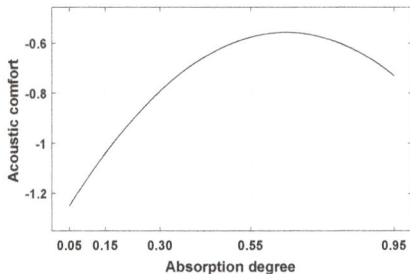

Figure 8. Effect of the absorption coefficient ($α_w$) on short-term acoustic comfort, estimated by a linear mixed-effects model.

Post hoc pairwise comparisons by LSD test (corrected by the Bonferroni method) revealed that **basketball 1** and **children 2** were rated as least and most comfortable sounds, respectively (all $p < 0.01$). No significant difference was found between the ratings for crying **baby** and for the **conversation 2** ($p > 0.05$). Furthermore, acoustic comfort was rated higher for **balcony 2** than for **balcony 0** ($p < 0.01$).

The repeated-measures ANOVA revealed a significant interaction between $α_w$ and sound source (F(7.3, 301.3) = 4.7) ($p < 0.001$), which can be observed in Figure 9. Whereas for **basketball 1** and **children 2** acoustic comfort was increased with increasing $α_w$ up to a saturation effect for $α_w > 0.55$, for crying **baby** and **conversation 2**, a strong parabolic relationship was found between $α_w$ and acoustic comfort.

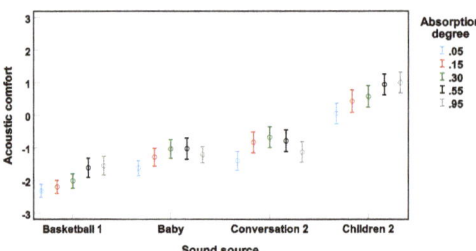

Figure 9. Significant interaction (Experiment 2) between $α_w$ and sound source. Mean acoustic comfort ratings across subjects and their 95% confidence intervals are depicted.

6. Experiment 3

In Experiment 3, possible effects of the absorption of balconies' ceilings on acoustic comfort was investigated. Thus, not only facade absorption was varied, but also every balcony ceiling.

6.1. Method

6.1.1. Hypotheses

In Experiment 3, the following three experimental hypotheses were investigated:

- Short-term acoustic comfort depends on the absorption coefficient ($α_w$).
- Short-term acoustic comfort depends on the sound source.
- Using absorbing materials on the balcony ceiling affects short-term acoustic comfort.

6.1.2. Experimental Design

Three design variables were considered in the design of Experiment 3: facade $α_w$ (three levels), source type (three levels), and balcony ceiling $α_w$ (three levels). $α_w$ was varied for Experiment 3 between

0.05, 0.30, and 0.95 for the absorption of the facade, as well as the balcony ceiling. Three sound sources were used: a bouncing ball (**basketball 2**), **conversation 1**, and **children 1**. The observer was placed at the second floor balcony.

6.1.3. Stimuli

Based on the combination of three facade absorption degrees, three sources, and three balcony ceiling absorption degrees, a total number of 27 stimuli were prepared for Experiment 3: 3 × 3 × 3 = 27. ODEON outputs were cut down to 10 s with fade-in and -out ramps of 400 and 800 ms, respectively. A-weighted equivalent continuous sound levels, L_{Aeq}, were between 49 to 59 dB(A) (mean L_{Aeq} = 56 dB(A)).

6.1.4. Subjects

Experiments 2 and 3 were conducted in one experimental session (see Section 3.5). The same subjects as in Section 5.1.4 participated in Experiment 3.

6.2. Results

Figure 10 shows the results of Experiment 3. A repeated-measures three-way ANOVA (corrected by the Greenhouse–Geisser method) revealed significant main effects of facade α_w ($F(1.4, 56.6) = 9.5$) and sound source ($F(2.0, 80.0) = 105.7$) on short-term acoustic comfort (all $p < 0.01$). α_w at the balcony ceiling was not found to be significantly affecting acoustic comfort ($F(2.0, 80.3) = 2.8$) ($p = 0.07$).

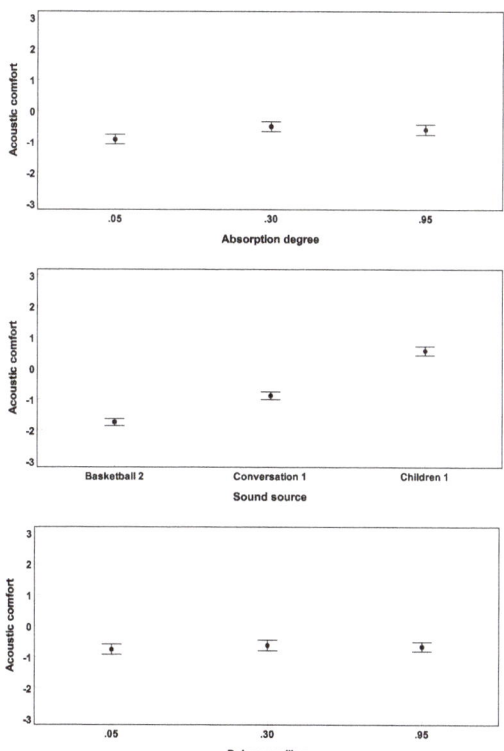

Figure 10. Results of Experiment 3: Mean acoustic comfort ratings across subjects and their 95% confidence intervals are shown for different absorption degrees α_w (**above**), sound sources (**middle**), and absorption degrees of the balcony ceiling α_w (**below**).

A linear mixed-effect model was established considering the covariate facade α_w (and $\alpha_w{}^2$), and the categorical variable sound source, as well as random intercept. Contribution of balcony ceiling α_w (and/or $\alpha_w{}^2$) in the model were not significant. Even though only three absorption degrees were tested in Experiment 3, the model estimate was very similar to the estimate in Experiment 2. Regarding sound source, post hoc pairwise comparisons revealed that **basketball 2** and **children 1** were rated as "least" and "most" comfortable sounds, respectively (all $p < 0.001$).

No interactions between the independent variables were found to be significant in predicting acoustic comfort. However, the authors would like to note that similar to the tendency for the main effect of balcony ceiling α_w ($p = 0.07$; see above), there was a tendency for an interaction between α_w at the facade and at the ceiling ($p = 0.09$). Thereby, for facade α_w of **0.05** (reflecting facade), usage of absorber at the balcony ceiling tended to increase acoustic comfort (see Figure 11). That is, only if there were no absorption on the walls, the absorbing material on the ceiling tended to be effective, however non-significant.

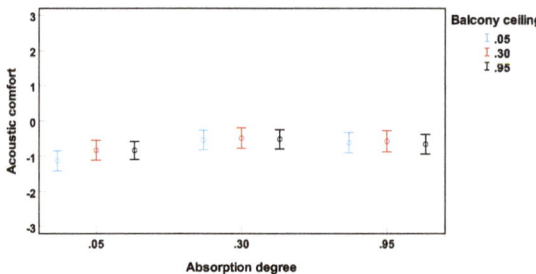

Figure 11. Non-significant interaction (Experiment 3) between α_w on the facade and α_w on the balcony ceilings. Mean acoustic comfort ratings across subjects and their 95% confidence intervals are depicted.

7. Discussion

The results of Experiment 1 revealed that the inner yards with absorbing building facades were acoustically more comfortable than the inner yards with reflecting building facades (see Section 4.2). Using a complete **glass facade** instead of the original brickwork and glass mix (in the **reference**) did not lead to significant changes in the acoustic comfort ratings. Similarly, an **exaggerated absorption** was not found to be significantly more effective than a simple **absorbing facade**. The results of Experiment 2 showed a similar pattern, whereby acoustic comfort increased with increasing α_w, however only up to $\alpha_w = 0.55$. Stronger absorption led to even lower acoustic comfort ratings (see Section 5.2).

Including $\alpha_w{}^2$ in the regression model and the resulting parabolic predicting relationships between α_w and short-term acoustic comfort seem to have provided a reasonable fit to the data (see Section 5.2). For the data presented here, only one point ($\alpha_w = 0.95$) fell on the right side of the parabolic curve. One should be careful about whether one point justifies such a model suggestion. However, not only could a similar curve be fitted to the data from Experiment 3 (see Figure 10 (above)), but also the results of a pilot test (not presented here), which included $\alpha_w = 1.00$, confirmed the parabolic shape. Thus, it is to assume that using absorbing materials on the facade would improve acoustic comfort, but only up to a point (for Experiment 1: the inner yard with **absorbing facade**; for Experiment 2: $\alpha_w = 0.55$), beyond which the effect on acoustic comfort would saturate (Experiment 1) or drop (Experiments 2 and 3). It can be concluded that, whereas some absorption is desirable, too much absorption—causing higher costs—might yield no further improvement, or may even decrease it (presumably because at some point the inner yard would lose its room acoustic quality; i.e., its "roominess").

With respect to the sound sources, all three experiments led to a consistent distinction between relatively unpleasant (e.g., **basketball**) and relatively pleasant (e.g., **children**) sound sources. Whereas in each experiment the unpleasant and the pleasant sounds were associated with lower and higher acoustic comfort ratings, the exact rating range was not robust between the three experiments. That might have to do with the SPL. The mean L_{Aeq} for Experiments 1, 2, and 3 was 52, 60, and 56 dB(A), respectively. Acoustic comfort rating histograms for the three experiments are shown in Figure 12. Although the median rating in all three experiments was −1, the mean rating was −0.4, −0.9, and −0.7 for Experiments 1, 2, and 3, respectively. That is, with increasing mean L_{Aeq} of the experiments, mean acoustic comfort decreased.

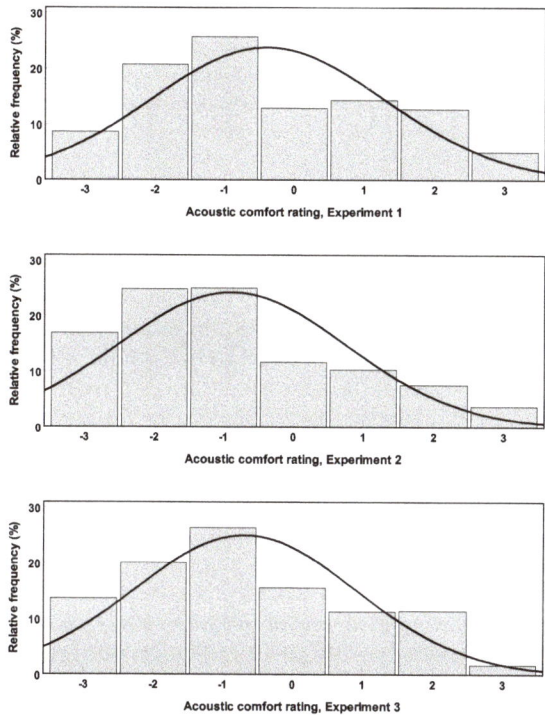

Figure 12. Acoustic comfort rating histograms for the data from Experiments 1 (**above**), 2 (**middle**) and 3 (**below**). Relative frequency is shown in percent.

This is consistent with the fact that, for almost all sources and experiments, a tendency was observed, whereby increased L_{Aeq} (caused by reflection or by the distance to the observer) was associated with lower comfort ratings. Only for Experiment 1 (with the lowest mean L_{Aeq}), and only in the case of the two rather pleasant **children** sounds, acoustic comfort increased with increasing L_{Aeq}, which is similar to observations by Yang and Kang [15] for pleasant sounds. The results indicate that pleasant sounds can be used to increase perceived comfort in inner yards. It should be noted, however, that no definitive pleasant or unpleasant sounds exist. Pleasantness or unpleasantness is a subjective perceived quality of a sound, which can only be interpreted in the context under investigation [5]. Therefore, the pleasantness or unpleasantness of the sound in this study might be judged differently in other contexts and by other subjects.

In addition to the playing **children** sounds used in this study, Kang and Zhang [16] reported that natural and culture-related sounds (e.g., music) were preferred compared to artificial sounds. Furthermore, Hong and Jeon [42] reported that, in particular, water and bird sounds have been usually evaluated as the most effective and favorable sounds to improve urban sound environments [37,51].

The above discussion (on L_{Aeq}) suggests three points for such experiments:

- Generally, increasing L_{Aeq} would be associated with decreased acoustic comfort.
- In order to use the bipolar scale appropriately, it is important that an appropriate (moderate) L_{Aeq} range is chosen. Too many stimuli with high L_{Aeq} (or equivalently a high mean L_{Aeq}) can cause positive skewness and would not allow subjects to use the scale properly.
- If a high mean L_{Aeq} is not avoidable, it might be more appropriate to switch to a unipolar (negative) scale, such as the 11-point ICBEN annoyance scale [49]. This might be more practical, as subjects would more likely experience discomfort (rather than comfort).
- Although using a lower L_{Aeq} range (e.g., mean L_{Aeq} = 45 dB(A)) might be tempting and would probably lead to higher acoustic comfort, the ecological validity of the experiment should be taken into account. Note that the stimuli of this study were not calibrated, but normalized to the A-weighted level of the signal with the largest maximum absolute amplitude and this marks one of the limitations of this study.

With respect to observer position, Experiments 1 and 2 did not reveal a clear picture. Whereas balcony 2 was rated as the least comfortable observer position in Experiment 1, it was rated as more comfortable than balcony 0 in Experiment 2. Nevertheless, a few conclusions can be made based on the results. First, there are differences in acoustic comfort in distinct observer positions. This is in accordance with observations by Calleri et al. [27], in which different SPLs and different perceived wideness were reported in different observation positions and facades (including interactions similar to those in Experiment 1). Second, one factor for this is the SPL at the point of observation (see the discussion above). Third, post hoc listening to the stimuli revealed that stimuli with too much echo and flutter echo were rated significantly lower (i.e., more negatively) than those with low or moderate echo. That is, observer positions which were subject to echo and flutter echo were least comfortable.

Covering balcony ceilings with absorbers was not found to significantly affect acoustic comfort. However, a non-significant tendency was found, whereby, in the absence of absorbers on the facade, absorbing ceilings were more comfortable than reflecting ceilings. One explanation for this could be that, in comparison to the large facade surface, balcony ceilings are small. Hence, when absorbers were installed on the facade, possible benefits from additional absorption of balcony ceilings were marginal. In the presence of reflecting facades, however, a low-cost absorption on the balcony might not only be helpful to reduce noise level [29,30,35,52], but also to improve acoustic comfort. This should be subject to further investigations.

While interpreting the results and making conclusions, it is important to consider limitations of this study. While controlled laboratory experiments are suitable for comparisons (such as for this study), on-site studies offer a more natural, realistic and complex picture of the existing soundscape. Furthermore, as the subjects were seated in the laboratory, no visual modelling of the buildings and the inner yards was offered to them. It should be noted that visualizations and aural-visual interactions can affect sound and noise perception as well as perceived acoustic comfort [17,53–57]. Whereas with the chosen setup such visual effects were not included in the design, at the same time, this enabled an investigation of the perceptual quality of acoustical characteristics without any visual confounders. A further limitation of this study is that, for each stimulus, a single source was present. The experimental design can (and should) be extended in further works with mixtures of background (e.g., vegetation and birds) sounds and foreground inner yard sounds and/or with mixtures of several (foreground) sound sources. Lastly, it should be noted that—other than changes in balconies' absorption coefficient in Experiment 3—balconies' geometry and design were not changed systematically in this study. Interesting information about influences of balconies on acoustics can be found in [29–35].

In the analysis of the experimental results, a discussion of room acoustical parameters (beyond the SPL; i.e., early decay time, reverberation time, speech transmission index, clarity index, and etc.) has been avoided here. However, it is possible (and planned) to carry out a post hoc analysis of the associations between the room acoustical parameters and acoustic comfort, e.g., by means of correlations between each room acoustical parameter and the observed acoustic comfort. It is expected that room acoustical parameters can describe or predict the acoustic comfort to some degree [26,27,58,59].

8. Conclusions

Three laboratory experiments were reported which investigated short-term acoustic comfort and discomfort in housing complexes when relatively pleasant and unpleasant everyday life sound sources were present in virtual inner yards. The results showed that moderate absorption of the building facade increased acoustic comfort. Different sound sources and distinct observer positions were associated with different acoustic comfort. While relatively pleasant sounds were associated with comfort, discomfort was observed in the presence of relatively unpleasant sounds. Observer positions with strong echo and/or flutter echo and those at which high sound pressure levels were registered were found to be least comfortable. The results indicate that a careful acoustic design of the facades of housing complexes might be helpful to improve acoustic comfort of the residents. A further analysis of the results is needed and planned with regard to room acoustical parameters to identify which room acoustical parameters are good indicators of acoustic comfort.

Author Contributions: Conceptualization, K.E. and A.T.; Methodology, A.T.; Software, A.T. and T.S.; Validation, T.S. and A.T.; Formal Analysis, A.T. and T.S.; Investigation, T.S. and A.T.; Resources, K.E.; Data Curation, A.T.; Writing—Original Draft Preparation, A.T.; Writing—Review and Editing, A.T., T.S., and K.E.; Visualization, A.T. and T.S.; Supervision, K.E. and A.T.; Project Administration, A.T.; Funding Acquisition, K.E.

Funding: This research received no external funding.

Acknowledgments: The authors are very grateful to the participants of the preliminary and main experiments of this study. They would like to thank Matthias Blau for the co-supervision of the first experiment [45]. A special thank goes to Reto Pieren for preparing the listening test software. The authors would also like to thank Oliver Scheuregger for his helpful comments regarding the English language.

Conflicts of Interest: The authors declare no conflict of interest.

Abbreviations

The following abbreviations are used in this manuscript:

AIC	Akaike information criterion
ANOVA	Analysis of variance
BIC	Bayesian information criterion
H0	Null hypothesis
ICBEN	International Commission on Biological Effects of Noise
L_{Aeq}	A-weighted equivalent continuous sound pressure level
L_{AFmax}	A-weighted FAST response maximum sound pressure level
LSD	Fisher's protected least significant difference
SPL	Sound pressure level

References

1. ISO 1996-1:2016. *Acoustics—Description, Measurement and Assessment of Environmental Noise—Part 1: Basic Quantities and Assessment Procedures*; International Organization for Standardization: Geneva, Switzerland, 2016.
2. ISO 1996-2:2017. *Acoustics—Description, Measurement and Assessment of Environmental Noise—Part 2: Determination of Sound Pressure Levels*; International Organization for Standardization: Geneva, Switzerland, 2017.
3. WHO. *Environmental Noise Guidelines for the European Region*; WHO Regional Office for Europe: Copenhagen, Denmark, 2018. Available online: http://euro.who.int/__data/assets/pdf_file/0008/383921/noise-guidelines-eng.pdf?ua=1 (accessed on 15 January 2019).
4. ISO 12913-1:2014. *Acoustics—Soundscape—Part 1: Definition and Conceptual Framework*; International Organization for Standardization: Geneva, Switzerland, 2014.

5. ISO 12913-2:2018. *Acoustics—Soundscape—Part 2: Data Collection and Reporting Requirements*; International Organization for Standardization: Geneva, Switzerland, 2018.
6. Kang, J. *Urban Sound Environment*, 1st ed.; Taylor & Francis Group: Milton Park, Oxfordshire, UK, 2017; pp. 1–304.
7. Schafer, R.M. *The Soundscape: Our Sonic Environment and the Tuning of the World*, 1st ed.; Destiny Books: Rochester, VT, USA, 1993; pp. 1–320.
8. Brown, A.L.; Gjestland, T.; Dubois, D. Acoustic Environments and Soundscapes. In *Soundscape and the Built Environment*; Kang, J., Schulte-Fortkamp, B., Eds.; CRC Press: Boca Raton, FL, USA, 2016; pp. 1–16.
9. Battaglia, P.L. Achieving acoustical comfort in restaurants. In Proceedings of the 168th Meeting of the Acoustical Society of America, Indianapolis, IN, USA, 27–31 October 2014.
10. Thomas, P.; Aletta, F.; Vander Mynsbrugge, T.; Filipan, K.; Dijckmans, A.; De Geetere, L.; Botteldooren, D.; Petrovic, M.; De Vriendt, P.; Van De Velde, D.; et al. Evaluation and improvement of the acoustic comfort in nursing homes: A case study in Flanders, Belgium. In Proceedings of the Euronoise 2018, Crete, Greece, 27–31 May 2018.
11. Xiao, J.; Aletta, F. A soundscape approach to exploring design strategies for acoustic comfort in modern public libraries: A case study of the Library of Birmingham. *Noise Mapp.* **2016**, *3*, 264–273. [CrossRef]
12. Brown, A.L.; Kang, J.; Gjestland, T. Towards standardization in soundscape preference assessment. *Appl. Acoust.* **2011**, *72*, 387–392. [CrossRef]
13. Coelho, J.L.B. Approaches to Urban Soundscape Management, Planning, and Design. In *Soundscape and the Built Environment*; Kang, J., Schulte-Fortkamp, B., Eds.; CRC Press: Boca Raton, FL, USA, 2016; pp. 197–214.
14. Sturm, U.; Bürgin, M. *Stadtklang—Wege zu Einer Hörenswerten Stadt. Report, Kompetenzzentrum Typologie und Planung in Architektur (CCTP)*; vdf Hochschulverlag AG: Zurich, Switzerland, 2016.
15. Yang, W.; Kang, J. Acoustic comfort evaluation in urban open public spaces. *Appl. Acoust.* **2005**, *66*, 211–229. [CrossRef]
16. Kang, J.; Zhang, M. Semantic differential analysis of the soundscape in urban open public spaces. *Build. Environ.* **2010**, *45*, 150–157. [CrossRef]
17. Iachini, T.; Maffei, L.; Ruotolo, F.; Senese, V.P.; Ruggiero, G.; Masullo, M.; Alekseeva, N. Multisensory Assessment of Acoustic Comfort Aboard Metros: A Virtual Reality Study. *Appl. Cogn. Psychol.* **2012**, *66*, 757–767. [CrossRef]
18. Schulte-Fortkamp B. The quality of acoustic environments and the meaning of soundscapes. In Proceedings of the 17th International Conference on Acoustics (ICA), Rome, Italy, 2–7 September 2001.
19. Yang, W.; Kang, J. Acoustic Comfort and Psychological Adaptation as a Guide for Soundscape Design in Urban Open Public Spaces. In Proceedings of the 17th International Conference on Acoustics (ICA), Rome, Italy, 2–7 September 2001.
20. Vardaxis, N.-G.; Bard, D.; Persson Waye, K. Review of acoustic comfort evaluation in dwellings—Part I: Associations of acoustic field data to subjective responses from building surveys. *Build. Acoust.* **2018**, *25*, 151–170. [CrossRef]
21. Vardaxis, N.-G.; Bard, D. Review of acoustic comfort evaluation in dwellings: Part II—Impact sound data associated with subjective responses in laboratory tests. *Build. Acoust.* **2018**, *25*, 171–192. [CrossRef]
22. Vardaxis, N.-G.; Bard, D. Review of acoustic comfort evaluation in dwellings: Part III—Airborne sound data associated with subjective responses in laboratory tests. *Build. Acoust.* **2018**, *25*, 289–305. [CrossRef]
23. Maag, T.; Kocan, T.; Bosshard, A. *Klangqualität für Offentliche Stadt-und Siedlungsräume*; Baudirektion Kanton Zurich: Zurich, Switzerland, 2016. Available online: https://tba.zh.ch/internet/baudirektion/tba/de/laerm/formulare_merkblaetter.html (accessed on 15 January 2019).
24. Maag, T.; Kocan, T.; Bosshard, A. The sonic public realm—Chances for improving the sound quality of the everyday city. In Proceedings of the INTER-NOISE and NOISE-CON Congress and Conference 2016, Hamburg, Germany, 21–24 August 2016.
25. Maag, T. Integrated urban sound planning—From noise control to sound quality for the everyday city. In Proceedings of the INTER-NOISE and NOISE-CON Congress and Conference 2017, Hong Kong, China, 27–30 August 2017.
26. Yang, H.-S.; Kim, M.-J.; Kang, J. Acoustic characteristics of outdoor spaces in an apartment complex. *Noise Control Eng. J.* **2013**, *61*, 1–10. [CrossRef]

27. Calleri, C.; Shtrepi, L.; Armando, A.; Astolfi, A. On the influence of different facade materials on the auditory perception of urban spaces. In Proceedings of the INTER-NOISE and NOISE-CON Congress and Conference 2017, Hong Kong, China, 27–30 August 2017.
28. Yu, C.-J.; Kang, J. Environmental impact of acoustic materials in residential buildings. *Build. Environ.* **2009**, *44*, 2166–2175. [CrossRef]
29. Lee, P.K.; Kim, Y.H.; Jeon, J.Y.; Song, K.D. Effects of apartment building façade and balcony design on the reduction of exterior noise. *Build. Environ.* **2007**, *42*, 3517–3528. [CrossRef]
30. Yeung, M. Adopting specially designed balconies to achieve substantial noise reduction for residential buildings. In Proceedings of the INTER-NOISE and NOISE-CON Congress and Conference 2016, Hamburg, Germany, 21–24 August 2016.
31. Tang, S.-K. A review on natural ventilation-enabling façade noise control devices for congested high-rise cities. *Appl. Sci.* **2017**, *7*, 175. [CrossRef]
32. Tang, S.-K. Noise screening effects of balconies on a building facade. *J. Acoust. Soc. Am.* **2005**, *118*, 213–221. [CrossRef]
33. Hossam El Dien, H.; Woloszyn, P. The acoustical influence of balcony depth and parapet form: Experiments and simulations. *Appl. Acoust.* **2005**, *66*, 533–551. [CrossRef]
34. Wang, X.; Mao, M.; Yu, W.; Jiang, Z. Acoustic performance of balconies having inhomogeneous ceiling surfaces on a roadside building facade. *Build. Environ.* **2015**, *93*, 1–8. [CrossRef]
35. Hossam El Dien, H.; Woloszyn, P. Prediction of the sound field into high-rise building facades due to its balcony ceiling form. *Appl. Acoust.* **2004**, *65*, 431–440. [CrossRef]
36. Hermida, L.; Pavón, I. Spatial aspects in urban soundscapes: Binaural parameters application in the study of soundscapes from Bogotá-Colombia and Brasília-Brazil. *Appl. Acoust.* **2019**, *145*, 420–430. [CrossRef]
37. Jeon, J.Y.; Lee, P.J.; You, J.; Kang, J. Perceptual assessment of quality of urban soundscapes with combined noise sources and water sounds. *J. Acoust. Soc. Am.* **2010**, *127*, 1357–1366. [CrossRef]
38. Laso, C.V.; Asensio, C.; Pavón, I. Design and Validation of a Simulator Tool Useful for Designers and Policy Makers in Urban Sound Planning. *Acoust. Aust.* **2017**, *45*, 515–527. [CrossRef]
39. Rey Gozalo, G.; Trujillo Carmonaand, J.; Barrigón Morillas, J. M.; Vílchez-Gómez, R.; Gómez Escobar, V. Relationship between objective acoustic indices and subjective assessments for the quality of soundscapes. *Appl. Acoust.* **2015**, *97*, 1–10. [CrossRef]
40. Schäffer, B.; Schlittmeier, S.J.; Pieren, R.; Heutschi, K.; Graf, R.; Hellbrück, J. Short-term annoyance reactions to stationary and time-varying wind turbine and road traffic noise: A laboratory study. *J. Acoust. Soc. Am.* **2016**, *139*, 2949–2963. [CrossRef] [PubMed]
41. Schäffer, B.; Pieren, R.; Schlittmeier, S.; Brink, M. Effects of Different Spectral Shapes and Amplitude Modulation of Broadband Noise on Annoyance Reactions in a Controlled Listening Experiment. *Int. J. Environ. Res. Public Health* **2013**, *15*, 1029. [CrossRef]
42. Hong, J.Y.; Jeon, J.Y. Designing sound and visual components for enhancement of urban soundscapes. *J. Acoust. Soc. Am.* **2013**, *134*, 2026–2036. [CrossRef] [PubMed]
43. Ribe, R.G.; Manyoky, M.; Wissen Hayek, U.; Pieren, R.; Heutschi, K.; Grêt-Regamey, A. Dissecting perceptions of wind energy projects: A laboratory experiment using high-quality audio-visual simulations to analyze experiential versus acceptability ratings and information effects. *Landsc. Urban Plan.* **2018**, *139*, 131–147. [CrossRef]
44. Ruotolo, F.; Maffei, L.; Di Gabriele M.; Iachini, T.; Masullo, M.; Ruggiero, G.; Senese, V.P. Immersive virtual reality and environmental noise assessment: An innovative audio-visual approach. *Environ. Impact Assess. Rev.* **2013**, *41*, 10–20. [CrossRef]
45. Sievers, T.; Eggenschwiler, K.; Taghipour, A.; Blau, M. Untersuchungen zur raumakustischen Aufenthaltsqualität in Innenhöfen von Wohnbauten. In Proceedings of the DAGA 2018—44 Jahrestagung für Akustik, Munich, Germany, 19–22 March 2018.
46. Moosbrugger, H.; Kelava, A. *Testtheorie und Fragebogenkonstruktionen*, 2nd ed.; Springer: Berlin, Germany, 2012; pp. 28–72.
47. Akaike, H. Information theory and an extension of the maximum likelihood principle. In Proceedings of the 2nd International Symposium on Information Theory, Tsahkadsor, Armenia, 2–8 September 1973; pp. 267–281.
48. Schwarz, G. Estimating the dimension of a model. *Ann. Stat.* **1978**, *6*, 461–464. [CrossRef]

49. ISO/TS 15666. *Technical Specification: Acoustics—Assessment of Noise Annoyance by Means of Social and Socio-Acoustic Surveys*; International Organization for Standardization: Geneva, Switzerland, 2013.
50. ISO 11654. *Acoustics—Sound Absorbers for Use in Buildings—Rating of Sound Absorption*; International Organization for Standardization: Geneva, Switzerland, 1997.
51. Guastavino, C. The Ideal Urban Soundscape: Investigating the Sound Quality of French Cities. *Acta Acust. Acust.* **2006**, *92*, 945–951.
52. Naish, D.A.; Tan, A.C.C.; Demirbilek, F. Simulating the effect of acoustic treatment types for residential balconies with road traffic noise. *Appl. Acoust.* **2014**, *79*, 131–140. [CrossRef]
53. Ernst, M.O.; Bülthoff, H.H. Merging the senses into a robust percept. *Trends Cogn. Sci.* **2014**, *8*, 162–169. [CrossRef]
54. Maffei, L.; Masullo, M.; Aletta, F.; Di Gabriele M. The influence of visual characteristics of barriers on railway noise perception. *Sci. Total Environ.* **2013**, *445–446*, 41–47. [CrossRef]
55. Maffei, L.; Iachini, T.; Masullo, M.; Aletta, F.; Sorrentino, F.; Senese, V.P.; Ruotolo, F. The effects of vision-related aspects on noise perception of wind turbines in quiet areas. *Int. J. Environ. Res. Public Health* **2013**, *10*, 1681–1697. [CrossRef] [PubMed]
56. Viollon, S.; Lavandier, C.; Drake, C. Influence of visual setting on sound ratings in an urban envoironment. *Appl. Acoust.* **2002**, *63*, 493–511. [CrossRef]
57. Zhang, M.; Kang, J. Towards the Evaluation, Description, and Creation of Soundscapes in Urban Open Spaces. *Environ. Plan. B* **2007**, *34*, 68–86. [CrossRef]
58. Fuda, S.; Aletta, F.; Kang, J.; Astolfi, A. Sound perception of different materials for the footpaths of urban parks. *Energy Procedia* **2015**, *78*, 13–18. [CrossRef]
59. Yang, H.-S.; Kang, J.; Kim, M.-J. An experimental study on the acoustic characteristics of outdoor spaces surrounded by multi-residential buildings. *Appl. Acoust.* **2017**, *127*, 147–159. [CrossRef]

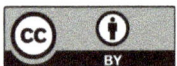

© 2019 by the authors. Licensee MDPI, Basel, Switzerland. This article is an open access article distributed under the terms and conditions of the Creative Commons Attribution (CC BY) license (http://creativecommons.org/licenses/by/4.0/).

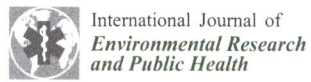

Article

A Cross-Sectional Survey on the Impact of Irrelevant Speech Noise on Annoyance, Mental Health and Well-being, Performance and Occupants' Behavior in Shared and Open-Plan Offices

Sonja Di Blasio *, Louena Shtrepi, Giuseppina Emma Puglisi and Arianna Astolfi

Department of Energy, Politecnico di Torino, Corso Duca degli Abruzzi 24, 10129 Torino, Italy; louena.shtrepi@polito.it (L.S.); giuseppina.puglisi@polito.it (G.E.P.); arianna.astolfi@polito.it (A.A.)
* Correspondence: sonja.diblasio@polito.it; Tel.: +39-011-090-4519

Received: 22 November 2018; Accepted: 15 January 2019; Published: 19 January 2019

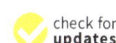

Abstract: This cross-sectional survey has compared subjective outcomes obtained from workers in shared (2–5 occupants) and open-plan (+5 occupants) offices, related to irrelevant speech, which is the noise that is generated from conversations between colleagues, telephone calls and laughter. Answers from 1078 subjects (55% in shared offices and 45% in open-plan offices) have shown that irrelevant speech increases noise annoyance, decreases work performance, and increases symptoms related to mental health and well-being more in open-plan than in shared offices. Workers often use headphones with music to contrast irrelevant speech in open-plan offices, while they take a break, change their working space, close the door or work from home in shared offices. Being female, when there are more than 20 occupants, and working in southern cities without acoustic treatments in the office, make it more likely for the occupants to be annoyed by irrelevant speech noise in open-plan offices. While, working in southern cities and with acoustic treatments in the office makes it more likely that noise annoyance will be reported in shared offices. Finally, more than 70% of the interviewed in open-plan offices were willing to reduce their voice volumes when advised by a noise monitoring system with a lighting feedback.

Keywords: irrelevant speech noise; noise annoyance; productivity; mental health; well-being; cross-sectional survey; open-plan offices; shared offices; occupants' behavior

1. Introduction

Irrelevant speech noise (ISN) is the noise that is generated from conversations between colleagues, telephone calls and laughter [1,2]. Office workers have mentioned that irrelevant speech is the most disturbing source of noise [1,3–6] in open-plan offices, due to the overall noise level and intelligible conversations [7–9]. A large number of cross-sectional surveys have been carried out on the theme of noise and comfort in open plan offices, but none has focused on ISN, although it has been reported to be the main source of annoyance and dissatisfaction. Moreover, no investigation on noise perception and its effects in offices with different sizes has been performed yet. In fact, the investigations so far performed have been aimed at considering the differences between open-plan and cellular offices, the latter with from one to two people, but shared offices that seat from two to five people, which can be alternatives to very noisy open-plan offices, have not been considered.

Given the relevance of the consequences of noise in offices with more than two occupants, several studies have investigated solutions for its mitigation, one of which is the room acoustic treatment.

The background on annoyance, loss of performance, mental health and well-being, due to noise in different types of offices is summarized hereafter, together with information on the effectiveness of acoustic interventions in rooms.

1.1. Background on Annoyance, Loss of Performance and Mental Health, and Well-Being from Noise in Offices

Several studies have dealt with the effects of noise annoyance in offices. Noise annoyance has been defined as a multi-faceted concept that includes behavioral noise effects, such as disturbance, and interferes with intended activities and evaluative aspects, such as nuisance, unpleasantness and getting on one's nerves [10]. In their semantic study, Guski et al. [10] demonstrated that the concept of noise annoyance was closely associated with disturbance and nuisance concepts. Therefore, the term "annoyance" has been used in the present study to indicate one effect of ISN.

Based on subjective assessments, a self-estimated loss of performance, due to ISN, was found in open-plan offices [1,5]. This outcome was then confirmed from the results of laboratory studies where subjective perception was considered and tests over several cognitive tasks were performed [8,11–13].

A considerable amount of literature has been published on the relationships between the presence of office noise, mental health and well-being. According to the WHO [14], mental health is a state of well-being in which the individual realizes his or her own abilities, can cope with the normal stresses of life, can work productively and fruitfully, and is able to make a contribution to his or her community. Mental wellbeing has instead been defined simply as feeling good and functioning well [15]. The consequences of mental health problems in the workplace can be depression, stress, burnout, but also headaches, ulcers, high blood pressure, reduction in productivity and output, loss of motivation and commitment, tension and conflicts between colleagues, etc. [16]. Several studies have investigated the typical symptoms and feelings associated with mental health and well-being in open-plan offices. Numerous symptoms, such as fatigue and headaches [1,17], difficulties in concentration [1,4,17], physiological stress [18], loss of motivation and tiredness [8] and increased cognitive workload [19], have been perceived in open-plan offices. Jahncke et al. [8] showed that the self-rating of the tiredness and motivation of subjects decreases for high noise levels compared to low noise levels. Pejtersen et al. [17] specified that fatigue, headaches and difficulties in concentration are related to the office size. De Croon et al. [19] highlighted that the cognitive workload increases as a result of the openness of a workplace and the distance between workstations. Moreover, Pejtersen et al. [17] and Denielsson [20] reported an increased sickness absence in open-plan offices.

1.2. Surveys on the Effects of Noise in Different Types of Office

A large number of studies have conducted subjective surveys on the effect of noise in open-plan offices [2,6,11,19], while others have performed comparisons between private and open-plan offices [1,5], but only a few have dealt with comparisons between different sized offices [17,20,21]. Moreover, about half of them carried out subjective surveys rather than objective ones, such acoustical measurements and cognitive tasks. Indeed, as affirmed by Frontczak et al. [22], occupants are the best source of information in terms of needs and comfort requirements.

In a cross-sectional survey on over 2300 workers, Pejtersen et al. [17] showed that noise was significantly related to the size of an office. They pointed out that occupants' complaints about noise increased tenfold in open-plan offices, compared to cellular offices. Denielsson [20] also found that noise disturbance was higher in large open-plan offices than in cellular ones. In a questionnaire survey carried out in office buildings, Sakellaris et al. [23] found that noise inside the building was closely related to the occupants' overall comfort, which in turn was affected by gender and age, and by building features, such as office size and building location.

1.3. The Influence of Room Acoustics on the Reduction and Perception of Noise in Offices

Some studies have focused on how to apply room acoustic solutions, such as sound absorption materials, screens between workstations [9,11,24,25] and sound masking systems [9,11,26,27] in offices in order to improve the acoustic conditions and reduce noise. As Hongisto et al. [22] declared, very little is currently known about the effects of room acoustics on the reduction of ISN, while Haapakangas et al. [11] found that disturbance, due to intelligible background speech, can be reduced by an optimal and accurate acoustic design of the office when the speaker and listener are at least four-to-six meters away from each other.

The present study is the first to have carried out a cross-sectional survey in order to specifically explore the impact of ISN on annoyance, performance, mental health and well-being, and occupants' behavior through a self-assessment questionnaire in two types of office, that is, shared and open-plan offices. Furthermore, it explores the willingness of office occupants to reduce ISN through their active involvement, which means lowering their voice volume when advised to do so by a noise monitoring system with lighting feedback, for example, Speech and Sound SEMaphore (SEM) [28] or SoundEar [29]. This research question arises from the studies of Hongisto et al. [25], who affirmed that one of the ways to reduce the disturbance of speech is to lower the voice effort. In addition, Bradley [30] considered that office etiquette was a successful way of encouraging the use of low voice levels in open-plan offices, and Schlittmeier and Liebl [9] affirmed that social conventions, such as defined silent times and phone times, can help to limit noise levels resulting from speech in open-plan offices.

Three research aims have been addressed in this work: (i) to evaluate the effects of ISN on annoyance, performance, mental health and well-being, and occupants' behavior in shared and open-plan offices; (ii) to investigate the relationships between perceived noise annoyance and personal characteristics (age, gender and professional sector) and office characteristics (city, number of people in the office and room acoustic design); (iii) to evaluate the attitude of workers toward the use of a noise monitoring system with lighting feedback to encourage new adaptive behavior in open-plan offices, such as controlling voice level.

2. Materials and Methods

2.1. Subjects and Offices

Nineteen companies, including eleven small and eight large companies, five research centers and one university in Italy were involved in the cross-sectional survey. The selected offices differed in terms of city, type of activity carried out by the workers, office layout and room acoustic design. The location of the cities was considered, since there is evidence of the multiple socio-economic-cultural variables that characterize the north-south differential [31]. A total of 1180 employees were recruited, through an online questionnaire, from September to November 2017. A response rate of 17% was achieved, which is in line with the response rate of online questionnaires [32]. Since the survey was aimed at investigating the effects of ISN inside offices, the responses of 102 employees who worked in private offices were excluded because the source of noise was mainly related to speech sound coming from outside the office and useful speech from colleagues visiting the office. Consequently, 1078 out of the 1180 subjects were considered for the analysis based on completed questionnaire, which were only registered in the database. The total sample (N = 1078) was divided into two samples according to the classification of the offices based on layout. Sample (S) included answers from subjects working in shared offices (from two to five workers), while sample (O) referred to open-plan offices (more than five people) [25]. Therefore, the corresponding percentages were about 55% (597 subjects) in the shared offices and about 45% (481 subjects) in the open-plan offices. As far as the total sample is concerned, 55% of the subjects worked in university, 3% in research centers, 41% in companies and 1% of the subjects were freelance workers; 28% of the workers came from engineering sectors, 21% from technical sectors and 27% from the administration sector. Background information, related to the city where the office was located, age, gender, professional sectors and number of workers in the office, is shown in Table 1. The respondents were 58% male and 42% female. A total of 78% of the subjects worked in Turin. The total sample was mainly distributed into three age ranges: 26–35 (33%), 36–50 (26%) and

51–65 years old (36%). The percentage of subjects that worked in shared, medium and large open-plan offices was about 55%, 43% and 1%, respectively.

Table 1. Main characteristics of the total sample (N = 1078) subdivided into shared and open-plan offices. The percentages of the two samples are indicated in square brackets.

	Background Information	Shared Offices	Open-Plan Offices
Gender	Female	269 (45)	188 (39)
	Male	328 (55)	293 (61)
City	Milan	11 (2)	28 (6)
	Turin	464 (78)	378 (79)
	Cuneo	5 (1)	10 (2)
	Rome	27 (5)	31 (6)
	Naples	88 (15)	34 (7)
	Other	2 (0)	0 (0)
Age range	18–25	23 (4)	26 (5)
	26–35	170 (28)	182 (38)
	36–50	187 (31)	98 (20)
	51–65	212 (36)	175 (36)
	65+	5 (1)	0 (0)
Professional sector	Technical	118 (20)	104 (22)
	Engineering	177 (30)	124 (26)
	Management	42 (7)	37 (8)
	Administration	152 (25)	139 (29)
	Creative, design and architecture	46 (8)	30 (6)
	Sales and public affairs	9 (2)	20 (4)
	Teaching	4 (1)	2 (0)
	Other	49 (8)	25 (5)
Number of people in the offices	From 2 to 5 (shared)	597 (55)	-
	From 6 to 20 (medium open-plan)	-	467 (43)
	From 21 to 200 (large open-plan)	-	14 (1)

2.2. Questionnaire

The questionnaire was prepared through Google Forms [33] and administrated through an online link distributed by email. It was designed according to the ethical code of the authors' university. The head of the human resources of each company approved the questionnaire. An accompanying letter was added to the email to invite workers to voluntarily participate in the survey. The subjects were also informed, in the letter, about the confidential treatment of their personal data and about the anonymity of the answers.

The online questionnaire included 17 questions, and it was available in Italian and English. Less than 5 min was needed to fill it in, a time that was chosen in order to avoid overtaxing and high dropout rates because of boredom.

The questionnaire was composed of three sections: (1) an explanation of the aim of the survey and response time (2) background questions (3) subjective opinions. The aim of the study was explained in the accompanying letter of the first section and the definition of ISN was provided, i.e., "the noise generated from conversations between colleagues, telephone calls and laughter" [1,2]. The term "chatting noise" was used in the questions instead of "Irrelevant Speech Noise" as it is a more common term and it is easier to understand by lay respondents. The seven background questions were submitted in order to collect general information about the gender, age, nationality, company and professional sector of the respondents.

The 10 questions in the third section are shown in Table 2. The following topics were investigated: annoyance (Q1), mental health and well-being (Q2 and Q6), productivity (Q3–Q5), occupants' behavior (Q7 and Q10) and the presence of acoustic treatments (Q8 and Q9). Several feelings and symptoms related to mental health and well-being were presented to the subjects in Q2 [14,16,34]. This list of feelings and symptoms can be divided as follows: (1) mental illness, such as stress, (2) loss of concentration, (3) emotional and social feelings, such as feeling displeased, loss of motivation, anger, negative feelings towards colleagues, and (4) physical symptoms, such as tiredness, overstrain and headaches. In addition, since mental health and well-being are closely related to interpersonal relationships [16], this aspect was investigated in Q6.

Occupants' behavior adopted to cope with ISN was assessed in Q7 and Q10. The personal strategies used to reduce annoyance resulting from people chatting were investigated in Q7 considering the following items: (1) use of technological tools, such as headphones with music and noise cancelling headphones, and (2) use of adaptive behavior [35,36], such as taking a break, changing working space, changing work task, working from home and closing the office door, and (3) asking colleagues to reduce their voice levels. The willingness of workers to be actively involved in ISN reduction, by lowering their voice volume when advised by a light-system device, was investigated in Q10 as a further feature of the occupants' behavior.

The content of the questionnaire was explicitly defined according to the purpose of the study. The wording of the questions, as well as the Likert scale ranking and the list of alternatives was drawn up on the basis of previous studies. Q1 and Q3–Q6 were based on questions presented in [25] and [26], respectively. The single choice questions, Q2 and Q7, were included according to [37,38], with the aim of investigating the main feeling or symptom and the main personal strategy adopted with regard to ISN, respectively. The lists of alternatives were defined according to [1,16,17] for Q2 and to [1] for Q7. Q8, Q9 and Q10 are new, compared to previous studies, and the list of alternatives in Q9 were designed considering the acoustic treatments generally used in offices. The options in Q2, Q7 and Q9 were randomized to change the order in which they were presented to the subjects.

Table 2. Questionnaire layout.

Topic	ID	Question	Scale	Labels
Annoyance	Q1	How much does people chatting in your office annoy you?	5	Not at all (1)–Extremely (5)
Mental health and well-being (Feelings and symptoms)	Q2	What is the main feeling (or symptom) related to people chatting during your work tasks?	Single choice	○ Loss of concentration ○ Loss of motivation ○ Tiredness and overstrain ○ Stress ○ Anger ○ Negative feelings such as feeling displeased ○ Negative feelings toward other colleagues ○ Headache ○ None ○ Other
Work productivity	Q3	How much do you agree with the following statement? "People chatting around me often interrupts me during my work tasks"	5	Strongly disagree (1)–Strongly agree (5)
	Q4	How much do you agree with the following statement? "People chatting does not allow me to work as much as I would like to"		
	Q5	How much do you agree with the following statement? "People chatting around me significantly reduces my work performance"		
Mental health and well-being (Interpersonal relationships)	Q6	How much do you agree with the following statement? "People chatting compromises the harmony of the entire office"	5	Strongly disagree (1)–Strongly agree (5)

Table 2. *Cont.*

Topic	ID	Question	Scale	Labels
Occupants' behavior (Personal strategies)	Q7	What is the main strategy that you use to reduce the annoyance resulting from people chatting?	Single choice	○ Change working space/room ○ Headphones with music ○ Noise cancelling headphones ○ Ask people to reduce voice ○ Change work task ○ Work from home ○ Take a break ○ Close the office door ○ None ○ Other
Presence of acoustic treatment	Q8	Are there any design strategies in your office aimed at the reduction of noise resulting from people chatting (sound absorption on ceiling or walls, partitions between desks, carpet, ecc.)?	Yes/No	
	Q9	If yes, what are the main strategies that are applied? (sound absorption on ceiling or walls, partitions between desks, carpets, ecc.)?	Multiple choice	○ Sound absorption on ceiling ○ Sound absorption on walls ○ Sound absorption on ceiling and walls ○ Partitions between desks ○ Carpets ○ None ○ Other
Occupants' behavior (with reference to a warning system with lighting feedback)	Q10	Would you pay attention to a light-system that advises you and your colleagues to control your voice volume in order to reduce noise resulting from people chatting in your workplace?	Yes/No	

2.3. Statistical Analysis

A statistical analysis was carried out with SPSS (IBM Statistics20, IBM, Armonk, NY, USA). According to Siegel and Castellan [39], non-parametric methods should be used to analyze data measured with ordinal and nominal scales, as in the case of this study. The significance of the differences between shared and open-plan offices, related to several factors such as noise annoyance, mental health and well-being, and work productivity, was assessed with the Mann-Whitney U Test (MWU), a test that is used for two groups of independent observations. This test was also applied for both types of office to investigate how noise annoyance varied according to gender, location of the city, and the presence or absence of acoustic treatments. The Kruskal-Wallis (KW) test, which is an extension of the MWU test for more than two groups, was applied in order to investigate how noise annoyance is related to different age ranges, professional sectors and number of people in an office. Subsequently, when a significant difference was found between groups, the Mann-Whitney U Test was applied between paired groups.

A logistic regression analysis was then performed in order to investigate the personal and office characteristics that affect noise annoyance, such as gender, age, city, professional sector, acoustic treatment and number of people in the office, in both shared and open-plan offices. Significant covariates were identified in the models on the basis of the "forward" variable selection procedure [40]. The "noise annoyance" response variable was dichotomized into "no annoyance" (1 = not at all; 2 = slightly) and "annoyance" (3 = fairly; 4 = highly; 5 = extremely).

Finally, the significance of the differences between shared and open-plan offices was detected by the z-test for proportions [41] when a nominal scale was used to gather data, as for Q2 and Q7.

3. Results

3.1. Effects of ISN on Annoyance, Productivity, Mental Health and Well-Being

Table 3 shows lower mean and mode values of Q1 to Q6 in shared offices compared to open-plan ones and significant differences between the two office types, according to the MWU Test. The workers in shared offices perceive ISN as less annoying than the workers in open-plan offices, and ISN compromises work performance and interpersonal relationships between colleagues less in shared offices than in open-plan ones. Significant positive correlations, with Spearman coefficients ≥ 0.5 and p-values < 0.01, were also found between the noise annoyance scores for Q1 and the scores for Q3 to Q6 in both shared and open-plan offices.

Table 3. Mean (Mn) and mode (Mo) values of the answers on noise annoyance, work productivity, and mental health and well-being related to ISN, for shared offices and open-plan offices, and two-tailed p-values of significance for the differences between the two office types, according to the MWU Test. Any statistically significant differences, with p-value < 0.05, are reported in bold.

Topic	ID	Shared Offices (N = 597)		Open-Plan Offices (N = 481)		MWU p-Value
		Mn	Mo	Mn	Mo	
Noise annoyance	Q1	2.54	2.00	3.07	3.00	**0.00**
Work productivity	Q3	3.06	3.00	3.44	4.00	**0.00**
	Q4	3.05	3.00	3.40	4.00	**0.00**
	Q5	2.98	3.00	3.22	4.00	**0.00**
Mental health and well-being (Interpersonal relationships)	Q6	2.71	2.00	2.98	3.00	**0.00**

3.2. Effects of ISN on Mental Health and Well-being, and Occupants' Behavior

Figure 1a shows the percentages of the feelings and symptoms indicated by the employees as a consequence of ISN, in shared and open-plan offices. It emerged that 69% and 66% of the employees declared that a loss of concentration is the main feeling consequence of ISN in shared and open-plan offices, respectively, while 4% and 6% of the workers self-estimated mental illness, such as stress, as the main feeling consequence of ISN in office types S and O, respectively. Emotional and social feelings, such as feeling displeased, less motivated, angry and negative feeling toward colleagues, were found to be the main consequence of ISN for 6% and 9% of the workers in office types S and O, respectively. Similarly, 4% and 9% of the workers related ISN with physical symptoms, such as tiredness, overstrain and headaches, in office types S and O, respectively. Significant differences were found between shared and open-plan offices, according to the z-test for proportions, for emotional and social feelings and physical symptoms (z equal to 2.06 and 3.63, respectively; p-value = 0.05).

Figure 1b shows the percentages related to different strategies adopted by the workers in order to cope with ISN in shared and open-plan offices, respectively. The use of technological tools, such as headphones with music and noise cancelling headphones, was the main solution for 22% and 32% of the workers in the S and O office types, respectively. Taking a break, changing working space or work task, working from home and closing the office door were the main strategies, in the form of adaptive behavior, adopted by 34% and 23% of the workers in S and O, respectively. Furthermore, 22% and 20% of the employees preferred asking colleagues to reduce their voice levels in office types S and O, respectively. Significant differences, with lower p-values than 0.05, were found between shared and open-plan offices, according to the z-test for proportions, but only related to the technological tools and adaptive behaviors (z equal to 3.81 and −4.08, respectively; p-value = 0.05) used by workers to cope with ISN.

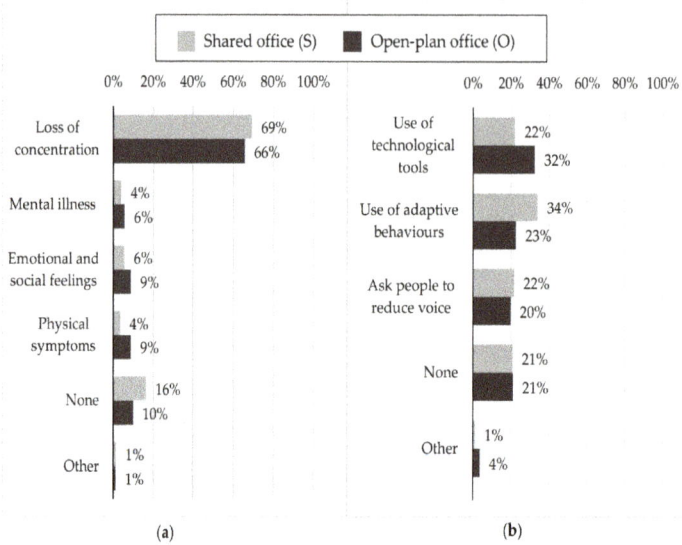

Figure 1. Percentages related to the effects of ISN on mental health and well-being, and occupants' behavior in shared (S) and open-plan (O) offices: (**a**) Subjective ratings on feelings and symptoms attributed by occupants to ISN; (**b**) Subjective ratings on personal strategies used by occupants to cope with ISN.

A total of 62% of the workers in shared offices and 72% in open-plan ones declared they were willing to reduce their voice levels when advised by a light-system device, which monitors the ISN level in shared and open-plan offices, as shown in Figure 2. Such a difference between offices was found to be statistically significant, according to the z-test for proportions (z equal to 3.37; p-value = 0.05).

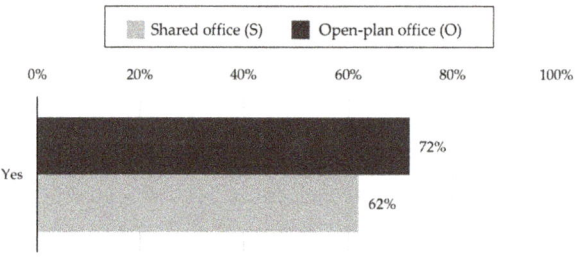

Figure 2. Percentages related to the willingness of the occupants to be influenced by a noise monitoring system with lighting feedback that encourages behavioral changes, such as the decrease of the voice volumes in order to reduce ISN.

3.3. Noise Annoyance, and Personal and Office Characteristics

3.3.1. Gender, Age Range, Professional Sectors and City

Table 4 shows the mean and mode values of the noise annoyance scores divided according to gender, age range, professional sector and city location, for both shared and open-plan offices, together with the significance of the differences between groups, according to the MWU or KW Test.

Table 4. Mean (Mn) and mode (Mo) values of the answers on noise annoyance related to gender, age range, professional sector and city latitude, for shared (S) and open-plan (O) offices, and two-tailed p-values of significance of the differences according to the MWU or KW Test. Statistically significant differences with p-values < 0.05 are reported in bold. The following abbreviations are used for the professional sectors: TEC for "Technical", EN-TE for "Engineering and Teaching", MA-AD for "Management and Administration", CR-DE-AR for "Creative, design and architecture", SPA for "Sales and public affairs", and OT for "Other". The northern cities are Milan, Turin and Cuneo, and southern cities are Rome and Naples.

	Sample	Descriptive Statistics	Shared Offices (N = 597)	Open-Plan Offices (N = 481)
Gender	Female N(S) = 269, N(O) = 188	Mn Mo	2.51 2.00	3.19 3.00
	Male N(S) = 328, N(O) = 293	Mn Mo	2.58 2.00	2.99 2.00
		MWU p-value	0.30	**0.04**
Age range	18–35 N(S) = 193, N(O) = 208	Mn Mo	2.36 2.00	2.92 3.00
	36–50 N(S) = 187, N(O) = 98	Mn Mo	2.62 2.00	3.12 3.00
	51–65+ N(S) = 217, N(O) = 175	Mn Mo	2.65 3.00	3.21 3.00
		KW p-value	0.08	**0.03**
Professional sector	TEC N(S) = 118, N(O) = 104	Mn Mo	2.62 3.00	3.18 3.00
	EN-TE N(S) = 181, N(O) = 126	Mn Mo	2.38 2.00	2.90 2.00
	MA-AD N(S) = 194, N(O) = 176	Mn Mo	2.60 2.00	3.10 3.00
	CR-DE-AR N(S) = 46, N(O) = 30	Mn Mo	2.57 3.00	2.93 3.00
	SPA N(S) = 9, N(O) = 20	Mn Mo	3.00 2.00 and 4.00	3.30 3.00
	OT N(S) = 49, N(O) = 25	Mn Mo	2.65 2.00	3.16 3.00
		KW p-value	0.18	0.28
City location	North N(S) = 480, N(O) = 416	Mn Mo	2.46 2.00	3.02 3.00
	South N(S) = 115, N(O) = 65	Mn Mo	2.90 3.00	3.77 3.00
		MWU p-value	**0.00**	**0.01**

The analyses yielded no significant difference between genders, according to the MWU Test, in the shared offices. This trend is also supported by the fact that the same mode value emerged for both genders. Conversely, a significant difference was found in open-plan offices, when observing the highest mean and mode values, with women being more annoyed by ISN than men.

Significant differences were observed between the three age ranges, that is, 18–25, 26–35 and 51–65+, although only in open-plan offices, according to the KW Test. A significant difference was observed between the first range, 18–35 years, and the last range, 51–65+ years, according to the MWU Test, with older subjects being more annoyed, i.e., with higher mean values.

No significant differences between professional sectors emerged, according to the KW Test, between the shared offices and the open-plan offices. However, the highest and lowest mean values were found for the subjects that work in the sales and public affairs sector (SPA) and in the engineering and teaching sector (EN-TE), in both types of office. However, the low number of subjects involved in the public affairs sector affected the statistical results of this sector, and further investigations are required.

The cities were divided in northern and southern cities based on their location. The analyses provided significant differences between the two locations of the cities in both shared and open-plan offices, with higher mean values for the subjects who work in southern cities than those who work in northern cities.

3.3.2. Number of People in the Office

Significant differences between shared (S), medium open-plan (MO) and large open-plan (LO) offices were obtained from the KW Test, as shown in Table 5, and significant differences between each paired office type were also found for the MWU Test. The mean values generally show that workers are more annoyed by ISN as the number of people in offices increases.

Table 5. Mean (Mn) and mode (Mo) values of the answers on noise annoyance related to the number of people in offices, and two-tailed p-value of significance of the difference between the number of people in offices, according to the KW Test. Statistically significant difference with $p\text{-value} < 0.05$ is reported in bold. The following abbreviations were used to indicate the type of office, on the basis of the number of people: S for "Shared office for two to five people", MO for "Medium Open-plan office for six to 20 people", LO for "Large Open-plan office for 21 to 200 people".

Descriptive Statistics	Number of People in the Office			KW p-Value
	S (2–5) N = 597	MO (6–20) N = 467	LO (21–200) N = 14	
Mn	2.54	3.05	3.71	**0.00**
Mo	2.00	3.00	3.00	

3.3.3. Presence of Acoustic Treatments

The subjects were asked to indicate whether any acoustic treatments were present in their office, after a visual inspection. As shown in Figure 3a, according to the respondents, 7% and 20% of the shared and open-plan offices were acoustically treated. As can be observed in Figure 3b, setting screens between workstations (SW) is the most commonly adopted acoustic treatment, and this is followed by the application of sound absorption materials on the ceiling (SAMC).

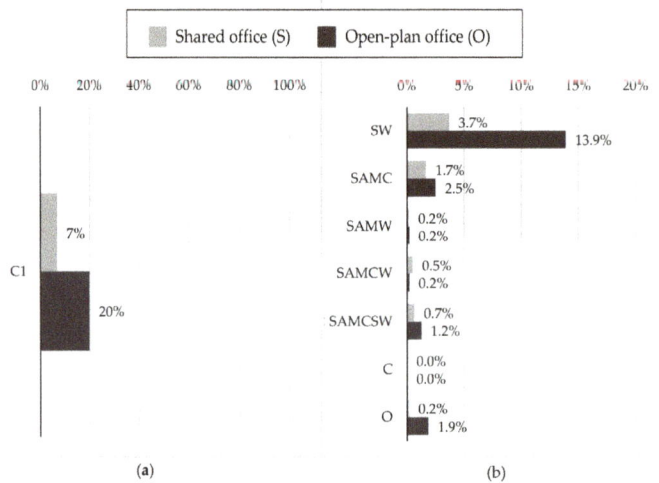

Figure 3. (a) Percentages of acoustic treatments self-estimated by the subjects for the shared and open-plan offices: (a) Subjective ratings on the presence (C1) of acoustic treatments; (b) Subjective ratings on the acoustic treatment types. The following abbreviations were adopted: SW for "screens between

workstation", SAMC for "sound absorption materials on ceiling", SAMW for "sound absorption materials on walls", SAMCW for "sound absorption materials on ceiling and walls", C for "carpets", SAMCSW for "sound absorption materials on ceiling with screens between workstations" and O for "other".

As can be observed in Table 6, significant difference emerged between the noise annoyance scores for the workers who self-estimated the presence (C1) or absence (C2) of acoustic treatment in open-plan offices, according to the MWU Test. Workers were found to be significantly more annoyed by ISN when open-plan offices were not acoustically treated, as shown by the higher mean and mode values.

Table 6. Mean (Mn) and mode (Mo) values of the answers on noise annoyance related to the self-estimated presence of acoustic treatment in shared and open-plan offices, and two-tailed p-values of significance of the difference between the presence and absence of treatment, according to the MWU Test, for both types of offices. Any statistically significant differences, with p-values < 0.05, are reported in bold.

Sample	Descriptive Statistics	Presence of Acoustic Treatment		MWU p-Value
		Yes	No	
Shared Offices		N = 41	N = 556	
	Mn	2.64	2.54	0.30
	Mo	3.00	2.00	
Open-Plan Offices		N = 96	N = 385	
	Mn	2.86	3.12	0.02
	Mo	2.00	3.00	

3.3.4. Personal and Office Characteristics that Affect Noise Annoyance

Table 7 shows the Odds Ratio (OR) of the effects of a number of covariates that significantly affect noise annoyance, according to the logistic regression analysis, for both types of office. The included variables are categorial, and the reference categories are the ones with the lowest mean noise annoyance score shown in Tables 4–6.

The regression model identified the location of the city, and the acoustic treatment as the significant covariates that affect noise annoyance in shared offices. Office workers in southern cities and workers with acoustic treatments in the office are about two times more likely to report annoyance from ISN than subjects who work in northern cities and in offices without acoustic treatments.

In addition to the location and the acoustic treatment, the regression model related to open-plan offices identified the gender and the number of people in the office as further significant covariates. Being female and working in southern cities, without acoustic treatment in the office, makes it about two times more likely to be annoyed by ISN than being male, working in northern cities and with acoustic treatment in the office. Furthermore, when there are more than 20 people in the office, it is about nine times more probable that the workers will be annoyed by ISN than when there are from 6 to 20 occupants.

The outcome related to the acoustic treatment condition in the office was found to be the opposite for the two office types, in agreement with the mean values shown in Table 6. The occupants of shared offices are less annoyed by ISN when the office is without any acoustic treatment, while the occupants of open-plan offices are less annoyed when the office has acoustical treatment.

Table 7. Odds Ratio (OR) and 95% oconfidence interval (CI) of the covariates that significantly (p-values < 0.05) affect noise annoyance in shared and open-plan offices according to the logistic regression analysis.

Covariates (Reference Category)	Shared Offices (N = 597)			Open-Plan Offices (N = 481)		
	OR	95% CI	p-Value	OR	95% CI	p-Value
Gender (Male)	-	-	-	1.79	1.19–2.70	0.00
City location (North)	2.52	1.65–3.86	0.00	2.26	1.18–4.33	0.01
Acoustic treatment (Absence for shared offices and Presence for open-plan offices)	2.17	1.11–4.22	0.02	1.70	1.06–2.72	0.03
Number of people in the office (6–20)	-	-	-	8.70	1.11–68.20	0.04

4. Discussion

Using data from the survey, which was administrated in eleven small and eight large companies, five research centers and one university in Italy, the present study has investigated the effects of irrelevant speech noise (ISN) in shared (two to five employees), and open-plan offices (more than five employees).

Although many surveys have been conducted on noise annoyance and acoustic comfort in open-plan offices, this study is the first that has specifically explored the impact of ISN on annoyance, performance, mental health and well-being and occupants' behavior. Moreover, this is the first study that has compared subjective assessments of shared offices with those of open-plan offices. The associations between perceived noise annoyance and personal characteristics (age, gender and professional sector) and office characteristics (city, number of people and room acoustics design) have also been evaluated. In addition, the study has investigated the willingness of office occupants to reduce ISN by lowering their voice levels when a noise monitoring system with lighting feedback advises them that high noise levels have been reached.

4.1. Effects of ISN on Noise Annoyance, Productivity, and Mental Helath and Well-Being

This study highlights that ISN generated by conversations between colleagues, telephone calls and laughter was more annoying in open-plan offices than in shared ones, and workers showed an increased annoyance with ISN according to the office size, i.e., in shared, medium and large open-plan offices. This result is in line with Danielsson [20], who found that noise due to conversation, equipment and other office noise sources was more annoying in open-plan offices than in smaller ones.

The perceived decrease in work productivity as a result of ISN was higher in open-plan offices than in shared offices. Workers were often interrupted by ISN and consequently they were not able to maximize their performance in larger offices. This comparison between shared and open-plan offices has not been investigated in the previous studies. However, it is coherent with the results of Kaarlela-Tuomaala et al. [1], who showed that the self-estimated waste of working time, due to noise, doubled when workers moved from private to open-plan offices. This result is important, in terms of office layout, since shared offices can be considered as an alternative to open-plan offices when the work productivity has to be increased.

About 70% of the workers in both office types declared difficulties in concentration as the self-estimated main feeling caused by ISN, with no significant difference between the types of offices. On the other hand, the feelings and symtoms related to mental health and well-being, such as emotional and social feelings (feeling displeased, less motivated, angry and feeling negative toward colleagues) and physical symptoms (tiredness, overstrain and headaches), were in general mentioned less frequently by the workers as the main consequences of ISN, but a significant increase was found for open-plan offices compared to shared offices. The pattern of results is in line with previous studies that demonstrated an association between the noise of different types of office and difficulties in concentration [1,4,17], and other feelings and symptoms related to mental health and well-being, such as tiredness and motivation [8], fatigue and headaches [1,17]. Moreover, the results are in agreement with those of Pejtersen et al. [17], who observed a significant increase in the prevalence of physical symptoms, such as fatigue and headaches, according to the size of the office.

In addition, mental health and well-being, related to interpersonal relationships between colleagues, was found to be more affected by ISN in open-plan offices than in shared ones. This finding is coherent with that of Brennan et al. [21], who underlined a worsening of satisfaction in co-worker relationships when they moved from private to shared offices.

4.2. Effects of ISN on Occupants' Behavior

One finding of the present work is that there was a significant difference between shared and open-plan offices, in terms of strategies adopted to cope with ISN, thus highlighting important implications for the design and management of offices. The use of technological tools, such as headphones with music, was the main solution used by workers to contrast ISN in open-plan offices, while adaptive behaviors, such as taking a break, changing working space or work task, working from home and closing the office door were the main strategies used in shared offices. Similar outcomes were also highlighted by Kaarlela-Tuomaala et al. [1], who found that workers adopted more coping strategies in open-plan offices than in private offices.

An important finding of this study is that about 70% of the workers in the open-plan offices and about 60% in the shared offices were willing to reduce ISN through their active involvement, if a noise monitoring system, with lighting feedback, advised them to reduce their voice volumes. The percentage was significantly higher for open-plan offices than shared offices, perhaps as a result of the higher perceived noise annoyance. According to these outcomes, it is possible to state that since an accurate room acoustic design is not enough to reduce the distraction and annoyance generated by nearby speech sounds [11,25], the use of a noise monitoring system, with lighting feedback, could be an effective complementary method. In this way, a positive behavior of the occupants would be promoted, such as lowering their voice levels or changing the room where they chat. In addition to the already experimented passive measures introduced to reduce ISN, such as the room acoustic design [9,11,24,25] or sound masking [9,26,27], this system may be able to reinforce and promote office etiquette and a behavioral code.

4.3. Effects Of Personal and Office Characteristics on Noise Annoyance

Women were found to be significantly more annoyed than men in open-plan offices, while no differences were found for shared offices. This outcome is in line with those of Kaarlela et al. [1] and Danielsson et al. [42], who found that women were more disturbed by noise than men in open-plan offices. Significant differences between noise annoyance scores for three age ranges were also obtained, although only in open-plan offices. A significant difference between the first range of 18–35 years and the last range of 51–65+ years was found, with the older subjects being more annoyed. In line with this finding, Pierrette et al. [6] found a significant positive correlation between age and perceived annoyance due to ISN, while Sakellaries et al. [23] documented that noise was an important factor for the oldest workers in open-plan offices.

No significant differences between professional sectors was obtained for the shared and open-plan offices related to noise annoyance due to ISN, even though the highest and lowest mean values of noise annoyance were found for subjects that worked in the sales and public affairs sector (SPA) and in the engineering and teaching sector (EN-TE). Since it is possible to hypothesize that engineers tend to carry out counting tasks, this result is in line with a previous finding by Logie [43], who showed that people who did mathematical tasks suffered a great deal from speech noise.

Significant differences between location of the cities were obtained for both the shared and open-plan offices. The results showed that subjects working in southern cities were more annoyed than subjects working in northern ones.

According to the workers' assessments, a small percentage of offices were acoustically treated in the study sites. The respondents identified screens between workstations as the most frequently used acoustic treatment in open-plan offices. Nevertheless, workers were found to be significantly more annoyed by ISN when open-plan offices were not acoustically treated, while the opposite emerged for shared offices. Seddigh et al. [24] showed that improved room acoustics was associated with lower perceived disturbances and cognitive stress in open-plan offices; however, in order to prove this aspect in the present study, it would be necessary to conduct objective measurements of noise levels and obtain further information about the introduced acoustic treatments.

When all the above-mentioned characteristics were considered together in the evaluation of the most important factors that affect noise annoyance in shared and open-plan offices, some of them resulted to be more significant. Office location and the room acoustic design were the most significant factors that affected the perception of noise annoyance in both office types, while gender and the number of people in the office also significantly affected noise annoyance in open-plan offices. It is important to underline that the acoustic treatment of rooms affects noise annoyance in open-plan and shared offices in different ways. Noise annoyance was reduced as the result of an acoustical treatment in the former and without any acoustical treatment in the latter. The ISN level is generally lower in shared offices than in open-plan offices, due to the presence of fewer people, but speech privacy can also be reduced. Speech privacy increases when reverberation increases [44], and for this reason the occupants could have identified a more reverberant environment as less annoying, because it resulted in a less intelligible speech.

In order to investigate these aspects, future research will deal with the same type of investigation inside the same offices types, but with the addition of acoustic measurements in both acoustically treated and untreated offices, and with or without the presence of a light system that advises people to reduce their voice volumes.

4.4. Limitations

The present study suffers from some limitations. Caution is needed when comparing the results of this work with the findings of previous studies, since the self-assessment questionnaire has not been suitably validated according to e.g., [37,38,45]. Nevertheless, an exploration stage was introduced according to [38], where people with special expertise in acoustics and architecture and people from the target population were involved in order to identify any ambiguities in the questions and to determine the list of possible responses for the proposed alternatives. Moreover, some questions were taken from distinguished literature that used validated questionnaires. Another limitation is that other factors that can affect noise annoyance, such as noise sensitivity [46], personal attitudes and psychosocial factors [10], were not taken into consideration. Another weakness is related to the cross-sectional study method, which does not allow the causality of the identified association between ISN and several of the investigated factors to be established [1]. Furthermore, certain limitations can be highlighted as a result of resorting to an online survey [47]. The nonresponse bias, in particular, cannot be investigated online, since the identity of non-respondents is generally unknown [48]. There is also a self-selection bias, i.e., subjects that were more annoyed by ISN in their offices may have been more likely to complete the questionnaire than those who were not so annoyed. This bias could be particularly marked duo to the low response rate. Moreover, the multiple responses of subjects cannot be excluded.

5. Conclusions

This cross-sectional study has compared the subjective outcomes of shared offices (2–5 workers) and open-plan offices (+5 workers) related to "irrelevant speech noise", which is the noise generated from conversations between colleagues, telephone calls and laughter. Answers from an online questionnaire were collected in nineteen companies, five research centres and one university in Italy, from 1078 subjects, of which 55% worked in shared offices and 45% in open-plan offices.

Irrelevant speech noise was found to be more annoying in open-plan offices and it compromise performance, mental health and well-being more than in shared offices. In open-plan offices, being female, and working in the southern cities without any acoustic treatment in the office, made it more likely for the respondents to be annoyed by irrelevant speech noise than being male and working in the northern cities with acoustic treatment in the office. Furthermore, having more than 20 occupants in an office made being annoyed more probable than having from 6 to 20 occupants. Moreover, working in the southern cities and with acoustic treatment in the office made it more likely that noise annoyance will be reported in shared offices.

Headphones with music was found to be the main solution adopted by workers to contrast irrelevant speech noise in open-plan offices, while adaptive behaviors, such as taking a break, changing working space or work task, working from home and closing the office door were the main strategies used in shared offices. A high percentage of workers stated they were willing to reduce irrelevant speech noise if a noise monitoring system with lighting feedback advised them to reduce their voice volumes.

Author Contributions: S.D.B. and A.A. designed and developed the questionnaire; S.D.B., L.S., A.A. and G.E.P. defined the formal analysis; S.D.B. managed the diffusion of the questionnaire, collected data and applied the formal analysis; L.S. and G.E.P. supervised the first analyses; S.D.B. and A.A. wrote the article; L.S. and A.A. reviewed the article drafts; A.A. supervised the research activity. All the authors revised the final manuscript.

Acknowledgments: The authors are grateful to Antonella Castellana and Cristina Calleri for the comments on the topics of the questionnaire. Particular thanks are extended to Prof. Franco Pellerey for his supervision of the statistical analysis. The kind collaboration of the management area of each company and the participation of the workers have made this work possible. The authors are also thankful to Alessia Griginis of "Onleco S.r.l." and Stefano Cerruti of "Bottega Studio Architetti" for their collaboration in the project of the warning system with lighting feedback.

Conflicts of Interest: The authors declare no conflict of interest.

References

1. Kaarlela-Tuomaala, A.; Helenius, R.; Keskinen, E.; Hongisto, V. Effects of acoustic environment on work in private office rooms and open-plan offices—Longitudinal study during relocation. *Ergonomics* **2009**, *52*, 1423–1444. [CrossRef] [PubMed]
2. Kang, S.; Ou, D.; Ming Mack, C. The impact of indoor environmental quality on work productivity in university open-plan research offices. *Build Environ.* **2017**, *124*, 78–89. [CrossRef]
3. Hedge, A. The open-plan office: A Systematic Investigation of Employee Reactions to Their Work Environment. *Environ. Behav.* **1982**, *14*, 519–542. [CrossRef]
4. Banbury, S.P.; Berry, D.C. Office noise and employee concentration: Identifying causes of disruption and potential improvements. *Ergonomics* **2005**, *48*, 25–37. [CrossRef]
5. Haapakangas, A.; Helenius, R.; Keskinen, E.; Hongisto, V. Perceived acoustic environment, work performance and well-being—Survey results from Finnish offices. In Proceedings of the 9th International Congress on Noise as a Public Health Problem, Foxwoods, CT, USA, 21–25 July 2008; pp. 21–25.
6. Pierrette, M.; Parizet, E.; Chevret, P.; Chatillon, J. Noise effect on comfort in open-space offices: Development of an assessment questionnaire. *Ergonomics* **2015**, *58*, 96–106. [CrossRef] [PubMed]
7. Hongisto, V. A model predicting the effect of speech of varying intelligibility on work performance. *Indoor Air* **2005**, *15*, 458–468. [CrossRef] [PubMed]
8. Jahncke, H.; Hygge, S.; Halin, N.; Green, A.M.; Dimberg, K. Open-plan office noise: Cognitive performance and restoration. *J. Environ. Psychol.* **2011**, *31*, 373–382. [CrossRef]
9. Schlittmeier, S.J.; Liebl, A. The effects of intelligible irrelevant background speech in offices—Cognitive disturbance, annoyance, and solutions. *Facilities* **2015**, *33*, 61–75. [CrossRef]
10. Guski, R.; Felscher-Suhr, U.; Schuemer, R. The concept of noise annoyance: How international experts see it. *J. Sound Vib.* **1999**, *223*, 513–527. [CrossRef]
11. Haapakangas, A.; Hongisto, V.; Hyönä, J.; Kokko, J.; Keränen, J. Effects of unattended speech on performance and subjective distraction: The role of acoustic design in open-plan offices. *Appl. Acoust.* **2014**, *86*, 1–16. [CrossRef]

12. Varjo, J.; Hongisto, V.; Haapakangas, A.; Maula, H.; Koskela, H.; Hyönä, J. Simultaneous effects of irrelevant speech, temperature and ventilation rate on performance and satisfaction in open-plan offices. *J. Environ. Psychol.* **2015**, *44*, 16–33. [CrossRef]
13. Martellotta, F.; della Crociata, S.; Simone, A. Laboratory study on the effects of office noise on mental performance. In Proceedings of the Forum Acusticum 2011, Aalborg, Denmark, 27 June–1 July 2011; pp. 1637–1642. [CrossRef]
14. Public Health England. *North West Mental Wellbeing Survey 2012/13*; PHE: London, UK, 2013.
15. Keyes, C.L.M. The mental health continuum: From languishing to flourishing in life. *J. Health Soc. Behav.* **2002**, *43*, 207–222. [CrossRef] [PubMed]
16. World Health Organization. *Mental Health and Work: Impact, Issues and Good Practices*; World Health Organization: Geneva, Switzerland, 2000.
17. Pejtersen, J.; Allermann, L.; Kristensen, T.S.; Poulsen, O.M. Indoor climate, psychosocial work environment and symptoms in open-plan offices. *Indoor Air* **2006**, *16*, 392–401. [CrossRef] [PubMed]
18. Evans, G.W.; Johnson, D. Stress and open-office noise. *J. Appl. Psychol.* **2000**, *85*, 779–783. [CrossRef] [PubMed]
19. De Croon, E.M.; Sluiter, J.K.; Kuijer, P.P.; Frings-Dresen, M. The effect of office concepts on worker health and performance: A systematic review of the literature. *Ergonomics* **2005**, *48*, 119–134. [CrossRef] [PubMed]
20. Danielsson, C.B. *Office Environment, Health & Job Satisfaction. An Explorative Study of Design's Influence*; School of Architecture, KTH Royal Institute of Technology: Stockholm, Sweden, 2005.
21. Brennan, A.; Chugh, J.S.; Kline, T. Traditional versus open office design—A longitudinal field study. *Environ. Behav.* **2002**, *34*, 279–299. [CrossRef]
22. Frontczak, M.; Schiavon, S.; Goins, J.; Arens, E.; Zhang, H.; Wargocki, P. Quantitative relationships between occupant satisfaction and satisfaction aspects of indoor environmental quality and building design. *Indoor Air* **2012**, *22*, 119–131. [CrossRef] [PubMed]
23. Sakellaris, I.A.; Saraga, D.E.; Mandin, C.; Roda, C.; Fossati, S.; De Kluizenaar, Y.; Carrer, P.; Dimitroulopoulou, S.; Mihucz, V.G.; Szigeti, T.; et al. Perceived indoor environment and occupants' comfort in European "Modern" office buildings: The OFFICAIR Study. *Int. J. Environ. Res. Public Health* **2016**, *13*, 444. [CrossRef] [PubMed]
24. Seddigh, A.; Berntson, E.; Jönsson, F.; Danielson, C.B.; Westerlund, H. Effect of variation in noise absorption in open-plan office: A field study with a cross-over design. *J. Environ. Psychol.* **2015**, *44*, 34–44. [CrossRef]
25. Hongisto, V.; Haapakangas, A.; Varjo, J.; Helenius, R.; Koskela, H. Refurbishment of an open-plan office—Environmental and job satisfaction. *J. Environ. Psychol.* **2016**, *45*, 176–191. [CrossRef]
26. Haapakangas, A.; Kankkunen, E.; Hongisto, V.; Virjonen, P.; Oliva, D.; Keskinen, E. Effects of five speech masking sounds on performance and acoustic satisfaction. Implications for open-plan offices. *Acta Acust. (United Acust.)* **2011**, *97*, 641–655. [CrossRef]
27. Renz, T.; Leistner, P.; Liebl, A. Auditory distraction by speech: Comparison of fluctuating and steady speech-like masking sounds. *J. Acoust. Soc. Am.* **2018**, *144*, EL83–EL88. [CrossRef] [PubMed]
28. Di Blasio, S.; Vannelli, G.; Shtrepi, L.; Masoero, M.C.; Astolfi, A. A subjective investigation on the impact of irrelevant speech noise on health, well-being and productivity in open-plan offices. In Proceedings of the Euronoise 2018, Crete, Greece, 27–31 May 2018; pp. 1883–1890.
29. SoundEar. Available online: https://soundear.com/ (accessed on 15 October 2018).
30. Bradley, J.S. The acoustical design of conventional open plan offices. *Can. Acoust.* **2003**, *27*, 23–31.
31. Carboni, O.A.; Russu, P. Measuring and forecasting regional environmental and economic efficiency in Italy. *Appl. Econ.* **2018**, *50*, 335–353. [CrossRef]
32. Nulty, D.D. The adequacy of response rates to online and paper surveys: What can be done? *Assess. Eval. High. Ed.* **2008**, *33*, 301–314. [CrossRef]
33. Google Forms. Available online: https://www.google.com/forms/about/ (accessed on 16 January 2019).
34. World Health Organization. *Mental Health Policies and Programmes in the Workplace*; World Health Organization: Geneva, Switzerland, 2005.
35. De Dear, R.; Brager, G. Developing an adaptive model of thermal comfort and preference. *ASHRAE Trans.* **1998**, *104*, 145–167.
36. Nicol, J.F.; Humphreys, M.A. Adaptive thermal comfort and sustainable thermal standards for buildings. *Energy Build.* **2002**, *34*, 563–572. [CrossRef]

37. Ortalda, F. *La Survey in Psicologia ("The Survey in Psychology")*, 3rd ed.; Carocci: Roma, Italy, 1998; pp. 91–92, ISBN 9788843010899.
38. Converse, J.M.; Presser, S. *Survey Questions: Handcrafting the Standardized Questionnaire*; Sage University Paper Series on Quantitative Applications in the Social Sciences; No. 07-063; SAGE Publications: Thousand Oaks, CA, USA, 1986; ISBN 9780803927438.
39. Sigel, S.; Castellan, N.J. *Non Parametric Statistics for the Behavioral Sciences*, 2nd ed.; McGraw-Hill: New York, NY, USA, 1988; pp. 116–126, 184–194, ISBN-13: 978-0070573574, ISBN-10: 0070573573.
40. Bursac, Z.; Gauss, C.H.; Williams, D.K.; Hosmer, D.W. Purposeful selection of variables in logistic regression. *Source Code Biol. Med.* **2008**, *3*, 1–8. [CrossRef] [PubMed]
41. Fleiss, J.L.; Levin, B.; Cho Paik, M. *Statistical Methods for Rates and Proportions*, 3rd ed.; John Wiley & Sons: Hoboken, NJ, USA, 2003; ISBN 0-471-52629-0.
42. Danielsson, C.B.; Bodin, L.; Wulff, C.; Theorell, T. The relation between office type and workplace conflict: A gender and noise perspective. *J. Environ. Psychol.* **2015**, *42*, 161–171. [CrossRef]
43. Logie, R.H.; Baddeley, A.D. Cognitive processes in counting. *J. Exp. Psychol. Learn. Mem. Cogn.* **1987**, *13*, 310–326. [CrossRef]
44. ISO 3382-3:2012. *Acoustics—Measurement of Room Acoustic Parameters—Part 3: Open-Plan Offices*; International Organization for Standardization: Geneva, Switzerland, 2012.
45. Brisson, C.; Blanchette, C.; Guimont, C.; Dion, G.; Moisan, J.; Vézina, M.; Dagenais, G.R.; Măsse, L. Reliability and validity of the French version of the 18-item Karasek Job Content Questionnaire. *Work Stress* **1998**, *12*, 322–336. [CrossRef]
46. Schutte, M.; Marks, A.; Wenning, E.; Griefahn, B. The development of the noise sensitivity questionnaire. *Noise Health* **2007**, *9*, 15–24. [CrossRef]
47. Wright, K.B. Researching Internet-Based Populations: Advantages and Disadvantages of Online Survey Research, Online Questionnaire Authoring Software Packages, and Web Survey Services. *J. Comput. Mediat. Commun.* **2005**, *10*. [CrossRef]
48. Sax, L.J.; Gilmartin, S.K.; Bryant, A.N. Assessing response rate and nonresponse bias in web and paper surveys. *Res. High. Ed.* **2003**, *48*, 409–432. [CrossRef]

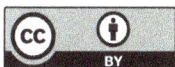

© 2019 by the authors. Licensee MDPI, Basel, Switzerland. This article is an open access article distributed under the terms and conditions of the Creative Commons Attribution (CC BY) license (http://creativecommons.org/licenses/by/4.0/).

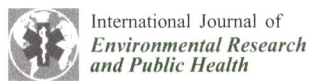

Article

Restorative Effects of Classroom Soundscapes on Children's Cognitive Performance

Shan Shu and Hui Ma *

School of Architecture, Tianjin University, Tianjin 300072, China; shan.shu@outlook.com
* Correspondence: mahui@tju.edu.cn; Tel.: +86-131-1480-1296

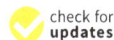

Received: 18 December 2018; Accepted: 17 January 2019; Published: 21 January 2019

Abstract: Previous studies have examined the restorative benefits of soundscapes on adults' cognitive performance, but it was unclear whether those benefits would be possible for children. In this paper, two experiments applied a before–after design to explore the restorative effects of different soundscapes on children's sustained attention and short-term memory, respectively, in a simulated classroom situation. In Experiment 1, 46 children aged 8–12 were first mentally fatigued by performing an oral arithmetic task and then were asked to conduct a sustained attention to response test (SART), in order to assess their attention fatigue. After that, a period of 3-min soundscape was presented, and SART was conducted again to examine their attention recovery. In Experiment 2, 45 children participated and the experiment procedure was the same as in Experiment 1, except that a digit span test (DST) was used instead to measure short-term memory. The results showed that music, birdsong, fountain sound, and stream sound facilitated greater recovery than other sounds in reaction time. Participants also showed better performance in short-term memory after exposure to fountain sound and stream sound, followed by music and birdsong. Those results confirmed the actual restorative effects of perceived restorative soundscapes on children's cognitive performance.

Keywords: restorative effect; children's cognitive performance; classroom soundscape; sustained attention; short-term memory

1. Introduction

Numerous studies have documented the positive effects of interacting with natural environments [1]. As an essential part of physical environments, emerging research has demonstrated that some pleasant soundscapes might have potential benefits on people's well-being and health [2–4].

The restorative benefits of soundscapes could be framed in terms of two prevailing theories of restorative environments: (1) Stress recovery theory (SRT) [5] and (2) attentional restoration theory (ART) [6]. SRT focuses primarily on the effects of environmental stimuli on emotional and physical responses, suggesting that interacting with nature could evoke positive responses indicative of stress reduction [7]. Indeed, numerous studies have provided some evidence for this by demonstrating an increase in pleasant mood [8], a decrease in heart rate [9–11], a reduced skin conductance level [12], and other stress-relieving measures. ART, which is commonly referenced to identify and restore a cognitive mechanism [13], draws on research demonstrating that attention can be separated into two components: Involuntary attention, in which attention is captured by salient stimuli, and voluntary or directed attention, in which attention is directed by cognitive-control processes [14]. According to ART, exposure to restorative stimuli with inherently fascinating quality could invoke involuntary attention, thereby allowing directed attention mechanisms a chance to replenish. Therefore, following an interaction with restorative stimuli, one is able to perform better on cognitive tasks that depend on directed attention abilities. This theory has been supported by numerous studies, including in-situ studies [15–17] and laboratory experiments [18], which focused on the comparison of various natural and urban scenes. However, there is still some uncertainty regarding which aspects of attention may be affected by exposure to restorative stimuli [19].

In accordance with ART, cognitive benefits from soundscape exposure have been frequently reported based on human perceptions. Most studies investigated the restorative qualities of soundscapes in terms of cognitive restoration using questionnaires. For instance, based on the four components that are highlighted in ART (fascination, being away, compatibility, and extent), which were important for producing a restorative environment, Payne developed a perceived restorativeness soundscape scale (PRSS) to assess perceptions of a soundscape's restorative potential [20] and further explored its construct validity [21]. This scale successfully differentiated the restorativeness of soundscapes from different urban parks and was thus used by other researchers [3,22]. In addition, a study involving semistructured interviews found that bird sounds were perceived as welcome distractions that effortlessly removed participants from cognitive fatigue [23]. Another laboratory experimental study showed a positive change in patients' cognitive response (i.e., interest and understanding) after exposure to hospital ward soundscape clips combined with bird singing and babbling stream [24]. A review paper referring to sound interventions in the clinic environment also suggested that pleasant natural sound intervention, which includes singing birds, gentle wind, and ocean waves, had benefits that contributed to perceived restoration of attention in patients and staff [25]. Therefore, the restorative potentials of soundscapes on cognition have been widely reported by previous research.

However, those studies were mainly based on the self-reported experience of cognitive restoration. Empirical studies involving cognitive benefits of sounds found mixed results: A few studies reported actual recovery of cognitive functioning after soundscape exposure [26,27], while others demonstrated no significant effects of restorative soundscapes on cognitive measures [28–30]. For example, a study used digit span backwards as a measure of cognitive performance to compare the restorative effects of different sounds and found that participants exposed to natural sounds did not perform better than those who were exposed to anthropogenic sounds [31]. Similarly, another laboratory study measured participants' task performance before and after sound exposure. Although results showed all sounds had positive effects on task performance, there was no significant difference between noise and natural sounds [32]. Those previous empirical studies applied quite different experiment stimuli, presentation methods, and measurements, thereby resulting in inconsistent outcomes. However, it is noteworthy that the research using audiovisual stimuli usually resulted in more restorative effects than those using only sound stimuli. In addition, various cognitive tests regarding attention and memory were mainly used as sensitive measures of cognitive restoration. Overall, even if some research has indicated the potential restorative effects of soundscapes, this theory still needs to be adequately tested by more evidence-based research with a systematic approach.

To date, however, not only does the evidence of soundscapes' cognitive benefits remain inconsistent, but it is also not clear whether these benefits could be generalized to children, since previous research primarily focused on adults. Given the widely reported academic burden in primary schools of China, which imposes increasing demands on children's cognitive resources and leads to fatigue and decline in cognitive performance, it may be a quite urgent task to explore the restorative stimuli that could facilitate cognitive recovery for children [33]. The cognitive capabilities needing restoration therein encompass sustained attention and short-term memory, which were often used as cognitive indicators of directed attention highlighted in ART [15,18]. Those two basic cognitive abilities are believed to underlie the emergence of a more complex cognitive progress and play an important part in children's education processes, such as learning, reading, and writing [34,35]. Therefore, these two cognitive capabilities should be considered first for investigation in the study of children's cognitive restoration.

Moreover, in contrast with annoyed ambient noise, which has been widely proven to have adverse effects on the two cognitive abilities in prior studies [36,37], pleasant soundscapes exhibited restorative potentials as perceived by children [22]. Thus, it seems reasonable to expect a positive effect on children's cognition after exposure to a restorative soundscape. In addition, considering the rapid development of children's cognitive functioning, which is less automatized and more easily influenced by surrounding environments compared to that of adults [38], the effects of restorative soundscapes on cognitive performance are likely to be different between children and adults.

The aim of this study was to explore the restorative benefits of various soundscapes on children's cognitive performance. Given that classrooms serve as a major educational environment for children's cognitive development [39], this study was carried out in a simulated classroom situation. Specifically, two experiments were carried out to examine the cognitive benefits of soundscapes: In Experiment 1, a sustained attention to response test (SART) was used as a measure of sustained attention, and in Experiment 2, a digit span test (DST) was used as a measure of short-term memory. We hypothesized that exposure to different classroom soundscapes has different restorative effects on children's sustained attention and short-term memory.

2. Materials and Methods

2.1. Participants

A total of 95 children aged 8–12 were recruited as participants in this study. Specifically, 46 children (mean = 10.25 years, SD = 1.33) participated in Experiment 1 (SART), and 45 children (mean = 10.31 years, SD = 1.40) participated in Experiment 2 (DST). Participants were recruited via social media and snowball sampling, from various primary schools in Tianjin, China. All the participants reported that they had normal hearing and normal vision. In addition, four participants were excluded during the data analysis, because their baseline cognitive scores were outliers.

The study was conducted in accordance with the Declaration of Helsinki. Ethical approval was obtained from the Academic Committee of School of Architecture, Tianjin University. All the children and their parents were informed about the study protocol, and they voluntarily participated in the study. Before the experiment, children gave oral consent, and parents gave written informed consent to the researchers.

In order to investigate the influence of demographic characteristics on children's cognitive restoration, participants were regrouped to simplify data analysis and interpretation. The variable 'age' was categorized to indicate the ranges: 7–8 years, 9–10 years, and 11–12 years. The baseline of CE (commission errors) was categorized to two levels: Fewer (≤ 9) and more (≥ 10) errors. The baseline of RT (reaction time) was categorized to three levels: Fast (<450), medium (450–500), and slow (>500). The baseline of DS (digit span) was categorized to two levels: Short (≤ 9) and long (≥ 10) sequence. Participants were grouped in order to have a similar sample size of each group. Sample demographics are shown in Table 1.

Table 1. Demographics characteristic of the participants in this study.

Variable	Characteristic	Experiment 1 (n)	Experiment 2 (n)
Gender	Boy	23	22
	Girl	23	23
Age (years)	7–8	14	14
	9–10	16	15
	11–12	16	16
Baseline (CE)	≤ 9	22	
	≥ 10	24	
Baseline (RT)	<450	18	
	450–500	13	
	>500	15	
Baseline (DS)	≤ 7		23
	≥ 8		22
Total		46	45

CE = Commission errors (number); RT = Reaction time (millisecond); DS = Digit span (length).

2.2. Experimental Stimuli

In order to provide a complete and realistic presentation of a classroom and avoid other distractions in the lab, an immersive virtual reality (VR) technology was employed in this study. A visual recording of the classroom was captured in a typical primary school of Tianjin, China. A panoramic camera consisting of six cameras (Insta360 Pro) arranged around a sphere was used to capture an omnidirectional picture of the classroom. The camera was placed on a tripod in the middle of the classroom with a height of 1.0m from the ground, to simulate the view of children when they were sitting. The panorama of the classroom was played in a VR head-mounted display (HMD) during the experiments, as shown in Figure 1.

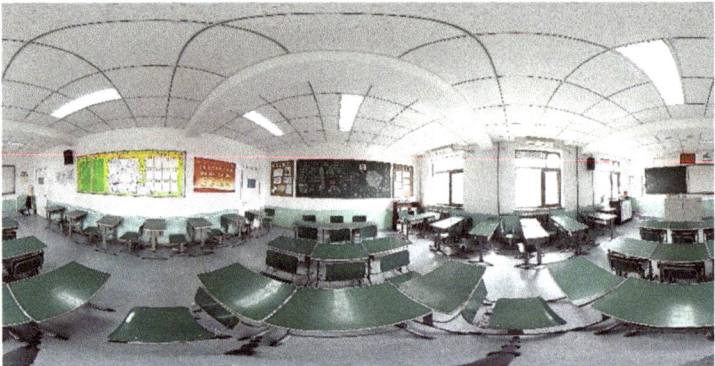

Figure 1. The panoramic view of a school classroom.

In this study, five environmental sounds (i.e., music, birdsong, fountain sound, bell ring, and stream sound) and ambient noise in the environment of classrooms were used to generate the sound stimuli. The five environmental sounds were selected for the following reasons: (1) They were assessed by children as the potential restorative sounds in a prior study [22] and (2) they are coherent with the classroom setting and could be easily added in a school classroom through corresponding soundscape design. Specifically, a typical classical piano music, named "Souvenirs d' enfance", was selected as the music stimulus, which was a piece of soft and relaxing music without lyrics. In addition, a series of chirps of sparrows and other few bird species were recorded in a park in Tianjin and used as the birdsong stimulus. The fountain sound was produced by an upward shallow jet and water falling along all sides of a square stone column, while the stream sound was recorded nearby a downwards stream consisting of slightly tilted stone steps and slowly flowing water. The sound of the bell ring was produced by irregularly striking a wind chime, which was constructed from a series of suspended mental bells. As for the ambient noise of the classroom, it was recorded in an unoccupied classroom with the window closed. The ambient noise included environmental sounds outside the classroom and noise from construction equipment in the building. The sound recordings were all collected over dual channels using a Sony PCM-D50 digital recorder equipped with two stereo microphones (set at 16 bit and 44,100 Hz sampling rate). A 30-s sample was extracted from each of the six sound recordings for audio reproduction.

To simulate the real-life settings of classrooms, five environmental sounds (i.e., music, birdsong, fountain sound, bell ring, and stream sound) were used as dominant sound signals, which were separately combined with the ambient noise of classrooms to generated five soundscape stimuli. Therefore, a preliminary test was carried out to identify the optimal restorative signal-to-noise (S/N) of dominant sounds and ambient noise. In the test, ambient noise in the classroom was set as 45 dBA according to the upper limit of noise standard in China primary school classrooms, and the S/N of five levels ($-5, 0, 5, 10, 15$) was used to simulate the sound environments in classrooms. Thirty children aged 8–12 were exposed to the soundscapes, and they were asked to evaluate each soundscape using a perceived restorative soundscape scale for children [22]. Results showed that children reported an S/N of 5 dB to be most restorative. Therefore, in this study, the A-weighted equivalent sound pressure level of five environmental sounds was set as 50 dBA, while the ambient noise was set as 45 dBA, with an S/N of 5 dB. Before the combination, the sound signals were normalized to the average sound level of 50 dBA (45 dBA for ambient noise) using a Norsonic Nor140 Class 1 sound level meter coupled to a reference class headphone AKG K702, whose high sensitivity could ensure the accuracy of the emitted signal with respect to the real sound. Both the adjustment of sound pressure level and the combination of soundscapes were processed by Adobe Audition software.

The psychoacoustic characteristics and restorative evaluation of the sound signals and combined soundscapes were analyzed using the Artemis software (HEAD acoustics), as shown in Table 2. As reported in a previous study, the Just Noticeable Differences (JNDs) of loudness, fluctuation strength, sharpness, and roughness were 0.5 sone, 0.012 vacil, 0.08 acum, and 0.04 asper, respectively [40]. It could be seen that the psychoacoustic values were quite scattered according to the types of sound signals and soundscapes. Thus, it was expected that the participants can perceive the difference of those parameters among soundscapes.

Table 2. Psychoacoustic characteristics and restorative evaluation of sound signals and combined soundscapes.

	Loudness (sone GF)		Fluctuation Strength (vacil)		Sharpness (acum)		Roughness (asper)		PRSS-C
	Sound signal	Soundscape	Sound signal	Soundscape	Sound signal	Soundscape	Sound signal	Soundscape	Soundscape
MS	8.54 (1.65)	14.80 (2.27)	0.058 (0.043)	0.046 (0.024)	1.31 (0.25)	2.05 (0.30)	0.74 (0.24)	1.53 (0.36)	3.71 (0.72)
BS	4.30 (1.23)	11.50 (2.11)	0.058 (0.044)	0.040 (0.022)	2.66 (0.60)	2.41 (0.33)	0.17 (0.22)	1.60 (0.43)	3.43 (0.78)
FS	7.92 (0.29)	13.00 (1.30)	0.005 (0.006)	0.012 (0.011)	2.76 (0.06)	2.79 (0.15)	1.61 (0.10)	1.92 (0.25)	3.29 (0.80)
BR	5.10 (1.90)	12.00 (2.10)	0.013 (0.008)	0.032 (0.020)	4.43 (1.02)	2.89 (0.58)	0.24 (0.20)	1.63 (0.43)	3.17 (0.82)
SS	7.14 (0.71)	13.40 (1.59)	0.031 (0.009)	0.033 (0.012)	2.39 (0.14)	2.54 (0.21)	2.34 (0.25)	2.76 (0.30)	3.12 (0.82)
AN	6.28 (1.28)		0.028 (0.018)		2.20 (0.31)		0.95 (0.42)		2.55 (0.63)

Mean values and standard deviation (SD) of psychoacoustics parameters for each sound signal and soundscape were presented in the table. MS = Music; BS = Birdsong; FS = Fountain sound; BR = Bell ring; SS = Stream sound; AN = Ambient noise. PRSS-C = Perceived restorative soundscape scale for children.

Altogether, six soundscapes, including music, birdsong, fountain sound, bell ring, and stream sound and ambient noise, were used as experimental sounds, while silence was used as a control stimulus in this study. Silence was widely reported to be an important factor in overall sound environment quality as perceived by adults. In addition, some prior studies have indicated the restorative potential of silence on human health [41]. The duration of each sound was set according to a preliminary test, in which the duration of each sound was set as five levels from 2 min to 6 min with a step of one minute. Ten children were exposed to the soundscapes and were asked their preference of the soundscapes on a five-point scale (from "not at all" to "extremely"). The results showed that a duration of 3 min was most preferred by children. Therefore, 3 min was set as the duration of each sound. Binaural signals of the soundscapes were delivered by computer through headphones (AKG K702) during the experiments.

2.3. Measures

In this study, two experiments were designed to explore the restorative benefits of soundscapes on children's sustained attention and short-term memory, respectively.

In Experiment 1, the sustained attention to response test (SART) was used to test the changes of participants' attentional capacity, as SART fits the definition of directed attention highlighted in ART.

SART is a computer-based go/no-go task which requires participants to withhold behavioral responses to an infrequent and unpredictable target during a period of rapid and rhythmic response to frequent nontargets [34]. The original SART were revised to be more suitable for children to operate, according to preliminary tests. The adapted SART version consisted of 135 digits from one to nine, including 15 targets (i.e., digit 3) and 120 nontargets (except digit 3). The SART was performed using a MATLAB program, and digits were presented to the participant on a computer screen every 1125 ms and remained on the screen for 250 ms. Participants needed to press the space bar every time a nontarget digit was seen and avoid pressing the space bar when viewing the target. Two indices were obtained in this test: (1) Reaction time: The mean response time in milliseconds that participants responded to nontargets; (2) commission errors: The number of times that participants inappropriately pressed the spacebar when the target was presented. The two indices measured response speed and response inhibition, respectively. Notably, participants were asked to give equal weight to responding as quickly as possible and to minimizing commission errors.

In Experiment 2, a digit span test (DST) was used to assess the changes of children's short-term memory, as there was wide evidence supporting the role of DST as a standardized measure of children's cognition [42]. DST has a large attentional component, as items must be moved in and out of the focus of attention. During the DST task, a list of random digits (e.g., "8, 3, 6") was presented on a computer screen at the rate of one every 800 milliseconds. Then, the participant was asked to immediately repeat the digits aloud in the same order they were presented. If they correctly recalled all of the digits, the next list with one digit longer would be presented (e.g., "9, 2, 4, 7"). The length of the list was increased until the participant failed to accurately recall a list of that length on two subsequent occasions. The index obtained in this test was the participant's digit span, indicating the length of the longest list a participant could remember.

2.4. Experimental Design

The experiments were performed in a semi-anechoic chamber in Tianjin University. Participants were accompanied by their parents, who waited in a room outside the chamber during the experiment. Participants took part in the experiment individually, supervised by a researcher.

Before the formal experiment, participants completed the baseline measure of the cognitive test. When the experiment started, they were first given a 5-min oral calculation task, which was assessed to be an effective way to induce attentional fatigue [32]. The difficulty of oral calculation was adapted to children of different age groups to ensure the same difficulty level for all children as much as possible. Specifically, participants aged 7–8 were asked to perform continuous subtraction from a number with three digits with a step of 3 accurately as soon as possible. If he/she did a miscalculation, they would be asked to stop and start their calculation from the beginning. Participants aged 9–10 performed the subtraction from a number with four digits with a step of 7, while participants aged 11–12 performed the subtraction from a number with four digits with a step of 13. Especially, a few children's oral calculation abilities were obviously better than those of their peers, so in those cases, a more difficult level of calculation was accordingly used. After that, participants were asked to perform the same cognitive test to assess attentional fatigue. The restoration period followed, when participants were exposed to an audiovisual soundscape for 3 minutes without any disturbance. Then, they were asked to perform the cognitive test again to examine whether their cognitive performance returned to normal level. Each experimental unit last around 13 minutes.

In order to control the whole experiment time within one hour, each participant could only experience four of seven soundscapes at most. Therefore, each participant performed the experimental unit four times, as shown in Figure 2. To ensure equal numbers of participants across soundscapes, the four soundscapes for each participant were randomly selected from seven soundscapes by computer. The four soundscapes were also counterbalanced in random order to minimize order effect. In total, each soundscape was experienced by 25 participants at least, which was a moderate sample size for statistical analysis. The sample size was set mostly based on the examples of other studies and our experience. In addition, data saturation was determined when the statistical values were rather steady with the addition of the last few participants. The cognitive baseline levels of participants in different soundscape groups would be examined to ensure no group differences across soundscapes.

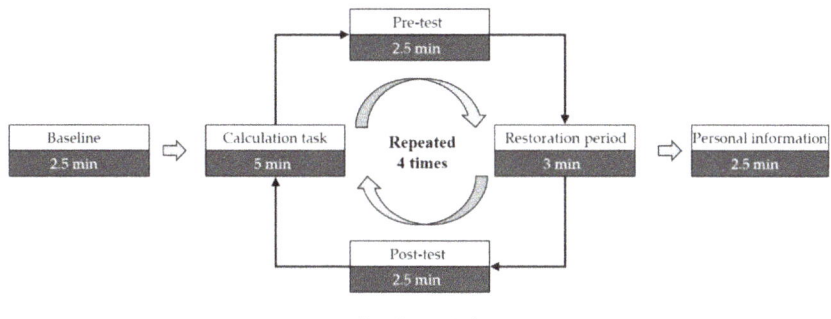

Figure 2. Diagram of experimental procedure.

Finally, the participants were also asked to provide their demographic information, including age in years and gender.

2.5. Data Analysis

The present study used SPSS 25.0 (IBM Corporation, Aemonk, NY, USA) to conduct all the statistical analysis. First of all, the baseline difference across soundscape groups was checked using a nonparametric Kruskal–Willis test, which was the prerequisite before the following analysis. Nonparametric tests were chosen for the following data analysis due to the non-normality of the collected data, which was examined by a Kolmogorov–Smirnov test. In both experiments, Wilcoxon signed-rank tests were first applied to compare children's cognitive performance before and after each soundscape exposure. Then, the Kruskal–Willis Test was used for the comparison of multiple soundscapes. The change values of variables before and after exposure to soundscapes was calculated as dependent variables, to accommodate individual difference. Additionally, the influence of demographic characteristics on restoration was explored using the Mann–Whitney U tests or Kruskal–Wills tests. In all analyses, an alpha value less than 0.05 was used as the criterion to determine significant differences.

3. Results

3.1. Restoration of Sustained Attention

The baseline levels of sustained attention demonstrated no significant difference among participants across different soundscapes. This was true for both measures: Commission errors and reaction time. The difference in sustained attention before and after the soundscape exposure was tested using a Wilcoxon signed-rank test.

Regarding the reaction time (Table 3), there was a significant improvement after exposure to music, birdsong, fountain sound, and stream sound. Additionally, the bell ring sound also showed a possible trend of reducing reaction time, while no difference in reaction time was shown after exposure to ambient noise and silence. After calculating the change values of sustained attention before and after the soundscape exposure, the Kruskal–Willis test yielded a significant difference between soundscapes in reaction time, $\chi^2(6) = 24.647$, $p = 0.000$. As shown in Figure 3, boxplots of before–after change values of reaction time were presented, showing mean, median, interquartile range, maximum, and minimum values, with higher change values indicating worse restorative effects. It can be seen that all five soundscapes showed restorative effects on reaction time. Specifically, the fountain sound and stream sound gave rise to the best restorative effects, followed by music and birdsong. Pairwise comparison showed that the change values of reaction time were significant lower for ambient noise than for fountain sound ($p = 0.004$) and stream sound ($p = 0.042$).

Table 3. The statistical scores of reaction time before and after exposure to each soundscape.

Soundscape	Before		After		Z (w)	p
	M (SD)	Median (IQR)	M (SD)	Median (IQR)		
MS	480.29 (83.21)	481.65 (105.4)	458.34 (77.41)	448.10 (118.4)	−3.264	0.001
BS	481.97 (93.35)	449.80 (110.6)	462.87 (80.72)	453.15 (98.0)	−3.238	0.001
FS	497.64 (86.14)	489.75 (161.5)	469.11 (79.60)	454.90 (127.8)	−4.203	0.000
BR	478.54 (88.35)	480.60 (117.0)	466.95 (81.25)	465.00 (129.4)	−1.898	0.058
SS	476.57 (88.37)	460.90 (138.3)	453.20 (78.51)	444.40 (96.2)	−3.628	0.000
AN	480.98 (77.34)	476.30 (114.4)	479.79 (86.04)	476.05 (124.2)	−0.063	0.949
SL	459.53 (86.22)	450.90 (113.3)	458.46 (90.02)	454.50 (101.3)	−0.902	0.367

MS = Music; BS = Birdsong; FS = Fountain sound; BR = Bell ring; SS = Stream sound; AN = Ambient noise; SL = Silence; IQR = Interquartile range.

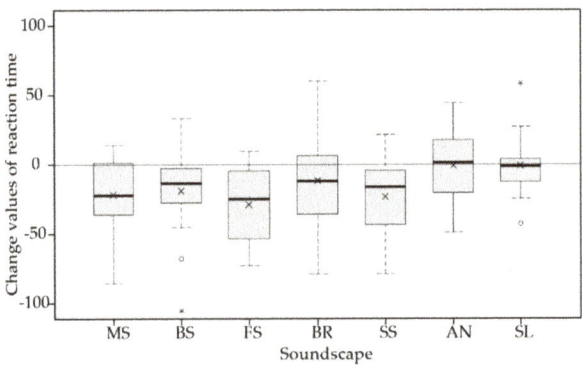

Figure 3. Boxplots of change values of reaction time between soundscapes, showing median, interquartile range, maximum, and minimum values. The crosses represent mean values. MS, BS, FS, BR, SS, AN, and SL represent music, birdsong, fountain sound, bell ring, stream sound, ambient noise, and silence, respectively.

Regarding the commission errors (Table 4), there was no significant reduction after each soundscape exposure. However, participants made fewer commission errors after exposure to birdsong and made more commission errors after exposure to music and bell ring, although the difference was not statistically significant. In addition, fountain sound, stream sound, and silence had almost no effects on the commission errors. Notably, a significant increase of commission errors was observed after exposure to ambient noise, that is, ambient noise showed adverse effects on children's ability of response inhibition, even if the sound pressure level (45 dBA) was lower than other soundscapes. The Kruskal–Willis test also yielded a significant difference between different soundscapes in commission errors, $\chi^2(6) = 15.315$, $p = 0.018$. As shown in Figure 4, boxplots of before–after change values of commission errors were presented, showing mean, median, interquartile range, maximum, and minimum values, with higher change values indicating worse restorative effects. The results showed that birdsong exhibited the best restorative effects, followed by fountain sound, stream sound, and silence. Pairwise comparison only found a significant difference between birdsong and ambient noise ($p = 0.013$).

Table 4. The statistical scores of commission errors before and after exposure to each soundscape.

Soundscape	Before		After		Z (w)	p
	M (SD)	Median (IQR)	M (SD)	Median (IQR)		
MS	8.85 (3.52)	8.50 (5.3)	9.50 (3.81)	10.00 (5.8)	−1.488	0.137
BS	9.69 (3.88)	10.50 (4.8)	8.85 (3.96)	8.50 (6.5)	−1.610	0.107
FS	9.73 (3.60)	10.00 (6.0)	9.72 (3.59)	10.00 (6.0)	−0.062	0.758
BR	8.52 (4.47)	9.00 (8.0)	9.67 (4.02)	10.00 (7.0)	−1.961	0.050
SS	9.37 (4.19)	10.00 (7.0)	9.22 (4.07)	10.00 (7.0)	−0.308	0.951
AN	8.42 (4.26)	8.00 (8.3)	10.12 (3.55)	10.00 (5.3)	−2.687	0.007
SL	9.81 (3.49)	10.00 (4.3)	10.00 (3.40)	10.00 (5.0)	−0.285	0.775

MS = Music; BS = Birdsong; FS = Fountain sound; BR = Bell ring; SS = Stream sound; AN = Ambient noise; SL = Silence; IQR = Interquartile range.

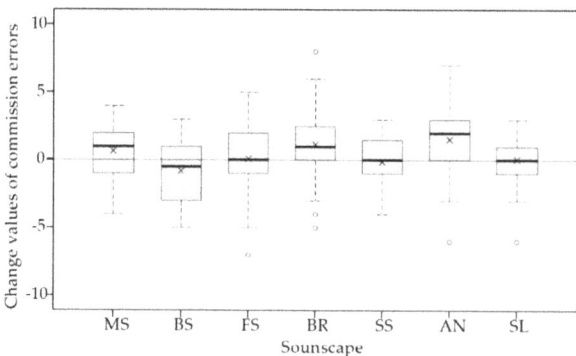

Figure 4. Boxplots of change values of commission errors between soundscapes, showing median, interquartile range, maximum, and minimum values. The crosses represent mean values. MS, BS, FS, BR, SS, AN, and SL represent music, birdsong, fountain sound, bell ring, stream sound, ambient noise, and silence, respectively.

In total, fountain sound and water sound demonstrated the best restorative effects on response speed (as measured by reaction time), while birdsong showed the best restorative effects on response inhibition (as measured by commission errors). In addition, bell ring and silence had almost no effects on children's sustained attention in terms of both response inhibition and response speed. However, ambient noise exhibited significantly adverse effects rather than restorative effects on children's sustained attention, at least in terms of response inhibition.

As for the influence of personal characteristics on the restoration of children's sustained attention, Mann–Whitney U tests showed that there was no significant difference between boys and girls in change values of both reaction time ($U = -0.609$, $p = 0.542$) and commission errors ($U = -0.458$, $p = 0.647$). Kruskal–Wallis tests also showed no significant influence of age on change values of reaction time ($\chi^2(2) = 0.909$, $p = 0.635$) and commission errors ($\chi^2(2) = 0.882$, $p = 0.643$). However, results indicated that participants who conducted more commission errors at baseline period performed better after the soundscape exposure, relative to participants who conducted fewer commission errors at baseline period ($U = -1.991$, $p = 0.047$). However, this difference between baseline levels was not achieved in the restoration of reaction time ($\chi^2(2) = 2.835$, $p = 0.242$).

3.2. Restoration of Short-Term Memory

The baseline scores of DST demonstrated no significant difference between the soundscapes. The Wilcoxon signed-rank test was used to assess the change values of digit span before and after exposure to the soundscape stimuli, as shown in Table 5. It can be seen that after exposure to music, birdsong, fountain sound, and steam sound, children's digit span was substantially improved, while bell ring, ambient noise, and silence showed no actual restorative effects.

Table 5. The statistical scores of digit span before and after exposure to each soundscape.

Soundscape	Before		After		Z (w)	p
	M (SD)	Median (IQR)	M (SD)	Median (IQR)		
MS	7.65 (1.41)	7.00 (2.0)	8.23 (1.38)	8.50 (2.0)	−2.251	0.024
BS	7.77 (1.34)	8.00 (2.0)	8.27 (1.34)	8.00 (2.0)	−2.053	0.040
FS	7.20 (1.53)	7.00 (5.0)	8.36 (1.80)	8.00 (1.0)	−3.699	0.000
BR	7.67 (1.47)	8.00 (2.0)	7.85 (1.70)	7.00 (2.0)	−0.700	0.484
SS	7.46 (0.99)	7.00 (1.0)	8.46 (1.50)	8.00 (3.0)	−3.214	0.001
AN	7.88 (1.48)	8.00 (2.0)	7.96 (1.84)	8.00 (4.0)	−0.254	0.799
SL	7.68 (1.44)	8.00 (2.0)	7.92 (1.44)	8.00 (2.0)	−1.039	0.299

MS = Music; BS = Birdsong; FS = Fountain sound; BR = Bell ring; SS = Stream sound; AN = Ambient noise; SL = Silence; IQR = Interquartile range.

The change values of digit span before and after exposure to different soundscapes were compared using Kruskal–Wallis tests. As shown in Figure 5, boxplots of before–after change values of digit span were presented, showing mean, median, interquartile range, maximum, and minimum values, with higher change values indicating better restorative effects. The results showed a main effect of soundscapes on the restoration of children's short-term memory ($\chi^2(6) = 19.876$, $p = 0.003$). Among the seven soundscapes, children's digit span improved to a significantly greater extent after exposure to fountain sound, relative to bell ring ($p = 0.029$) and ambient noise ($p = 0.018$), as indicated by a pairwise comparison. In addition, stream sound also showed a relatively good restorative effect on short-term memory, followed by music and birdsong, as shown in Figure 5.

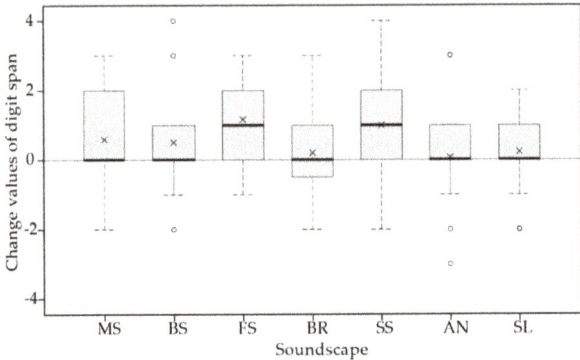

Figure 5. Boxplots of change values of digit span between soundscapes, showing median, interquartile range, maximum, and minimum values. The crosses represent mean values. MS, BS, FS, BR, SS, AN, and SL represent music, birdsong, fountain sound, bell ring, stream sound, ambient noise, and silence, respectively.

Regarding the influence of children's demographic characteristics, the nonparametric analysis showed that the change values of children's digit span did not differ between genders ($p = 0.962$), ages ($p = 0.128$), and baseline levels ($p = 0.149$).

4. Discussion

In this study, two experiments were conducted to examine the effects of restorative soundscapes on children's cognitive performance. In Experiment 1, children's sustained attention was measured by SART. Although the bell ring did not show any restorative effects on children's sustained attention, we did find evidence for the restorative effects of music, birdsong, fountain sound, and stream sound on children's response speed, as measured by reaction time. These findings not only provide empirical support for our previous study that explored restorative soundscapes based on children's perceptions [22], but also extend understanding of other works with adults, which only indicated the cognitive benefits of natural sounds in comparison with artificial sounds [26]. However, those soundscapes did not show significant restorative effects on response inhibition, as measured by commission errors. A possible reason was that response speed was reported to be negatively related to the performance of response inhibition [43], which was also confirmed in this study at the baseline levels ($p = 0.000$). Therefore, the results indicated that acute exposure to restorative soundscapes is not sufficient to cause positive effects on those two separate cognitive performances simultaneously. In addition, change values in reaction time did not correlate with changes in commission errors after soundscape exposure ($p = 0.918$), suggesting that the observed improvements in reaction time were not driven by the decrease in commission errors. In Experiment 2, short-term memory was measured by DST, in which digit span was used as the index of short-term memory. The results demonstrated that a brief exposure to fountain sound and stream sound could indeed help children to recover from a state of induced cognitive fatigue. As perceived restorative soundscapes, music and birdsong also have positive effects on children's short-term memory, although the effects were not significant. These results suggested that water soundscapes, such as fountain sound and stream sound, could be practically designed and played back during the intervals of classes for children who need various cognitive resources, including both sustained attention and short-term memory. Especially, music and birdsong could be mainly used for children who need restoration and improvement of response speed.

Comparing the change values of those three cognitive indices, it can be seen that the restorative effects of some soundscapes (such as fountain sound, stream sound, music and birdsong) were actually achieved in both children's response speed and digit span, rather than response inhibition. This might be explained according to previous studies on child psychology development, which suggested that response speed and memory span are usually viewed as a simple cognitive progress and could be improved easily in a short period. Response inhibition, however, is one of the integrative executive functions and a comparative complex progress for goal-directed behavior [44]. Therefore, the results in this study indicated that restorative soundscapes may affect different cognitive processes to a various extent. Although the restorative effects of soundscapes on children's basic cognitive functioning need further study with a larger sample size, this line of reasoning might lead to a number of intriguing research possibilities on various cognitive capabilities.

In addition, consistent with our hypothesis, the five potential restorative soundscapes as perceived by children in a previous study (i.e., music, birdsong, fountain sound, bell ring, and stream sound) showed significantly different effects on children's cognitive performance [22]. Generally, fountain sound and stream sound yielded the best restorative effects, followed by music and birdsong, while bell ring showed possible adverse effects instead. The results could be partly explained by the psychoacoustic characteristics of soundscapes. On one hand, as shown in Table 2, the psychoacoustic parameters (fluctuation strength, sharpness, and roughness) of music sound, birdsong, and bell ring changed to a greater extent compared with the fountain sound and stream sound after combination with the ambient noise. This indicated that children's perceptions of fountain sound and stream sound were less influenced by the noise relative to other sounds. This was also approved by previous studies, which suggested water sounds were more appropriate than other sounds for masking noise [45]. On the other hand, it is interesting to note that the soundscapes which were perceived as more restorative, such as music and birdsong, did not necessarily show better actual restorative effects compared to fountain sound and stream sound, which were perceived as less restorative by children, as shown by the PRSS-C evaluation in Table 2. One possible reason is that music sound and birdsong have much greater fluctuation strength than fountain sound and stream sound, and may thus lead to higher mood vibrancy [46]. By contrast, water sounds with smaller fluctuation strength might make it much easier for children to restore calm and stability during the cognitive task after the soundscape exposure. Another alternative explanation could be that children were more relaxed after exposure to music, which substantially lowered children's arousal levels, thereby reducing their cognitive performance instead. This tinterpretation is consistent with the Yerkes–Dodson Law [47]. In addition, the bell ring showed the least restorative effects on children's cognitive performance among the five potential restorative soundscapes. This might be because of its extremely high sharpness, which is caused by high-frequency components in the sound. Although sharpness was found to be essential for preference, it was not helpful in enhancing the calmness [45]. Moreover, it is important to note that there were only six soundscapes used in this study, and the psychoacoustic characteristics of those soundscapes were only used to partly explain the possible reason for the results. Future studies are still needed to confirm the correlation between the psychoacoustic parameters and soundscapes' cognitive effects on children.

Furthermore, this study provides more empirical support for previous research, which demonstrated that ambient noise in classrooms had significant adverse effects on children's cognitive performance [37,48,49]. It was apparent that the current noise level (45 dBA) is not sufficient to achieve the desired effects on children's cognition, thus raising the need for more effective noise reduction measures. However, there was only one fixed background noise level to simulate the real-life sound environment in school classrooms in this study. Therefore, more future studies should be performed to investigate the influence of different background noise levels on the restorativeness of soundscapes. It is also interesting to note that exposure to silence did not facilitate recovery on children's cognitive performance, which was quite different from previous studies with adults that suggested quietness has positive effects on adults' health and well-being [41,50]. Therefore, noise reduction is not necessarily sufficient to define a restorative acoustic environment in school classrooms. The environmental design of restorative soundscapes, such as fountain sound and stream sound, is essential for children's cognitive recovery.

Finally, although we found no significant effects of gender and age on children's cognitive restoration, future studies might be required to investigate whether children's personal characteristics may alter the restorative effects of soundscapes. However, it is worthy to note that children's self-reported normal hearing and vision were used as the measures of their perceptual abilities in this study. In order to exclude the possible influence of the individual difference in perceptual accuracy, a more accurate hearing and vision test should be performed in future studies. Moreover, we found that children with a lower baseline level of response inhibition were more restored after exposure restorative soundscapes than those of higher baseline level. This result is in line with previous studies, which suggested that acoustic environments affect cognitive performance differently depending on individual differences in cognition baseline [51]. Although the results are less conclusive and need examination through more research, they may imply that more attention should be given to the design of restorative soundscapes for children with poorer cognitive abilities.

5. Conclusions

In a simulated situation of a school classroom, two experiments were carried out to examine the restorative effects of soundscapes on children's cognitive performance. Based on children's performance of sustained attention and short-term memory, the following conclusions could be drawn.

1. Among the seven soundscapes, water sound and fountain sound showed the best restorative effects on children's cognitive performance, followed by music and birdsong. Bell ring and silence showed no significant restorative effects, while ambient noise showed adverse effects.

2. Regarding children's sustained attention, restorative soundscapes showed benefits in terms of response speed, except for bell ring. However, children's capability of response inhibition did not differ significantly before and after exposure to those soundscapes.

3. Regarding children's short-term memory, only fountain sound and stream sound showed significant restorative effects. Music and birdsong also had positive effects on short-term memory; however, the effects were not significant.

4. Children's gender and age had no influence on their restoration of cognitive performance. In addition, restorative soundscapes might have more restorative function on the response inhibition of children with lower attentional baseline level than those with higher attentional baseline level.

Author Contributions: Conceptualization, H.M. and S.S.; Methodology, H.M. and S.S.; Software, S.S.; Validation, H.M. and S.S.; Formal analysis, S.S.; Investigation, S.S.; Resources, H.M.; Data curation, S.S.; Writing—original draft preparation, S.S.; Writing—review and editing, H.M.; Visualization, S.S.; Supervision, H.M.; Project administration, H.M.; Funding acquisition, H.M.

Funding: This research was funded by the National Natural Science Foundation of China, grant number 51478303 and 51678401.

Acknowledgments: The authors are also grateful to Boya Yu for his support on experiment software, and sincere thanks to Kerstin Persson Waye for the comments on the draft of this manuscript.

Conflicts of Interest: The authors declare no conflict of interest. The funders had no role in the design of the study; in the collection, analyses, or interpretation of data; in the writing of the manuscript, or in the decision to publish the results.

References

1. Hartig, T. Restorative Environments. *Encycl. Appl. Psychol.* **2004**, 273–279. [CrossRef]
2. Aletta, F.; Oberman, T.; Kang, J. Associations between Positive Health-Related Effects and Soundscapes Perceptual Constructs: A Systematic Review. *Int. J. Environ. Res. Public Health* **2018**, *15*, 2392. [CrossRef]
3. Lee, P.J.; Park, S.H. Effects of exposure to rural soundscape on psychological restoration. In Proceedings of the Euronoise 2018 conference, Crete, Greece, 27–31 May 2018.
4. Kamp, I.V.A.N.; Kempen, E.V.A.N.; Klaeboe, R.; Kruize, H.; Brown, A.L.; Lercher, P. Soundscapes, human restoration and quality of life. In Proceedings of the Inter-Noise 2016 conference, Hamburg, Germany, 21–24 August 2016; pp. 1948–1958. [CrossRef]
5. Ulrich, R.S.; Simons, R.F.; Losito, B.D.; Fiorito, E.; Miles, M.A.; Zelson, M. Stress recovery during exposure to natural and urban environments. *J. Environ. Psychol.* **1991**, *11*, 201–230. [CrossRef]
6. Kaplan, R.; Kaplan, S. *The Experience of Nature: A Psychological Perspective*; Cambridge University Press: Cambridge, UK, 1989; ISBN 9780521341394.
7. Berto, R. The Role of Nature in Coping with Psycho-Physiological Stress: A Literature Review on Restorativeness. *Behav. Sci.* **2014**, *4*, 394–409. [CrossRef] [PubMed]
8. Benfield, J.; Taff, B.; Newman, P.; Smyth, J. Natural sound facilitates mood recovery. *Ecopsychology* **2014**, *6*, 183–188. [CrossRef]
9. Medvedev, O.; Shepherd, D.; Hautus, M.J. The restorative potential of soundscapes: A physiological investigation. *Appl. Acoust.* **2015**, *96*, 20–26. [CrossRef]
10. Hume, K.; Ahtamad, M. Physiological responses to and subjective estimates of soundscape elements. *Appl. Acoust.* **2013**, *74*, 275–281. [CrossRef]
11. Annerstedt, M.; Jönsson, P.; Wallergård, M.; Johansson, G.; Karlson, B.; Grahn, P.; Hansen, Å.M.; Währborg, P. Inducing physiological stress recovery with sounds of nature in a virtual reality forest—Results from a pilot study. *Physiol. Behav.* **2013**, *118*, 240–250. [CrossRef]
12. Alvarsson, J.J.; Wiens, S.; Nilsson, M.E. Stress Recovery during Exposure to Nature Sound and Environmental Noise. *Int. J. Environ. Res. Public Health* **2010**, *7*, 1036–1046. [CrossRef]
13. Kaplan, S. The restorative benefits of nature: Toward an integrative framework. *J. Environ. Psychol.* **1995**, *15*, 169–182. [CrossRef]
14. Kaplan, S.; Berman, M.G. Directed attention as a common resource for executive functioning and Self-Regulation. *Perspect. Psychol. Sci.* **2010**, *5*, 43–57. [CrossRef]
15. Berman, M.G.; Jonides, J.; Kaplan, S. The Cognitive Benefits of Interacting With Nature. *Psychol. Sci.* **2008**, *19*, 1207–1212. [CrossRef]
16. Faber Taylor, A.; Kuo, F.E. Children with Attention Deficits Concentrate Better after Walk in the Park. *J. Atten. Disord.* **2009**, *12*, 402–409. [CrossRef] [PubMed]
17. Berman, M.G.; Kross, E.; Krpan, K.M.; Askren, M.K.; Burson, A.; Deldin, P.J.; Kaplan, S.; Sherdell, L.; Gotlib, I.H.; Jonides, J. Interacting with nature improves cognition and affect for individuals with depression. *J. Affect. Disord.* **2012**, *140*, 300–305. [CrossRef] [PubMed]
18. Berto, R. Exposure to restorative environments helps restore attentional capacity. *J. Environ. Psychol.* **2005**, *25*, 249–259. [CrossRef]

19. Ohly, H.; White, M.P.; Wheeler, B.W.; Bethel, A.; Ukoumunne, O.C.; Nikolaou, V.; Garside, R. Attention Restoration Theory: A systematic review of the attention restoration potential of exposure to natural environments. *J. Toxicol. Environ. Health Part B* **2016**, *19*, 305–343. [CrossRef] [PubMed]
20. Payne, S.R. The production of a Perceived Restorativeness Soundscape Scale. *Appl. Acoust.* **2013**, *74*, 255–263. [CrossRef]
21. Payne, S.R.; Guastavino, C. Exploring the Validity of the Perceived Restorativeness Soundscape Scale: A Psycholinguistic Approach. *Front. Psychol.* **2018**, *9*, 1–17. [CrossRef]
22. Shu, S.; Ma, H. The restorative environmental sounds perceived by children. *J. Environ. Psychol.* **2018**, *60*, 72–80. [CrossRef]
23. Ratcliffe, E.; Gatersleben, B.; Sowden, P.T. Bird sounds and their contributions to perceived attention restoration and stress recovery. *J. Environ. Psychol.* **2013**, *36*, 221–228. [CrossRef]
24. Mackrill, J.; Jennings, P.; Cain, R. Exploring positive hospital ward soundscape interventions. *Appl. Ergon.* **2014**, *45*, 1454–1460. [CrossRef]
25. Iyendo, T.O. Sound as a supportive design intervention for improving health care experience in the clinical ecosystem: A qualitative study. *Complement. Ther. Clin. Pract.* **2017**, *29*, 58–96. [CrossRef]
26. Gould Van Praag, C.D.; Garfinkel, S.N.; Sparasci, O.; Mees, A.; Philippides, A.O.; Ware, M.; Ottaviani, C.; Critchley, H.D. Mind-wandering and alterations to default mode network connectivity when listening to naturalistic versus artificial sounds. *Sci. Rep.* **2017**, *7*. [CrossRef]
27. Zhang, Y.; Kang, J.; Kang, J. Effects of Soundscape on the Environmental Restoration in Urban Natural Environments. *Noise Health* **2017**, *19*, 65–72. [CrossRef]
28. Emfield, A.G.; Neider, M.B. Evaluating visual and auditory contributions to the cognitive restoration effect. *Front. Psychol.* **2014**, *5*, 548. [CrossRef]
29. Benfield, J.A.; Bell, P.A.; Troup, L.J.; Soderstrom, N. Does Anthropogenic Noise in National Parks Impair Memory? *Environ. Behav.* **2010**, *42*, 693–706. [CrossRef]
30. Jahncke, H.; Hygge, S.; Halin, N.; Green, A.M.; Dimberg, K. Open-plan office noise: Cognitive performance and restoration. *J. Environ. Psychol.* **2011**, *31*, 373–382. [CrossRef]
31. Abbott, L.C.; Taff, D.; Newman, P.; Benfield, J.A.; Mowen, A.J. The Influence of Natural Sounds on Attention Restoration. *J. Park Recreat. Admin.* **2016**, *34*. [CrossRef]
32. Ma, H.; Shu, S. An Experimental Study: The Restorative Effect of Soundscape Elements in a Simulated Open-Plan Office. *Acta Acust. United Acust.* **2018**, *104*, 106–115. [CrossRef]
33. Sun, J.; Dunne, M.P.; Hou, X.; Xu, A. Educational stress among Chinese adolescents: Individual, family, school and peer influences. *Educ. Rev.* **2013**, *65*, 284–302. [CrossRef]
34. Manly, T.; Robertson, I.H.; Galloway, M.; Hawkins, K. The absent mind: Further investigations of sustained attention to response. *Neuropsychologia* **1999**, *37*, 661–670. [CrossRef]
35. Passolunghi, M.C.; Siegel, L.S. Short-Term Memory, Working Memory, and Inhibitory Control in Children with Difficulties in Arithmetic Problem Solving. *J. Exp. Child Psychol.* **2001**, *80*, 44–57. [CrossRef]
36. Clark, C.; Paunovic, K. WHO Environmental Noise Guidelines for the European Region: A Systematic Review on Environmental Noise and Cognition. *Int. J. Environ. Res. Public Health* **2018**, *15*, 285. [CrossRef]
37. Lercher, P.; Evans, G.W.; Meis, M. Ambient Noise and Cognitive Processes among Primary Schoolchildren. *Environ. Behav.* **2003**, *35*, 725–735. [CrossRef]
38. Evans, G.W. Child Development and the Physical Environment. *Annu. Rev. Psychol.* **2006**, *57*, 423–451. [CrossRef]
39. Edwards, D.; Mercer, N. *Common Knowledge (Routledge Revivals): The Development of Understanding in the Classroom*; Routledge: Abingdon, UK, 2013; ISBN 9780203095287.
40. You, J.; Jeon, J.Y. Just noticeable differences in sound quality metrics for refrigerator noise. *Noise Control Eng. J.* **2008**, *56*, 414–424. [CrossRef]
41. Shepherd, D.; Welch, D.; Dirks, K.N.; McBride, D. Do quiet areas afford greater health-related quality of life than noisy areas? *Int. J. Environ. Res. Public Health* **2013**, *10*, 1284–1303. [CrossRef]
42. Rosenthal, E.N.; Riccio, C.A.; Gsanger, K.M.; Jarratt, K.P. Digit Span components as predictors of attention problems and executive functioning in children. *Arch. Clin. Neuropsychol.* **2006**, *21*, 131–139. [CrossRef]
43. Logan, G.D.; Cowan, W.B. On the Ability to Inhibit thought and Action: A Theory of an Act of Control. *Psychol. Rev.* **1984**, *91*, 295–327. [CrossRef]

44. Luna, B.; Garver, K.E.; Urban, T.A.; Lazar, N.A.; Sweeney, J.A. Maturation of cognitive processes from late childhood to adulthood. *Child Dev.* **2004**, *75*, 1357–1372. [CrossRef]
45. Jeon, J.Y.; Lee, P.J.; You, J.; Kang, J. Acoustical characteristics of water sounds for soundscape enhancement in urban open spaces. *J. Acoust. Soc. Am.* **2012**, *131*, 2101–2109. [CrossRef]
46. Aletta, F.; Kang, J. Towards an urban vibrancy model: A soundscape approach. *Int. J. Environ. Res. Public Health* **2018**, *15*. [CrossRef]
47. Yerkes, R.M.; Dodson, J.D. The relation of strength of stimulus to rapidity of habit-formation. *J. Comp. Neurol. Psychol.* **1908**, *18*, 459–482. [CrossRef]
48. Klatte, M.; Spilski, J.; Mayerl, J.; Möhler, U.; Lachmann, T.; Bergström, K. Effects of Aircraft Noise on Reading and Quality of Life in Primary School Children in Germany: Results from the NORAH Study. *Environ. Behav.* **2017**, *49*, 390–424. [CrossRef]
49. Klatte, M.; Bergström, K.; Lachmann, T. Does noise affect learning? A short review on noise effects on cognitive performance in children. *Front. Psychol.* **2013**, *4*, 1–6. [CrossRef]
50. Haapakangas, A.; Hongisto, V.; Varjo, J.; Lahtinen, M. Benefits of quiet workspaces in open-plan offices—Evidence from two office relocations. *J. Environ. Psychol.* **2018**, *56*, 63–75. [CrossRef]
51. Ljung, R.; Israelsson, K.; Hygge, S. Speech intelligibility and recall of spoken material heard at different signal-to-noise ratios and the role played by working memory capacity. *Appl. Cogn. Psychol.* **2013**, *27*, 198–203. [CrossRef]

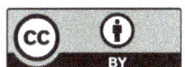

© 2019 by the authors. Licensee MDPI, Basel, Switzerland. This article is an open access article distributed under the terms and conditions of the Creative Commons Attribution (CC BY) license (http://creativecommons.org/licenses/by/4.0/).

MDPI
St. Alban-Anlage 66
4052 Basel
Switzerland
Tel. +41 61 683 77 34
Fax +41 61 302 89 18
www.mdpi.com

International Journal of Environmental Research and Public Health Editorial Office
E-mail: ijerph@mdpi.com
www.mdpi.com/journal/ijerph

www.ingramcontent.com/pod-product-compliance
Lightning Source LLC
LaVergne TN
LVHW071937080526
838202LV00064B/6625